Eye Tracking

Eye Tracking
A Comprehensive Guide to Methods and Measures

Kenneth Holmqvist
Humanities Laboratory
Lund University
Sweden

Marcus Nyström
Humanities Laboratory
Lund University
Sweden

Richard Andersson
Humanities Laboratory
Lund University
Sweden

Richard Dewhurst
Humanities Laboratory
Lund University
Sweden

Halszka Jarodzka
Centre for Learning Sciences and Technologies
Heerlen
the Netherlands

Joost van de Weijer
Humanities Laboratory
Lund University
Sweden

OXFORD
UNIVERSITY PRESS

OXFORD
UNIVERSITY PRESS

Great Clarendon Street, Oxford OX2 6DP

Oxford University Press is a department of the University of Oxford.
It furthers the University's objective of excellence in research, scholarship,
and education by publishing worldwide in

Oxford New York

Auckland Cape Town Dar es Salaam Hong Kong Karachi Kuala Lumpur
Madrid Melbourne Mexico City Nairobi New Delhi Shanghai Taipei Toronto

With offices in

Argentina Austria Brazil Chile Czech Republic France Greece
Guatemala Hungary Italy Japan Poland Portugal Singapore
South Korea Switzerland Thailand Turkey Ukraine Vietnam

Oxford is a registered trade mark of Oxford University Press
in the UK and in certain other countries

Published in the United States
by Oxford University Press Inc., New York

British Library Cataloguing in Publication Data

Data available

Library of Congress Cataloguing in Publication Data

Data available

Prelims Typeset in Nimbus
by Glyph International, Bangalore
Printed and bound by
CPI Group (UK) Ltd, Croydon, CR0 4YY

ISBN 978-0-19969708-3

10 9 8 7 6

Whilst every effort has been made to ensure that the contents of this book are as complete,
accurate and up-to-date as possible at the date of writing, Oxford University Press is not able to
give any guarantee or assurance that such is the case. Readers are urged to take appropriately
qualified medical advice in all cases. The information in this book is intended to be useful to the
general reader, but should not be used as a means of self-diagnosis or for the prescription of medication.

Why we Wrote this Book

This book is written by and for researchers who are still in that part of their careers where they are actively using the eye-tracker as a tool; those who have to deal with the technology, the signals, the filters, the algorithms, the experimental design, the programming of stimulus presentation, instructions to participants, working the varying tools for data analysis, and of course, worrying about all the different things that *must not* go wrong!

A central theme of the book concerns the wide range of fields eye tracking covers. Suppose an educational psychologist wishes to use eye tracking to evaluate a new software package designed to support learning to read. She may have an excellent idea as a starting point, and some understanding of the kind of results eye tracking could provide to tackle her research question, but unless she and the group around her are also adept in computer science, it is unlikely she will know how the eye movement data she collects is generated: How raw data samples are converted into fixations and saccades using event detection algorithms, how the different representations of eye movement data are calculated, and how all the measures of eye movements relate to these processes. All this is important because subtleties involved in working with eye-tracking data can have large consequences for the final results, and thus whether our educational psychologist can confidently conclude that her software package is effective or not in supporting the development of reading skills.

This is not to say that hard-core computer science skills are the crux of good eye-tracking research, for this is certainly not the case. One can equally envisage a situation where an expert in programming and the manipulation of data plans and executes an eye-tracking study poorly, simply because she is not trained in the principles of experimental design, and the associated literature on the visual system and oculomotor control.

There are many contrasts between the diverging schools of thought which use eye tracking; practices and preferences vary, but certainly experts in different fields do not draw on each other's strengths enough. We felt there was a need to pinpoint the relative merits of adopting methods based in one field alone, whilst highlighting that the lack of synergy between different disciplines can lead to sub-optimal research practices, and new advancements being overlooked.

Besides technical details and theory, however, the heart of this book revolves around practicality. At the Humanities Laboratory at Lund University we have been teaching eye-tracking methodology regularly since 2000. We commonly see newcomers to the technique run aground when encountering just the sort of issues raised above, but beginners struggle with problems which are even more practical in nature. Hands-on advice for how to actually use eye-trackers is very limited. Setting up the eye camera and performing a good calibration routine is just as important as the design of the study and how data is handled, for if the recording is poor your options are limited from the outset.

There are fundamental methodological skills which underpin *using* eye-trackers, but at the other end of the spectrum there is also the vast choice of measures available to the eye-tracking researcher. For the present text to be complete, therefore, we felt a requirement should also be to draw together eye-tracking measures, as well as methods, into an understandable structure. So, starting around 2005, we began producing a taxonomy of all eye-movement methods and measures used by researchers, examining how the measures are related to each other, what type of data quality they rely on, and previous data processing they require. Our classification work thus consisted of searching the method sections from thousands of journal papers, book chapters, PhD theses and conference proceedings. Every measure and method we found was catalogued and put into a growing system. Some of the measures were extremely elusive, as they are known by different names, not only between research fields, but even within, and often the precise implementations are missing in the published texts. At first, we were very unclear how to classify measures. Some varieties of taxonomic structures that we rejected can be found on p. 463. We ended up with a classification structure where the operational definitions are at the centre.

Users of eye-trackers often lack proficient training because there is little or no teaching community to rely on. As a result people are often self taught, or depend on second-hand knowledge which may be out of date or even incorrect. When they participate in our eye-tracking methodology courses, we find that many new users are very focused on their research questions, but are surprised how much time they need to invest in order to master eye tracking properly. Often people attending have just purchased an eye-tracker to compliment their research, or for use in their company to tackle ergonomic and marketing-related questions. Our aim for this book is to make learning to use eye-trackers a much easier process for these readers. If you have a solid background in experimental psychology, computer science, or mathematics you will often find it straightforward to embrace the technologies and workflows surrounding eye tracking. But whatever your background, you should be able to achieve the same level of knowledge and understanding from this book as you would from training on eye tracking in-house in a fully competent laboratory.

More specifically, this book has been written to be a support when:

1. Evaluating or acquiring a commercial eye-tracker,
2. Planning an experiment where eye tracking is used as a tool,
3. About to record eye-movement data,
4. Planning how to process and interpret the recorded data, before carrying out statistical tests on it,
5. Reading or reviewing eye-movement research.

In our efforts to classify eye-tracking methods and measures, combined with useful practical hints and tips, we hope to provide the reader with the first comprehensive textbook on methodology for new users of eye tracking, but which also caters for the advanced researcher. Previous versions of this book have been used in eye-tracking education in Lund. Also, colleagues of ours in Potsdam, Tübingen, and Helsinki have used earlier manuscripts of the book when teaching and training masters and PhD level students in eye tracking. Lastly, although not the target audience, manufacturers have already shown a great interest in the book at the manuscript stage, which we hope may lead to even better eye-trackers in the future.

How to submit suggestions

Please send comments and suggestions to etbook@humlab.lu.se.

Acknowledgements

Many people have helped us with this book. First of all, the eye-tracking seminar in Lund has debated previous manuscripts many times over. In particular, the authors would like to thank Kerstin Gidlöf, Paulina Lindström, Nils Holmberg, Roger Johansson, Jana Holsanova, Janna Spanne, Lenisa Brandão, Linnea Larsson, Johan Pihel, and Philip Pärnamets.

Another weekly seminar on book chapters was given during winter and spring 2009, when the author Kenneth Holmqvist visited KMRC Tübingen as a guest professor. The comments from that seminar group were invaluable for a variety of reasons. A great many thanks to Peter Gerjets, Katharina Scheiter, Gabriele Cierniak, Birgit Imhof, Yvonne Kammerer, Tim Kühl, Kim Stalbovs, Frank Papenmeier, Vera Bauhoff, Daniel Wessel, Susana Ruiz-Fernandez, Daniel Bratzke, Tanja Seifried, Katrin Giel, Anne Schüler, and Anne Rau.

Well over a hundred students have read and given feedback on earlier drafts while taking the 7.5 ECTS eye-tracking courses given in Lund since 2000, and at the LETA crash course in eye-tracking methods that we have organized since 2008.

We would also like to thank the many colleagues that have contributed by reviewing draft chapters. Ignace Hooge, Benjamin Tatler, and Pieter Blignaut for their thorough comments on many chapters of the book. Dan Witzner Hansen for his insightful methodological comments on Chapter 2 and elsewhere. Tamara van Gog for her knowledgeable comments on the use of verbal retrospection from eye-movement data. Tim Smith for reviewing Chapter 6, and Marc Pomplun for reading Chapter 7 and suggesting many points of improvement. Tom Foulsham and Andrew Duchowski for insightful comments on Chapter 8. Marc-Antoinne Nüssli and David Hardoon for their thorough reviews of a previous version of Chapter 11, and Michael Dorr for kindly reviewing Chapter 10. Others for reading and suggesting improvements on parts of the text: Jarkko Hautala, Sarah Lukas, Jaana Simola and her students, Cristian Sminchisescu, and Kristina Magnusson. Thanks also to David Dewhurst for checking some of the chapters when the book was in its final stages.

This book would have been difficult to write without close discussions with manufacturers. In particular, we would like to thank Martin Pötter of SMI for generously sharing with us years of experiences from the manufacturer's perspective, and Jan Hoffman of SMI for sharing his solutions for customer relations and support handling. William Schmidt of SR Research provided excellent feedback on earlier drafts of Chapter 2. Gunnar Troili and Henrik Eskilsson of Tobii Technology for reviewing Chapters 2, 5, and 7. Walter Nitico of SMI for checking our precision measurements and pointing out an error in previous drafts.

Thousands of participants in ours and other studies have contributed by providing data and eye-images that we have selected. Although anonymous, their participation has provided us with the examples in many of the chapters, and we extend our thanks to them also. Furthermore, we are grateful too to Roger Johansson, Nils Holmberg, Paulina Lindström, and Kerstin Gidlöf for giving us access to their data for use in this book.

This book was written while two of the authors built up the technological infrastructure that is now extensive at the Humanities Laboratory at Lund University. We are thankful to the Swedish Research Council, the Crafoord foundation, and the Knut and Alice Wallenberg foundation for funding the eye-tracking and other equipment we use in our lab. On our road to building up a large-scale eye-tracking laboratory we encountered several practical policy issues surrounding lab access, computer security, data integrity, and support for different workflows, which needed coordinating with our University administration. We are grateful to Marianne Gullberg for helping us implement an actual solution to them.

We are indebted to Florian Hug for letting us use the Subversion server at his department, which has been invaluable to the collaborative writing process. Thanks to Nils Holmberg for setting up and managing our own Subversion server. Not having to bother with who works with what version made writing this book so very much easier.

Finally, without electronic access to journal papers, this book would have been much more difficult to write. The authors want to thank all the libraries, publishing houses and scholars who have given (or sold our universities) access to thousands of peer-reviewed journal papers on eye-tracking-based research.

Contents

II DETECTING EVENTS AND BUILDING REPRESENTATIONS

About the Authors

Writing this book has been a collaborative effort. No chapter has been written by a single author alone. No author has written in only one chapter. Instead we have taken turns writing on chapters, so that more than one of us have worked through each chapter as a whole. This said, there are many passages where the competence of one author dominates.

Kenneth Holmqvist is an associate professor in Cognitive Science at Lund University. Kenneth founded the eye-tracking laboratory in 1995, which later grew into the large Humanities Laboratory. He has worked in a large variety of eye-tracking-based research stretching from reading research and scene perception, over to newspaper reading, advertisement studies, and gesture recognition in face-to-face interaction. Kenneth also has expertise in eye tracking used in applied areas, including decision making in supermarkets and research on safety in car driving and air traffic control. In 2000, Kenneth initiated regular masters courses in eye-tracking methodology. In 2006, he founded the Scandinavian Conference on Applied Eye Tracking, and in 2008, the international LETA training courses in eye-tracking methodology. Kenneth is the initiator and main author of this book.

Marcus Nyström received his PhD in Information Theory from the department of Electrical and Information Technology at Lund University, Sweden, in 2008, working with foveated video compression and scene perception. His research interests span eye-tracking methodology in general and analysis of eye-tracking data in particular. Marcus is the second author of this book, and has been central to its development throughout, but he has given particular attention to Chapters 2, 5, 7, 8, 10, and 11.

Richard Andersson is a PhD student in Cognitive Science at Lund University. He has far too many research interests, to his supervisors' dismay, but is especially involved in the interaction of language and vision, and general eye-tracking methodology, including eye tracking on great apes. Richard also works as a laboratory assistant and serves as technical staff on all things eye tracking in the Humanities Laboratory. Furthermore, he teaches at the LETA intensive eye-tracking course. Richard has made contributions to Chapters 3, 4, 6, and 12.

Richard Dewhurst is a post-doctoral researcher at Humanities Laboratory. He completed his PhD on training eye movements at the University of Nottingham in 2009, as part of the Cognition and Language research group. Prior to this he also obtained an MSc in psychological research methods from the University of Nottingham, and a BSc in psychology from the University of Wales, Bangor. His research focuses on attentional mechanisms and eye movements. More specifically how eye movement control changes with learning and experience, and how to devise and implement procedures for improving visual skills through training eye movements. Richard made significant contributions to Chapters 3, 8, 11, and 12.

Halszka Jarodzka is assistant professor at the Center for Learning Sciences and Technologies of the Open University of the Netherlands. She holds a Masters degree in Psychology and a PhD from the Knowledge Media Research Center, both at the Eberhard-Karls University of Tübingen. Halszka's research focuses on the use of eye tracking in educational psychology, in particular the diagnosis of expertise differences through eye tracking and verbal protocols, as well as the training of classification and diagnostic processes with eye movement modelling examples. Halszka has made significant contributions to Chapters 3, 4, 8, and 9.

Joost van de Weijer defended his PhD thesis at the Max Planck Institute for Psycholinguistics in 1998. Thereafter he worked as a postdoc researcher at Johns Hopkins University, Baltimore, and at the Department of Linguistics and Phonetics in Lund. Currently, he is affiliated to the Centre for Languages and Literature and the Humanities Laboratory, both at Lund University. His major contributions to this book concern the methodological issues that are involved in experimental research using eye tracking (Chapters 3, 10, 11, 12, and 13).

1   Introduction

Eye tracking as a research tool is more accessible than ever, and is growing in popularity amongst researchers from a whole host of different disciplines. Usability analysts, sports scientists, cognitive psychologists, reading researchers, psycholinguists, neurophysiologists, electrical engineers, and others all have a vested interest in eye tracking for different reasons. There is no doubt that it is useful to record eye movements, it advances science and leads to technological innovations. The growth of eye tracking in recent years, however, also presents a variety of challenges, most pressing of which is how to support the rapidly increasing number of users of eye-trackers. To address this concern this book follows the pipeline of empirical investigation with eye tracking from beginning to end, providing detailed advice and discussion of the issues that can be encountered en route.

1.1   The structure of this book

This book is about how to record high quality eye-tracking data from commercially available video-oculographic eye-tracking systems, and how to derive and use measures that give insights into oculomotor, cognitive, and neurobiological processes. Part I presents the technology and skills needed to perform high quality research with eye-trackers. Part II covers the predominant methods applied to the data which eye-trackers record. These include the parsing of raw sample data into oculomotor events, and also how to calculate other representations of eye-movements such as heat maps and transition matrices. Part III gives a comprehensive outline of the measures which can be calculated using the events and representations described in Part II. This is a taxonomy of the measures available to eye-tracking researchers, sorted by type of movement of the eyes and type of analysis.

In this chapter, we will introduce the overarching concepts of the book and how they have been laid out into parts and chapters.

1.1.1   Technical and methodological skills

Eye-tracking technology, experimental design, and data recording are *technical and methodological skills* that require practical and theoretical training over several years. Part I thus outlines the prerequisites of doing eye tracking efficiently. This begins with selecting an eye-tracker that fits your needs, so Chapter 2 covers the technical properties of eye-tracking systems and associated effects on data quality in detail. Chapter 3 takes the overall perspective of the process of an experiment, from a vague idea to the analysis of data. In short, an eye-tracking experiment must both tackle your research question appropriately, *and* produce data which you can analyse statistically. Remember that perfect data quality from a high-end eye-tracker can never compensate for an inadequate experimental design. In Chapter 4 we address the practicalities of actually recording data, using example eye images from real participants. We demonstrate how different eye colours and physiologies, glasses, contact lenses, mascara, and other factors are dangers to data quality.

1.1.2 Events and representations

Part II describes the methods for constructing and calculating *events and representations* from the recorded data. We define an event as a countable entity in eye-movement data: you can say how many of them there are. There are events that can be seen in a plot of the raw eye-movement data (saccades, blinks, and square-wave jerks, to mention a few), and there are complex events that require additional conditions in their definition (transitions, look-aheads, and regression scanpaths). Events have properties that researchers use in their analyses, such as onset, duration, direction, and velocity, and each such property has a single numerical value. In Part II, we define and discuss more than 20 of the most general events in eye-movement data.

We define a representation as a recalculation of a set of data, from one or several trials, one or several participants, or simply the whole of the data. Forming a transition matrix, a heat map, a proportion-over-time curve, a main sequence diagram, or simply a histogram are all examples of building representations of data. A very particular type of representation is to use verbal retrospection, and let recorded speech represent the eye-movement data. Representations are not countable, so it is of little use to ask your colleague how many transition matrices she has in her data. Nor do representations have obvious properties with straight-forward numerical values, as do events. The entropy of a transition matrix, for instance, is mathematically nontrivial and also not easy to interpret.

The five methods for building events and representations are given one chapter each. The event-detection algorithms of Chapter 5 detect and measure oculomotor events such as fixations and saccades in the raw data stream, but they require thresholds and produce artefacts that call for a deep understanding on the part of the user. The area of interest (AOI) tool in Chapter 6 lets the user segment space and define and measure events such as dwells, and representations such as transition matrices. AOIs are probably the most used tools in eye-tracking research, but when using them, the same questions re-occur: what is the smallest possible size of an AOI? Can I use AOIs with animated stimuli? Can I have a single AOI with disconnected parts? The heat maps and attention maps of Chapter 7 produce not only questionable visualizations, but also very useful Gaussian and matrix representations, showing the distribution of eye-movement data according to set parameters. Analysing scanpaths (Chapter 8) allows the detection of events such as backtracks and regressions, of great importance in reading and usability research. Moreover, abstract representations of different scanpaths may also be compared, revealing similarities in oculomotor behaviour which are otherwise unmeasurable. Finally, Chapter 9 describes the principles for co-analysis with auxiliary data types (mouse and keyboard logging, motion tracking, fMRI, EEG, and speech data). Each of these gives a variety of latency and distance measures; moreover, co-analysing speech data allows the re-represention of eye-movements as cued retrospective verbal protocols.

Each event and representation chapter to a certain extent builds on, contrasts against, and abstracts from the previous ones. You will find that each chapter is slightly more conceptual than the one before, and precise calculations are progressively replaced by examples of principles. This reflects how mature each means of analysis is today.

Also, event and representations are abstractions that reduce the amount of information compared to raw data, and this is necessary because the eye-tracking measures employed in the experimental design can only give us the values we need for statistical analysis on the basis of abstracted and reduced events, but virtually never from raw data itself. The events of each new chapter have abstracted and reduced information to a larger degree compared to the events of the preceding chapter.

1.1.3   Measures and their operational definitions

Part III is a taxonomy of about 120 eye-tracking measures. We have extracted them from a vast search of published research, and interpreted and evaluated each measure with respect to its value to research overall. We disentangle the relationship between different measures, to provide a structured account of the micro-universe that is eye-movement measures. Thus, four large classes of eye-tracking measures are described in this book, namely:

Movement measures which are concerned with a whole variety of eye-*movements through space*, and the properties of these movements.

Position measures which deal only with *where* a participant has or has not been looking, and the properties of eye-movements at spatial locations.

Numerosity measures which pertain to the number, proportion, or rate of any *countable* eye-movement event.

Latency measures which express the *duration from the onset of one event to the onset of a second event*. Measures of this type also appear in the form of spatial distances.

Finally, Chapter 14 takes a step back, reflecting on the collective body of eye-tracking measures, and proposes a structured model of measures and their operational definitions.

1.2   How eye-movement measures are described in this book

There are so many eye-movement measures that we wanted to assist the reader with a quick conceptual tool to navigate between the measures available to them. In order to find and understand eye-movement measures more easily, therefore, use the target question and summary boxes at the start of each measure section. This will help you evaluate the suitability of each measure for your study.

1.2.1   The target question and the summary box

Measures are identified by their *target question*, as in the example below. Select a measure that has a target question which corresponds to the operationalization in your experimental design. The *input representation* shows what data you need in order to calculate values for this measure, in the case below, either raw data samples or fixations, the position of the AOI, and the onset time of the stimulus. The summary box below relates to entry time, a common latency measure. You will find such summary boxes throughout Part III.

Target question	*How soon after stimulus onset is the AOI entered?*
Input representation	*Raw data samples or fixations, AOI location, and onset time of stimulus*
Output	*Entry time in AOI in milliseconds*

From time to time, we will refer to the *variable type* to which a measure belongs, that is whether a measure gives nominal, ordinal, interval, or ratio data. This information may be used to select an appropriate statistical analysis which can be performed on the output values (see p. 87–95). In many cases, for instance measures that express time or distance, the variable type is clear. For others, which are more complex, the choice of variable type is much less apparent.

1.2.2 The name(s)

The initial text for a given measure will first describe all of the measures' varying names. For some measure, there are many names which are used interchangeably in the literature. For established measures, we stick to the most logical name from the perspective of all fields of eye-movement research, even if the name deviates from one or two research traditions. For measures that are newly established and little used, we use the original name from the paper, unless it has potential for misunderstanding, in which case we give it a name that most closely corresponds to the overall terminology and best describes its properties.

1.2.3 The operational definitions

Next, we describe the operational definitions of the measure, i.e. how the measure is calculated, in precise terms. Definitions will sometimes require mathematical descriptions, which we provide, often complemented by an illustration of the main principles behind the measure. We present mathematical and statistical methods at the first necessary occurrence, and later only refer to these, if, for instance, they are reused within the scope of other measures.

Operational definitions typically have a host of methodological considerations accompanying them. Sometimes these concern the type of eye-tracker, filters, or the settings in the detection algorithms, and sometimes the task or the participants themselves.

1.2.4 Typical values and histograms

We report values of measures from the literature and from our own research projects. Histograms are provided for normal data when possible, and can be used to decide which steps to take for statistical processing. Methodological issues often appear here, too.

1.2.5 Usage

Many measures contain a list of examples of research in which they have been used, such as:

Saccadic latency: When asked to react quickly, participants respond with a decreased saccadic latency (Kapoula, 1984).

Consider these references to research as *possible factors to take into consideration when designing your experiment*. Use them to support rather than substitute a literature search. Remember that if you use the measure in your study, the precise definitions of the measure must work for the experimental design and in particular the predictions in your hypotheses. In the selection of cited papers, we have aimed at breadth in method and applications rather than depth into theoretical questions. Measures in the position chapter have fewer such references, and instead, we summarize position research relevant to experimental design in the last section of this chapter.

1.3 Terminology and style

For a variety of reasons, terms on eye-tracker properties and measures are far from standardized. Thus, the precision of an eye-tracker is sometimes called 'spatial resolution', 'jitter', or 'inherent noise level' in product brochures and journal papers, and there has been no consensus on how it should be measured. For some measures, the many names originate from the divided research fields. In reading, for instance, there is a measure called 'gaze duration', which in human factors is called 'dwell time'. 'Dwell time' is often confused with 'total

dwell time', and 'gaze' has a completely different meaning outside of the reading community compared to within. In fact, the operational definition we give of the measure dwell time
in this book has at least eight alternative names in the literature. When two measures are
conceptually similar, such as 'dwell time' and 'fixation duration', they are often confused
with one another, even in some peer-reviewed publications. A few measures are christened
by the software engineer programming the manufacturer's analysis toolbox, so Areas of Interest (AOIs) may also be called LookZones or Interest Areas (IAs) depending on your brand
of eye-tracker. 'Raindrop analysis', 'Bee swarm', and 'Sinnbild' are three other examples of
data analysis terms chosen by programmers. The mysterious term 'main sequence', for the
relation between saccadic amplitude and peak velocity, was copied from the astronomical
term for the relation between the brightness and colour of small stars (Bahill, Clark, & Stark,
1975b). Other terms, such as 'scanpath', are so loaded with theoretical baggage that some
researchers refuse to use them, and invent alternative names, adding to the confusion.

Although most research papers are internally consistent in their use of terms, searching for
eye-movement measures and comparing between papers is made much more difficult by the
lack of overall standardization. Because previous publications have used a myriad of terms,
and future researchers need to know these when searching for and comparing to old research,
in the text, we list the major alternative names that have been used for eye-tracking concepts,
algorithms, events, representations, and measures. To the extent possible, the book adheres to
our preferred terminology, but quotations and figures from other authors retain their original
terminology.

Researchers in many fields use eye-trackers, and the terminology from their papers have
followed into this book. Although we have tried to adapt to the language of each application
field, mistakes may remain that are only visible to the insider.

1.4   Material used in the book

We have repeatedly used data from the following studies in examples:

1. 318 native speakers of Swedish read 16 pages from an English book on marketing, and
   160 of these came back two years later to read a very similar text. The first recording
   was made monocularly at 1250 Hz using the SMI HiSpeed system, and the second
   binocularly at 500 Hz using the same eye-trackers. Data are described in Nyström and
   Holmqvist (2010).
2. 24 speakers of Swedish read four texts from the standardized *Högskoleprovet* (Swedish
   Scholastic Aptitude test), either in silence, with cafeteria noise, while listening to music
   they like to listen to while studying, or while listening to music that they would never
   consider studying with. Recordings were made monocularly at 1250 Hz using the SMI
   HiSpeed system. Data description in Johansson, Holmqvist, Mossberg, and Lindgren
   (2011).
3. 68 people who were on their way into a supermarket were asked to wear the monocular
   SMI HED 200/25 Hz system while buying their groceries. Data are described in Gidlöf,
   Wallin, Dewhurst, and Holmqvist (in progress).
4. 23 engineering students and 21 students of the Humanities were asked to solve 43 mathematical problems of three different kinds, while their eye-movements were monitored
   using the SMI HiSpeed 1250 Hz system. Data are described in Holmqvist, Andrà, et
   al. (2011).

5. 24 ninth-graders browsed the web for 15 minutes using the SMI RED 4, 60 Hz system, with a set of 20 starting links to choose from, but with an instruction to browse freely. Data description in Sandberg, Gidlöf, and Holmberg (2011).

Ideally, we would have liked to have collected our examples from all 20+ manufacturers of eye-trackers, but this has proven practically impossible. The vast majority of examples in this book have been collected with SMI, Tobii, and SR Research systems in our lab, or in the labs of colleagues. We use the examples we have, because we think they are very general to many eye-trackers, and not specific to a single system or manufacturer. Softwares used and described are versions used during 2006–2010, the period during which we wrote the book, and are included to describe principles. We refer to manufacturer manuals for current versions.

By definition, a book on eye-tracking methodology will have to contain many examples of what works well and what can go wrong in eye-tracking research. Thus, during a few years, we have collected many examples of successes and mishaps in our own lab and the labs of colleagues, that we have used in the book as warnings and eye-openers. Our examples are not considered as an endorsement or critique of a particular eye-tracker, but the illustrated property should be critically evaluated against any eye-tracker you consider using.

Part I

Technical and Methodological Skills

Part I introduces the three central competence areas needed in any eye-tracking study: the hardware, the experimental design, and the actual recording of the data from participants. Mastering these skills is the key to producing high-quality eye-movement data.

2   Eye-tracker Hardware and its Properties

This chapter introduces the machines that we call *eye-trackers*, their properties, and the people manufacturing and using them. It provides a minimal level of technological detail for researchers who record and use eye-movement data. Earlier drafts have been reviewed by staff from SR Research Ltd., SMI GmbH, and Tobii AB, and by independent researchers with expertise in developing eye-trackers. The chapter is structured like this:

- First, a brief historical look back on how eye-trackers were built and used.
- Manufacturer customer relations are the focus of Section 2.2 (p. 12).
- In Section 2.3 (p. 16), we present a list of issues important to consider before acquiring an eye-tracker, and before setting up an eye-tracking laboratory.
- Section 2.4 (p. 17) focuses on the properties of the environment where you make your records (the 'lab'), and the competences needed in it.
- Section 2.5 (p. 21) gives a very condensed overview of the eye movements measured by an eye-tracker, and then describes the dominating measuring principle: the pupil-and-corneal-reflection method.
- In Section 2.6 (p. 29), we review the quality of recorded data. Methods for measuring data quality are discussed here.
- Section 2.7 (p. 51) covers the set-up of eye cameras and infrared illumination. This set-up differs depending on your chosen hardware, and your particular research question. These issues will be addressed with various pictures taken from our lab to illustrate the types of problems you might encounter, and solutions to them.

If you plan to buy an eye-tracker, read the entire chapter before ordering, considering how the different technical aspects described will impact the specific type of research that you wish to carry out. If you are just now beginning with an eye-tracking project, read only the summary checklist given in Table 2.2, and then go to Chapter 3. If you already have an eye-tracking lab up and running, you may find this chapter useful for organizational and technical background. Or if you only require a quick introduction to the technical terms used to describe eye-tracker properties, read from Section 2.5 in this chapter.

2.1   A brief history of the competences around eye-trackers

The earliest eye-trackers were built in the late 1800s. They were technically difficult to build, mostly mechanical, and not very comfortable for the participants. Huey (1898) used a bite-bar with partially cooled sealing-wax attached to the mouth-piece; this ensured participants kept their heads still. Delabarre (1898) anaesthetized the eyeball by applying a solution of two to three per cent cocaine; a Paris ring was then attached to the eye which connected it to a mechanical level. Only at the beginning of the twentieth century did Dodge and Cline (1901) introduce the principle of photographing the reflection of an external light source from the fovea. This is much less invasive and in recent years has become the dominating technique for recording eye movements.

From around 1950, individual researchers developed a number of different techniques, the most common of which are the following:

- Lens systems with mirrors (some protruding, making blinking difficult) were used by Yarbus, Ditchburn and others in the 1950s to 1970s. Having a very high precision, these highly uncomfortable contact lenses made possible the recording of very detailed movements of the eye.
- Electromagnetic coil systems, which measure the electromagnetic induction in a silicon contact lense placed on the anaesthetized eye, were long considered the most precise method of measuring any eye movements (Collewijn, 1998), but are now known to alter the saccades of participants who wear them (Frens & Van Der Geest, 2002; Träisk, Bolzani, & Ygge, 2005). Contact lenses had to be modelled individually for each participant, and even then often remained uncomfortable.
- Electrooculography (EOG) systems measure the electromagnetic variation when the dipole of the eyeball musculature moves. Also, EOG systems typically only measured horizontal movements, and suffered from the electromagnetic noise of surrounding muscles. They still exist as a low-cost variety of eye tracking, having a high sampling frequency, although accuracy is poor due to drift.
- The Dual Purkinje systems from Fourward Technology were very expensive, difficult to maintain, had a very small visual field of recording, but were also extremely precise and accurate without having to place something directly onto the participants eye. Using video, they recorded data using both the first and the fourth Purkinje reflections (Crane & Steele, 1985). However, Deubel and Bridgeman (1995) presented data indicating that saccade endings are inadequately measured with this technique, due to the fourth reflection.

For a closer review of these and other early technologies, see Duchowski (2007, pp. 51–59), Rötting (2001, pp. 41–53), Ciuffreda and Tannen (1995, pp. 184–205), L. R. Young and Sheena (1975), or Ditchburn (1973, pp. 36–77). Additionally, Wade and Tatler (2005) offer an excellent historical overview of eye-movement research.

Throughout most of the twentieth century, eye-movement researchers were required to build their own systems before using them to do research. Ready-made, over-the-counter eye-trackers were simply not an alternative. Even in relatively recent times, they have had to build their own eye-trackers themselves, from electronics that had to be understood in detail, as the following methods section from Heywood and Churcher (1981) clearly exemplifies:

> The experiments were carried out in a darkened room. Participants sat, their heads fixed by a dental bite and a forehead rest, facing a Tektronix 604 display CRT (31 phosphor) 51 cm away at eye level. The movements of their right eyes were recorded using an infrared photoelectric technique modified from those described by Wheeless et al. (1966) and Jones (1973). An image of the eye, lit with partially collimated infrared light from a GaAs LED (Texas Instruments, TIXL 16), was formed on a perspex screen, in which were mounted two infrared sensitive photodiodes (Texas Instruments, TILSI). The system was constructed so that with appropriate positioning of the two photodiodes, subtraction of their output signal yielded a signal linearly related to horizontal eye rotation over the central ±15° of the visual field, and addition of their output gave a similar signal related to vertical eye rotations linear over the central ±10°. In the present experiment we were concerned only with horizontal eye movements. The signals were amplified and were sampled by a computer (CAI Alpha LSI 2) that also controlled the participants' displays and recorded the movements of the target. The entire system had a half-power bandwidth of 330 Hz: the sample rate in the present experiment was 500 Hz, and the resolution of the system was better than 6 min arc.

Being required to build their own hardware had several disadvantages for scientists: Above all, it slowed down their research. It made eye tracking more exclusive and often completely impractical. However, running self-built eye-trackers had advantages, too: a researcher who has also built the system is more likely to know the properties of the data, and what filters and settings are necessary. Eye-movement behaviour can be more readily differentiated from the artefacts of the measurement system. Algorithms can be more closely attuned to actual eye-movement behaviour. Errors are easy to diagnose; and maintenance operations do not risk data quality as easily.

Beginning in the mid 1970s, this situation changed profoundly. Companies driven by engineers, such as ASL (Applied Science Laboratories), were beginning to build and sell eye-tracking systems to researchers. Ten years later, there were many companies offering eye-tracking hardware. Being able to buy eye-trackers made eye tracking more accessible and versatile. Suddenly researchers could focus on their research, leaving the technical issues to the manufacturer.

Of course, having one group of people *building* eye-trackers and another group *using* them gives rise to an unfortunate split of competencies. It is unfortunate for the researcher, because it is difficult to interpret (with absolute confidence) the data output from a system which they did not design. Likewise, researchers are often not trained in the technical skills required to maintain the system, and influence the technology and its development. Conversely, this situation is unfortunate for the manufacturer, because it is harder to build a system if you do not know exactly what it is going to be used for. It is uncommon for manufacturers to be trained in the principles of experimental design and statistical analysis, therefore the software and hardware requirements of researchers may not be met.

The number of researchers and others who use eye-trackers has grown enormously over the past 20 years. Current-day users of eye-trackers can choose between a large number of different systems from many competing manufacturers. Many of these strive to make it (seem) easy and effortless to do eye tracking. In fact, one line of current commercial development is going towards eye-tracking systems that require almost no system knowledge on the part of the user. In marketing research, some users are asking for eye-tracking systems that are so easy to use that it allows them to show a number of advertisements to any groups of participants, and then just press one button to get a diagnosis of the advertisement, without thinking about any of the technical properties of the eye-tracker, let alone experimental design.

In reality, eye-trackers are advanced physiological measuring systems, and they are produced in small series. Not enough people have tested and given feedback on them for you to be able to trust their functionality like you trust a DVD player, a microwave oven, or even a laptop computer. There will be difficulties in measurements, data quality issues and even bugs, and the diagnoses and workarounds will require system knowledge. We can use one DVD player for all disks, but not one eye-tracker for all studies. There are many technical aspects to eye-trackers that decide whether your particular study will be feasible with a particular eye-tracker. Researchers who understand their systems are much more likely to produce reliable results, and knowledgeable customers are much more likely to get a system they can actually use for the intended purpose.

Therefore, in this chapter, we will spend some time reviewing current types of eye-trackers and their properties, but also where eye-trackers should be located for optimal recordings and usability, and what sort of infrastructure is needed around them. First, however, we must discuss the current manufacturers and their complex relation to the researchers and others who buy equipment from them.

2.2 Manufacturers and customers

Before the 1980s, most researchers both built *and* did research with their eye-tracking system. Today, that single role is divided into two principal parties: the manufacturer and the researcher. Manufacturers have different origins. Some were founded by researchers, like SR Research with the EyeLink family of eye-trackers, co-founded by Dave Stampe and Eyal Reingold of the Department of Psychology at the University of Toronto, or Interactive Minds which grew from a group at the Department of Applied Psychology in Dresden. Others sprung out of engineering research work, for instance ASL (Applied Science Laboratory), which originates from MIT research in the 1960s and 1970s, and SMI (SensoMotoric Instruments), which spun off from an engineer's PhD thesis (Teiwes, 1991) on torsional eye tracking in neurological applications in the early 1990s.

In spring 2009, we could find 23 companies prepared to sell video-based eye-tracking systems to us. A handful of companies sell eye-trackers based on now less common principles, for instance coil systems, EOG systems, and diode-sensor systems. Of the 23 manufacturers of video-based eye-trackers, three were founded before 1985, and more than 50% after 2000. Most of them only sell one or two products, and several of those appear to have only a small customer group. The vast majority of companies have been founded by engineers and applied physicists, and very few of the companies had a psychologist in the group of founders.[1]

Over the past twenty years, several other manufacturers started but never grew large, and finally vanished. All the time, new people reinvent the wheel, possibly oblivious of the market situation, and this gives rise to media reports of "a new fantastic invention that can measure where people are looking", with predictions of the many applications such a tool could have. These inventions are seldom long-lived.

A few researchers continued building their own eye-trackers to give them the precise properties they required for their research. Mike Land's portable head-mounted eye-tracker from the mid-1990s is a good example, and Jeff Pelz and colleagues at Rochester also customize eye-trackers with similar goals in mind: to investigate eye movements in natural environments and when performing everyday tasks.

Sometimes a specific line of research develops its own eye-trackers, which is the case with the Visagraph, a series of family-based low-cost eye-trackers that have been used in diagnostic optometric reading tests in schools for several decades, but not in any other research. Similarly, the company Verify International, before going out of business in 2007, built their own eye-trackers for consumer research (known through publications such as Pieters & Wedel, 2004).

There is also an ongoing effort to develop smaller, less expensive, and more accessible eye-trackers, coordinated in the academic network COGAIN,[2] and it may not be long until it is technically feasible for each laptop to have a simple built-in eye-tracking function. Today, it is even possible to turn your webcamera into a simple eye-tracker.[3]

In the following bulleted list we cover the main customer groups, focusing on the large manufacturers who supply them. We have first-hand knowledge of these companies, their eye-trackers, and the support which they offer.

- The academic researcher group is definitely the oldest, and probably the largest of the customer groups. It is fairly stable over time, but also very heterogenous in research themes. Dispersed over almost all disciplines of science, they are united by a desire to

---

[1] The exact number is not easy to determine, but it is safe to say that psychologists are part of the founders/owners in at least four of these 23 companies.

[2] http://www.cogain.org/

[3] e.g., http://www.gazegroup.org

use proper experimental set-ups and statistics, often also emphasizing precise timing, accuracy, precision, and high sampling frequency in data. Researchers usually buy their eye-trackers as part of building or expanding a lab, or after having received funding for a project. In the authors' experience, for more than a decade, the leading manufacturers that provide for this demanding customer group are SR Research with the EyeLink system, SensoMotoric Instruments (SMI), and Applied Systems Laboratory (ASL), with Tobii Technology opening up and taking a leading role in some applied parts of academia.[4]

- Another large but much more recent group of eye-tracker customers is the media and advertisement consultants, who ask for eye-trackers that are simple to use. These consultants often want to rent the eye-tracker for a specific project, rather than buy it. They use eye-trackers as a method, among others, to decide whether to say "no" or "go" to an advertisement campaign, and they are often happy with heat map representations of data (see Chapter 7). Experimental designs and statistical significance tests typically do not give any added value to media or advertisement consultants. Also, some non-academic usability testers share methods and requirements with this user community. Many of the companies compete to sell to these users, but Tobii has dominated this customer category since the mid 2000s.

- Human factors researchers make up a small group that has existed for a long time. They have specific demands to be able to use eye-trackers in the field: in cars, nuclear plants, aeroplanes etc. Applied sports psychologists and consumer researchers can also have the same type of requirements, along with a few 'real-world' academic researchers. ASL, SMI, Smart-Eye, and Seeing Machines have traditionally had a focus on these users, but several others are also selling to this varied group.

- There is a group of clinical users of eye-trackers who are not interested in gaze positions per se, but are more concerned with movement patterns such as nystagmus, deviant saccadic forms, oculomotor dynamics, and torsional movements of the eye. Calibration must be possible even for participants who cannot fixate properly. The eye-trackers used for these purposes and the studies carried out, are often designed for diagnosing individual participants, or identifying core functional deficits of a visual disorder, rather than for testing large groups to find generalizable results.

- A previously small, but in later years very rapidly growing, group is the users of gaze-guided computer interfaces. They cannot operate a computer by other means, because of a disability or because the task requires their hands for other jobs. LC Technology was an early player in this group, now followed by Tobii and a few small companies. For this group, low price is often prioritized over high data quality. They want to interact with their computers using the eye-tracker on a one-to-one basis, and do not usually work with precise experimental designs and statistics over several users. Knowing the technical details of the system is often of little interest.

- Eye laser surgeons comprise a user group for which the primary interest is an accurate, precise, and quick eye-movement signal, that can be used to move a laser knife to compensate for the signal change when an eye movement occurs. Hardware and software requirements, as well as gaze estimation method, differ between this user group and all others.

---

[4]The strength of each company can be measured differently, for instance taking into account: 1) the number of peer-reviewed journal publications where their system was used, divided by research area and impact factors, 2) the number of systems sold, 3) the number of employees (divided into developers versus sales), 4) the presence of the manufacturer at conferences and meetings, and 5) the image they have in the community.

The users of eye-trackers, such as those listed above, also differ very much in their technical competence. Some labs, and some branches of research as a whole, have better skills than others to evaluate the technical properties of an eye-tracker before purchasing. Programming stimulus presentation, carrying out successful recordings, and developing algorithms and software for data analysis are all important considerations before buying an eye-tracker; proficiency in these abilities differs a lot between the user groups mentioned above, and this can effect the choice of which eye-tracker to buy and the validity of the studies carried out with it. Variance in the competencies required to evaluate and run eye-trackers, and program auxiliary software which compliments their use, exist both within academia and outside of it.

The *diversity* of customer groups has lead to manufacturers producing very different kinds of eye-trackers. Some of the manufacturers have a long history of providing eye-trackers of multiple types, for instance ASL and SMI, and to some extent SR Research (by offering optional extensions), while most of the others have concentrated on the specifics of their main target group.

Not only hardware and recording software, but also stimulus and presentation tools vary between manufacturers. The simple rule seems to be: the more a manufacturer provides for the academic community, the more versatile and powerful is their stimulus presentation tool, simply because the (predominantly academic) customers of those manufacturers have asked for solutions that support a large range of experimental designs. Manufacturers who mostly cater for the advertisement and usability customer group, typically offer slide shows with limited support for running sophisticated empirical studies; they rather emphasize web support in their stimulus tools.

The analysis software from manufacturers also reflects which customer groups they have. Many customers investigating applied domains (e.g. website usability) mainly care about *visualizations* of eye-tracking data (heat maps and scanpaths, see Chapters 7 and 8 for a thorough discussion), rather than graphs and appropriate statistical comparisons. The analysis software, and the way the salespeople present it, will then focus on visualizations that look good in demos, but will only have limited options for exporting data (other than raw data, fixation sequences, and area of interest hits). The researcher, however, is trained to trust a result *only* if it comes from a correctly performed experiment, with statistically significant effects. Therefore, the manufacturers with more academic researchers as customers have analysis software that allows for a variety of different experimental designs, and which can export a rich range of outcome measures (dependent variables).

The background of the manufacturers' *sales people* differs wildly. Before you take advice from any salesperson, find out what their *background and motivation* is: are they newly graduated engineers who know very little about eye-tracking research, or do they have comprehensive experience and know-how? If you press them on a technical issue, will they simply guess that their system handles it, or can they tell you about the technical properties of the system and the motivation behind it? How well do they understand the scientific aspects of eye-tracking research, and the role of their equipment and software in your workflow? What is their contact network in the scientific and applied fields of eye-tracking, and will they make it available to you? Can their claims about the role of their company and products among researchers and practitioners be supported by independent sources? Their prime motivation will always be to sell you a system, but does the salesperson have additional motivations that are beneficial to you: to maintain good relations to you as a customer, using you as a reference for future customers, to assist you in publishing papers in scientific journals; perhaps they are only interested in adding you as an additional node in their network clients to help them gain future sales.

Many customers over-estimate the *scientific competence of the manufacturers*, thinking that they not only produce the systems, but also know exactly how to use eye-trackers to do research, which settings to use for algorithms, and how to interpret the many metrics which can be derived from the data eye-trackers produce. All manufacturers know a lot about which cameras to use, the algorithms and filters used to process the video image, and the mathematics underlying gaze estimation, but too few staff of manufacturers are academics who publish research results. For a lot of the staff of manufacturers eye-trackers are products rather than research tools. Eyal Reingold of SR Research is a notable exception—with vast research experience in vision and eye movements he is a co-founder of the EyeLink system, arguably the most dominant eye-tracker on the market for the academic user group.

As competence in how to use eye-trackers for research still resides in the research laboratories, manufacturers will always need close collaboration with researchers who are well acquainted with the requirements and workflow of real eye-tracking studies when they make decisions about how to develop their hard- and software. When you talk to a manufacturer, try to find out how they gain access to scientists' experiences.

Sales people from the companies with a strong position in the academic world invariably say two things that are important to consider. First, they do not want to sell you something that you cannot use. This is a sign of normal business ethics. Second, if you want a property or functionality that they do not currently have, but which is interesting also for other customers, they will try to implement it and add it not only to the system that you buy, but to the future product line of the company. This is not only salespeople's talk; the authors of this book have witnessed several joint development projects with the three leading companies and researcher groups at universities. Customer requirements are a major factor behind product development, and it is important to evaluate a company in terms of how well they integrate requests (and bug reports) without compromising the integrity and overall consistency of their system.

If employees in a manufacturer company are often exchanged, there is a risk that their competence is lower than in a company where key staff have worked longer. Both technical development and customer relations are competencies that take time to form.

Evaluate the manufacturer's history of software upgrades. Are the upgrades coming at a reasonable rate? Do upgrades solve or address important issues? Is upgrading easy to perform? Are the upgrades done in such a way as to support comparability of results across software versions (for instance, when a new event detection algorithm is introduced)?

The manufacturer's *support line* is often the only remaining link between the manufacturer and the researcher. As an eye-tracker is a piece of equipment that often requires its owner to contact support, evaluate manufacturer support before acquiring the system. Be aware that the different manufacturers have very different reputations with respect to their support line. Some are extremely helpful, specific and quick, inviting discussion with a dedicated company representative who focuses on finding a solution that works for you as customer, and gives you feedback on how your request is being processed.

There is *no standardization* between systems. Terms for measurement quality differ, as well as the methods manufacturers use to calculate reported performance figures for their systems. Many of the concepts of recording and analysis also differ between manufacturers. Thus, comparing the webpages and specification sheets between several manufacturers and using that as a basis for acquiring an eye-tracker is often confusing and of little use.

Technological transparency and openness varies between manufacturer companies. There are several important aspects to this:

- Manufacturers vary in *how they record, calculate, and report performance values* such as precision. If you want to be sure, make your own tests.
- Some have developed *technically transparent recording software*, so that the user can see and control virtually everything. Several companies, for instance SMI, SR Research and ASL, have had this policy for a long time. The direct opposite is to hide the record-

ing settings, eye-video, and data viewers and only supply as little control as possible to the user. These opposing strategies obviously address the more versus less technical user groups. Technological transparency does require more of the user, in terms of getting over a competence threshold, but in the authors' experience, gives better and more easily comprehensible data.

- The *analysis software* of some manufacturers allows direct control over filter and algorithm settings, while other software has reduced access to or even makes settings inaccessible defaults. Again, having access to both allows and requires an understanding of the analysis tools, and increases your chances of performing a good, valid study.

Some customers would like their eye-tracking systems to be plug-and-play, with technical detail well hidden. Other customers are deeply suspicious of hidden details, knowing that the 'clean' data emerging may have lost the effect they looked for or introduced artefacts. In 2007, for example, a group of some 20 dissatisfied European academic users wrote a common letter to one manufacturer, demanding to have the source code for their fixation detection algorithm. In the long run, technological transparency and openness give better customer relations.

Still, relatively few users switch between manufacturers. *Long-term customer–manufacturer relationships* are common, for many reasons. The users are acquainted with the hardware, the stimulus and analysis software, and the way to work with them. In particular for users with lower technical competence, learning to use a second system, and having two manufacturers to talk to, is seen as a cost, which must be outweighed by the perceived improvement in the newly acquired technology, be it better precision or improved functionality.

To summarize so far, if you plan to use or even buy a particular eye-tracker:

- Find out who the manufacturers are and what competences the salespeople have that advise you to buy their system.
- Contact representatives of the manufacturer's customer group. Read their publications (or reports), talk to them at conferences, and visit their labs. If you need other things in your eye-tracker than what they make use of (or know about), check that these specifications are actually met. If their eye-trackers require other technical competences than those that you have, is it likely that you can gain the required skills?
- Take an academic course in eye-tracking methodology.
- Borrow a system and test it. The properties that we describe in Chapters 2–9 can mostly be turned into a test of hardware, algorithms, stimulus, and analysis tools.
- When talking to the manufacturers, bring the checklist in Table 2.2, and add your own points. Do not forget to ask them which variety of the algorithms and filters described in Chapters 2–9 they have implemented, and why.

2.3 Hands-on advice on how to choose infrastructure and hardware

In Tables 2.1 and 2.2, we provide condensed advice on the topics of the chapter. If you are setting up an eye-tracking laboratory, or if you let an established eye-tracking laboratory host your study, you might be interesting in checking Table 2.1. Table 2.2 is a list of which hardware and system properties addressed above should be checked before you buy an eye-tracker, or in any other way decide to use an eye-tracker in a study. Note that some properties concern only one type of eye-tracker, and that some are more fundamental than others.

Table 2.1 Properties of the recording environment and skills of those who run it.

Property to check	Risks if you ignore the property
Cramped recording space	Uncomfortable participant
Lab availability	Difficult to get participants to show up
Sunlight, lamps and lighting conditions	Optic artefacts, imprecision, and data loss
Electromagnetic fields	Optic artefacts, inaccuracy, and data loss (magnetic headtracking systems)
Vibrations	Variable noise, low precision
Scientific competence of technical staff	Invalid, unpublishable results; time-consuming studies
Recording experience of staff	Data quality low
Programming experience of staff	Data analysis very time-consuming
Statistical experience of staff	Invalid, unpublishable results; confusion

2.4 How to set up an eye-tracking laboratory

An eye-tracking laboratory needs both physical space for the eye-tracker and the experiments, and an infrastructure that keeps the laboratory up to date and running.

2.4.1 Eye-tracking labs as physical spaces

There is not one single solution for designing an eye-tracking laboratory. Every place where there are active people can be made into a place where researchers eye-track people. Take a car with a built-in eye-tracker and other measurement systems, or the mobile eye-trackers that we used in supermarkets for a study of consumer decision making. Neither are labs in the traditional sense. So, what is an eye-tracking lab, and how should it be designed? Most researchers work with single monitor stimuli, rather than real-life scenes. They then, in the authors' experience, prefer sound and light isolated rooms, minimizing the risk of distracting participants' attention from the task. They also tend to put their eye-tracker in very cramped locations (cubicles), where there is little room to turn around, let alone rebuild the recording environment for the needs of different studies.

In our lab, we found it useful to make the windowless recording rooms large enough (around 20–25 m^2) to be able to rebuild their interior depending on the varying needs of different projects (see Figure 2.1). Many labs—including our own—have also built one-way mirror windows between recording rooms and a central control room. This allows the researcher controlling the experiment to leave the participant(s) alone with their task, whilst still being able to monitor both recording status on the eye-tracking computer, and the participant through the one-way mirror. Having several recording rooms allows for multiple simultaneous recordings. At our lab in Lund, this has proved valuable more than once, when large data collections are to be made in a short period of time.

It is useful to minimize direct and ambient sunlight (i.e. to have few or no windows), and to illuminate the room with fluorescent lighting (the best are neon lights), which both emits less infrared light and vibrates less than incandescent bulbs (the worst are halogen lamps). Figure 4.15(a) on page 126 shows what a halogen lamp can do—note, do not make the room too dark, as this makes the pupil large (and variable), affecting data quality for most eye-trackers. A bright room keeps the pupil small even with a variable-luminance stimulus, which generally makes the data quality better. Also, in darker rooms the participant may

Table 2.2 Eye-tracker properties to ask manufacturers about.

Property to check	Risks if you ignore the property	Page
Manufacturer staff and openness policy	Poor support; strange errors in the system that are not explained to you	15
Manufacturer major user groups (publications; visits)	System properties that you need may be lacking	12
Software upgrade cycles and method	No improvement in software for years; a lot of hassle with software details	-
What eye movements can the system measure?	Study impossible to operationalize	23
Bi- or monocular	*Small* differences in fixation data go unnoticed	24
Averaging binocularity	Large offsets when one eye is lost	60
The quality of the eye camera	Noise (low precision)	38
Can the eye image be seen?	More difficult to record some participants; poorer understanding of system	116
The gaze estimation algorithm	Low data quality (precision and accuracy)	27
Frequency of infrared used	Poor data outdoors and in total darkness	-
Sampling frequency	You *may* need to record much more data; velocity and acceleration values invalid	29
Accuracy	Spatial (area of interest) analyses will be invalid	41
Drift (accuracy drops over time)	Constant recalibration; experimental design changes	42
Precision	Fixation and saccade data will be invalid; gaze contingency difficult; small movements not detectable	34
Filters used in velocity calculations	Fixation and saccade data will be imprecise	47
Headbox (remotes)	Data and quality loss when participant moves	58
Head movement compensation algorithm	Noise (low precision); spatial inaccuracy	-
Recovery time	Larger data loss just after participant moves or blinks	53
Latencies (in both recording and stimulus software)	Invalid results; gaze contingency studies impossible	43
Camera and illumination set-up	Data recording difficult or not possible with glasses	53
Robustness, the versatility for recording on more difficult participant populations	Data loss and poorer data for many participants	57
Portability of mobile system	Cannot be used out of laboratory	-
Connectivity	Difficult or impossible to add auxiliary stimulus presentations or data recordings	-
Tracking range	Data loss when participant looks in corners	58
Reference system for output coordinates	Data analysis very time consuming for some head-mounted systems	61
Parallax	Small and systematic offset in gaze-overlaid video data	60

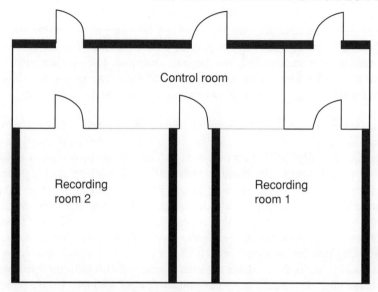

Fig. 2.1 Layout of one recording area in the Humanities Laboratory at Lund University. Each recording studio is 25 m². Ante-chambers allow for reception of participants, storage, and a space for the researcher to work between participants. We also have several additional recording rooms for minor studies, technical maintenance, and storage.

see the infrared illumination reflected in the mirror, although this depends somewhat on the wavelength of light emitted from the illumination.

Sounds will easily distract your participant's visual behaviour, so it is advisable to use a soundproof room if you can. For sensitive measurements, place the eye-tracker on a firm table standing on a concrete floor. Do not allow the participant to click the mouse or type on the keyboard on the same table where the eye-tracker is located. Also minimize vibrations from nearby motion of people or outside traffic. If you are using magnetic systems for head-tracking, also minimize various sources of electromagnetic noise (lifts, fans, some computers) in the recording and neighbouring rooms. Stabilized electrical current is an advantage for some measurements, but not critical.

If you are recording eye-tracking data in fMRI systems, the strong magnetic fields require optimized eye-tracking equipment to be used, typically built to film the eye from a safe distance with long-range optics and mirrors near the face. With MEG systems, no auxiliary electromagnetic field may be introduced, and therefore long-distance eye-trackers are also used.

If possible, have your laboratory close to a participant population, or at least make it easy for your participants to reach your lab. That makes it easier to set up a 'production line' where participants arrive one after the other to large recordings.

2.4.2 Types of laboratories and their infrastructure

There are labs that have done eye tracking for 20 years or more, and there are others that have just started. There are labs that only serve a few researchers around the owner of the system, and there are labs that actively invite others to use their equipment, against a cost. There are some eye-tracking companies that conduct studies on a commercial basis.

The largest *commercial* eye-tracking labs have 20–50 eye-trackers to test advertisement campaigns. They are connected to, and sometimes part of, the largest, well-known consumer product companies, and have gathered the necessary technical and scientific competence in their groups. Unfortunately, they do not publish their work, and they are reluctant to talk about how they use eye tracking and how they are structured. The smallest commercial eye-tracking labs are often media consultants, consisting of one or two people, who often have no previous experience in any of the competence areas necessary to do high-quality eye-tracking work.

Many *academic* eye-tracking laboratories consist of a professor and one or two graduate students and/or post-doctoral researchers, who between them can mostly provide the *scientific* competence needed in their own studies, and who can—if needed—also read up on previous eye-movement research and its technicalities. Some labs quickly grasp the technology of their eye-tracker. If the research group is less technically inclined, the necessary *technical* maintenance is often thought to be a task for the computer technician in the department, the one who is also responsible for email, servers, web, and some programming. However, unless the computer technician learns how to operate and design studies with the eye-tracker, such a division of competences is, in our experience, an unfortunate organization of labs. It typically forces the graduate students to take full charge of the eye-tracker, solve technical issues, upgrade the software, and maintain contact with the manufacturer's support line. The graduate students do this because anyone who makes a change in hardware or the settings of the recording system must also understand that system well enough to be able to make a recording, and see that the data quality requirements for the next study in line are satisfactorily met. Since data quality issues are central throughout the research process, from data recording, over the various stages of data analysis, to the responses from reviewers to submitted manuscripts, satisfactory diagnosis and maintenance of an eye-tracker can only be done by a person confident in *all* aspects of this research process. It can be difficult to find an employee who is sufficiently competent in every one of these skills, and inevitably mistakes will be made as graduate students learn.

Ideally, a *larger lab* is headed by a person who has both technical and research background, someone who can bridge the competence gap that originates from the time when eye-trackers began to be manufactured and sold. This means knowing the recording technology in enough detail to know what a good signal is, to diagnose and remedy errors, to be able to record and analyse data, and follow the research process all the way from hypothesis formulation to reviewer comments and publication.

Since recording high-quality eye-tracking data requires expertise that they can only get from experience, it is important for the staff doing the actual recording work to take part in many recordings with different participants, stimuli, and tasks. As the quality of recorded data is important for subsequent data analysis, it is easier if the same person does both recording and analysis; it is better if the researcher with the highest incentive to get good data takes part in the recordings, so she can influence the many choices made during eye-camera set-up and calibration (pp. 116–134). The exception is when the analysis is subjective in nature and needs to be performed by a person naive to the purpose of the experiment. Any staff who meet and greet participants should have appropriate professionalism for the job; they should be able to answer questions relating to the experimental procedure which the participant is about to undergo.

It is very useful if laboratory staff are also knowledgeable in programming, both for stimulus presentation and for data coding/analysis. Matlab, R, and Python are the preferred software in our and many other labs. If you have scientific ambitions—following the standards of peer-reviewed journals, rather than having heat maps as deliverables—it is also very useful to have a dedicated methodological and statistical specialist in your laboratory.

Since it may be difficult to find all these qualities in one person, you may need several staff members in your lab. Finally, whether you alone carry the full responsibility of your eye-tracking laboratory, or you share it with others, it is very useful to be part of a laboratory network, sharing experiences, knowledge, and software.

2.5 Measuring the movements of the eye

This section introduces the major eye-movement measuring method in use today, the pupil-and-corneal-reflection method. To better understand the principles of this measurement technique, we will begin with a very brief survey of the eye, and its basic movements.

2.5.1 The eye and its movements

The human eye lets light in through the *pupil*, turns the image upside down in the lense and then projects it onto the back of the eyeball–the *retina*. The retina is filled with light-sensitive cells, called *cones* and *rods*, which transduce the incoming light into electrical signals sent through the optic nerve to the visual cortex for further processing. Cones are sensitive to what is known as high spatial frequency (also known as visual detail) and provide us with colour vision. Rods are very sensitive to light, and therefore support vision under dim light conditions.

There is a small area at the bottom of Figure 2.2(a), called the *fovea*. Here, in this small area, spanning less than 2° of the visual field, cones are extremely over-represented, while they are very sparsely distributed in the periphery of the retina. This has the result that we have full acuity only in this small area, roughly the size of your thumb nail at arm's distance. In order to see a selected object sharply, like a word in a text, we therefore have to move our eyes, so that the light from the word falls directly on the fovea. Only when we *foveate* it can we read the word. Foveal information is prioritized in processing due to the cortical magnification factor, which increases linearly with eccentricity, from about 0.15°/mm cortical matter at the fovea to 1.5°/mm at an eccentricity of 20° (Hubel & Wiesel, 1974). As a result, about 25% of visual cortex processes the central 2.5° of the visual scene (De Valois & De Valois, 1980).

For video-based measurement of eye movements, the pupil is very important. The other important, and less known, element on the eyeball is the *cornea*. The cornea covers the outside of the eye, and reflects light. The reflection that you can see in someone's eyes usually comes from the cornea. When tracking the eyes of participants, we mostly want only one reflection (although in some systems two or more reflections are used), so we record in infrared, to avoid all natural light reflections, and typically illuminate the eye with one (or more) infrared light source. The resulting *corneal reflection* is also known as 'glint' and the '1st Purkinje reflection' (P1). One should also be aware that light is reflected further back as well—both off the cornea and the lens—as illustrated in Figure 2.2(b). The corneal reflection is the brightest, but not the only reflection.

Human eye movements are controlled by three pairs of muscles, depicted in Figure 2.3. They are responsible for horizontal (yaw), vertical (pitch), and torsional (roll) eye movements, respectively, and hence control the three-dimensional orientation of the eye inside the head. According to Donder's law (Tweed & Vilis, 1990), the orientation uniquely decides the direction of gaze, independent of how the eye was previously orientated. Large parts of the brain are engaged in controlling these muscles so they direct the gaze to relevant locations in space.

The most reported event in eye-tracking data does not in fact relate to a movement, but to the state when the eye remains still over a period of time, for example when the eye temporarily stops at a word during reading. This is called a *fixation* and lasts anywhere from some tens

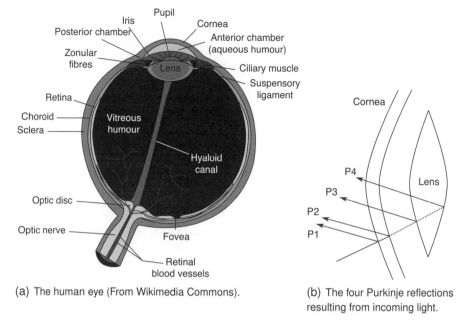

(a) The human eye (From Wikimedia Commons).

(b) The four Purkinje reflections resulting from incoming light.

Fig. 2.2 For eye tracking, the important parts in the order encountered by incoming light are: the *cornea*, the *iris* and *pupil*, the *lens*, and the *fovea*.

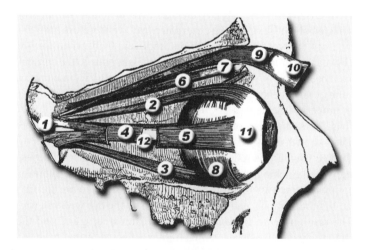

Fig. 2.3 The human eye muscles. The muscle pair (2)–(3) generate the vertical up-down movements, while (4)–(5) generate horizontal right-left movements. The pair (7)–(8) generate the torsional rotating movement. (9)–(10) control the eyelid. Reprinted from Gray's Anatomy of the Human Body, Henry Gray, Copyright (1918).

of milliseconds up to several seconds. It is generally considered that when we measure a fixation, we also measure attention to that position, even though exceptions exist that separate the two.

The word 'fixation' is a bit misleading because the eye is not completely still, but has three distinct types of micro-movements: *tremor* (sometimes called physiological nystagmus), *microsaccades* and *drifts* (Martinez-Conde, Macknik, & Hubel, 2004). Tremor is a small movement of frequency around 90 Hz, whose exact role is unclear; it can be imprecise

Table 2.3 Typical values of the most common types of eye movement events. Most eye-trackers can only record some of these.

Type	Duration (ms)	Amplitude	Velocity
Fixation	200–300	–	–
Saccade	30–80	4–20°	30–500°/s
Glissade	10–40	0.5–2°	20–140°/s
Smooth pursuit	–	–	10–30°/s
Microsaccade	10–30	10–40'	15–50°/s
Tremor	–	< 1'	20'/s (peak)
Drift	200–1000	1–60'	6–25'/s

muscle control. Drifts are slow movements taking the eye away from the centre of fixation, and the role of microsaccades is to quickly bring the eye back to its original position. These intra-fixational eye movements are mostly studied to understand human neurology.

The rapid motion of the eye from one fixation to another (from word to word in reading, for instance) is called a *saccade*. Saccades are very fast—the fastest movement the body can produce—typically taking 30–80 ms to complete, and it is considered safe to say that we are blind during most of the saccade. Saccades are also very often measured and reported upon. They rarely take the shortest path between two points, but can undergo one of several shapes and curvatures. A large portion of saccades do not stop directly at the intended target, but the eye 'wobbles' a little before coming to a stop. This post-saccadic movement is called a *glissade* in this book (p. 182).

If our eyes follow a bird across the sky, we make a slower movement called *smooth pursuit*. Saccades and smooth pursuit are completely different movements, driven by different parts of the brain. Smooth pursuit requires something to follow, while saccades can be made on a white wall or even in the dark, with no stimuli at all.

Typical values for the most common types of eye movements are given in Table 2.3. While these eye movements are the ones most researchers report on, especially in psychology, cognitive science, human factors, and neurology, there are several other ways for the eye to move, which we will meet later in the book.

Rather than mm on a computer screen, eye movements are often measured in *visual degrees* (°) or *minutes* ('), where $1° = 60'$. Given the viewing distance d and the visual angle θ, one can easily calculate how many units x the visual angle spans in stimulus space. The geometric relationships between these parameters are shown in Figure 2.4, and can be expressed as

$$\tan \frac{\theta}{2} = \frac{x}{d} \tag{2.1}$$

Note, however, that this relationship holds only when the gaze angle is small, i.e. when the stimulus is viewed in the central line of sight. For large gaze angles, the same visual angle θ_1 may result in different displacements (x_1 and x_2) on the stimulus, as illustrated in Figure 2.4.

If your stimulus is shown on a computer screen, you may want to use pixels units instead of e.g. mm. If $M \times N$ mm denotes the physical size of a screen with resolution $r_x \times r_y$ pixels, then 1 mm on the screen corresponds to r_x/M pixels horizontally and r_y/N pixels vertically.

When measuring eye-in-head movement, visual angle is the only real option to quantify eye movements, since the movements are not related to any points in stimulus space. Visual angle is also suitable for head-mounted eye tracking in an unconstrained environment, e.g. a supermarket, since the distance to the stimulus will change throughout the recording.

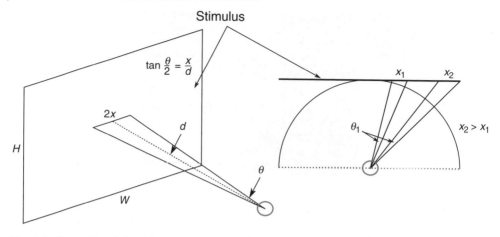

Fig. 2.4 Geometric relationship between stimulus unit x (e.g., pixels or mm) and degrees of visual angle θ, given the viewing distance d. Notice that on a flat stimulus, the same visual angle (θ_1) gives two different displacements (x_1, x_2).

2.5.2 Binocular properties of eye movements

An important aspect of human vision is that both eyes are used to explore the visual world. When using the types of movements defined in the previous section, the eyes sometimes move in relation to each other. *Vergence* eye movement refers to when the eyes move in directly opposite directions, i.e. converging or diverging. These opposite movements are important to avoid double vision (diplopia) when the foveated object moves in a three-dimensional space.

For most participants, both eyes look at the same position in the world. But many people have a dominant eye, and one which is more passive. If the difference is large, the passive eye may be directed in a different direction from that of the dominant one, and we say colloquially that the participant is *squinting*. The technical term is either *binocular disparity* or *disjugacy*.

In reading, disparity can be in the order of one letter space at the onset of a new fixation, and can occur in more than half of the fixations. Liversedge, White, Findlay, and Rayner (2006) found that disparity decreased somewhat over the period of the fixation, but not completely, and was of both crossed (right eye to the left of the average gaze position and vice versa) and uncrossed nature. In a non-reading 'natural' task, Cornell, MacDougall, Predebon, and Curthoys (2003) reported disparities of up to $\pm 2°$, but also noticed that disparities of $5°$ were present (but rare) in the data. All these results were found for normal, healthy participants.

While it is commonly believed that the eyes move in temporal synchrony, binocular coordination varies over time. During the initial stage of a saccade, for example, the abducting eye (moving away from the nose) has been found to move faster and longer than the adducting eye (moving towards the nose) (Collewijn, Erkelens, & Steinman, 1988). At the end of the saccade this misalignment is corrected, both through immediate glissadic adjustments, and slower post-saccadic drift during the subsequent fixation (Kapoula, Robinson, & Hain, 1986).

2.5.3 Pupil and corneal reflection eye tracking

The dominating method for estimating the point of gaze—where someone looks on the stimulus—from an image of the eye is based on pupil and corneal reflection tracking (see D. W. Hansen & Ji, 2009, Hammoud, 2008, and Duchowski, 2007 for technical details and

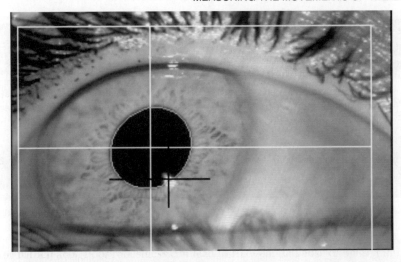

Fig. 2.5 A pupil–corneal reflection system has properly identified the pupil (white cross-hair) and corneal reflection (black cross-hair) in the video image of a participant's eye.

an overview of other methods).

A picture of an eye with both pupil and corneal reflection correctly identified can be seen in Figure 2.5. While it is possible to use pupil-only tracking, the corneal reflection offers an additional reference point in the eye image needed to compensate for smaller head movements. This advantage has made video-based pupil and corneal reflection tracking the dominating method since the early 1990s.

The pupil can either appear dark in the eye image, which is the most common case, or bright, as with some ASL (Applied Science Laboratory), LC Technology, and Tobii systems. The bright pupil is bright because of infrared light reflected back from the retina, through the pupil. Such a system requires the infrared illumination to be co-axial with the view from the eye camera, which puts specific requirements on the position of cameras and illumination (Figure 2.6(a)). As long as the pupil is large, a bright-pupil system operates in approximately the same way as a dark-pupil system, but for small pupil sizes (when there is a lot of ambient light), a bright-pupil system may falter. The original motivation behind bright-pupil systems appears to have been to compensate for poor contrast sensitivity in the eye camera by increasing the difference in light emission between pupil and iris, but with new improved camera technology, contrast between iris and pupil is often also very good for most dark-pupil systems, as can be seen in Figure 2.5. At least one eye-tracker has been built that switches between bright and dark tracking mode, which requires the turning on and off of several infrared illuminators depending on how well tracking works in the current state (Figure 2.6). No studies have systematically investigated which of the two tracking modes gives better data quality over large populations, but in the authors' experience, data quality rather depends on the quality of the eye camera and other parts of the eye-tracker.

Noteworthy is that the methods used for image analysis and gaze estimation can vary significantly across different eye-trackers, both freely available and commercial. Therefore it may be difficult to compare systems between different manufacturers. To complicate the issue even further, some eye-tracking manufacturers keep many key technical details about the system secret from the user community. Sometimes the user is not allowed to see how the eye image is analysed, for instance, but only a very simplified representation of the position of the eyes is given. Figure 2.7 shows the eye image and the simultaneous simplified representation of the eyes, on a *remote system* (p. 51). If the recording software allows the operator to see

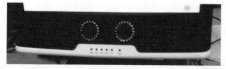

(a) Bright pupil mode: A ring of infrared diodes around the two eye cameras, making illumination almost co-axial with camera view.

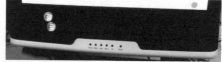

(b) Single side dark-pupil mode: Diodes off-axis to the left.

(c) Dual side dark-pupil mode: Diodes off-axis on both sides.

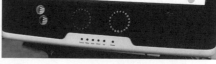

(d) Searching: Rapidly switching between dark- and bright-pupil illumination.

Fig. 2.6 Four illumination states of the Tobii T120 dual mode remote eye-tracker. This particular eye–tracker changes to another tracking mode when tracking fails in the current mode.

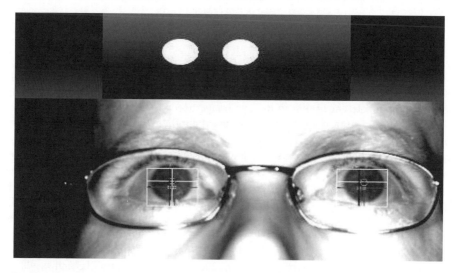

Fig. 2.7 Eye image in bottom half; and simplified representation of the eyes at the top.

the eye image, it is easier to set up the eye camera to ensure that tracking is optimal. Access to the eye image also makes it easier to anticipate and detect potential problems before and during data collection (pp. 116–134).

Figure 2.8 shows a schematic overview of a video-based eye-tracker, where the operations required to calculate where someone looks have been divided in three main blocks: *image acquisition*, *image analysis*, and *gaze estimation*.

In the acquisition step, an image of the eye is grabbed from the camera and sent for analysis. This can usually be done very quickly, but if head movement is allowed (as in remote eye-trackers), the first step of the analysis is to detect where the face and eyes are positioned in the image, whereafter image-processing algorithms segment the pupil and the corneal reflection from a zoomed-in portion of the eye. Geometrical calculations combined with a calibration procedure are finally used to map the positions of the pupil and corneal reflection to the data sample (x, y) on the stimulus.

While the pupil is a part of the eye, the corneal reflection is caused by an infrared light

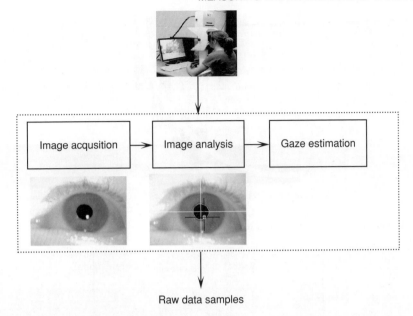

Raw data samples

Fig. 2.8 Overview of a video based eye-tracking system.

source positioned in front of the viewer. The overall goal of image analysis is to robustly detect the pupil and the corneal reflection in order to calculate their geometric centres, which are used in further calculations. This is typically done using either *feature-based* or *model-based* approaches. The feature-based approach is the simplest where features in the eye image are detected by criteria decided automatically by an algorithm or subjectively by the experimenter. One such criterion is thresholding, which finds regions with similar pixel intensities in the eye image. Having access to a good eye image where the pupil (a dark oval) and the corneal reflection (smaller bright dot) are clearly distinguishable from the rest of the eye is important for thresholding approaches. Another feature-based approach looks for gradients (edges, contours) that outline regions in the eye image that resemble the target features, e.g. the pupil.

To increase the precision of the calculation of geometric centres, the algorithms typically include sub-pixel estimation of the contours outlining the detected features. The principal calculation is illustrated in Figure 2.9.

The major weakness of feature-based pupil–corneal reflection systems is that the calculation of pupil centre may be disturbed by a descending eyelid and downward pointing eye lashes. Lid occlusion of the pupil may cause—as we will see on pages 116–134 on camera set-up—*offsets* (incorrectly measured gaze positions) and increased *imprecision* in the data in some parts of the visual field. Figure 2.10 shows a participant with a drooping eyelid and downward eyelashes. The pupil is covered and cannot be identified, while the corneal reflection is dimly seen among the lashes.

A second weakness of feature-based systems concerns extreme gaze angles, at which the corneal reflection is often lost, but as we explain on pages 116–134, this can often be solved by moving the stimulus monitor, eye cameras, or infrared sources.

A third and mostly minor weakness is that the measured gaze position may be sensitive to variations in pupil dilation. In recordings where accuracy errors are not tolerated—as in the control systems for the lasers used in eye surgery—another technology called limbus-tracking is used. The limbus is the border between the iris and the sclera. It is insensitive to variations

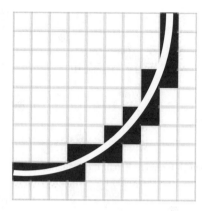

Fig. 2.9 Increasing precision by sub-pixel estimation of contours.

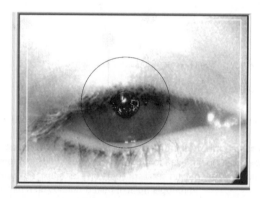

Fig. 2.10 In model-based eye tracking, the recording computer uses a model of the eye to calculate the correct position of the iris and the pupil in the eye video, even if parts of them are occluded by the eyelids. Rings indicate features of the model.

in pupil dilation, but very sensitive to eyelid closure, and is therefore fairly impractical except in specific applications such as laser eye surgery.

Model-based solutions can alleviate the weakness of feature-based pupil–corneal reflection systems by using a model of the eye that fits onto the eye image using pattern matching techniques (Hammoud, 2008). A useful eye model would assume that both iris and pupil are roughly ellipsoidal and that the pupil is in the middle of the iris. For example, using an ellipsoidal fit of the pupil would prevent the calculated centre of the pupil moving downward when the upper eyelid occludes the top part of the pupil, something that happens in the beginning and at the end of each blink, or when the participant gets drowsy.

Another model assumption is that the pupil is darker than the iris, which is darker than the sclera. When the model knows this, it can position the iris and pupil circles onto the most probable position in the image.

Moriyama, Xiao, Cohn, and Kanade (2006) implemented and tested a model-based iris detector that could be used for eye tracking. Although it does solve many eyelid problems known from feature-based pupil–corneal reflection systems, the model-based eye-tracker still sometimes misplaces the iris due to shadows in the eye image. While having the potential to provide more accurate and robust estimations of where the pupil and corneal reflection centres are located, model-based approaches add significantly to the computational complexity since they need to search for parts of the eye image that best fit the model. Without a good initial guess of where the pupil and corneal reflections are located, the time it takes the algorithm to find the indented features (often called *recovery time*) may be unacceptably long. Fortunately, a full search is needed only in the first frame, since feature positions in subsequent frames can be predicted from previous ones. Note that recovery time is very individual, since the algorithm will find some participants' eyes much faster than others. As feature-based approaches can provide this first guess, eye-tracking approaches that combine feature- and model-based approaches will probably become even more common in the future.

Now assume that the centres of both pupil and corneal reflection have been correctly identified, that the head is fixed and that we have a complete geometrical model of the eye, the camera, and the viewing set-up; then the gaze position could be calculated mathematically (Guestrin & Eizenman, 2006). However, this is usually not done in real systems, mainly due to the difficulty in obtaining robust geometric models of the eye. Instead, the majority of current systems use the fact that the relative positions of pupil and corneal reflections change systematically when the eye moves: the pupil moves faster, and the corneal reflection more slowly. The eye-tracker reads the relative distance between the two and calculates the gaze position on the basis of this relation. For this to work, we must give the eye-tracker some examples of how points in our tracked area correspond to specific pupil and corneal reflection relations. We tell this to the eye-tracker by performing a *calibration*, which typically consists of 5, 9, or 13 points presented in the stimulus space that are fixated and sampled one at the time. The practical details of calibration are described on pages 128–134.

While using one camera and one infrared source works quite well as long as the head is fairly still, more cameras and infrared sources can be used to relax the constraints on head movement and calibration. Using two infrared sources gives another reference point in the eye image, and is in theory the simplest system that allows for free head movement, which is desirable in remote eye-trackers. Using multiple cameras and infrared sources, it is theoretically possible to use only one point to calibrate the system (Guestrin & Eizenman, 2006). However, using another light source complicates the mathematical calculations.

The most common commercially available eye-trackers are those with one or two cameras and one or multiple infrared light sources that work best with 5, 9, and 13 point calibrations. More on different types of eye-camera set-ups can be found on pages 51–64.

2.6 Data quality

Data quality is a property of the sequence of raw data samples produced by the eye-tracker. It results from the combined effects of eye-tracker specific properties such as sampling frequency, latency, and precision, and participant-specific properties such as glasses, mascara, and any inconsistencies during calibration and in the filters during and after recording.

Some eye-trackers also output pupil and corneal reflection positions, calculated directly from the eye image prior to gaze estimation. We will not talk about the quality of this position data as they are not used very often; however, the reader should observe that they have properties common to the sequence of raw data samples.

Data quality is of the utmost importance, as it may undermine or completely reverse results. Already McConkie (1981) argues that every published research article should list measured values for the quality of the data used, but this has not yet become the standard.

2.6.1 Sampling frequency: what speed do you need?

The sampling frequency is one of the most highlighted properties of eye-trackers by manufacturers, and there is a certain competition in having the fastest system. You do need some speed in your system to be able to calculate certain eye-tracking measures, but high-speed eye-trackers are typically more expensive, more restrictive for the participants, and also produce larger data files.

Sampling frequency is measured in *hertz* (Hz), a unit we will frequently use throughout the book. A 50 Hz eye-tracker records the gaze direction of participants 50 times per second. This may sound like often enough, but a 50 Hz eye-tracker is generally considered a slow system.

So what speed do you need in your eye-tracker? For oscillating eye movements, we can use the Nyquist-Shannon sampling theorem to argue that a sampling frequency at least twice as large as the recorded movement is needed. For instance, for a tremor at 150 Hz, the necessary minimal sampling rate for detection is 300 Hz. Generally, the required sampling frequency depends on what you need to detect or measure, and how precisely you want to measure it. The faster the eye movement, the faster your system has to be.

However, most statements on required sampling frequency are not based on scientific or mathematical investigation. For instance, the border between low speed and high speed is often considered to be around 250 Hz. Why 250 Hz? There are only a few, little-cited studies to support this, and they all deal with the calculation of saccadic peak velocity. Nevertheless, it has gradually become accepted that the statistical effect sizes most studies report would be undermined by using a system which records at a frequency less than 250 Hz. But does this mean that data recorded with systems slower than 250 Hz will suffer from a temporal inaccuracy that renders statistical conclusions invalid? This depends on your outcome measure/dependent variable and your desired effect size. In the literature on reading research, differences below 20 milliseconds in fixation durations are claimed; at the limit of your system's capabilities one might reasonably question the validity and replicability of these effects.

Existing eye-trackers cover a spectrum of sampling frequencies from a few Hz up to more than 1000 Hz.

25–30 Hz These are the slowest systems sold, and typically record data only as gaze-overlaid videos (p. 61). The sampling rates 25 and 30 Hz (or more precisely 29.97 Hz) originate respectively from the European television PAL-standard and the NTSC-standard used in the United States. Only web-cam based eye-trackers are slower.

50–60 Hz Many remote systems and head-mounted eye-trackers run at this speed, because it was the most common frequency in camera technology for a long time.

120 Hz This range of sampling frequencies gradually became more common from around 2007.

250 Hz The low end of the higher speed systems, set here because this was the speed of the 1990s eye-tracker SMI EyeLink I, running at 250 Hz.[5]

500 Hz Midsection of sampling frequencies that was reached by pupil-corneal reflection eye-trackers around the year 2000. Not many manufacturers provide this speed, and those that do typically offer eye-trackers that are *tower-mounted contact systems* (defined on p. 51).

1000–2000 Hz The highest sampling frequencies available in 2010. Before these high-speed video-based eye-trackers arrived around 2006, only coil-based and dual Purkinje systems had this speed.

The higher the speed of the eye-tracker, the more infrared illumination is needed, since each eye camera sample is collected for a shorter interval (like camera shutter speed and ISO in traditional photography). Also notice that sampling may be different between the two eyes. Some dual camera systems such as the remote eye-tracker EyeFollower from LC

---

[5]Up until August 2001, SMI manufactured and sold the EyeLink eye-trackers.

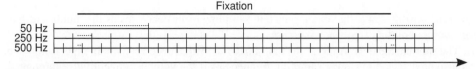

Fixation

50 Hz		
250 Hz		
500 Hz		

Fig. 2.11 A hypothetical fixation recorded at sampling frequencies 50, 250, and 500 Hz. At each small peg along the time line, the eye camera photographs the eye, and a gaze position is calculated, and we have a sample. As the fixation starts and ends anywhere between samples, and is not recorded until the subsequent sample, we will have errors on the calculated fixation duration at both start and end. Errors—indicated with dashed lines—will be larger for slower systems, but when averaging over many durations, these errors to a large extent become equal (R. Andersson, Nyström, & Holmqvist, 2010).

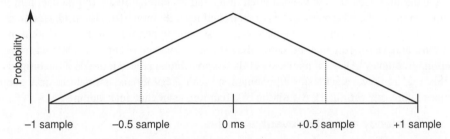

Fig. 2.12 The probability function for fixation duration measurement error at a given sampling frequency.

Technologies are particular in that they can output 120 Hz data, but every sample is taken alternately from the opposite eye, requiring only 60 Hz sampling from cameras.

Samples, and what happens between them

When a *single* photo is taken of the eye and processed by gaze estimation, it results in a *sample*. For a 50 Hz system, there are 50 samples recorded per second. Each sample is ideally momentous; but even in real 50 Hz systems, it is not 20 ms long. It is the intermediary window of no sampling that is 20 ms long. Figure 2.11 illustrates samples and the intermediary windows of no sampling, along a time line for three different sampling frequencies.

A fixation that we recognize in a sample can have started anytime between the previous sample (when we saw there was no saccade) and the current sample. If you have a 50 Hz system, you have 20 ms between samples, so the saccade can start anywhere within that window of no sampling (of 20 ms). If instead you have a 500 Hz eye-tracker, the window of no sampling is only 2 ms. This means that with a higher sampling frequency, we can more precisely measure the start and end ('on-' and 'offset') of saccades, fixations, and other events of the eye.

Fixation durations and other event durations

Given a low-speed eye-tracker, can we reliably measure, e.g. fixation durations? R. Andersson et al. (2010) quantified the effect of sampling frequency on event durations such as fixation durations in a series of simulations and tests on real data. Since the probability of error in sampled event durations follows the distribution shown in Figure 2.12, the central limit theorem can be used to deduce the relationship between sampling frequency (f_s), number of data points (e.g. fixation durations) (n) and the resulting error,

$$\bar{\varepsilon} \sim N(0, \frac{1}{18nf_s^2})$$ (2.2)

This relationship shows that the variance in sampling error decreases as the number of fixations or the sampling frequency increases.

The simulations in R. Andersson et al. (2010) show that even very small effect differences can also be detected at slower sampling frequencies if the number of recorded data points is large enough. There is a quadratic relation between the sampling frequency and the number of fixations needed. This means that, for example, if you are choosing between a 50 and a 250 Hz system, if all else is equal, you will need 25 times $((\frac{250}{50})^2)$ as many data points with the 50 Hz system to achieve the same low variance in the average as with the 250 Hz system. In other words, for most event durations, it is always possible to compensate for the effect of a low sampling frequency with more data. Equation (2.2) is generally true for all eye-tracking duration measures with a sampled onset and a sampled offset. In practice, however, not all sampling-related errors can be compensated for with more data. Event-detection algorithms, like fixation detection, may introduce biases and uncertainty in the estimation of the durations, and these error may be larger than the sampling-related error calculated from the sampling frequency. Also, in many cases it is not possible to record more data to compensate for this, e.g. if you work with special populations such as babies and animals, or only get one chance to correctly estimate the duration of a fixation, as in gaze interfacing.

Saccadic latency and other event latencies

R. Andersson et al. (2010) distinguish between event durations, which were described in the previous section, and event latencies. Latencies consist only of a single sampled onset or offset, and the other point is given by a sampling-independent point in time, such as the start of a trial. The fact that latencies only consist of a single sampled point has the effect that the temporal error caused by the limited sampling frequency does not even out, even given large amounts of data. Fortunately, this error is predictable given enough data, and has the expected mean of half a sample of time. That is, if the sampling frequency is 50 Hz, then the expected error is $\frac{1000}{50} = 20$ ms. This error is either an overestimation or an underestimation, depending on whether the sampled point is the onset or the offset of the event. For a latency where the latency is counted from the start of the trial, a sampling-independent point, then the latency is over-estimated. For a measure where the event offset is given, e.g. by a trial end, then the latency is underestimated.

Saccadic velocity and acceleration

A high sampling frequency is required to accurately capture fast eye movements such as saccades. In reading, saccades are around 30–40 ms, which means the motion will be registered only by 1–2 samples with a 50 Hz system.

The smaller the saccades, the higher the required sampling frequency. For instance, Enright (1998) suggests that saccadic peak velocity can be estimated using 60 Hz pupil–corneal reflection eye-trackers, but only if the saccades are larger than 10°. If the saccades are shorter than 10°, e.g. saccades from reading research, then the peak velocity calculation will not be accurate from 60 Hz systems. Juhola, Jäntti, and Pyykkö (1985), who used EOG- and photoelectric eye-tracking systems to study 20° saccades, provide evidence that sampling frequency should be higher than 300 Hz in order to reliably calculate the maximum saccadic velocity. Inchingolo and Spanio (1985), using a 200 Hz EOG system, found that saccadic duration and velocity data were equivalent to data recorded with a 1000 Hz system, albeit only if the saccades are larger than 5°. The lowest bid is given by Wierts, Janssen, and Kingma (2008), who argue that a 50 Hz eye-tracker can be accurately used to measure peak velocities as long as saccades are at least 5°.

Acceleration values are even more sensitive to sampling frequency than velocity. A 50 Hz eye-tracker cannot provide accurate peak acceleration/deceleration values (Wierts et al., 2008).

Table 2.4 Sampling frequencies and the number of microsaccade studies having used them according to the overview in Martinez-Conde et al. (2009).

Sampling frequency	Number of studies
<200	1
200–300	9
500	25
1000	2

Microsaccades

As the average microsaccade has the same dynamic characteristics as a saccade, only around a factor 50 smaller (Engbert, 2006), correctly measuring it requires a higher sampling frequency than does measuring saccades. The durations of microsaccades are only somewhat smaller than saccadic durations, however, which means that the requirement on sampling frequency would only slightly exceed that for saccade measurements. There appear to be no systematic investigations of these requirements, but in practice eye-trackers used in microsaccade research have sampling frequencies no lower than 200 Hz. Table 2.4 presents sampling frequencies from microsaccade studies in the overview by Martinez-Conde, Macknik, Troncoso, and Hubel (2009).

Gaze contingency

In gaze-contingent experiments, the stimulus display changes online in relation to how the eyes move (p. 49). The stimulus is typically manipulated during a saccade when visual intake is significantly impaired. To maximize the time available for such a computationally costly stimulus manipulation, it is important to quickly and accurately detect the offset and, in particular, the onset of a saccade. In this case a high sampling frequency is very desirable.

2.6.2 Accuracy and precision

While the *accuracy* of an eye-tracker is the (average) difference between the true gaze position and the recorded gaze position, *precision* is defined as the ability of the eye-tracker to reliably reproduce a measurement. The difference between accuracy and precision is illustrated in Figure 2.13. Obviously, a good eye-tracker should have both high accuracy and high precision. Beware that these two properties of eye-trackers are often confused.

This section only deals with *spatial* precision. There is also *temporal* precision, which we describe on page 43.

Other much-used eye-tracking concepts that draw on the definition of accuracy and precision include:

Offset Formally, angular distance between calculated fixation location and the location of the intended fixation target, i.e. an operational definition of accuracy. Informally, an acceptable precision in combination with a poor accuracy, examplified in the left part of Figure 2.13.

Drift A gradually increasing offset, common in older eye-trackers.

System-inherent noise Best possible precision you can get with a given eye-tracker, also known as *spatial resolution*. This is typically measured with artificial eyes, which are absolutely still, so we know for certain that spatial variance comes from the eye-tracker itself.

Oculomotor noise Traditionally refers to the fixational eye movements tremor, microsaccades, and drift, even though microsaccades have been linked to cognitive functions (Martinez-

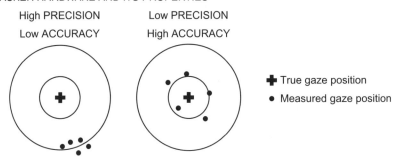

Fig. 2.13 Precision and accuracy.

Conde et al., 2009). Oculomotor noise is often called *jitter* (Martinez-Conde et al., 2004; Jacob, 1991).

Typical precision The average precision as measured from a large participant population with a wide spectrum of eye physiologies and iris colours. The typical precision is the precision that can be expected of a system in a standard eye-tracking experiment.

Optic artefacts False, i.e. physiologically impossible, high-speed movements, often with a much larger amplitude than other types of noise, and caused by interplay between the optical situation (such as glasses, contact lenses, additional reflections and shadows, and varying ambient light conditions) and the gaze estimation algorithm.

Environmental noise Variation in the gaze position signal caused by external mechanical and electromagnetic disturbances in the recording environment.

Noise (general) The combination of system-inherent, oculomotor, and environmental noise and sometimes also including optic artefacts.

Resolution is a common term related to precision, usually referring to 'the smallest movement that can be detected'. It is sometimes defined as the standard deviation of the pupil position in the eye video, but to the vast majority of users, this is less relevant than precision in gaze position.

Both accuracy and precision can—after some training—be evaluated in data visualizations such as scanpath plots with raw data, and space–time diagrams where data samples are plotted against time.

Precision and how to measure it

Spatial precision is one of the most important technical properties of an eye-tracker. Precision is important for everyone who wants to calculate fixation or saccade measures, and perhaps unexpectedly even for your heat map visualizations. Also, if you need to measure the very small fixational eye movements known as tremor, drift, and microsaccades, you need very high precision. While precision is vital for such measurements, accuracy is not of critical importance. Several types of gaze-contingent studies require both a very high precision and a high accuracy.

Precision should be calculated from data samples recorded when the eye is fixating on a stationary target, such that sample variation originating from eye movement is excluded to as large an extent as possible. The only way to completely disregard eye movement is to use an artificial eye positioned in front of an eye-tracker. There are two common ways to calculate precision: standard deviation of data samples and root mean square (RMS) of inter-sample distances.

The most straightforward way to calculate precision for n data samples is perhaps to use the standard deviation,

Artificial eye,
no vibration

Artificial eye,
mouse click

Human eye,
mouse click

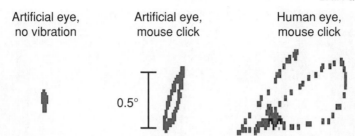

0.5°

Fig. 2.14 Raw data samples in (x,y)-space. The recording with an artificial eye on this 250 Hz remote eye-tracker has an RMS of 0.02° when everything is still, but clicking a mouse on the same table where the eye-tracker is standing causes vibrations in the data large enough to be mistaken for small saccades. The RMS will remain small across all these low-frequency vibrations, but standard deviation will respond to the movement.

$$s_x = \sqrt{\frac{1}{n}\sum_{i=1}^{n}(x_i - \bar{x})^2} \qquad (2.3)$$

This can be computed separately in the horizontal and vertical dimensions, and measures how dispersed samples are from their mean value.

Precision can also be calculated using angular distances θ_i (in degrees of visual angle) between successive data samples $((x_i, y_i)$ to $(x_{i+1}, y_{i+1}))$. It is then typically computed as the root mean square (RMS) of such distances,

$$\theta_{RMS} = \sqrt{\frac{1}{n}\sum_{i=1}^{n}\theta_i^2} = \sqrt{\frac{\theta_1^2 + \theta_2^2 + \cdots + \theta_n^2}{n}} \qquad (2.4)$$

Note that precision calculated from data samples directly and that calculated from inter-sample distances capture variation in the eye-movement signal in slightly different ways; since inter-sample distances only compare temporally adjacent samples, they are less sensitive to a large overall spatial dispersion of the data. Figure 2.14 gives an example where standard deviation and RMS will differ significantly in the rightmost measurement, but not in the measurement to the left. θ_{RMS} seems to be the choice of most eye-tracking manufacturers and practitioners to quantify precision, and it is also the measure we will use in this book.

Poorer eye-trackers have RMS values up to 1°, while manufacturers of high-end eye-trackers typically report a precision that is better than 0.10°, although precisions down to 0.01° are sometimes reported.[6] A 0.01° RMS would mean that the average sample to sample movement due to noise in the eye-tracker is around 0.0001°, far below the amplitude of microsaccades, even below the level of the oculomotor noise originating from eye muscles. Not all manufacturers report precision, and only some calculate the reported value using an artificial eye, which exhibits no physical movements at all, so that all measured movements can be attributed to the system-inherent noise of the eye-tracker.

For microsaccade and gaze-contingent studies, a rule of thumb is that the eye-tracker should have an RMS lower than about 0.03°. For very accurate calculation of fixation durations and saccadic measures, see to it that your eye-tracker has a RMS lower than around 0.05°. Any further increase in RMS always introduces noise in your measures of all these events.

[6]For instance, SR Research (2007) and www.smivision.de

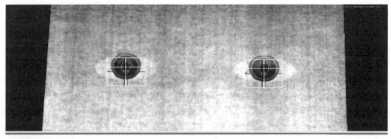

(a) Artificial eyes as seen from the scene camera of the SMI RED X remote.

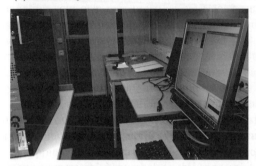 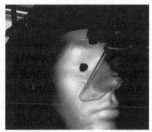

(b) Set-up of artificial eyes in precision test of SMI RED X remote eye-tracker. The eyes are on the grey patch on the black computer to the left. Make sure the eyes are properly attached and do not vibrate.

(c) Set-up of an artificial eye in a precision test of SMI HED X.

Fig. 2.15 Artificial eyes used for testing the (spatial) precision of eye-trackers.

Figure 2.15 shows how we use a pair of artificial eyes to test the precision of two SMI systems. The procedure is simple: first of all, calibrate on a human so that you can get coordinate data.[7] Then put one or a pair of artificial eyes where the human eye(s) would have been, and make sure the artificial eyes are properly attached (Figure 2.15(b)). Beware of vibration movements from the environment, which should not be part of your precision measurement. See to it that the gaze position of the artificial eye(s) is somewhere in the middle of the calibration area, and then start the recording. Export the raw data samples, use trigonometry and the eye-monitor distance with the physical size and resolution of the monitor to calculate sample-to-sample movement in visual degrees. Then select a few hundred samples or more where the gaze position appears to be still, and calculate the RMS from these samples.

Testing only with an artificial eye may be misleading, however. The artificial eyes do not have the same iris, pupil, and corneal reflection features as human eyes, and may be easier or more difficult for the image analysis algorithms to process. Also, in actual eye-tracking research, real eyes tend to exhibit a large variation in image features that cannot be simulated with artificial eyes. Therefore some manufacturers complement the artificial eye test with a precision test on a human population with a large variation in eye colour, glasses, and contact lenses, as well as ethnic background, having them fixate several positions across the stimulus monitor. The distribution of precision values from such a test, examplified in Figure 2.16, is an important indicator of what precision you can expect in actual recordings, and its average defines the *typical precision*. Its drawback is that this data includes oculomotor noise, and

---

[7]Calibration on a human *may* introduce some small noise, so if you have a system where you can get data without first calibrating, you may do that, but be aware that the RMS will not be comparable to systems that require calibration before data recording.

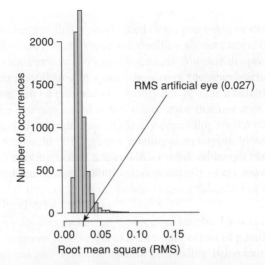

Fig. 2.16 Histogram over RMS values calculated from 165 people looking at 13 validation points just after calibration and again after 10–20 minutes of reading, using a high-end tower-mounted eye-tracker. The arrow pointing to 0.027° indicates the RMS value calculated from data recorded with an artificial eye. This indicates that the eye-tracker is optimized for human eyes rather than for our artificial eye.

therefore both human and artificial eyes are needed.

Also note that different artificial eyes give slightly different RMS values for the same eye-tracker. We found RMS values of 0.021° and 0.032° on the same eye-tracker when using two different artificial eyes. Also different specimens of the same eye-tracker may exhibit different RMS values, which would indicate a difference in build quality.

It is easy to do the test on human eyes yourself. Calibrate the system, and record the human as he is staring at a single point as steadily and for as long as possible. Export the raw data, and use samples in the beginning of the long fixation, blinks excluded, to calculate the RMS value. In our tests, an artificial eye often gave on average data 2–10 times as precise as a real human eye during fixation, but exceptions such as in Figure 2.16 were also found.

Factors that influence precision

Precision is influenced by the eye-tracking hardware and software, participant-specific properties, and the recording environment. In the following section, we will discuss the influence of these factors in relation to our own observations from measuring RMS values from almost 20 different eye-trackers from several manufacturers, using both artificial eyes and real eyes[8] making prolonged fixations. We only made 1–5 measurements per eye-tracker and setting/condition, but found a strong consistency in RMS values across similar recordings. These values are presented so as to explain the properties of the hardware, and should not be seen as an absolute property of a specific eye-tracker or a specific manufacturer. Precision varies with a number of factors, so these values may deviate somewhat from the ones in your recording.

It is possible to improve precision by modifying or adjusting the hardware components of the eye-tracker. Precision is for example closely related to the *resolution of the eye camera*. In particular, the camera should view the pupil and corneal reflection with many pixels, in high quality, and be able to robustly segment them from their backgrounds in order to have a high precision output (see Figure 2.17). As the number of pixels spanned by the eye image

---

[8]The same person (one of the authors), with no mascara, downward eye lashes, glasses or contact lenses, and good lighting conditions.

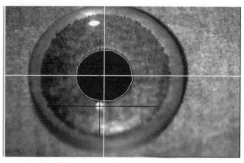
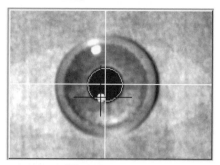

(a) The pupil spans 77 pixels.   (b) The pupil spans 39 pixels.

Fig. 2.17 The measured RMS value in eye-tracker (a) is 5–10 times better than the RMS value for eye-tracker (b). In general, the resolution of the eye camera is one major factor behind precision. The more pixels used for the pupil, and in particular for the corneal reflection, the better.

decreases as the camera moves further away from the eye, long-range eye-trackers such as those used in fMRI studies typically have lower precision than tower-mounted eye-trackers that film the eye from a shorter distance. One way to artificially increase the size of the corneal reflection is to *reduce the focus of the eye camera*. This should theoretically increase precision, but the measurements we have made indicate the opposite. It is unclear why. The free head motion in remote eye-trackers is often combined with *autofocusing eye cameras*, i.e. the focus of the eye video changes back and forth, which is very likely to give a precision that varies with time. High-end eye-trackers sometimes allow for binocular recording with a single camera by zooming out to film both eyes simultaneously. According to the above argumentation, this should reduce the precision.

Eye cameras differ both within and between manufacturers, and the competitive market sometimes forces many to use less expensive cameras, which may have difficulties clearly distinguishing iris and pupil for a large spectrum of participants with differing pigmentation. For instance, Kammerer (2009) showed that the eye camera of a common remote eye-tracker gives significantly poorer data quality for participants with bright-coloured irises (and that glasses give poorer data than contact lenses). Another reason why low-quality eye cameras increase noise levels in data is the slower pixel updating, which makes pixels retain some of the brightness of the passing corneal reflection, leaving a bright trace behind the real reflection (Droege & Paulus, 2009). A camera with a high-quality sensor simply gives better data (when all else is equal).

When manufacturers choose what eye cameras to put in their eye-tracker, there is often a tradeoff between precision and sampling frequency. Since sampling frequency is currently the most pronounced sales argument, it is often prioritized over precision. This appears to be the case both for remote eye-trackers and tower-mounted systems. Furthermore, for a longer sampling time, that is, if the eye camera is open for a longer period for each sample, the movement of the eye during that period smears the sampled eye image as a natural lowpass filter, which may additionally increase precision for lower sampling frequencies.

There are several software-related factors that influence precision. Simultaneous binocular and separate recordings of two artificial eyes on those remote eye-trackers that allowed it gave on average an 8-fold increase in RMS, compared to calculating a single average from the two eyes. If you have a system with a higher than necessary sampling frequency, it is possible to trade a lower sampling frequency against higher precision. For instance, replace every four samples in a 2000 Hz recording with a single average of those four, and you will have a more precise 500 Hz recording.

Precision can be increased by *filtering*, and many manufacturers indeed filter the data in the system they sell. Turning off the default filter in one of the most precise remote systems increases the low RMS 0.01° value to 0.03°. Check what filters there are and note that some filters improve precision at the cost of an increased latency.

In practice, the eye image is processed so that the border between the pupil and the iris is not represented by the pixels we see in Figure 2.17 but by the *sub-pixel estimation* exemplified in Figure 2.9. A sub-pixel estimation of the border curve responds more smoothly to very small movements of the eye. The sample-to-sample motion in the data stream will be smaller, and the eye-tracking software delivers better precision levels than a pixel-based border calculation would give.

Another way to increase precision is to turn off the corneal reflection and make a *pupil-only* recording, which is possible with some of the systems we tested. The increase in precision when recording without corneal reflection is usually dramatic, but it comes at a cost of poorer accuracy and lower tolerance to head movements, and is therefore best suited for studies where accuracy is of less relevance (studies of fixational eye movements such as microsaccades, for instance), and for systems that have a fixed head-camera position (head-and tower-mounted contact systems).

When the head is allowed to move freely relative to the eye camera, as in remote eye tracking, an additional layer of *head position calculations* is added to the gaze estimation algorithm. Consequently, precision drops (Kolakowski & Pelz, 2006). The precise calculation and update frequency for head position, seen as eye position in the eye camera, varies with manufacturers but is not generally revealed.[9] We know that many of the possible technical solutions decrease precision, however. It is quite possible that remote eye-tracking can only give a high precision if the positions of the head and eye are *measured* using optical reflectors or magnetic sensors, but few remote systems have been produced that add sensors to the participants.

Bite bars lock the distance and position between eye and camera. This can be particularly useful when studying very small eye movements, such as microsaccades, but bite bars are hardly ever used today. For the remote system with the poorest precision, the RMS value decreased after we put the participant in a head support system.

The poorest RMS value we noted in our investigation was 1.03°, measured on a human eye in one of the most popular 50 Hz remote eye-trackers. The best precision we found was 0.0012°, using an artificial eye in a high-end tower-mounted system from one of the manufacturers with an academic user group. In comparison, the Dual-Purkinje eye-trackers were reported to have precision of about 0.005° (Crane & Steele, 1985). Table 2.5 lists the range of RMS values found when measuring precision on different systems with both human and artificial eyes.

While tower-mounted and head-mounted eye-trackers in our test scored very well, remote eye-trackers were more variable. Also, the *exact position* of the participant affects precision in remote eye-tracking. In one of these, we got RMS values as low as 0.01° when we positioned artificial eyes so as to minimize the online cursor movement in the recording software. When instead we positioned the artificial eyes without this position adjustment, RMS increased to 0.08°. Figure 2.35 (p. 59) shows how precision varies with distance from the monitor for another commercial remote eye-tracker.

Note that the manufacturer value reported—irrespective of brand of eye-tracker—may very well be for an eye position that gives the lowest precision value possible. Real partici-

---

[9]If you fear that change in pupil size is part of the calculation of head position (which would degrade data quality) and want to test this, put a participant in a chinrest at a fixed distance and vary light conditions so that the pupil changes, and see if the eye-tracker reports distance changes.

Table 2.5 Ranges of RMS values in the three classes of eye-trackers (described on page 51), according to our measurements. Included eye-trackers were manufactured by Tobii, SMI, SR Research, ASL, and SmartEye.

Set-up	Artificial eye	Human eye
Remote	0.0100°–0.3060°	0.0300°–1.0300°
Head-mounted	0.0013°–0.0067°	n/a
Tower-mounted	0.0012°–0.0300°	0.0100°–0.0500°

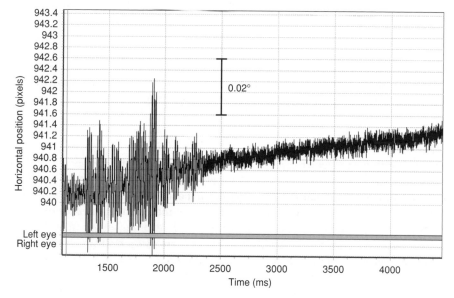

Fig. 2.18 Vibration noise from walking past the table where the eye-tracker is placed, followed by system-inherent noise. 1 vertical unit corresponds to less than 0.02° of visual angle. Raw *x* coordinates over time as recorded with a high-end eye-tracker on an artificial eye.

pants may sit very differently, and move around. Therefore, place your artificial eyes at different positions in front of the eye-tracker, so you can measure the full spectrum of RMS values throughout the region known as the 'headbox' (p. 58).

Variation in the amount of light that hits the eye changing the contrast in the eye video is a likely factor for precision decrease.

Noise may also result from movements in the immediate vicinity of the eye-tracker. Figure 2.18 shows data from a pupil-only recording of an artificial eye. At the beginning of the plot, there is a series of sinusoidal patterns that resulted from a person getting up from a chair next to the table where the eye-tracker was placed. Having participants click a mouse on the same table where the eye-tracker is placed can induce low-frequency noise with amplitudes up to 1°, as shown in Figure 2.14. For sensitive recordings of microsaccades and drifts, movement vibrations in the eye-tracker should be avoided, whether resulting from people moving next to the eye-tracker, clicking a mouse or typing a keyboard, or from heavy lorries driving by.

In some remote systems with poor eye cameras, precision can be so low that even *fixation and saccade analysis* should not be done without first reviewing the data and removing sections with very poor data. Figure 2.19 shows eye movements recorded by a popular commercial eye-tracker; precision is so poor that even a coarse fixation-saccade analysis does not

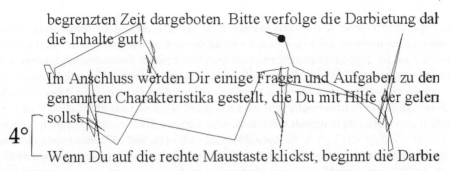

begrenzten Zeit dargeboten. Bitte verfolge die Darbietung daß
die Inhalte gut!

Im Anschluss werden Dir einige Fragen und Aufgaben zu den
genannten Charakteristika gestellt, die Du mit Hilfe der geleru
sollst.

4°

Wenn Du auf die rechte Maustaste klickst, beginnt die Darbie

Fig. 2.19 Poor precision as seen in the raw data scanpath (gaze replay) view. Notice that there are (probably) 4–5 fixations here, but that within each possible fixation, there are movements as big as many normal saccades. RMS within fixations (saccades and blinks excluded) for this recording of a real eye is 2.92°. Recorded 2009 with a common remote 50 Hz system and standard settings. Participant without glasses, contact lenses, and other noise-increasing physical properties.

Table 2.6 Factors that influence precision, assuming all else equal, and effects found (* indicate our own investigation).

Factor	Effect on RMS
Eye position in camera	Large variations *
Filtering	Up to 4 times better *
Averaging data from two eyes	Up to 7 times better *
Eye camera resolution	Large, higher is better *
Sensor refresh time in eye camera	n/a
Head compensation method	Large
Autofocus eye camera	Probably worse
Reducing focus in eye camera	Small *
Binocular recording	Small *
Pupil-only recording	Up to 3 times better *
Participant eye colour	Can be large
Bite bars and head support	Generally better *
Long range (fMRI eye-trackers)	Worse

seem worthwhile.

A summary of factors that influence precision can be found in Table 2.6.

Accuracy

Accuracy is calculated as the average angular offset (distance) θ_i (in degrees of visual angle) between n measured fixation locations and the corresponding locations of the fixation targets,

$$\theta_{\text{Offset}} = \frac{1}{n} \sum_{i=1}^{n} \theta_i \qquad (2.5)$$

Although accuracy is straightforward to calculate given the position of a fixation, there is little consensus on exactly how to define the fixation (see Chapter 5). It is also not clear where on the monitor accuracy should be measured.

The technical key to high accuracy lies in a robust *gaze estimation algorithm*. Given the geometric set-up and the position of the pupil and corneal reflection from the eye image, gaze estimation is used to calculate the actual gaze direction of the viewer. In a series of simulations, Guestrin and Eizenman (2006) found the main sources of error in gaze estimation to be derived from noise in pupil/corneal reflection locations and a mismatch between the assumed spherical shape of the corneal reflection compared to its true shape.

Accuracy is vital in all studies that use area of interest analysis or gaze contingency, that is, those that need to know exactly where a participant is looking. A pertinent example of this comes from the reading research community, where debate has revolved around the accuracy of the saccade targeting system versus the accuracy and precision of commercially available eye-trackers. The quote below from Rayner, Pollatsek, Drieghe, Slattery, and Reichle (2007) illustrates this point clearly:

> ...there can be a discrepancy between the word that is attended to even at the beginning of a fixation and the word that is recorded as the fixated word. Such discrepancies can occur for two reasons: (a) inaccuracy in the eye tracker and (b) inaccuracy in the eye-movement system. ... Kliegl, Nuthmann, and Engbert (2006) attempted to rule out the first hypothesis by using only fixations in which their eye-tracking device agreed that both eyes were on the same word. (p. 522)

In contrast, accuracy is often less important for the calculation of stimulus-independent events such as fixations, saccades, and microsaccades.

Theoretically, accuracy is limited by the size of the fovea, the area of high visual acuity, which spans some 1.5–2° of the visual field. At a standard recording distance of 70 cm distance, this area corresponds to around 2 cm. You might think that accuracy cannot be better. However, accuracy is also decided by the precise position of the eye during calibration (p. 128). If eyes are directed so that each calibration point is projected onto the same position of the fovea for each point, then accuracy can be at the level of < 0.5°, or half a centimetre at a 70 cm distance, which is what manufacturers state in their product fliers. Beware that many researchers report accuracies such as "the eye tracker is binocular, sampling at 50 Hz with 0.5° accuracy", which is virtually always a reiteration of information from manufacturer fliers rather than accuracy measured in the researcher's own experiment.

Accuracy tends to be poorest in the corners of the stimulus monitor, it exhibits a systematic variation across the entire field of recording, and furthermore it depends strongly on the particular characteristics of the individual participant (Hornof & Halverson, 2002).

Accuracy, furthermore, depends on the particular system used, with tower-mounted eye-trackers giving the best accuracy, followed by head-mounted systems, followed by remote eye-trackers. *Drift* means that the measured data samples move slowly away from the true gaze position, as physical conditions change after calibration. The experimenter is then forced to do regular recalibrations during the experiment. Today, most eye-trackers are less likely to drift, but even some high-end eye-trackers were very drift-prone long into the 2000s.

However, accuracy is also influenced by a number of factors that the operator of the eye-tracker must learn to work with:

- What happens during and just after calibration. For instance, many participants are alerted by the importance of the calibration, opening their eyes, tensing a little, and this is the state that you calibrate. If your participant later relaxes, changes position, and perhaps closes his eyes a little, accuracy may soon drop. Setting up the eye camera correctly before calibrating is the practical key to high accuracy. In some systems, typically the remote ones, the eye–video set-up is done automatically, while other systems rely on manual set-up. Whether your system has an automatic set-up or not, it is very useful to understand how a particular eye–video configuration relates to recorded data quality, so we will delve deeply into this on pages 116–134.

- All the individual participant and environmental properties that degrade eye-tracking data also influence accuracy: glasses, contact lenses, eye colour, varying eye physiologies, varying levels of sunlight, tears etc. all introduce an added inaccuracy averaging to 0.1–0.3° but sometimes much larger. Even variations in pupil dilation due to changes in stimulus brightness can increase inaccuracy with up to 1.5°.

- Head movements (e.g. due to an active task requiring speech or arm movements) may decrease accuracy in some remote eye-trackers, but the forehead and chin support of the high-end systems appear to stabilize the head enough to retain very good accuracy in all tasks.

Reported measured accuracy values range from 0.3° to around 2°. For instance, Jarodzka, Balslev, et al. (2010) found a 0.3° average accuracy in a tower-mounted eye-tracker, while Komogortsev and Khan (2008) accepted data with inaccuracies below 1.7°. Other researchers simply re-calibrate until the desired level of accuracy is reached. Tatler (2007) and Foulsham and Underwood (2008), for instance, do not begin to record data until the measured accuracy is below 0.5°. Van Der Geest and Frens (2002, p. 193) remark that results from video-based eye-trackers "should be treated with care when the accuracy of fixation position is required to be smaller than 1°". In comparison, Deubel and Schneider (1996) report an accuracy better than 0.1° on their Dual-Purkinje-Image eye-tracker. Practical within-participants comparisons of accuracy in commercial eye-trackers have been made by Komínková, Pedersen, Hardeberg, and Kaplanová (2008) (SMI RED and HED 50 Hz) and Nevalainen and Sajaniemi (2004) (ASL 501, ASL 504 and Tobii 1750).

Several approaches have been suggested to maintain high accuracy after the initial calibration. They include online monitoring of data quality so as to trigger recalibrations when accuracy is low (Hornof & Halverson, 2002). Einhäuser, Rutishauser, and Koch (2008), for example, performed an additional drift correction when participants failed to look within 1.4° of a centrally located fixation cross within five seconds. Manual or automatic offset compensation can also be performed during the analysis phase, although this should generally be avoided (p. 224).

2.6.3 Eye-tracker latencies, temporal precision, and stimulus-synchronization latencies

Latency and temporal precision are two properties that both have to do with the minute timing of the samples recorded by an eye-tracker. Although important to all realtime, gaze-contingent studies, and for studies that require precise synchronization to external equipment such as EEG, fMRI, and motion tracking, these timing issues are remarkably little discussed. Latency and synchronization issues are also crucial when recording auxiliary data channels which complement eye movement recordings (pp. 95–108, pp. 134–139, and Chapters 9 and 13 address the combination of auxiliary data with eye-tracking).

If your study only concerns showing stimuli and recording data for offline analysis, the latency between the stimulus presentation and the eye-tracker is a much more important danger to your results; nevertheless, this source of temporal error is also little discussed in the literature.

Eye-tracker latency

Eye-tracker latency is defined as the average end-to-end delay from an actual movement of the tracked eye until the recording computer signals that a movement has taken place. Having a low eye-tracker latency is a crucial property in gaze-contingent research, but in most other types of study, the stimulus-synchronization latency of page 45 is much more important.

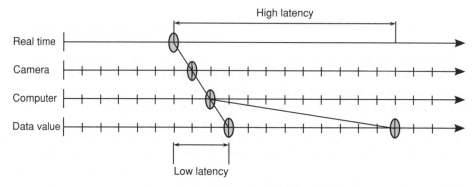

Fig. 2.20 The time from eye movement ('real time') until the data value is available from the eye-tracker defines the latency. Capturing the eye image, transferring it to the computer, and calculating the gaze direction should not take longer than three samples to achieve a low latency. However, factors such as heavy CPU loads on the computer can lead to higher latencies, as indicated at the top of the figure.

Eye-tracker latency can be measured by having the recording computer (of the eye-tracker) trigger a movement in an artificial eye, and measure the time until a change occurs in the data sample output from the gaze estimation algorithm (and filters). In order to avoid additional latencies due to mechanical movements, produce an artificial movement in the artificial eye by switching off the real infrared illumination and switching on a second infrared illumination somewhere else. When the altered position of the corneal reflection is seen by the eye camera and travels through the gaze estimation algorithm, it will be registered by the recording software as a change in sample data. The time from change in infrared illumination until change in sample data is the eye-tracker latency.

An alternative but less exact measuring method is to use a mirror and a high-speed camera. The mirror is positioned next to the participant, and the high-speed camera films the participant's eye and, through the mirror, the recording software where the current raw data sample is displayed. The monitor used should have the lowest possible refresh time, and the spatial precision of the eye-tracker should be reasonably good.

Theoretically, a high-quality eye-tracking system should have a constant latency of less than three samples (i.e. 3 ms on a 1000 Hz system). This means that the eye image is being analysed and transformed into a data sample in less than three samples. The first sample is for stabilizing the eye image in the camera, the second sample is for moving the eye image to the computer buffer, and the third is for calculating the gaze data. Figure 2.20 shows the principle of latency and the path over time from the oculomotor event to the data coordinate value in the recording software. Measuring as described above, SMI and SR Research report similar average latencies for their high-end systems: slightly less than 2 ms for 1000/1250 Hz.

When working with offline analysis, if you have a *constant* latency and can measure or calculate it, you can mostly move or subtract it from the timestamp in your data, and correct for it. Unfortunately, latencies are often variable.

Temporal precision

Temporal precision is defined as the standard deviation of eye-tracker latencies. A high temporal precision means that even if the samples arrive with a latency, the interval between successive samples remains almost constant. If the temporal precision is low, you have a variable latency and a variable delay in the synchronization to external software such as stimulus programs or auxiliary recordings such as EEG.

```
Recording date: 09.12.2008
Recording time : 12:40:37:484 (corresponds to time 0)
Study: XXXXXXX_S2_gazereplay
Subject: G_grt-a_90
Recording: G_grt-a_90
Screen resolution: 1280 x 1024
Coordinate unit: Pixels


Timestamp      Found   GazepointX      GazepointY

...

7261    Both    516      451
7281    Both    513      448
7301    Both    560      452
7660    None    -1280    -1024
7680    Both    533      454
7700    Both    528      465

...
```

Fig. 2.21 After timestamp 7301, there are 360 ms not accounted for. Either timestamps are erronous, which causes a negative latency, or samples are just not registered, which only means a loss of data. Excerpt from raw data file originating from a common 50 Hz eye-tracker used in actual research.

The cause behind variable latencies is usually that the recording computer allows processes—such as hard disk operations—to take up processor time and even get priority over the gaze data calculations. Again, for gaze-contingent tasks such as boundary crossing or simulated scotoma experiments, it is enough that the processor is occupied for a short instance, and the participant will detect an anomaly in the experiment.

The authors have recently tried a 50 Hz remote eye-tracker from a major manufacturer where latencies increased from 40 ms up to 2300 ms when increasing the load on the processor (as in the 'high latency' path in Figure 2.20). Latencies then decreased over a period of a few seconds until it was back to an acceptable value. Variable latencies of this size undermine several of the eye-tracking measures in Part III, including all duration measures (such as fixation duration, saccade duration, dwell time etc.). If these measures are important to you, and you have a system with variable latency, there is not much you can do, except to acquire a better system.

Equally important to eye-tracker latency is that samples are not lost from the data file. Figure 2.21 shows a loss of 360 ms of sample time, noticed by accident in the raw data mode, and not visible after fixation analysis has been done.

High-end eye-trackers have built in technical solutions to the latency problem. Absolutely foolproof solutions include placing the image and gaze estimation calculations on a dedicated computer board or in a real-time operating system, so they can have a processor entirely to themselves. Another solution often implemented in commercial systems, and which works for all post-processing of data, is to keep all eye images and their time code in a buffer. This makes the gaze data timestamp in the data file correct, even if the processor needs to prioritize other calculations. If you are doing gaze-contingent studies, such a system may build up the size of the buffer, and feedback to the participant may be too late. However, system tests of a high-end eye-tracker that the authors have carried out, show that such latencies are so rare that they are likely to play no role in your results.

Stimulus-synchronization latencies

Another type of much larger latencies arises in the interplay between stimulus presentation and recording software. Stimulus presentation software sends synchronization signals to the

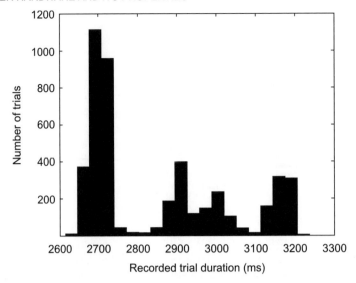

Fig. 2.22 Histogram of actual trial durations in a film viewing task. Bin size 30 ms. The films all had a 3300 ms duration. Could be related to the latency problem in Figure 2.21, or caused by latencies in the video playback. Recorded 2008 with a very common remote 60 Hz eye-tracker and manufacturer presentation software. From Wiens, Moniri, Kerimi, and Juth (2009).

recording software in order to keep the two in synchrony, typically at the onset of a new stimulus. However, clocks on the two computers may run differently, and signals may be delayed at ports for a variety of reasons. Running both stimulus and recording software on the same computer increases the danger of latencies, because the processor and hard disk must share time between recording and demanding operations such as video replay and internet browsing.

When using video stimuli, there is a latency not only at the onset of the video, but at every single frame. This is because video players typically run slightly faster or slower than the recording of data samples, so that at every frame in the video, the data sample resulting from a participant looking at that frame is in fact stored earlier or later in the data file (than the time of the frame in the video). Sending regular synchronization messages throughout the video playback gives a certain control over these variations. Another way is to use hardware time-locks, which however require advanced low-level programming.

Poor synchronization is fairly common, and can be disastrous to a study. Figure 2.22 shows data from an actual study where the stimulus presentation program failed to present videos in real time. Such timing errors then propagate through the subsequent analysis steps. This particular synchronization error was discovered as the expected statistical effect at the beginning of the film appeared to be significant even *before* the onset of the stimulus (Wiens et al., 2009). Several video-playing stimulus programs have this problem. When playing videos with a commercial presentation software, we have seen latencies up to 1500 ms for 20 second videos, relative to the recorded eye-tracking data.

In some cases, inadequacies in software may cause large latencies. For example, in tests we have made with a specific software version of a very common recording software, after a few recordings, the software lagged behind (due to memory leaks, probably). This can be seen in the sluggish response to mouse clicks. In data we recorded just before this behaviour, we found latencies up to 3 seconds between onset of stimulus images and recording. Since eye-tracking software is always developing and is shipped in small series that few people give feedback on, latencies like these may suddenly appear in data after a software upgrade, and disappear again after the next upgrade.

2.6.4 Filtering and denoising

Filtering and denoising of eye-tracking data is a little-discussed issue, but most manufacturers do it to decrease variations that derive from sources other than eye movements themselves.[10] All types of filtering have an effect on subsequent analysis; in particular event detection, which is discussed in Chapter 5.

There are two places where filters can be found:

- Data are often already filtered while recording, and the recording software typically has settings for filtering, which are not always easy to understand for the typical user (and often not even for the experienced user). Filtering in real time during recording imposes a certain latency, which is typically around 1–2 samples (1–2 ms in a 1000 Hz system).
- There is usually a second (hidden or visible) filtering option in the analysis software used to calculate velocities and accelerations.

Beware of what types of filter your analysis software uses, since the choice can significantly affect your results. If possible, try to understand what the filters do; test a few filter settings in your software and see how they affect velocity and acceleration data.

Denoising and artefact removal

Noise reduction optimally aims to remove all variation in the recorded data that does not derive from true eye movement. It can be done online during recording or offline after all data are recorded. For some applications, such as gaze interaction, online analysis is the only option since data are used in real time to control an interface. In other applications, offline processing of data is done in preparation for subsequent analyses.

One type of noise among data samples is the *optic artefacts*. These can derive from recording imperfections due to, e.g. downward eyelashes or an erroneously detected pupil or corneal reflection. These unphysiological movements often appear as sudden spikes in the data and can rather easily be identified and removed. Stampe (1993) distinguishes between *impulse* and *ramp* noise. The former is characterized by a one sample spike, whereas the latter comprises a plateau with two deviating samples. Stampe (1993) proposes a heuristic filter design for detecting and replacing such artefactual samples with neighbouring sample values. Since access to the next sample is necessary to decide whether the current sample is impulse noise, the filtering process adds a one sample delay. Similarly, detection of ramp noise adds a two sample delay. The amplitudes of the artefacts are typically checked against a threshold such that only samples deviating more than a threshold value from their neighbouring samples are removed.

Another type of noise is the low-amplitude, high-frequency noise that occurs due to eye-tracker imprecision as well as oculomotor noise. Filters targeting precision are harder to design, because the noise and real eye movement are tightly intertwined, and the filter thus stands a risk of removing authentic eye movements.

A challenge in the design of filters for eye-movement data is to retain high-frequency information necessary to accurately describe saccadic waveforms, while removing similar high-frequency information from fixations. Kumar, Klingner, Puranik, Winograd, and Paepcke (2008) proposed a solution where fixation samples were detected and lowpass filtered online,

---

[10]Some manufacturers let you choose what filters to use; others filter for you without telling what they do.

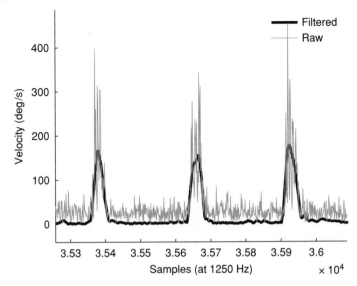

Fig. 2.23 The effect of filtering on velocity. 'Raw' velocity is generated from sample-by-sample differences of adjacent data samples, whereas the 'filtered' velocity represents the same data after lowpass filtering.

leaving saccade samples unprocessed. They found that this improved interaction in systems where gaze was used as an input.

Filtering when calculating velocity and acceleration values

Filtering is important when calculating velocity and acceleration. Velocity calculation is done by a process called *numerical differentiation*, which in its simplest form finds the eye velocity $\dot{\theta}$ by calculating the angular distance θ between two adjacent pairs of data samples, and multiplies this distance by the sampling frequency of the eye-tracker $f_s = 1/\Delta t$. Formally, this can be expressed as

$$\dot{\theta} = \frac{\theta}{\Delta t} \tag{2.6}$$

This way we get the velocity in its most common representation: degrees of visual angle per second (denoted $°/s$). Acceleration can be calculated by performing the same operations on the velocity samples. Notice that each time we perform a differentiation using this simple method, the noise will be magnified. Unless the precision of the eye-tracker is exceptionally high, filtering is required to produce velocity and acceleration data that are of use in subsequent analyses.

Figure 2.23 illustrates the unfiltered, noisy velocity curve, and the much smoother lowpass filtered curve, which is what you typically see in your manufacturer's software, and which is used for detecting events such as fixations and saccades. It is still possible to see the saccades in the unfiltered version, but separating fixations from saccades by means of thresholding becomes difficult.

There is a range of filters that can be used when generating velocity and acceleration data from raw data samples. The most careful investigations on this issue were made by Inchingolo and Spanio (1985) and Larsson (2010), who showed how saccade parameters (e.g. duration and peak velocity) change as a function of filter type and threshold. Many of the design criteria of filters seem to be guided by heuristics, or 'rules of thumb' motivated by visual inspection of the data (e.g. Stampe, 1993). Be aware that pattern matching filters, such as Stampe (1993) and Duchowski (2007) amplify parts of the eye-movement signal with similar appearance as the filters while attenuating other portions. Investigating the effect of filters on

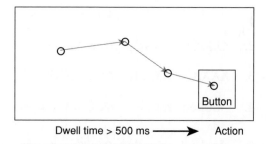

Fig. 2.24 Gaze-sensitive button. If looked at (dwelled upon) for more than e.g. 500 ms, an action is performed: changing stimulus, starting music, etc.

eye-movement velocity and acceleration, Larsson (2010) concluded that the Savitzky–Golay filter used by Nyström and Holmqvist (2010) and the differential filter by Engbert and Kliegl (2003) produced the most physiologically reasonable values. Unlike the pattern-matching filter, these two filters make no strong assumptions on the overall shape of the velocity curve.

The application imposes constraints on the design of a filter. Gaze-contingent experiments, for example, require short filters that do not introduce excessive latencies in the data, whereas offline analyses can use longer, more complex filters.

2.6.5 Active and passive gaze contingency

Gaze contingency means that the stimulus display changes depending on where or at what a participant is looking. There are two different ways to do this: *(inter)active gaze contingency*, which is technically easier, and *passive gaze contingency* which demands more of your system.

Active gaze contingency refers to the process of actively and consciously controlling an interface by means of gaze input. Figure 2.24 illustrates the principle for selecting an item, and therefore initiating an action. The gaze position from the eye-tracker basically replaces the mouse position, and this allows the user to perform actions such as open menus, click on buttons, select music, or operate an entire interface just by looking at appropriate items. Items are typically selected when they are looked at for longer than a certain duration, but can also be combined with enveloping menu hierarchies to allow for easy undoing and avoidance of the so-called Midas touch problem (Jacob, 1991). A 50 Hz eye-tracker is enough, since this is not a time critical process, but precision and accuracy must be high, so that data samples remain inside the button area for as long as the user looks there.

During passive gaze contingency, in contrast, participants are not required to actively control the appearance of a stimulus display. In fact, most gaze-contingent experiments of this kind assume that participants are not consciously aware that the display is updated contingent on where they look. In the typical situation, the display has a high level of detail only directly where the participant looks, whereas peripheral parts of the display are reduced in detail, but not so much that it can be detected by the participant. The display is then updated during each saccade, such that the display change is completed before visual intake begins at the beginning of the next fixation.

Passive gaze contingency has been implemented more for theoretical than applied purposes; it has long been used in research on vision, reading, and psycholinguistics. In reading alone, there are several types of gaze contingency, as Figure 2.25 shows. Reading researchers design gaze-contingent manipulations in order to investigate how much information we pick up from the word to the right of the fixated word. All such manipulations require very good timing on the part of the eye-tracker. In the boundary paradigm, for example, a word must be

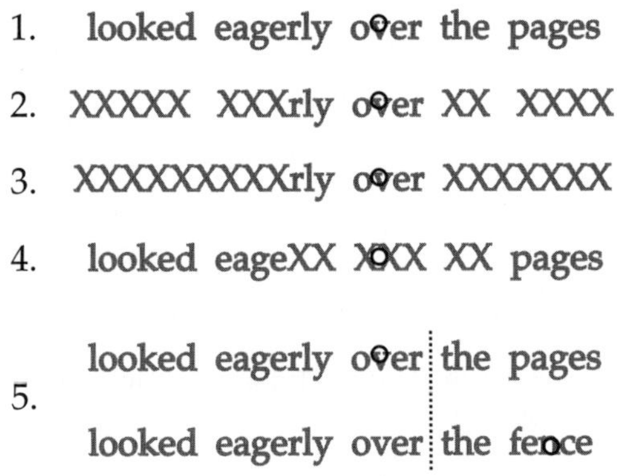

1. looked eagerly over the pages

2. XXXXX XXXrly over XX XXXX

3. XXXXXXXXXrly over XXXXXXX

4. looked eageXX XXX XX pages

5.
looked eagerly over the pages

looked eagerly over the fence

Fig. 2.25 Different varieties of passive gaze contingency in reading research: 1. Gaze cursor over text. 2. Moving window with spaces visible. 3. Moving window without visible spaces. 4. Foveal mask with spaces visible. 5. Boundary paradigm. An invisible boundary is placed in the stimulus. When gaze passes the boundary, the word or picture on the other side changes, and the eye lands on a word contrary to what was visible before the eye movement was directed there. (Note, the small black circles indicate fixation position, shown to illustrate the technique; this may or may not be shown on screen to participants depending on your choice of gaze-contingent paradigm)

changed instantly when the saccade to it has just started. If we take the current sentence as an example; while you were fixating 'current', the next word was still 'sentence', but with a boundary paradigm, as soon as you start to move your eye, we can change 'sentence' to some other word, such as 'technology', which is what your eye will land on.

Since saccades are very short during reading, only some 20–40 ms, the gaze data must be first calculated (which takes up to three samples, see Figure 2.20), and then fed back to the stimulus program very quickly, within no more than some 10–15 ms, so that the stimulus program can update the monitor image (preferably CRT, so refresh time is low) before the end of the saccade and the saccadic blindness.

The foveal mask, case 4 in Figure 2.25, is often called 'simulated scatoma' (compare 'macular scatoma'); it artificially creates a blind spot in foveal vision which resembles the scatoma caused by physiological disorders of the eye such as macular degeneration. In healthy participants this blurring of foveal vision can help answer questions both about visual processing in physiological disorders which cause scatoma, and about visual processing per se in areas such as reading and scene perception.

The ability to make passive gaze-contingent studies of the demanding kind depends on how quickly a data sample, or the beginning saccade, can be fed back to the stimulus program so that the stimulus can be changed without the participant noticing an anomaly. Foveal masks and moving windows move in close to real time with the eye, which means that both latency and stimulus update time of the system must be very low. Only if the whole system is very fast does the illusion work, that the monitor changes without the participant noticing that a change has taken place. It is enough for the participant to notice once for his behaviour to change— once the gaze-contingent manipulation is spotted the participant will constantly remain aware of it. Thus, the eye-tracking system must have a high accuracy, a low and constant latency, a high sampling frequency, online saccade detection, and a very tight connection between recording system and stimulus presentation.

2.7 Types of eye-trackers and the properties of their set-up

Even if they all use the same video-based pupil-to-corneal reflection measurement technology, eye-trackers are very different among themselves. If you want to do both gaze-contingent reading research and study the eye movements of soccer players during games, you will most likely need two different eye-trackers.

The eye-trackers shown in this section are *examples of basic hardware set-ups* and their consequences on data. In real life, manufacturers offer *hardware combinations* that extend each of these basic types to more functions or allow the user to build more than one type of eye-tracker from the same set of basic hardware, but the basics are always the same.

2.7.1 The three types of video-based eye-trackers

Basically, a video-based eye-tracker has an infrared illumination and an eye video camera, and typically an additional scene camera for head-mounted eye-trackers. Illumination(s) and camera(s) can be put on a table in front of the participants, or on their heads. Sometimes head-tracking is added to head-mounted systems. This gives us three types of eye-trackers that differ not only with respect to the position of cameras and illumination, but more importantly in the type of data they produce and how we can analyse the output.

1. The most common set-up is the *static eye-tracker*, which puts both illumination and eye camera on the table, in front of the participant. There are two sub-types; *tower-mounted* eye-trackers that are in close *contact* with the participant, restraining head movements, and those that view from a distance, known as *remote* eye-trackers, with nothing or very little attached to the head. In practice, stimuli are almost always presented on a monitor, although wall projections and real scenes can easily be used with static eye-trackers.
2. Another common set-up is the *head-mounted eye-tracker*, which has put both illumination and cameras on the head of the participant, mounted on a helmet, cap, or a pair of glasses. A scene camera takes the role of recording the stimulus—the scene of view.
3. The third type of set-up adds a *head-tracker* to the head-mounted eye-tracker in order to calculate the position of the head in space. For reasons soon to be explained, this addition makes the analysis of data from head-mounted systems much easier. Not many manufacturers offer this combination, however.

These three different ways to combine illumination and camera give eye-trackers with very different properties. We will use the terms 'remote', 'tower-mounted', 'head-mounted', and 'head-tracking' throughout the rest of the book. We will now describe the three types in detail.

Static eye-trackers come in two varieties; those that restrict the participant's head less, and those that restrict it more. For a number of reasons, you get better data if you restrict the participant's head more. Previously, bite-bars were used to immobilize participants' heads. Today, the video-based eye-trackers with the best precision have forehead and chin rests that gently restrict the participant's head movements, like at the optician, as in Figures 2.26(a) and 2.26(b). The camera and illumination are hidden inside the box on top of the eye-tracker. The gentle head restriction is the price you pay for high precision and accuracy.

Eye-trackers that restrict the head less place the camera near the stimulus (monitor), without contact to the participant. These 'remote' eye-trackers are capable of viewing the participant's eye from a distance, and even keep track of the eye as it moves within a certain volume (Figure 2.27). Because of imperfections in gaze estimation models during head movement, and because the eye is typically filmed at a lower resolution, data from remote systems are

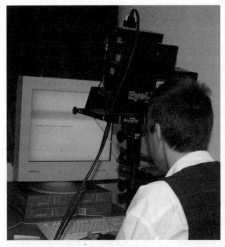 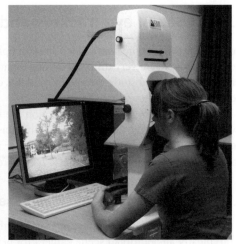

(a) The SR EyeLink 1000 Hz tower-mounted eye-tracker.

(b) The SMI 1250 Hz HiSpeed tower-mounted eye-tracker.

Fig. 2.26 Two types of static tower-mounted contact eye-trackers with high sampling frequency, precision, and accuracy. Both film the eye via a mirror.

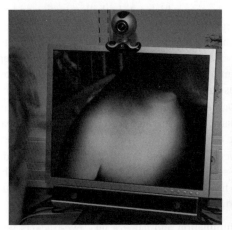 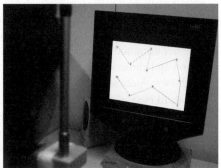

(a) SMI RED 4, a 50 Hz remote system. Here with an additional web camera to observe participants' facial expressions during diagnosis of neuropaediatrics cases.

(b) Tobii 1750 remote system at 50 Hz. One of the most sold eye-trackers in the mid 2000s. The participant is using a chin rest to increase precision.

Fig. 2.27 Remote eye-trackers: illumination and eye camera are hidden in the dark ledge below each monitor. Nothing is attached on the participant.

almost invariably of a poorer quality than data from those eye-trackers that restrict or measure the participant's head movements. Research is intense in improving the data quality of remote eye-trackers, however.

Knowing the position of the head is again the key to sufficient accuracy and precision. One particular variety of remote eye-trackers solves the geometrical problem by putting an infrared reflector on the forehead of the participant and measuring exactly where he is. Others that use magnetic head tracking have also been on the market. Their low market share indicates that many users prefer not having to add any markers or sensors to the participant's

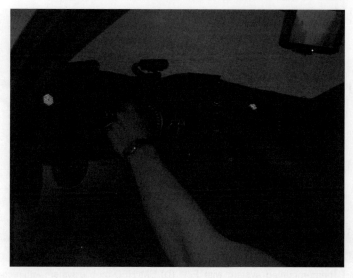

Fig. 2.28 A four-camera SmartEye system set-up in a car simulator. Infrared illumination is seen as white hexagons on either side of the steering wheel, and two of the cameras are seen as dark silhouettes on top of the dashboard.

head, even if it is at the cost of a somewhat lower data quality.

Remote eye-trackers are generally easier to operate, however, and the participants more easily tend to forget that the eye-tracker exists. They are the only practical alternative to record on infants, and allow additional measuring equipment to be added to the participant's head without too much interference. Remote systems also exist in multi-camera versions, which can be built into workplaces (such as cars and flight simulators) where participants need to turn their head a lot. Figure 2.28 shows a four-camera set-up.

There is a hypothesis—sometimes used as a sales argument—that participants behave more naturally in a remote system than in tower- and head-mounted systems, which would mean that data would be ecologically more valid. Such a superiority of remotes remains to be proven, however. In the authors' experience, participants feel only moderately restrained even in tower-mounted systems: in our lab we have had participants speak, type with the keyboard, and even play intense first-person-shooter games, and we have still recorded highly accurate data from participants who claim to have behaved naturally.

When a participant moves his eyes out of reach of the eye camera, and then returns to his initial position, the remote eye-tracker typically takes some time—known as *recovery time* and sometimes 'pickup time'—to resume tracking, which is of extra importance if you have very mobile participants, such as infants. Recoveries are also made after long blinks, and tend to be longer with remotes than with systems that know where the eye is. If your system has a long recovery time you lose a corresponding portion of data during each recovery.

Static eye-tracking systems, whether tower-mounted or remote, can be used with one stimulus plane, typically a monitor, but also a magazine, or just the monitor-less field of view above the camera housing. A static eye-tracker gives a data file with coordinates in the coordinate system of that plane, i.e. that monitor magazine or field of view. This coordinate system is defined and positioned as part of the set-up and calibration, which we will look at in Section 4.5. Giving coordinates in a fixed coordinate system is an important property that makes analysis much simpler, and it is by no means a self-evident one. The reason that it works is that the eye camera, the illuminations, and the stimulus (the monitor looked at) are fixed spatially, and the head of the participant is fixed or at least fairly well measured.

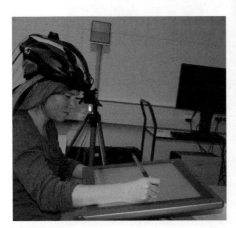 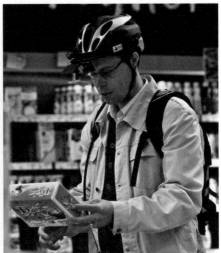

(a) SMI HED head-mounted system with Polhemus headtracking. The device generating the magnetic field is located in the upper part of the figure. Sensors are mounted on the helmet.

(b) SMI HED-mobile system with recording computer in rucksack (from 2008). Photo used courtesy of Gunnar Menander and Petra Francke.

Fig. 2.29 Head-mounted systems with (a) and without (b) head tracking.

Head-mounted systems as in Figure 2.29(a) have cameras and illuminations mounted on top of a helmet, cap, head-band, or a pair of glasses. They allow the participants maximum mobility, in particular if the recording computer is small and lightweight. If the mounting is steady, the participant can take part in many different real life activities, such a driving, riding a bicycle, buying food in a supermarket, playing tennis etc. Traditional head mounted systems are likely to be the most versatile eye-trackers when it comes to glasses, contact lenses, drooping eyelids, mascara and steep viewing angles. This is because the eye camera angle towards the eye can—in principle—be shifted and adapted to the individual participant and task—an important property that we will cover in detail on pages 116–134. A notable exception are the Tobii eye-tracker glasses from 2010, where no parts can be adapted.

Head-mounted systems also have a scene camera mounted on the helmet, filming in the line of sight, as in Figure 2.30. The recording computer overlays the gaze coordinate onto the scene video, which is endowed with a moving marker that shows where the participant is looking. The result is known as a *gaze-overlaid video*, and for reasons that we will discuss on page 61, this is (mostly) all you can use. Even if there is a data file, the coordinates of the data file will refer only to positions in the scene video, not to positions in the surrounding world. We will have a closer look at the consequences of this property on data analysis in pages 60, 175, and 227.

In order to associate objects in stimulus space with collected data samples, some head-mounted eye-trackers can be combined with magnetic head tracking. The head-tracking system calculates all (absolute) motion of the head, and adds that onto the (relative) motion of the eye in the head. The resulting combined head–eye gaze vector is expressed in the coordinate system of the recording environment. Surfaces in the environment can be measured up, and given their own reference systems. With such a combined system, the eye-tracker will give both gaze-overlaid video *and* a very useful data file, that allows for automatized data analysis, while still allowing for very large head movements.

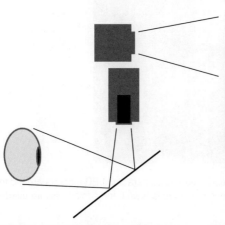 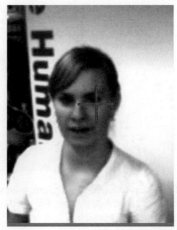

(a) Head-mounted eye-trackers have an additional scene camera; here placed above eye camera and illumination. The scene camera films forward, while the eye camera in this case films through a mirror.

(b) Scene camera view with gaze-overlaid haircross cursor at the gaze position.

Fig. 2.30 The scene camera of head-mounted systems.

Another method to get data coordinates that are meaningful in analysis is to attach (large enough) object markers with specific patterns onto the stimulus. These markers are captured as part of the scene video, and four markers define the corners of a rectangular object. When the participant is within a certain range, the recording software finds the markers, and can relate gaze to the objects even with lots of head movements. Putting markers in a natural stimulus risks altering the participant's visual behaviour, however.

There are also head-mounted eye-trackers with a more restricted version of head tracking. The most well known is the SMI EyeLink I 250 Hz system and its follow-up, the SR EyeLink II 250/500 Hz, which has a small camera on top of the headgear and four light emitting diodes (LEDs) at the corners of the single plane (see Figure 2.31). On the basis of the positions of LED corners in the camera image, the software calculates the position of the head relative to the monitor, and thus compensates for head movement. This works fairly well, but the plane must largely be perpendicular to the line of gaze and cannot for instance be tilted to lie down on a table. Also, with this technical solution, it is not possible to get data samples from more than one plane. In fact, this type of eye-tracker much resembles tower-mounted eye-trackers in its high precision, but still allowing for some degree of head movements. Accuracy, however, sometimes has the tendency to drop over time, if the eye-tracker slips relative to the head. Data consists of a file of co-ordinates in one plane, just like the static eye-trackers.

There are other human interfaces, such as fMRI (functional magnetic resonance imaging) eye-trackers, VR (virtual reality) goggles with built-in eye tracking, and even primate eye-trackers. For the purpose of this section, it suffices to say that they are all versions of static eye-trackers: The stimulus is fixed in relation to the eye camera and the participant's head.

In addition to gaze direction, many of these eye-trackers output the pupil and corneal reflection positions in the eye-video, which can—assuming there is software to support this—in principle be used to extend the area from which data is collected to beyond the area calibrated. Some systems even output these gazes outside of the calibration plane as coordinates, but for a variety of reasons, the quality of this data is typically much poorer than within the calibration

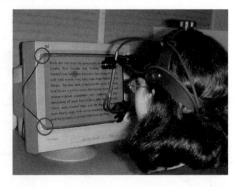

Fig. 2.31 The EyeLink I 250 Hz system, with head-mounted camera and LED markers around the stimulus to define the coordinate system. For clarity, two of the LEDs have been circled. Picture used with kind permission from SR Research.

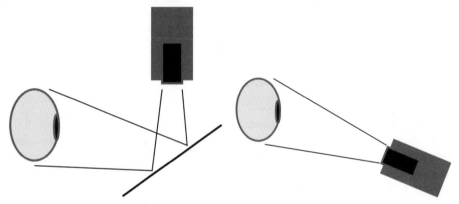

(a) Contact and head-mounted eye-trackers with mirror.

(b) Remote eye-trackers and mirrorless head-mounted eye-trackers.

Fig. 2.32 Eye camera viewing angle towards the eye. The grey and black boxes are the infrared illumination and camera.

plane.

Also note that contact eye-trackers and (most) head-mounted eye-trackers film the eye through a mirror, while the remote eye-trackers film directly, as in Figure 2.32. On pages 116–134, when we describe how to set up the eye camera to get an optimal viewing angle and the best possible data quality, we will often manipulate the camera angle towards the eye to adjust it to our participant's individual physiology, glasses etc.

All current high-end systems have mirrors, but the ideal eye-tracker is mirrorless, because the mirror introduces edges in the visual field of the participant. This may change the wavelengths of the light reaching the participant's eye and introduce reflections from overhead illumination. Nevertheless, the advantages of having camera and illumination in a fixed position to the participant's eye, and the increased data quality this means, still outweigh the disadvantages of introducing a mirror. Eye image quality is high with current mirrors, and with the stimulus display at a distance much larger than that of the mirror, in our experience, participants are no more disturbed by the mirror than by wearing glasses.

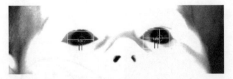 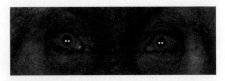

(a) Eye-video from participant aged 48 days successfully tracked with dark-pupil remote eye-tracker.

(b) Eye-video of an orangutan from Lund University Primate Research Station at Furuvik Zoo, recorded using a remote dark-pupil system.

Fig. 2.33 Two representatives of uncommon groups of participants recorded with the same remote eye–tracker.

2.7.2 Robustness

Robustness (also known as *versatility*) refers to how well an eye-tracker works for a large variety of participants. Poor robustness can lead to frequent data loss of up to a third of the participants (p. 141) and poorer data quality. Some eye-tracking systems have a hard time with glasses, and contact lenses are also a problem that some eye-trackers handle better than others. Participants also vary in their eye physiology: some eye-trackers may produce poorer data for certain eye colours, and another common obstacle to good data recording is drooping eyelids, which of course vary between participants.

In order to handle as many participants as possible, your eye-tracker should allow you to vary the angle of the eye camera to the eye. As we will see on pages 116–134, adjusting the eye-camera angle solves many problems. This is often more difficult on remote systems than on head-mounted ones, but the design of the head-mounted system also plays an important role to its robustness. If you can also vary the position of the infrared illumination, your system will be even more versatile, especially for people wearing glasses. The major problem with contact lenses can easily be solved, as we will later see, if you can adjust the focus of the eye camera. The current manufacturer trend is to remove these options from the operator of the eye-tracker, and thereby prioritize ease of usage over robustness.

Technological components that manufacturers use to automatize robustness reflect what the researchers would manipulate: increased resolution and sensitivity of the eye camera(s), number of eye cameras, the quality of the camera sensors, the number of and precise positioning of illuminators, and the implementation of image processing algorithms, which together have a major impact on the robustness of an eye-tracking system whether or not the researcher has access to camera settings and positions of illumination.

Infants are a special class of participants, for whom remote eye tracking is most suited. Infants may move about a lot, and can hardly be restricted using chin rests or bite bars. Before they can sit, they can be placed lying in a tight hammock that gently restricts sideward head movements, with the eye-tracker and stimulus monitor overhead. Light should be turned down in the room, so the stimulus monitor appears more salient to the infant. When sitting in a parent's lap, holding their head gently mimimizes large head movements. Figure 2.33(a) shows a very young human participant recorded on a remote eye-tracker.

Our primate relatives would disassemble the eye-tracker if they could, so they have historically always been more or less restricted when being eye-tracked. New attempts are made to track through protective glass, and remotes are then the common choice among video-based trackers. The orangutan in Figure 2.33(b) was tracked through a 20 mm polymethyl methacrylate glass at 50 cm distance.

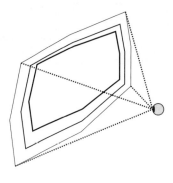

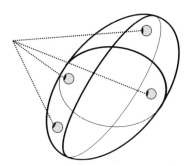

(a) Tracking range: how far to the side can a participant look and we still get (good) data. Towards the edge, data will be gradually poorer.

(b) Head box: how large is the volume in which the participant can move and we still get (good) data. Towards the edge, data will be gradually poorer.

Fig. 2.34 Illustration of tracking range and headbox.

2.7.3 Tracking range and headboxes

The *tracking range* (also known as *visual field of recording*) is a measure of how far to the side your participant can look and you still get data. The *headbox* is the volume relative to the eye-tracker in which a participant can move without compromising the quality of recorded data. Figure 2.34 illustrates both concepts. There is currently no generally accepted definition of either that could be used to compare different eye-trackers.

Most eye-trackers will have problems with extreme *gaze angles*, that is when the line of gaze deviates very much from the direction of the head, because the corneal reflection degrades or either pupil or corneal reflection are covered by the eyelid (p. 131).

The tracking range is particularly important with large stimuli. If you have a broadsheet newspaper as a stimulus, and an eye-tracker that does not allow your participant to move his head, then looking at the texts in the corners of the pages will require him to turn his eyes very much to the side. If your participant is a car driver, he will make very large eye (and head) movements when alternating between the rear-view mirror, pedestrians on each side of the car, the GPS on the dashboard etc. If instead you have a very small stimulus, such as a cellular telephone, your participant does not have to make very large eye movements to look at all of it.

Single-camera video-based eye-trackers can measure gaze on a stimulus within a horizontal gaze span of around 40°, and around 25° in the vertical direction, relative to the head direction. For a static eye-tracker (the common one-camera remote, for instance) at a viewing distance of 70 cm, the horizontal 40° corresponds to a width of approximately 50 cm. Tracking range is not an absolute property of the eye-tracker, but depends on participant physiology, with borders of decreasing data quality in all extreme gaze angles (p. 116–134).

A large headbox is important when participants move around in front of a remote eye-tracker, for instance infants, monkeys, and some clinical groups. For many remote systems, data quality shows considerable variation within the headbox, and may be much worse towards the extremes, as the precision measurement in Figure 2.35 exemplifies.

Multi-camera remote systems can measure gaze in the entire 360°, because another camera takes over when the first one falters. This is very useful when participants rotate on an office chair in front of a large control board, or if they drive a car. The increased headbox often

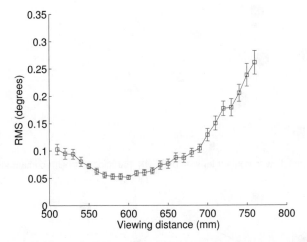

Fig. 2.35 Precision versus viewing distance in a specific remote eye-tracker. For each distance from the monitor, 24 recordings were made on a pair of artificial eyes positioned in the middle of the eye video, and average RMS was calculated over those recordings. Precision varies significantly and is at its best at a smaller distance than recommended by the manufacturer. Data collected 2011 in collaboration with Pieter Blignaut.

comes at the cost of a time consuming calibration of the environment and head of the participant, and therefore suits experiments with few participants and long trials. There are also remote eye-trackers with single eye cameras that mechanically move with the participant's head, also creating larger headboxes.

2.7.4 Mono- versus binocular eye tracking

Monocular eye-trackers record from one eye only, while a binocular eye-tracker takes data from both eyes. The vast majority of eye-tracking research is done monocularly, for mainly two reasons. First, it is commonly believed that both eyes make the same movement at approximately the same time, and also look at roughly the same position. It would therefore give no additional value to measure both eyes simultaneously. As we saw on page 24, however, this is not always a valid assumption. Second, monocular eye-trackers are cheaper to acquire. These two reasons combined make it tempting to buy a system that can measure only from one eye at a time.

Binocular eye tracking may be particularly relevant in some situations:

- When recording from children, who have a larger distance between gaze positions of the left and right eyes—known as *disjugacy* or *disparity*—than adults.
- It you have an experiment where double vision due to the misalignment of the two eyes relative to each other—known as *diplopia*—may occur.
- If you plan to perform clinical studies on participants with neurological dysfunctions affecting vergence (see Leigh & Zee, 2006, p. 367).
- If small differences in saccade measures matter to your study.

The purpose of recording binocular data often differs between high-end and low-end eye-trackers. High-end eye-trackers output one data stream for each eye with a quality high enough to address the situations above. Low-end eye-trackers typically give you only one data stream (a cyclopean view), even if both eyes are used. In this case, binocularity is used only to increase the accuracy and precision of the data from a remote eye-tracker by cal-

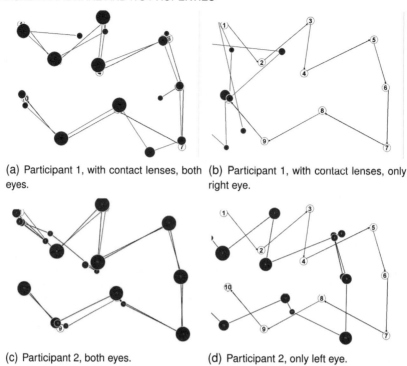

(a) Participant 1, with contact lenses, both eyes.

(b) Participant 1, with contact lenses, only right eye.

(c) Participant 2, both eyes.

(d) Participant 2, only left eye.

Fig. 2.36 The effect on accuracy of concealing one eye. Data from two participants looking at the numbers 1 to 10 in order, recorded 2009 on a very common but slightly outdated remote 50 Hz eye-tracker. Solid circles represent detected fixations. The small fixations next to the large ones are artefacts from low precision in combination with a dispersion-based fixation algorithm.

culating averages between the two data samples, or using the eye with currently better data quality. The precision increase can be considerable (Cui & Hondzinski, 2006). Conversely, if an averaging remote system temporarily loses track of one eye, there can be a dramatic loss of accuracy in the data, as Figure 2.36 very clearly shows. If you plan to buy a remote system, this is one property to test.

2.7.5 The parallax error

A head-mounted system with a scene camera will exhibit a larger or smaller *parallax error*; that is: the gaze cursor, which we saw as a cross in Figure 2.39, will be misaligned with the actual line of gaze for certain distances from the object looked at. Figure 2.37 shows the principle for parallax error. The size and direction of the parallax error varies systematically with the distance to the object looked at. If the fixated object is at the same distance as the calibration plane, *when the participant was calibrated*, then the parallax error will be zero. At larger or smaller viewing distances the parallax error grows, being at its worst at very close distances.

In the gaze-overlaid scene video for the right eye, the parallax error always follows a line, slightly tilted as the scene camera is above eye level, with far away errors to the left and close object errors to the right, assuming the head-camera configuration in Figure 2.37 (the reverse case for the left eye). The error is so systematic that if you are coding the resulting gaze-overlaid videos manually, it is possible—with a little training and an understanding of the principle behind parallax—to directly estimate the parallax error, and subtract it from the

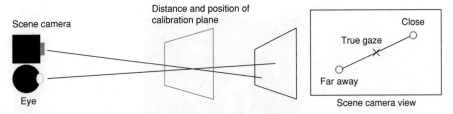

Fig. 2.37 Parallax error. The grey plane is the position of the original calibration screen. The dark plane is the true stimulus. The scene camera view shows a frame from the overlaid scene video. The cross marks the true gaze position, and the two dotted rings mark where the eye-tracker will put the overlaid gaze marker in relation to the true gaze position, depending on the distance to the object looked at. A far away stimulus pulls the error in one direction, and a close stimulus pulls it in the other direction. The gaze cursor is only perfectly positioned for stimuli at the same distance as the calibration plane during calibration. This figure assumes the scene camera is mounted above the eye level between both eyes, and the displayed error is true for measurements on the right eye.

gaze position shown while coding.

The cause of the parallax error is the fact that the scene camera and the eye look at the scene from slightly different angles. The two gaze lines of the eye and the scene camera cross at the distance at which the calibration screen was, but are misaligned elsewhere. There are several hardware solutions to parallax:

- A few eye-trackers are built so that the line of sight coincides perfectly with the scene camera direction, but at the cost of difficult and endurable mechanical solutions.
- Adding head tracking and measuring the position of the eye and scene camera allows a mathematical solution to parallax, but head tracking limits the mobility of the participant.
- Binocular head-mounted eye-trackers can use a depth calibration and linear depth correction.
- Another alternative with a binocular eye-tracker is to simply average data samples from the two eyes.

When these solutions are not available, the eye and scene cameras should be placed as closely together as possible on the headgear.

2.7.6 Data samples and the frames of reference

The vast majority of all eye-tracking research today consists of showing participants sequences of still images (possibly with sound), and having the observing participant sit more or less still in front of a static (remote or contact) eye-tracker. Virtually all analysis software is written for this particular set-up. The data file that you get will be a sequence of coordinates with time stamps, and the coordinates will be meaningful in the coordinate system of your stimulus. For instance, if you show a face, as in Figure 2.38, any raw data sample with coordinates $(x = 262, y = 291)$ will *always* be the coordinate of the pearl earring in that face image, because everything is still and kept in place. This association between the coordinate of a raw data sample and a semantic object is necessary later, in the analysis software. It makes it possible to calculate the duration that a participant gazes at the object (known as 'dwell time') and how many times he looks there (known as 'entries'). Also fixation and saccade analysis becomes easier. The association between sample coordinates and stimulus positions is established during *calibration*, typically quite a fast set-up carried out for each participant individually (p. 128).

(0,0)

x

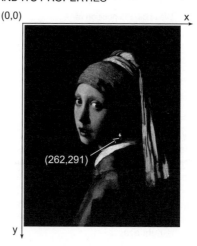

(262,291)

y

Fig. 2.38 The coordinate system in eye-tracking studies typically has the origin (x=0, y=0) in the upper left corner. For as long as this picture is shown, the data coordinate (x=262, y=291) will be a point on the pearl earring; that is, we have a link between a coordinate and a semantic object. The stimulus is the painting 'Het Meisje met de Parel' by Johannes Vermeer, circa 1665.

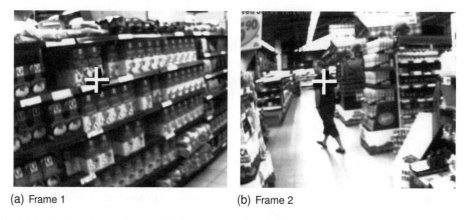

(a) Frame 1   (b) Frame 2

Fig. 2.39 Head motion and motion in the stimulus dissociate the link between gaze coordinates and semantic objects. Pictures show how the two data samples with identical coordinates indicate two entirely different objects at two instances separated by only a couple of seconds. Two frames from a gaze-overlaid video recorded with the SMI HED mobile system.

There are two large obstacles to the desired connection between gaze direction and a meaningful portion of the stimulus viewed: either *the participant's head moves*, or *the scene changes*, in ways the system cannot measure (we will overlook for now the errors stemming from moving the infrared emitters or the camera, adding glasses to the participant after calibration etc.). Suppose the researcher has a participant walking in a supermarket with a mobile head-mounted eye-tracker. Coordinates in the data file would indicate different positions at different times, because the participant moves. The coordinates $(262, 291)$ may at one moment be a box of pasta on the product shelf, and only seconds later be one of the other customers in the supermarket (see Figures 2.39(a) and 2.39(b)). Since the coordinate reference $(262, 291)$ changes in meaning all the time, adding up gaze data at this position over a whole trial (a round in the supermarket) would simply not give a value that refers to one single object, and many types of analyses would make no sense.

The same dissociation of coordinates and stimulus content occurs if you have animated stimuli: web pages with scrolling, video clips, and various multimedia products. As an object moves across the screen, its coordinate values change continuously with its position. First of all, this stimulus motion may make coordinate based analysis such as area of interest (AOI) analysis much more difficult, unless you use dynamic AOIs (see pages 209 and 227). Second, when viewing slowly moving objects, the eye makes what is known as a *smooth pursuit motion*, and this makes fixation analysis invalid with some of the current methods for event detection (p. 169).

There are notable technical solutions to parts of the problem with gaze coordinates lacking a permanent association to semantic objects.

- If you have a head-mounted system, the simplest solution is to *lock the head* relative to the stimulus. It works for single monitor stimuli, making a tower-mounted system out of the head-mounted system.
- If you do not want to fasten the head-mounted system (and the participants) in a tight construction, you may instead *measure the precise positions and movements of the head*, and add that measurement to the eye-tracker position to get a resulting *gaze vector* that is meaningful in the environment of the head-tracker. Both magnetic and camera-based head tracking can be used, but magnetic is the common choice.
- If you do not use a head-mounted system, but your coordinate problem is due to animation in the stimulus, the optimal solution is to *automatically detect and extract the coordinates of objects from the animated stimulus*. This is difficult in general, but feasible when the target object is known and very different from other objects in the environment, such as an overhead information board at a train station or an airport. Scrolling on web pages was a problem until two manufacturers made their own browsers that could read the scroll distance, and add it to the gaze coordinate. Placing markers on the stimulus and filming them with a scene camera (Figure 2.31) can give coordinates in the space spanned by the markers. In a similar manner, you may add radar and GPS measurements onto your car, so it calculates the precise position of your own and neighbouring cars, of pedestrians and buildings, and immediately calculate what object the driver's gaze hits.

With a head-mounted or a remote eye-tracker, if you record only gaze-overlaid video, but want to calculate numbers for the data, for instance how much time each participant looked at each type of pasta, then you have to extract this information manually from the video. If you have 20 minute recordings on video, and want to code fixation durations and dwell time (two central measures for how long people look), throughout the recording—for instance by requiring the gaze marker to be still for three frames which equal 120 ms for a 25 Hz video system—you may spend several days coding each participant. If your task requires you to code only portions of the recordings, an eye-tracker that only delivers gaze-overlaid video is more acceptable. Skipping large portions and coding only small time windows is reasonable in face-to-face interaction studies as well as consumer visual behaviour in supermarkets, assuming that the question is "What did they look at during the 10 seconds before they selected what to buy?", or "What did they look at during the 5 seconds after the interlocutor uttered a pronoun?". See pp. 227–229 for different methods for coding gaze-overlaid video data.

In conclusion, an eye-tracker produces streams of data samples, either in the coordinate system of the scene video camera attached to the participant's head, or in the coordinate system of the stimulus. As we noted, an area of interest can be placed on the stimulus to give a portion of the (x, y)-values a semantic value like 'the pearl'. The recorded eye-movement data can then be expressed as a sequence of semantically meaningful areas, such as PPMMPPH, where P, M, and H refer to the pearl, mouth, and headscarf in Figure 2.38. This is also known as an AOI string. An alternative to letting the researcher decide what values (x, y) coordinates should be given, is to use values calculated from the (x, y) points in the stimulus. For instance, we can calculate the luminosity at each position and get a string of numerical luminosity values, or produce a string of pasta prices by replacing each gaze hit on a pasta package by the price of that particular pasta. These are called feature values and feature strings, because luminosity and price are features of the stimulus. While semantic AOIs can only be used when the researcher defines the AOIs in accordance with the experimental design, feature values can be extracted algorithmically from the stimulus. Chapter 6 explains these uses of eye-movement data in detail.

2.8 Summary

This chapter introduced properties and varieties of video-based eye-trackers, which produce an output consisting of:

- often **the position of the pupil** and **corneal reflection** from the eye camera,
- always **raw data samples** with time stamps and (x, y) coordinates,
- sometimes **velocity** and rarely **acceleration** values,
- sometimes **gaze-overlaid videos**,
- in many eye-trackers, **pupil size** is a free extra.

Eye-trackers are built for different purposes and have a number of hardware and software related properties that should be taken into account when designing an experiment. The resolution of the eye camera and sampling frequency are examples of important hardware properties that influence what types of eye movements that can and cannot be measured. Software accompanying the eye-trackers contain algorithms that perform, for example, image analysis to find pupil and corneal reflections in the eye video, gaze estimation, and calculation of eye-movement velocity and acceleration from raw data samples.

Together with the participants and the recording environment, such properties decide the quality of the recorded data, and thus largely constrain the research questions that can be addressed, and the type of analyses that can be performed on the data. It is therefore important to have a basic understanding of how your eye-tracker works, in order to successfully design an experiment, record data, and analyse the recorded data.

3 From Vague Idea to Experimental Design

In Chapter 2, we described the competencies needed to build, evaluate, use and manage eye-trackers, as well as the properties of different eye-tracking systems and the data exiting them. In Chapter 3 we now focus on how to initially set up an eye-tracking study that can answer a specific research question. This initial and important part of a study is generally known as 'designing the experiment'.

Many of the recommendations in this chapter are based on two major assumptions. First, that it is better to strive towards making *the nature of the study experimental*. Experimental means studying the effect of an *independent variable* (that which, as researchers, we directly manipulate—text type for instance) on a *dependent variable* (an outcome we can directly measure—fixation durations or saccadic amplitude for instance) under tightly controlled conditions. One or more such variables can be under the control of the researcher and the goal of an experiment is to see how systematic changes in the independent variable(s) affect the dependent variable(s). The second assumption is that many eye-tracking measures—or dependent variables—*can be used as indirect measures of cognitive processes that cannot be directly accessed*. We will discuss possible pitfalls in interpreting results from eye-tracking research with regard to such cognitive processes. Throughout this chapter, we will use the example of the influence of background music on reading (p. 5). We limit ourselves to issues that are specific to eye-tracking studies. For more general textbooks on experimental design, we recommend Gravetter and Forzano (2008); McBurney and White (2007), and Jackson (2008).

This chapter is divided into five sections.

- In Section 3.1 (p. 66) we outline different considerations you should be aware of depending on the rationale behind your experiment and its purpose. There is without doubt huge variation in the initial starting point depending on the reason for doing the study (scientific journal paper or commercial report, for instance). Moreover, the previous experience of the researcher will also determine where to begin. In this section we describe different strategies that may be chosen during this preliminary stage of the study.
- In Section 3.2, we discuss how the investigation of an originally vague idea can be developed into an experiment. A clear understanding is needed of the total situation in which data will be recorded; you need to be aware of the potential causal relationships between your variables, and any extraneous factors which could impact upon this. In the subsections which follow we discuss the experimental task which the participants complete (p. 77), the experimental stimuli (p. 79), the structure of the trials of which the experiment is comprised (p. 81), the distinction between within-subject and between-subject factors (p. 83), and the number of trials and participants you need to include in your experiment (p. 85).
- Section 3.3 (p. 87) expands on the statistical considerations needed in experimental research with eye tracking. The design of an experiment is for a large part determined by the statistical analysis, and thus the statistical analysis needs to be taken into consideration during the planning stages of the experiment. In this section we describe

how statistical analysis may proceed and which factors determine which statistical test should be used. We conclude the section with an overview of some frequently used statistical tests including for each test an example of a study for which the test was used.

- Section 3.4 (p. 95) discusses what is known as *method triangulation*, in particular how auxiliary data can help disambiguate eye-tracking data and thereby tell us more about the participants' cognitive processes. Here, we will explore how other methodologies can contribute with unique information and how well they complement eye tracking. Using *verbal data* to disambiguate eye-movement data is the most well-used, yet controversial, form of methodological triangulation with eye-movement data. Section 3.4.8 (p. 99) reviews the different forms of verbal data, their properties, and highlights the importance of a strict method for acquiring verbal data.

3.1   The initial stage—explorative pilots, fishing trips, operationalizations, and highway research

At the very outset, before your study is formulated as a hypothesis, you will most likely have a loosely formulated question, such as "How does listening to music or noise affect the reading ability of students trying to study?". Unfortunately, this question is not directly answerable without making further operationalizations. The operationalization of a research idea is the process of making the idea so precise that data can be recorded, and valid, meaningful values calculated and evaluated. In the music study, you need to select different levels or types of background noise (e.g. music, conversation), and you need to choose how to measure reading ability (e.g. using a test, a questionnaire, or by looking at reading speed). In the following subsections, we give a number of suggestions for how to proceed at this stage of the study. The suggested options below are not necessarily exclusive, so you may find yourself trying out more than one strategy before settling on a particular final form of the experiment.

3.1.1   The explorative pilot

One way to start is by doing a *small-scale explorative pilot study*. This is the thing to do if you do not feel confident about the differences you may expect, or the factors to include in the real experiment. The aim is to get a general feeling for the task and to enable you to generate plausible operationalized hypotheses. In our example case of eye movements and reading, take one or two texts, and have your friends read them while listening to music, noise, and silence, respectively. Record their eye movements while they do this. Then, interview them about the process: how did they feel about the task—how did they experience reading the texts under these conditions? Explore the results by looking at data, for instance, look at heat maps (Chapter 7), and scanpaths (Chapter 8). Are there differences in the data for those who listened to music/noise compared to those who did not? Why could that be? Are there other measures you should use to complement the eye-tracking data (retention, working memory span, personality tests, number of books they read as children etc.). It is not essential to do statistical tests during this pilot phase, since the goal of the pilot study is to generate testable hypotheses, and not a *p*-value (nevertheless you should keep in mind what statistics would be appropriate, and to this end it might be useful to look for statistical trends in the data). Do not forget that the hypotheses you decide upon should be relevant to theory—they should have some background and basis from which you generate your predictions. In our case of music and eye movements whilst reading, the appropriate literature revolves around reading research and environmental psychology.

3.1.2 The fishing trip

You may decide boldly to run a larger pilot study with many participants and stimuli, even though you do not really know what eye-tracking measures to use in your analyses. After all, you may argue, there are many eye-tracking measures (fixation duration, dwell times, transitions, fixation densities, etc.), and some of them will probably give you a result. This approach is sometimes called *the fishing trip*, because it resembles throwing out a wide net in the water and hoping that there will be fish (significant results) somewhere. A major danger of the fishing trip approach is this: if you are running significance tests on many eye-tracking measures, a number of measures will be significant just by chance, even on completely random data. If you then choose to present such a selection of significant effects, you have merely shown that at this particular time and spot there happened to be some fish in the water, but another researcher who tries to replicate your findings is less likely to find the same results. More is explained about this problem on p. 94.

While fishing trips cannot provide any definite conclusions, they can be an alternative to a small-scale explorative study. In fact, the benefits of this approach are several. For example, real effects are replicable, and therefore you can proceed to test an initial post-hoc explanation from your fishing trip more critically in a real experiment. After the fishing trip, you have found some measures that are statistically significant, have seen the size of the effects, and you have an indication of how many participants and items are needed in the real study. There are also, however, several drawbacks. Doing a fishing-trip study involves a considerable amount of work in generating many stimulus items, recruiting many participants, computing all the measures, and doing a statistical analysis on each and every one (and for this effort you can not be *certain* that you will find anything interesting).

It should be emphasized that it is *not* valid to selectively pick significant results from such a study and present them as if you had performed a focused study using only those particular measures. The reason is, you are misleading readers of your research into thinking that your initial theoretical predictions were so accurate that you managed to find a significant effect directly, while in fact you tested many measures, and then formulated a post-hoc explanation for those that were significant. There is a substantial risk that these effects are spurious.

3.1.3 Theory-driven operationalizations

Ideally, you start from previous theories and results and then form corollary predictions. This is generally true because you usually start with some knowledge grounded in previous research. However, it is often the case that these predictions are too general, or not formulated as testable concepts. Theories are usually well specified within the scope of interest of previous authors, but when you want to challenge them from a more unexpected angle, you will probably find several key points unanswered. The predictions that follow from a theory can be specified further by either referring to a complementary theory, or by making some plausible assumptions in the spirit of the theory that are likely to be accepted by the original authors, and which still enable you to test the theory empirically.

If you are really lucky, you may find a theory, model, statement, or even an interesting folk-psychological notion that directly predicts something in terms of eye-tracking measures, such as "you re-read already read sentences to a larger extent when you are listening to music you like". In that case, the conceptual work is largely done for you, and you may continue with addressing the experimental parameters. If the theory is already established, it will also be easier to publish results based on this theory, assuming you have a sound experimental design.

3.1.4 Operationalization through traditions and paradigms

One approach, similar to theory-driven operationalizations, is the case where the researcher incrementally adapts and expands on previous research. Typically, you would start with a published paper and minimally modify the reported experiment for your own needs, in order to establish whether you are able to replicate the main findings and expand upon them. Subsequently you can add further manipulations which shed further light on the issue in hand. The benefits are that you build upon an accepted experimental set-up and measures that have been shown in the past to give significant results. This methodology is more likely to be accepted than presenting your own measures that have not been used in this setting before. Furthermore, using an already established experimental procedure will save you time in not having to run as many pilots, or plan and test different set-ups.

Certain topics become very influential and accumulate a lot of experimental results. After some time these areas become *research traditions* in their own right and have well-specified *paradigms* associated with them, along with particular techniques, effects, and measures. A paradigm is a tight operationalization of an experimental task, and aims to pinpoint cause and effect ruling out other extraneous factors. Once established, it is relatively easy to generate a number of studies by making subtle adjustments to a known paradigm, and focus on discovering and mapping out different effects. Because of its ease of use, this practice is sometimes called 'highway research'. Nevertheless, this approach has many merits, as long-term systematicity is often necessary to map out an important and complex research area. You simply need many repetitions and slight variations to get a grasp of the involved effects, how they interact, and their magnitudes. Also, working within an accepted research tradition, using a particular paradigm, makes it more likely that your research will be picked up, incorporated with other research in this field, and expanded upon. A possible drawback is that the researcher gets too accustomed to the short times between idea and result, and consequently new and innovative methods will be overlooked because researchers become reluctant of stepping outside a known paradigm.

It should be noted that it is possible to get the benefits of an established paradigm, but still address questions outside of it; this therefore differentiates paradigm-based research from theory-driven operationalizations. Measures, analysis methods, and statistical practices, may be well developed and mapped out within a certain paradigm designed for a specific research tradition, but nothing prohibits you from using these methods to tackle other research questions outside of this area. For example, psycholinguistic paradigms can be adapted for marketing research to test 'top-of-the-mind' associations (products that you first think of to fulfil a given consumer need).

In this book, we aim for a general level of understanding and will not delve deeper into concerns or measures that are very specific to a particular research tradition. The following are very condensed descriptions of a few major research traditions in eye tracking:

- *Visual search* is perhaps the largest research tradition and offers an easily adaptable and highly informative experimental procedure. The basic principles of visual search experiments were founded by Treisman and Gelade (1980) and rest on the idea that effortful scanning for a target amongst distractors will show a linear increase in reaction time the larger the set size, that is, the more distractors present. However, some types of target are said to 'pop out' irrespective of set size; you can observe this for instance if you are looking for something red surrounded by things that are blue. These asymmetries in visual search times reflect the difference between *serial* and *parallel* processing respectively—some items require focused attention and it takes time to bind their properties together, other items can be located pre-attentively. Many manipulations of the basic visual search paradigm have been conducted—indeed any experiment where you have to find a pre-defined target presented in stimulus space is a form of visual search—and from this research tradition we have learned much about the tight coupling between attention and eye movements. Varying the properties of targets and distracters, their distribution in space, the size of the search array, the number of potential items that can be retained in memory etc. reveals much about how we are able to cope with the vast amount of visual information that our eyes receive every second and, nevertheless, direct our eyes efficiently depending on the current task in hand. In the real world this could be baggage screening at an airport, looking for your keys on a cluttered desk, or trying to find a friend in a crowd. Although classically visual search experiments are used to study attention independently of eye movements, visual search manipulations are also common in studies of eye guidance. For an overview of visual search see Wolfe (1998a, 1998b).

- *Reading research* focuses on language processes involved in text comprehension. Common research questions involve the existence and extent of parallel processing and the influence of lexical and syntactic factors on reading behaviour. This tradition commonly adopts well-constrained text processing, such as presenting a single sentence per screen. The text presented will conform to a clear design structure in order to pinpoint the exact mechanisms of oculomotor control during reading. Hence, 'reading' in the higher-level sense, such as literary comprehension of a novel, is not the impetus of the reading research tradition from an eye movement perspective. With higher-level reading, factors such as genre, education level, and discourse structure are the main predictors, as opposed to word frequency, word length, number of morphemes etc. in reading research on eye-movement control. The well-constrained nature of reading research, as well as consistent dedication within the field has generated a very well-researched domain where the level of sophistication is high. Common measures of interest to reading researchers are first fixation durations, first-pass durations and the number of between- and within-word regressions. Unique to reading research is the stimulus lay-out which has an inherent order of processing (word one comes before word two, which comes before word three...). This allows for measures which use order as a component, regressions for instance, where participants re-fixate an already fixated word from earlier in the sentence. Reading research has also spearheaded the use of gaze-contingent display changes in eye-tracking research. Here, words can be changed, replaced, or hidden from view depending on the current locus of fixation (e.g. the next word in a sentence may be occluded by (x)s, just delimiting the number of characters, until your eyes land on it, see page 50). Gaze-contingent eye tracking is a powerful technique to investigate preview benefits in reading and has been employed in other research areas to study attention independently from eye movements. Good overview or milestone articles in reading research are Reder (1973); Rayner (1998); Rayner and Pollatsek (1989); Inhoff and Radach (1998); Engbert, Longtin, and Kliegl (2002).

- *Scene perception* is concerned with how we look at visual scenes, typically presented on a computer monitor. Common research questions concern the extent to which various bottom-up or top-down factors explain where we direct our gaze in a scene, as well as how fast we can form a representation of the scene and recall it accurately. Since scenes are presented on a computer screen, researchers can directly manipulate and test low-level parameters such a luminance, colour, and contrast, as well as making detailed quantitative predictions from models. Typical measures are number of fixations and correlations between model-predicted and actual gaze locations. The scene may also be divided into areas of interest (AOIs), from which AOI measures and other eye movement statistics can be calculated (see Chapter 6 and Part III of the book respectively). Suggested entry articles for scene perception are J. M. Henderson and Hollingworth (1999), J. M. Henderson (2003) and Itti and Koch (2001).

- *Usability* is a very broad research tradition that does not yet have established eye-tracking conventions as do the aforementioned traditions. However, usability research is interesting because it operates at a higher analysis level than the other research traditions, and is typically focused on actual real-world use of different artefacts and uses eye tracking as a means to get insight into higher-level cognitive processing. Stimulus and task are often given and cannot be manipulated to any larger extent. For instance, Fitts, Jones, and Milton (1950) recorded on military pilots during landing, which restricted possibilities of varying the layout in the cockpit or introducing manipulations that could cause failures. Usability is the most challenging eye-tracking research tradition as the error sources are numerous, and researchers still have to employ different methods to overcome these problems. One way is using eye tracking as an explorative measure, or as a way to record post-experiment cued retrospective verbalizations with the participants. Possible introductory articles are Van Gog, Paas, Van Merriënboer, and Witte (2005), Goldberg and Wichansky (2003), Jacob and Karn (2003), and Land (2006).

As noted, broad research traditions like those outlined above are often accompanied by specific experimental paradigms, set procedures which can be adapted and modified to tackle the research question in hand. We have already mentioned gaze-contingent research in reading, a technique that has become known as the *the moving-window paradigm* (McConkie & Rayner, 1975). This has also been adapted to study scene perception leading to Castelhano and Henderson (2007) developing the *flash-preview moving-window paradigm*. Here a scene is very briefly presented to participants (too fast to make eye movements) before subsequent scanning; the eye movements that follow when the scene is inspected are restricted by a fixation-dependent moving window. This paradigm allows researchers to unambiguously gauge what information from an initial scene glimpse guides the eyes.

The *Visual World Paradigm* (Tanenhaus, Spivey-Knowlton, Eberhard, & Sedivy, 1995) is another experimental set-up focused on spoken-language processing. It constitutes a bridge between language and eye movements in the 'real world'. In this paradigm, auditory linguistic information directs participants' gaze. As the auditory information unfolds over time, it is possible to establish at around which point in time enough information has been received to move the eyes accordingly with the intended target. Using systematic manipulations, this allows the researchers to understand the language processing system and explore the effects of different lexical, semantic, visual, and many other factors. For an introduction to this research tradition, please see Tanenhaus and Brown-Schmidt (2008) and Huettig, Rommers, and Meyer (2011) for a detailed review.

There are also a whole range of experimental paradigms to study oculomotor and saccade programming processes. The *anti-saccadic paradigm* (see Munoz and Everling (2004) and Everling and Fischer (1998)) involves an exogeneous attentional cue—a dot which the eyes are drawn to, but which must be inhibited and a saccade made in the *opposite* direction, known as an *anti-saccade*. Typically anti-saccade studies include more than just anti-saccades, but also pro-saccades (i.e. eye movements *towards* the abrupt dot onset), and switching between these tasks. This paradigm can therefore be used to test the ability of participants to assert executive cognitive control over eye movements. A handful of other well-specified 'off-the-shelf' experimental paradigms also exist, like the anti-saccadic task, to study occulomotor and saccade programming processes. These include but are not limited to: the *gap task* (Kingstone & Klein, 1993), the *remote distractor effect* (Walker, Deubel, Schneider, & Findlay, 1997), *saccadic mislocalization* and *compression* (J. Ross, Morrone, & Burr, 1997). Full descriptions of all of these approaches is not within the scope of this chapter; the intention is to acquaint the reader with the idea that there are many predefined experimental paradigms which can be utilized and modified according to the thrust of your research.

3.2   What caused the effect? The need to understand what you are studying

A basic limitation in eye-tracking research is the following: it is impossible to tell from eye-tracking data alone what people think. The following quote from Hyrskykari, Ovaska, Majaranta, Räihä, and Lehtinen (2008) nicely exemplify how this limitation may affect the interpretation of data:

> For example, a prolonged gaze to some widget does not necessarily mean that the user does not understand the meaning of the widget. The user may just be pondering some aspect of the given task unrelated to the role of the widget on which the gaze happens to dwell. ... Similarly, a distinctive area on a heat map is often interpreted as meaning that the area was interesting. It attracted the user's attention, and therefore the information in that area is assumed to be known to the user. However, the opposite may be true: the area may have attracted the user's attention precisely because it was confusing and problematic, and the user did not understand the information presented.

Similarly, Triesch, Ballard, Hayhoe, and Sullivan (2003) show that in some situations participants can look straight at a task-relevant object, and still no working memory trace can be registered. Not only fixations are ambiguous. Holsanova, Holmberg, and Holmqvist (2008) point out that frequent saccades between text and images may reflect an interest in integrating the two modalities, but also difficulty in integrating them. That eye-movement data are non-trivial to analyse is further emphasized by the remarks from Underwood, Chapman, Berger, and Crundall (2003) which detail that about 20% of all non-fixated objects in their driving scenes were recalled by participants, and from Griffin and Spieler (2006) that people often speak about objects in a scene that were never fixated. Finally, Viviani (1990) provides an in-depth discussion about links between eye movements and higher cognitive processes.

In the authors' experience, it is very easy to get dazzled by eye-tracking visualizations such as scanpaths and heat maps, and assume for instance that the hot-spot area on a webpage was interesting to the participants, or that the words were difficult to understand, forgetting the many other reasons participants could have had for looking there. Its negative effect on our reasoning is known under the term 'affirming the consequent' or more colloquially 'backward reasoning' or 'reverse inference'.

We will exemplify the idea of backward reasoning using the music and reading study introduced on page 5. This study was designed to determine whether music disturbs the reading process or not. The reading process is measured using eye movements. These three components are illustrated schematically in Figure 3.1. In this figure, all the *(m)*s signify properties of the experimental set-up that were manipulated (e.g. the type of music, or the volume level). The *(c)*s in the figure represent different cognitive processes that may be influenced by the experimental manipulations. The *(b)*s, finally, are the different behavioural outcomes (the eye movements) of the cognitive processes. Note that we cannot measure the cognitive processes *directly* with eye tracking, but we try to capture them indirectly by making manipulations and measuring changes in the behaviour (eye movement measures).[11]

---

[11] See Poldrack, 2006 for an interesting discussion regarding reverse inference from the field of fMRI.

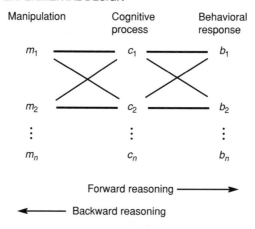

Fig. 3.1 Available reasoning paths: possible paths of influence that different variables can have. Our goal is to correctly establish what variables influence what. Notice that there is a near-infinite number of variables that influence, to a greater or lesser degree, any other given variable.

Each of the three components (the columns of Figure 3.1) introduce a risk of drawing an erroneous conclusion from the experimental results.

1. During data collection, perhaps the experiment leader unknowingly introduced a confound, something that co-occurred at the same time as the music. Perhaps the experiment leader tapped his finger to the rhythm of the music and disturbed the participant. This would yield the path $(m_2) \rightarrow (c_1) \rightarrow (b_1)$, with (m_2) being the finger tapping. As a consequence, we *do* get our result (b_1), falsely believing this effect has taken the path of $(m_1) \rightarrow (c_1) \rightarrow (b_1)$, while in fact it is was the finger tapping (m_2) that drove the entire effect.

2. We hope that our manipulation in stage one affects the correct cognitive process, in our case the reading comprehension system. However, it could well be that our manipulation evokes some other cognitive processes. Perhaps something in the music influenced the participant's confidence in his comprehension abilities, (c_2), making the participant less confident. This shows up as longer fixations and additional regressions to double-check the meaning of the words and constructions. Again, we do get our (b_1), but it has taken the route $(m_1) \rightarrow (c_2) \rightarrow (b_1)$, much like in the case with long dwell time on the widget mentioned previously.

3. Unfortunately, maybe there was an error when programming the analysis script, and the eye-movement measures were calculated in the wrong way. Therefore, we think we are getting a proper estimation of our gaze measures (b_1), but in reality we are getting numbers representing entirely different measures (b_2).

Erroneous conclusions can either be *false positives* or *false negatives*. A *false positive* is to erroneously accept the null hypothesis to be false (or an alternative explanation as correct). In Figure 3.1 above, the path $(m_1) \rightarrow (c_2) \rightarrow (b_1)$ would be such a case. We make sure we present the correct stimuli (m_1), and we find a difference in measurable outcomes (b_1), but the path of influence never involved our cognitive process of interest (c_1), but some other function (c_2). We thus erroneously accepted that (c_1) is involved in this process (or more correctly: falsely rejected that it had no effect). The other error is the *false negative*, where we erroneously reject an effect even though it is present and genuine. For example, we believe we test the path $(m_1) \rightarrow (c_1) \rightarrow (b_1)$, but in fact we unknowingly measure the wrong eye-movement variables (b_2) due to a programming error. Since we cannot find any differences in what we believe our measures to be, we falsely conclude that either our manipulation (m_1) had no effect, or our believed cognitive process (c_1) was not involved at all, when in fact if we had properly recorded and analysed the right eye-movement measures we would have observed a significant result. False negatives are also highly likely when you have not recorded enough data; maybe you have too few trials per condition, or there are not enough participants included in your study. If this is the case your experiment does not have enough *statistical power* (p. 85) to yield a significant result, even though such an effect is true and would have been identified had more data been collected.

How can we deal with the complex situation of partly unknown factors and unpredicted causal chains that almost any experiment necessarily involves? There is an old joke that a good experimentalist needs to be a bit neurotic, looking for all the dangers to the experiment, also those that lurk below the immediate realm of our consciousness, waiting there for a chance to undermine the conclusion by introducing an alternative path to (b_1). It is simply necessary to constrain the number of possible paths, until only one inevitable conclusion remains, namely that: "(m_1) leads to (c_1) because we got (b_1) and we checked all the other possible paths to (b_1) and could exclude them". Only then does backward reasoning, from measurement to cognitive process, hold.

There is no definitive recipe for how to detect and constrain possible paths, but these are some tips:

- As part of your experimental design work, *list* all the alternative paths that you can think of. Brainstorming and mind-mapping are good tools for this job.
- Read previous research on the cognitive processes involved. Can studies already conducted exclude some of the paths for you?
- The simpler eye-movement measures belonging to fixations (pp. 377–389) and saccades (pp. 302–336) are relatively well-investigated indicators of cognitive processes (depending on the research field). The more complex measures used in usability and design studies are largely unvalidated, independent of field of research. We must recognize that without a theoretical foundation and validation research, a recorded gaze behaviour might indicate just about any cognitive process.
- If your study requires you to use complex, unvalidated measures, do not despair. New measures must be developed as new research frontiers open up (exemplified for instance by Dempere-Marco, Hu, Ellis, Hansell, & Yang, 2006; Goldberg & Kotval, 1999; Ponsoda, Scott, & Findlay, 1995; Choi, Mosley, & Stark, 1995; Mannan, Ruddock, & Wooding, 1995). This is necessary exploratory work, and you will have to argue convincingly that the new measure works for your specific case, and even then accept that further validation studies are needed.
- Select your stimuli and the task instructions so as to constrain the number of paths to (b_1). Reduce participant variation with respect to background knowledge, expectations, anxiety levels, etc. Start with a narrow and tightly controlled experiment with excellent statistical power. After you have found an effect, you might have to worry about whether it generalizes to all participant populations; is it likely to be true in all situations?
- Use *method triangulation*: simple additional measurements like retention tests, working memory tests, and reaction time tests can help reduce the number of paths. Hyrskykari et al. (2008), from whom the quotes above came, argue that retrospective gaze-path stimulated think-aloud protocols add needed information on thought processes related to scanpaths. If that is not enough, there is also the possibility to add other behavioural measurements. We will come back to this option later in this chapter (p. 95).

3.2.1 Correlation and causality: a matter of control

A fundamental tenet of any *experimental* study is the operationalization of the mental construct you wish to study, using *dependent* and *independent* variables. Independent variables
are the causal requisites of an effect, the things we directly manipulate, $(m_i, i = 1, 2, \ldots, n)$
in Figure 3.1. Dependent variables are the events that change as a direct consequence of our
manipulations—our independent variables are said to *affect* our dependent variables. This terminology can be confusing, but you will see it used a lot as you read scientific eye-tracking
literature so it is important that you understand what it means, and the crucial difference between independent and dependent variables. In eye tracking your dependent variables are any
of the eye-movement measures you choose to take (as extensively outlined in Part III).

A perfect experiment is one in which no factors systematically influence the dependent
variable (e.g. fixation duration) other than the ones you control. The factors you control are
typically controlled in groups, such as 'listens to music' versus 'listens to cafeteria noise' or
along a continuous scale such as introversion/extroversion (e.g. between 1 and 7). A perfectly
controlled experimental design is the ideal, because it is only with controlled experimental
designs that we are able to make statements of causality. That means, if we manipulate one
independent variable while keeping all other factors constant, then any resulting change in
the dependent variable will be due to our manipulated factor, our independent variable (as it
is the only one that has varied).

In reality, however, all experiments are less than perfect, simply because it is impossible
to control for every single factor that could possibly influence the dependent variable. A
correlational study allows included variables to vary freely, e.g. a participant reading to music
could be influenced by the tempo of the songs, the genre, the lyrics, or simply the loudness
of the music. If all these variables correlate with each other, it is not possible to separate the
true influencing variable from the others. This results in the problem that we cannot know
anything about the *causality* involved in our experiment. Perhaps one factor influences the
dependent variable, or it could be that our dependent variable is actually causing the value of
one of our 'independent' variables. Or, both variables could be determined by a third, hidden,
variable. Lastly, they could be completely unrelated. Let us look at two examples from real
life.

A psycholinguist wants to investigate the effect of prosody on visual attention. The experiment consists of showing pictures of arrays of objects while a speaker describes an event
involving the objects. The auditory stimuli are systematically varied in such a way that one
half of the scenes involve an object that is mentioned with prosodic emphasis, while the other
half is not emphasized at all. A potentially confounding factor is the speaker making an audi-
ble inhale before any emphasis. This inhale is a signal to the participant to be on the alert for
the next object mentioned, but it is not considered a prosodic part of the emphasis (which in
this case includes only pitch and volume). In this example, the inhale *systematically* co-varies
with the manipulated, independent variable, and may lead to false conclusions. Confounding
factors may also co-vary in a random way with the independent variable. Such unsystematic
co-variation is cancelled out given enough trials.

As another example, consider an educational psychologist testing the readability of difficult and easy articles in a newspaper. The hypothesis is that easier articles have a larger
relative reading depth, because readers do not get tangled up with complex arguments and
difficult words. A rater panel has judged different articles as being more or less difficult, on
a 7-point scale. So we let the students read the real newspaper containing articles with both
degrees of difficulty. Our results show that the easier articles have a larger reading depth.
However, the readers are biased to spend more energy reading articles with interesting topics,
and read them with less effort. Therefore, interesting articles have a lower difficulty rating.

This is our first hidden factor. Furthermore, the most interesting articles are placed early in the newspaper, which the reader attends to when most motivated. As the reader reads on, he skips more and more. Because of this, the least interesting articles (misjudged as difficult), are skipped to a larger extent—not because they are difficult, but because they correlate with late placement order, our second hidden factor. The net result is that we end up with an experiment purporting to show an effect due to difficulty/ease of articles, while the real effect is driven by interest and placement.

The bottom line is that it is impossible to control all factors, but with the most important factors identified, controlled, and systematically varied, we can confidently claim to have a sound experimental design. The first scenario is such, because the stimuli are directly manipulated to include almost all relevant factors. The second example is more tricky. We are biased by the panel of raters and trust them to provide an objective measurement of a predictor variable, but the raters are only human. Experiments such as these are also typically presented as experimental in their design, although they are much more sensitive to spurious correlations than our first scenario. The key problem is that the stimuli are not directly controlled. The newspaper has the design it has, and the articles are not presented in a random and systematically varied manner. By allowing important factors to covary, we end up with a design that is susceptible to correlations and is more likely to produce false conclusions.

It should nevertheless be remembered that increasing experimental control tends to decrease ecological validity and generalizability of the research. Land and Tatler (2009) in their preface express concern over the "passion for removing all trace of the natural environment from experiments" they see with many experimental psychologists. Accepting the loss of some control may often be a reasonable price to pay to be able to make an ecologically valid study. In the end, we do want to say something about performance in the real world. An example of the difference between the real world and the laboratory is presented by Y. Wang et al. (2010), who found a greater number of dwells to in-car instruments during field driving compared to simulator driving.

3.2.2 What measures to select as dependent variables

Designing a study from scratch often involves the very concrete procedure of drawing the eye-movement behaviour you and your theories predict on print-outs of your stimuli, and matching the lines you draw with candidate measures from Chapters 10–13. Some of these measures are relatively simple, while others are complex. Often, you may inherit your measures from the paradigm you are working in, or the journal paper you are trying to replicate. Your study may also be so new that you need to employ rarely used, complex measures. After you have selected some measures, run a pilot recording and make a pilot analysis with those measures. In either case, you should strive to select your measures during the designing phase of the experiment, and make sure they work with your eye-tracker, the stimuli, your task, and the statistics you plan to use.

Note that as a beginning PhD student, you may have to spend up to a whole year until the experiment is successfully completed, but with enough experience the same process can be reduced to as little as a month. It is seldom the data recording experience, nor the theoretical experience that makes this difference, but the experience in how to design and analyse experiments with complex eye-movement measures. Making sure appropriate measures are used will certainly save you time during the analysis phase and possibly prevent you from having to redesign the experiment and record new data.

Frequently, the complex measures inherit properties of the simpler ones. For instance, transition matrices, scanpath lengths, and heat map activations depend on how fixations and saccades were calculated, which in turn depend on filters in the velocity calculation. It is not straightforward to decide which measures to choose as dependent variables, as this choice depends on many different considerations.

In addition, complex measures such as transition diagrams (p. 193), position dispersion measures (p. 359), and scanpath similarity measures (p. 346) have not yet been subjected to validation tests, or used over a number of studies to show to which cognitive process they are linked. Active validation work exists only for a few simple measures from within scene perception, reading, and parts of the neurological eye-tracking research, for instance smooth pursuit gain (p. 450) and the anti-saccade measures (p. 305). These measures have been used extensively, and we have gathered considerable knowledge about what affects their values in one or the other direction.

An initial factor concerns the possibilities and the limitations of the hardware that you use. Animated stimuli, for instance, invalidate fixation data from all algorithms that do not support smooth pursuit detection (p. 168). Second, the sampling frequency (p. 29) may limit what measures you can confidently calculate. Third, the precision of the system and partici-pants (p. 33) may exert a similar constraint. Fourth, relatively complex measures may require extensive programming skills or excessive manual work (in particular with head-mounted systems, p. 227), making them not a viable option for a study. Finally, some measures are more suitable for standard statistical analysis than others.

Therefore, in any type of eye-tracking project, part of the experimental design consists of selecting measures to be used for dependent variables, and to verify that the experimental set-up and equipment make it possible to calculate the measures. It is definitely advisable, in particular when using new experimental designs, to use the data collected in the pilot study (an essential check-point, described on p. 114) to verify that the method of analysis, including calculation of measures, actually works.

If you are at the start of your eye-tracking career, the approach of already thinking about the analysis stage when you are designing the experiment forces you to think through the experiment carefully and to design it so it answers your research question faster, more accur-ately, and with less effort. The eyes should always be on the research question, and eye-tracking is just a tool for answering it.

Question the *validity* and *reliability* of your measures. Validity is whether the dependent variable is measuring what you think it is measuring, for instance you may assume longer dwell time is a good index of processing difficulty in your experiment, but in fact this reflects preferential looking at incongruous elements of your stimulus display. Reliability refers to replicable effects; your chosen measure may give the same value over-and-over, in which case it is reliable, but note that a reliable measure is not necessarily a valid one (see page 463 for an extended discussion). You may find longer dwell times time and time again, which are not a measure of processing difficulty, as you thought, but rather a measure of incongruity. Below is a quick list on how to select your eye-tracking measures keeping the above issues in mind:

- Obviously, select the measure which fits your hypothesis best. If you think that your text manipulation will yield longer reading times, then first-pass duration or mean-fixation duration are likely measures, but number of regressions only an indirect (but likely correlated) measure. Unless of course your hypothesis is actually that reading times will be longer due to more regressions.
- Are you working within an established paradigm? Use whatever is used in your field to maximize the compatibility of your research.
- Identify other functionally equivalent measures for your research question. Are you interested in mental workload for example? Then find out what other measures are

used to investigate this, for instance using the index. Perhaps some of the alternative measures are better and completely missed by you and others in your paradigm.

- Prioritize measures that have been extensively tested, as there is better insight into potential factors affecting them. For example, first fixation durations in reading have been tested extensively and we know how they will react to changes in, for instance, word frequency. It would be less problematic to do a reverse inference with this kind of measure (using the first fixation durations to estimate the processing difficulty increase of a manipulation) than with other less well-explored measures.

- Select measures that are as fine-grained as possible, for example measures that focus on particular points in time rather than prolonged gaze sequences. This allows you to perform analyses where you identify points in time where the participant is engaged in the particular behaviour in which you are interested, e.g. searching behaviour, and then extract just the measures during just these points. This is more powerful than just extracting all instances of this measure during the whole trial, where the particular behaviour of interest is mixed with many other forms of gaze behaviour (which essentially just contribute noise to your results).

- To minimize problems during the statistical analysis, select measures that are either certain to generate normally distributed data, or measures that generate several instances per trial. In the latter case, if you cannot transform your data adequately or suffer from zero/null data, then you can take the mean of the measures inside the trials.[12] The implications of the central limit theorem are that a distribution of means will be normally distributed, regardless of the distribution of the underlying data. You will now have sacrificed some statistical power in order to have a well-formed data distribution which does not violate the criteria of your hypothesis tests. See Figure 3.2 for an example of different means to which you can aggregate. In this example, there is only one measurement value per trial, but repeated measurements within each trial would have provided even more data to either keep or over which to aggregate.

3.2.3   The task

Eye-tracking data is—as shown very early by Yarbus (1967, p. 174ff) and Buswell (1935, p. 136ff)—extremely sensitive to the task, so select it carefully. A good task should fulfil three criteria:

1. The task should be neutral with regard to the experimental and control conditions. The task should not favour any particular condition (unless used as such).
2. The task should be engaging. An engaging task distracts the participant from the fact that they are sitting in, or wearing, an eye-tracker and that you are measuring their behaviour.
3. The task should have a plausible cover story or be non-transparent to the participant. This stops the participant from second-guessing the nature of the experiment and trying to give the experimenter the answers that she wants. When the experiment itself causes the effects expected it is said to have *demand characteristics*.

If you are afraid to bias them, then give participants a very neutral task, but remember that weak and overly neutral tasks may also make each participant invent their own task. If you present an experiment with 48 trials and you do not provide a task, you are not to be surprised

---

[12]Note that if a level of averaging is severely skewed by outlying data points, it might be more appropriate to take a median at the trial or participant level.

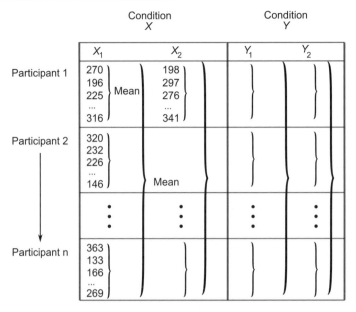

Fig. 3.2 A typical experimental design, and how means are calculated from it. Here we have two independent variables, X and Y, each with two factors, $X_{1,2}$ and $Y_{1,2}$. The conditions could be preferred and non-preferred music, each with high and low volume level, for instance. Each number represents an eye-movement measure from one trial.

if you find that the participants have been looking outside of the monitor, daydreaming, or falling asleep. Very general tasks such as "just look at the images" may require some mock questions to make the participants feel like they can provide answers/reactions to the stimuli. If you show pictures and want to make it probable that participants indeed scan the picture, a very neutral mock question could be "To what degree did you appreciate this image?". This question is neutral in the sense that it motivates participants to focus attention on the image presented, but still does not bias their gaze towards some particular part or object in the scene. Furthermore, if you add random elements, such as asking alternating questions and only at a random 30% of the trials, it reduces tediousness and predictability.

Tasks can also be used very actively in the experimental design, which was what Yarbus did, showing the same image to a participant but with differing instructions, thereby creating experimental conditions. In such a case the overt task starts and drives the experimental condition. A motivating task can also be the instruction to solve a mathematical problem, or to read so that the participants can answer questions afterwards. An engaging task can consume the full interest of the participants and surplus cognitive resources are aimed at more thoroughly solving the task. Additionally, an engaging task is not as exhausting for the participant, thus he can do more trials and provide you with more data. An important property of an engaging task is that it makes sense to the participant and allows him to contribute in a meaningful way.

In a general sense, the task starts when you contact potential participants, and talk to them about the experiment. When you recruit your participants, you must give them a good idea about what they are going to do in your experiment, but you should only tell them about the task you present to them. You should not reveal the scientific purpose of your study, since prior knowledge of what you want to study may make them behave differently. Suppose for instance that the researcher wants to show that people who listen to a scene description re-enact the scene with their eyes, as in Johansson, Holsanova, and Holmqvist

(2006). If a participant knows that the researcher wants to find this result, the participant is likely to think about it and to want to help, consciously or not, in obtaining this result, thus inflating the risk of a false positive. Such knowledge can be devastating to a study. For certain sensitive experiments, it may be necessary to include many distractor trials to simply confuse the participants about the hypotheses of the experiment. Additionally, our researcher should give participants a cover story, to be revealed at debriefing, that goes well with the kind of behaviour and performance she hopes participants will exhibit. For example:

> Throughout, participants were told that the experiment concerned pupil dilation during the retelling of descriptions held in memory. It was explained to them that we would be filming their eyes, but nothing was said about our knowing in which directions they were looking. They were asked to keep their eyes open so that we could film their pupils, and to look only at the white board in front of them so that varying light conditions beyond the board would not disturb the pupil dilation measurements (excerpt from Johansson et al. (2006), procedure section).

When you have settled on a task instruction that you feel fulfils the listed criteria sufficiently, then it is a good idea to write down the instructions. Written instructions allow you to give exactly the same task to all participants, rather than trying to remember the instructions by heart and possibly missing small but important parts of the task. Written instruction also help negate any *experimenter effects*: subtle and unconscious cues from the experimenter giving hints to the participant on how to perform.

3.2.4 Stimulus scene, and the areas of interest

Stimuli are of course selected according to the research question of the study in hand, and can be anything from abstract arrays of shapes or text, to scenes, web pages, movies, and even the events that unfold in real-world scenarios such as driving, sport, or supermarket shopping.

Scenes can roughly be divided up into two groups:

- Natural and unbalanced scenes, where objects are where they are and you do not control for their position, colour, shape, luminance etc. An example would be the real-world environment we interact with every day.
- Artificial and balanced scenes, which consist of objects selected and placed by the experimenter. For example, a scene constructed from clip arts, or a screen with collections of patches with different spatial frequency.

The two types offer their own benefits and drawbacks. Natural scenes, on average, will generalize better to the real world, as they are often a part of it or mimic it closely. If you find that consumers have a certain gaze pattern in a cluttered supermarket scene, you do not necessarily have to break down the scene into detailed features such as colour, shape, and contrast, but rather you can just accept that the gaze pattern works in this environment and not try to generalize outside of it. After all, the scene can be found naturally and this gaze pattern will at least work for this situation.

On the other hand, if you want to generalize across different scenes, you need a tighter control on all possible low-level features of the scene. This is where artificially constructed scenes work best, because you can manipulate the features and arrange them as you see fit.

In your efforts to control the scene, you should be aware of what attracts attention and consequently eye movements. This is especially challenging when you want to compare two types of natural scenes. Artificial scenes can be controlled on the detail level, but natural scenes usually cannot. If you want to compare two types of supermarket scenes to investigate which supermarket has the best product layout strategy, with varying products, it is impossible to completely control every low-level feature of the scenes. You just have to accept that colour, luminance, contrast, etc. vary, and try to set up the task so the layout strategy will be the larger effect which drives your results. Perhaps, you can add low-level features post-hoc as covariates in the analysis, by extracting them from the scene video, to at least account for their effect.

When selecting the precise stimuli, it is useful to consider what it is that generally draws our attention, so the effect of primary interest is not blocked or completely dominated by other larger effects. Below are a few examples of factors that are known to influence the allocation of visual attention, more can be found on pages 394–398:

- People and faces invariably draw the eyes, so if you want to study what vegetation elements in a park capture attention, you should perhaps not include people or evidence of human activity in the stimulus photos.
- If you use a monitor, the participants are likely to look more at the centre than towards the edges. They are also more likely to make more horizontal than vertical saccades, and very few oblique ones.
- Motion is likely to bring about reflexive eye movements towards it, irrespective of what is moving. Consider this if you want to conclude, for example, that bicycles capture drivers' attention more than pedestrians do; this may simply be because bicycles move faster, and nothing more.
- If you are looking at small differences in fixation duration, it matters whether you put stimuli in the middle or close to the edges of the monitor, because precision of samples will be lower at the extremities of the screen. The imprecision may force a premature end of the fixation by the fixation detection algorithm, and consequently cause your effect.
- Keep the brightness of your stimuli at approximately the same level, and also similar to the brightness of the calibration screen, or you may reduce data quality, as the calibration and measurement are performed on pupils with different sizes.

Stimulus images are often divided into AOIs, the 'areas of interest', which are sometimes also called 'regions of interest'. How to make this division is discussed in depth in Chapter 6. In short, the researcher chooses AOIs while inspecting potential stimulus pictures with the precise hypothesis and measures of the study in mind. Selecting AOIs while reviewing your already recorded data is methodologically dubious, because you may intentionally or subconsciously select your AOIs so that your hypothesis is validated (or invalidated). If you want to analyse what regions in your picture or film attracted participant gazes, but have the regions defined by the recorded data, you should use heat/attention map analysis (Chapter 7) rather than AOI analysis (Chapter 6).

As a very simple example of AOIs, you could show several pictures each with a matrix of objects in them, as in Figure 3.3(a), and determine whether visually similar items have more eye movements between them, than visually dissimilar objects. Simply construct an AOI around each object, and compare how many movements across categories versus within categories occur. Most eye-tracking analysis softwares allow for manual definition of AOIs as rectangles, ellipses, or polygons. AOIs are typically given names like 'SHEARS' and 'HAMMERS' to help keep track of the groups in the experimental conditions. This is also a perfect example of a case where it is easy to define the AOIs before the data recording, which should always be the preferred way.

When using film or animations as stimuli, as in Figure 3.3(b), where there are many moving objects, static AOIs are often of little use. Dynamic AOIs instead follow the form, size, and position of the objects as they move, which makes the data analysis easier. To the authors' knowledge, the first commercial implementation of dynamic areas of interest was

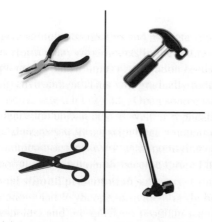 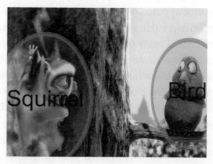

(a) Large square areas of interests with clear margins to compensate for minor offsets in data samples.

(b) Elliptical, but cropped, area of interest around the squirrel and the bird in the stimulus picture. Reproduced here with permission from the Blender foundation www.bigbuckbunny.org.

Fig. 3.3 Examples of AOIs.

made available in 2008, decades after the static AOIs began to be used. Dynamic AOIs come with their own set of methodological issues, however (p. 209).

3.2.5 Trials and their durations

A trial is a small, and most often, self-repeating building block of an experiment. In a minimal within-subjects design there may be as few as two trials in an experiment, for instance one trial in which participants look at a picture while listening to music, and another trial where they look at the picture in silence. The research question could be how music influences viewing behaviour. Or there may be several hundreds of trials in an experiment, for instance pictures of two men and two women, with varying facial expressions, hair colour, types of clothes, eye contact, etc., to see if those properties influence participants' eye movements.

In an experimental design, trials are commonly separated in time by a central fixation cross. For instance, you may have an experiment in which you first show a fixation cross in the middle of the screen, then remove the cross so as to have a blank screen while at the same time playing the word 'future' auditorily. The crucial period of time for eye-movement recording here is the blank screen, but it could equally be an endogenous spatial cue to the left or right or some other manipulation. The idea behind this experiment would be to see if time-related words such as 'future' or 'past' make participants look in specific directions. The trial sequence (fixation cross, stimulus presentation, and so on) will then iterate until the specified number of trials corresponding to that condition of the experiment has been fulfilled. Experimental trials are often more complex than this however, and may contain features like varying *stimulus onset asynchrony*, where the flow of stimulus presentation during the trial is varied according to specified time intervals. Taking the *flash-preview moving-window paradigm* outlined above as an example, the brief length of time for which the first scene picture is displayed, before the following gaze-contingent display, can be varied corresponding to different durations. Võ and Henderson (2010) have implemented such a manipulation to shed light on just how much of a glimpse is necessary to subsequently guide the eyes in scene viewing, and they found that 50–75 ms is sufficient.

Thus, the 'layout' of a trial is usually decided as part of the design of the experiment. In some cases, however, trials must be reconstructed afterwards. For instance, in a study of natural speech production, a trial may start anytime a participant utters a certain word. Post-recording trials are more difficult to create, and few eye-tracking analysis software packages have good support for them.

Typically, an eye-tracking study involves many participants, and many trials in which different stimuli are presented. It is not uncommon, to have say 40 participants looking at 25 pictures with a duration of 5 seconds each. Always design your experiment to extract the maximum amount of data. Add as many trials as you can without making it tedious for the participants.

Moreover, we do not want all participants to look at all stimuli in the same order, because then they may look differently at early stimuli compared to late ones; this could be due to a *learning effect* or an *order effect*. The former case refers to when participants have become better at the task towards the end of the experiment, the latter case is when there is something about the order of presentation which biases responses and eye-movement behaviour. To avoid such confounds trial presentation is randomized for all 40 of your participants, no two participants viewing the stimuli in the same order. Then, any effects of learning or order will be evenly spread out across all stimulus images, and will not interfere with the actual effect that we want to study. Presentation order can usually be randomized by the experimental software. This is easy and usually enough to eliminate learning/order effects. Otherwise, a separate distinct stimulus order is prepared for each participant beforehand. This takes more time, but is virtually foolproof as it can be counter-balanced and randomized with a higher degree of control.

An old problem with scrambling stimulus presentation order, was that in your data files the first 5 seconds of each participant were recorded from different trials. It is not possible to place the first 5 seconds of data next to one another, participant by participant, as you would typically want to do when you calculate the statistical results comparing 20 of your participants to the other 20. Until very recently, eye-tracking researchers had to unscramble the data files manually, or write their own piece of software to do it for them. This was a very time-consuming and rather error-prone way to work with the data. Today, most eye movement recording software communicates with the stimulus presentation program so as to record a reference to the presented stimulus (such as the picture file name) into the correct position in the eye movement data file. Thus, the information for how to *de*randomize is in the data file, and can be used by the analysis software. Some eye-tracking analysis programs today allow users to derandomize data files fairly automatically, immediately connecting the right portion of eye-tracking data to the correct stimulus image, which simplifies the analysis process a great deal.

When showing sequences of still images that are all presented at a constant duration, participants may learn how much time they have for inspection and adopt search strategies that are optimized for the constant presentation duration (represented by thoughts such as, for instance "I can look up here for a while, because I still have time to look at the bottom later"). If such strategies undermine the study, *randomized variable trial durations* can be used to reduce predictability and counteract the development of visual strategies (see also Tatler, Baddeley, & Gilchrist, 2005).

Precise synchronization between stimulus onset and start of data recording for a trial is very important. Many factors may disturb synchronization and cause latencies that make your data difficult to work with or your results incorrect (p. 43). One potential problem is the loading time of stimulus pictures in your stimulus presentation program. If for some reason you show large uncompressed images (e.g. large bitmaps) as stimuli, and send the start of a recording signal just before presenting the picture, the load time of the picture until it is

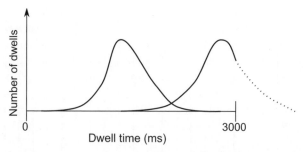

Fig. 3.4 Dotted line of one distribution of dwell times is outside of the fixed trial duration.

shown may be in the order of hundreds of milliseconds, which means that your participants do the first saccades and fixations not on the picture (which you will think when looking at data), but on the screen you showed before the picture was loaded. The solution to the loading problem is to pre-load images into memory before they are shown. Playing videos for stimuli requires an even more careful testing of synchronization. Additionally, synchronizing the eye-tracker start signal with the screen refresh is important to avoid latencies due to screen updates, especially when using newer but slower flat-screen monitors, which typically operate at 60 Hz. Ideally, these issues should be taken care of by your particular stimulus presentation package, and these low-level timing issues are beyond the scope of this book.

Fixed trial durations in combination with a small number of AOIs may complicate variance-based statistical analysis for a number of measures, for instance dwell time (p. 386), reading depth (p. 390), and proportion over time analysis (p. 197). Figure 3.4 shows the distribution of dwell time on a single AOI presented in two different conditions measured in trials of 3000 ms length. In one of the two conditions, the distribution nicely centres around 1500 ms, and both tails are within bounds. In the second condition, however, the top of the distribution is close to the 3000 ms limit that part of what would have been its right tail has been cut off by the time limit of the trial.

3.2.6   How to deal with participant variation

In the planning stage, participants appear as abstract entities with very little or no individual variation or personal traits. Later, during recording, real people come to the laboratory and fill the abstract entities with what they are and do. It is important to see participants as both. In this section, 'participants' refers only to the abstract entities that provide us with data points, while on pages 115–116 we discuss participants as people.

A large proportion of the eye-tracking measures that have been examined have proven to be *idiosyncratic*, which means that every participant has his or her own basic setting for the value. Fixation duration, one of the most central eye-tracking measures, is idiosyncratic. In Figure 3.5, participants 2, 9, and 21 have long individual fixation durations, while participants 6 and 12 have short individual fixation durations. This is like their baseline. The figure shows that the variation between participants is much larger than it is within the participants. The difference between trials completely drowns in these idiosyncratic durations, and it means that we are actually trying to find a small effect within a much larger effect.

How can we deal with participant variability and idiosyncrasy? Participants can be divided into groups and assigned tasks/stimuli in a variety of different ways. The two most common, used here only for exemplification, are the *within-* and the *between-subjects designs*. Table 3.1 shows these two varieties in our example with the four sound conditions. In a between-subjects design, the participants only read a text under one sound condition, either

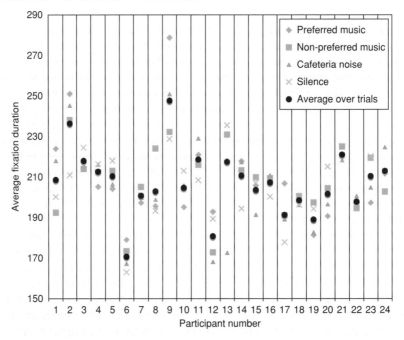

Fig. 3.5 Idiosyncracy: every participant has his or her own individual average fixation duration and exhibits it across different recordings. Individual participant variation is large, and the effect of the experimental conditions is small.

Table 3.1 Between- and within-subjects design in a task with four conditions (different sounds being
played, or silence). S1 to S16 are the different participants. In the between-subjects design everyone reads
one text to one type of sound, and then leaves the lab. In the within-subjects design, every participant has
to read in all four sound conditions.

Condition	Between				Within			
Preferred music	S1	S5	S9	S13	S1	S2	S3	S4
Non-preferred music	S2	S6	S10	S14	S1	S2	S3	S4
Cafeteria noise	S3	S7	S11	S15	S1	S2	S3	S4
Silence	S4	S8	S12	S16	S1	S2	S3	S4

listening to music liked, music disliked, noise, or silence. So when we compare preferred
music to unpreferred, we also compare two different participants to one another. In a within-
subjects design, on the other hand, each participant reads texts in all four conditions, which
means that a comparison between sound conditions is made within the same participant. It
does require every participant to read four texts, which takes longer and may introduce learning effects (the last text is read differently than the first), which forces us to randomize. The
within-subjects design also means that we must find four comparable texts so the effects we
find are not driven by text differences rather than the investigated sound conditions.

In most psychological research, the effects sought after are usually so small that we need
many trials to find them, making a within-subjects design the only practically available solution. Furthermore, this approach also lets us see to what extent the effect is representative in a
larger population of participants. In a within-subjects design, since we try to find the effect for
each individual, we can also see how many of the participants display the sought-after effect.
If all participants display it, then the effect is highly generalizable to a larger population.

However, this does not mean that participant idiosyncracy is not a problem for your data. Unexplained variance still shows up as noise in your models and your ultimate goal is often to provide as full an explanation as possible of what is going on. This also means explaining or at least reducing the impact of idiosyncratic factors so you can more clearly see the effect of your manipulation and accurately estimate its size (data analysis programs like SPSS give you the option to output the *effect size* of a significant result you obtain). Statistical approaches such as multilevel modelling are good for adding random factors (participants and items) and modelling them in order to explain their effect and contribution to the variance, for example by using random intercepts and slopes for every participant or item in the regression. Nevertheless, as a rule of thumb, it is a good idea to reduce the heterogeneity of your participants if you want to establish that your manipulations have a statistically significant effect on their performance. Both the task and the reception of the participants into the laboratory can be used for this.

So are there any benefits to using a between-subjects design? Yes, but they depend on the experiment in hand. Any within-subjects design has some problem of potentially allowing the participants to guess the manipulation. Given enough trials, the participant notices the pattern, e.g. the presentation of common words versus unusual words, and starts guessing the nature of the experiment. Once he has figured out the aim of the experiment, the participant is very likely to behave as expected to please the experimenter. This can be solved by introducing filler trials to throw the participant off his hypotheses, but for very sensitive experiments it will be best to use a between-subjects design.

Furthermore, consider an experiment where we test the impact of two different instructions on problem solving. We give participants a problem to solve and provide them with one type of information. We cannot then present them with the same problem again and supply them with another type of information, as they carry the experience from the first instance with them. In other words, we only have one try per participant, and we have to use a between-subjects design. Given enough participants, we will be able to tell whether one type of information had a larger impact than the other type.

Naturally, if we use participants that are part of a fixed category, for instance dyslexics, then we are forced to use a between-subjects design as we can never 'switch-off' the dyxlexia for a participant and use him as his own baseline. Pre-occuring variables like this, which exist in your participants and you cannot directly manipulate, are known as *quasi* independent variables.

3.2.7 Participant sample size

Only when you know the experimental design can you estimate the number of participants you need for your study, but even then it requires an estimation of the variance in the data you have not yet collected.

It is often the case that the journal in which you plan to publish requires that each condition has a sufficient number of participants, for instance 10 contributing to each cell mean, or maybe more. If you have a 2-by-2 design, as in Figure 3.2—two independent variables, each with two levels—-you have four basic cells. In this figure the design structure is entirely within-subjects, but could equally be between-subjects, with different people listening to preferred or non-preferred music.[13] If this is the case, as different individuals relate to different participant groups, we would need more participants in total to achieve the minimum requirement of a sample size of 10 for each cell mean. The reason for a minimum sample

---

[13] In this particular case, we would actually have a *mixed design* here, music type would be manipulated between participants, while volume level would be manipulated within subjects.

size per cell is that we want to make sure that we have used enough data so that we do not prematurely dismiss our results as null. More participants and trials prevents us from making this mistake, giving us better *statistical power*. Failure to find a significant effect due to too low power, even though an effect is present, is what statisticians call a Type II error—a false negative.

It is also worth bearing in mind that you might lose participants along the way. It is common practice to exclude participants from the analysis of eye-tracking data due to poor data quality of the recording, or perhaps they simply did not do the task properly because they struggled to fully understand the task instructions, in which case they should also be removed. Insufficient data due to sample attrition is an issue which we will also address when we come to data recording in the next chapter.

Conversely, there is such a thing as too much data, as well as too little. Consider an experiment where we let participants read two types of text, one technical and one more casual, and measure the average fixation duration. With 20 participants in each of the two cells, we find significant differences at the $p < 0.05$ level. If we instead record 500 participant in each cell, we will very likely find that the signal-to-noise ratio has been amplified so the test is now significant at a $p < 0.001$ level. In other words, the probability that our observed differences in fixation durations between the technical texts and casual texts are due to chance is 1 in 1000. More data has made our result stronger, but it was not necessary to record data from so many participants.

Caution is needed with regard to large sample sizes, therefore, as it is potentially possible to find positive effects in almost any experimental manipulation you do. With enough data, any effect, however trivial, will cut through the random noise. Now, consider an alternative experiment where we again use 20 participants per cell, but do not find the expected effect of our manipulation. If we keep recording until we have 500 participants per cell, and we then observe a significant effect at the $p < 0.05$ level, we now run the risk of a an error similar to, but not quite, a Type I error—a false positive. Given enough data, small effects will be amplified until they qualify as significant. For example, during our manipulation, we happened to pick two texts which had slight and barely visible differences in the font type. With enough data, we found significant effects, not in our intended manipulation of text genre, but rather in the type of font used. We risk falsely assuming an effect of text genre when in fact there is none (but an effect of font type).

The optimal number of participants to use varies, but there are various approaches to solve this. One way would be to follow the canonical research in your particular research field and journals, and just use the same number of participants and items. If you believe your effect size will deviate from previous research, then take earlier studies and calculate their statistical power (what is called the *retrospective power*). You can then use this power value together with the expected magnitude of your effect to generate the required number of participants needed for each cell. There is software for doing power calculations, but they still require an educated guess of the effect of magnitude and its variance. When the result of our hypothesis test is null, high statistical power allows us to conclude with greater confidence that this result is genuine, and that it is very unlikely that an effect of the hypothesized magnitude or larger was present.

Often, we accept a risk of a type II error (known as β) which is larger than the risk of a type I error (α), because the former can require large amounts of data to negate, which is not feasible in a standard eye-tracking experiment. The risk we take entails ending up with results that falsely show no effect of our manipulation. This is deemed less problematic than type I errors. This is not to say, however, that type I errors, i.e. spurious and invalid effects, do not show up in eye-tracking data. This probably happens all the time, but they only really pose a threat to the research tradition if they are not understood by the researcher, not questioned by the reviewer, or not replicated by the research community. The error can be one or a combination of many aspects of the experiment: poor precision and accuracy of the eye-tracking hardware, bad operationalizations of the mental construct and selection of dependent and independent variables, questionable synchronization between stimulus presentation and eye movement recordings. It is up to the researcher to decide whether it is more important to be confident that the effect is present, or if it is more important to be confident that the effect is not there. Statistical power is seldom reported as we are typically interested in positive effects and there is a publication bias for these effects. We should keep in mind though, that (failed) replications can be very interesting and then power becomes an important issue to correctly falsify previous findings.

It is beyond the scope of this book to discuss detailed power calculations, but two simple examples can be given to put power and sample size into perspective. These examples were calculated using the formulae and tables in Howell (2007) for simple one-way ANOVAs.

- If we want an α of 0.05 (we correctly accept 95% of all true effects) and a power of 0.80 (we correctly reject 80% of all false effects), then we need a sample size of 72 participants per cell (i.e. per experimental condition).
- Given an α of 0.05 and a power of 0.95, then we need a sample size of 119 per cell.

However, there is more to the discussion than just getting your results significant. For example, earlier studies may have just very few participants (Noton & Stark, 1971a: two and four participants; Gullberg & Holmqvist, 1999: five participant pairs), and even though the results may be significant, there is also the problem of generalizability. With four participants, it is likely that these people will deviate from the average person we want to generalize to. Typically, the hypothesis tests tell us how likely it is that a sample is drawn from a particular population or not. This assumes that the participants are randomly sampled from the population at large. In practice, this is never the case. It is a fact that the vast majority of academic research is carried out on university students; this is also true of eye tracking. Unfortunately, we cannot see that anybody will go through the challenge of doing completely randomized sampling of the population during the recruitment of participants to an experiment. We can only hope to be humble when drawing conclusions and making generalizations. However, a study with only four participants may still be interesting. Not because we can generalize from it (which we cannot), but because it may generate interesting hypotheses that we may proceed later to test with a full experiment. The point is to not present a case study as a full generalizable experiment, or vice versa.

3.3 Planning for statistical success

Once the data of your experiment have been collected, you will have one or several files with the raw data samples. At this point in the future, you should already have a clear idea what to do with this data. Typically, the subsequent analysis consists of four main steps, each of which is described in the following subsections.

3.3.1 Data exploration

Data exploration is not often discussed in textbooks, but is nevertheless an important part of the analysis. The main purpose of data exploration is to get to know the data in order to be able to account for choices that are made in later stages of the analysis. A secondary purpose, which is nevertheless also vital, is to check for possible errors in the data. It happens all too easily that data were coded erroneously or incorrectly measured when the experiment was carried out. Feeding the data into a data analysis without checking for errors may have devastating effects, either producing significant effects that do not exist, or hiding them.

The first goal of data exploration is to *check whether data quality is sufficient*. This can mostly be done in manufacturer software by inspecting the recorded data of individual participants. Position- and velocity-over-time diagrams, scanpath plots, and heat map visualizations are excellent tools to quickly inspect and judge the quality of data. For participants and trials who pass through this initial test, use event detection, AOI analysis, or the other methods in Chapters 5–9 to calculate values to those eye-movement measures that you have selected as so-called variables in your experiment.

Another main goal is to *look at the distribution of these variables*. A regular requirement for statistical tests is that the data are normally distributed (i.e. symmetrically distributed around the mean with values close to the mean being more frequent than values further away from the mean, compare the left part of Figure 3.6). As will become apparent in Part III of this book, many eye-tracking measures are not normally distributed. Eye-tracking measures, including fixation duration and most saccade measures, tend to have skewed distributions so that one tail of a histogram is thicker than the other tail, examplified in the right part of Figure 3.6. Skewed variables may become normally distributed after transformation, for instance, by computing the logarithm of the values, which may be the single most used transformation available. This transformation makes a positively skewed (typically right-skewed) distribution normal-looking by reducing higher values more than lower values. A distribution commonly log-transformed is human reaction time values, where there is a physical limit to how fast a human can respond to a stimulus, but no limit to how slow they can be. Therefore, the distribution typically has a fat positive tail consisting of the trials where the participant was fatigued, inattentive, or disrupted. A less common, but theoretically more powerful approach, is to analyse skewed distributions directly using methods developed for gamma distributions (if the untransformed values resemble this distribution). If the dependent variable is a proportion, especially outside the 0.3–0.7 range, then a log odds (logit) transformation is common. Navigating between transformations and methods for particular distributions becomes important during the analysis stage, especially so if you have limited data and cannot afford to aggregate it to produce a Gaussian distribution.

A third goal of exploratory data analysis is to *identify outliers*, that is, values that fall outside the normal range of measurements. These values need to be handled with care, as they may exert a disproportionately large influence on the results of the final analysis. Outliers may be the consequence of errors in the data recording or the event detection, or they may be actual rare measurements. In case they are errors, they need to be corrected or excluded. In case they are rare measurements, you may decide to leave them in or to exclude them. There are no strict guidelines about what to do with outliers. In some cases, it may be possible to predefine outliers. For instance based on previous experience and other research, one excludes all values that fall outside the range that is normally to be expected. In other cases this might not be possible and you need to decide which values are to be left out and which ones may stay in. This decision should ideally be made before the analysis is done. One strategy is to examine standardized values, and exclude values that are more than 3.29 standard deviations above or below the mean (Tabachnick & Fidell, 2000). Such rare values are not outliers by definition, however, since a few such extreme values are to be expected if the datafile is sufficiently large. Outliers may, finally, disappear spontaneously as a consequence of data transformation.

Plotting is also an indispensable tool in the later stages of data exploration. Particularly useful are box-and-whiskers plots, which give simultaneous information about the distribution as well as potential outliers (compare Figure 3.7). Additional plots that might be helpful are histograms (as in Figure 3.6), scatterplots, stem-and-leaf plots. In this stage of

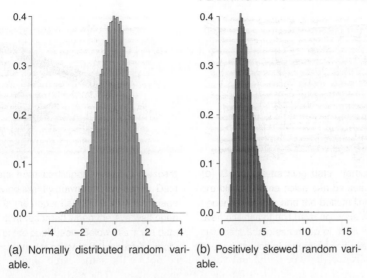

(a) Normally distributed random variable.

(b) Positively skewed random variable.

Fig. 3.6 Histograms, symmetric and skewed, respectively.

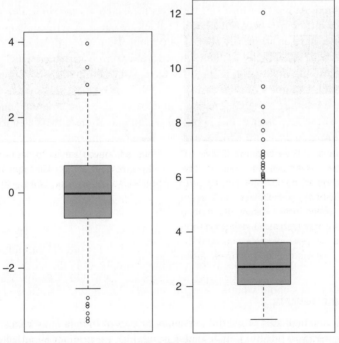

(a) Normally distributed random variable.

(b) Positively skewed random variable.

Fig. 3.7 Boxplots of the variables shown in Figure 3.6.

the analysis, it is wise to make a plot for each participant separately as well as for each item. In that way, it becomes possible to identify potentially deviant participants or items that need to be excluded from further analysis.

3.3.2 Data description

Data description means using summary statistics (mean, mode, variance, etc.) to present in a concise way the results of the study. In order to be able to present these statistics, the available data usually need to be formatted so that they are readable by the software package with which the analysis is carried out. Sometimes the manufacturer software can do part of this job, but more often than not, you may need to do additional work in the form of transposing, restructuring, or aggregating the raw data files. Since errors may steal into the data at this stage as well, it is wise not to do these transformations by hand, but to leave them as much as possible to the computer.

The choice of summary statistics depends on what is known as *the measurement scale* of the variables of interest. An often-made distinction is between four types of measurement scales. At the lowest level are *categorical* or *nominal* variables. These take different values, but the values are unordered. Examples are colours, professions, grammatical categories, and so on. At the next level are *ordinal* variables. The values that these can take may be ordered, but the differences between adjacent values need not be the same. An example is the order in which a participant looks at different AOIs in an image. The participant may, by way of illustration, first look for a long while at one AOI, and then only briefly at the next before going on to a third AOI. These time differences are not visible when only the order of the AOIs is measured. At the next level are variables measured at *interval* scale. Values may be ordered and the differences between adjacent values are equal. A further characteristic is that interval variables have an arbitrarily chosen zero point. Typical examples of interval variables are temperature and IQ. Finally, at the highest level are *ratio* variables which are similar to interval variables with the exception that they have a true zero point, i.e. zero means that the variable is absent. Examples of ratio variables are dimension variables such as height, width, and time. In eye-tracking research, interval and ratio variables are common, and many of the measures to be described later in this book fall within one of these two categories.

The descriptive analysis often focuses on two aspects of the data, usually termed measures of central tendency (the mean, median, or the mode) and measures of dispersion (the range, the variance, or the standard deviation). The former summarize the value that is in a way the most representative of the sample, whereas the latter summarize the amount of variability in the sample. An explanation of these measures can be found in any introductory textbook on statistics.

Which measure to choose from depends largely on the measurement scale of the variables. All measures may be used for interval and ratio variables; for ordinal variables, the median, the mode, and the range may be used; for nominal variables, only the mode may be used.

3.3.3 Data analysis

The choice of statistical analysis should be as much part of the planning of a study as any of the other considerations given in this chapter. Statistical tests cannot be adapted so that they fit any kind of experimental design. Rather, the design of the study needs to be adapted so that the data can be analysed by an existing statistical test. If the choice of the test is not taken into account during the planning stages of the study, there is a risk that the results cannot be analysed properly, and, consequently, that drastic data transformations severely reduce the statistical power or, ultimately, that all the effort that was taken to run the study has been in vain.

The principle behind statistical testing is the following. The participants (and the materials) constitute a sample that is taken from some population of interest, for example, normal-reading adults, dyslectic children, second-language learners, and so on. A population is usually large, making it impossible to measure all of its members. The sample, thus, is a non-perfect image of reality, and consequently there is some degree of uncertainty in the results. Note that this uncertainty is smaller for large samples than for small samples. This uncertainty is also known as 'sampling error'. Sampling error is the variability that is for instance the consequence of measuring different participants, or the same participants on different occasions, or the same participants with different stimulus material (see also page 83). The purpose of inferential statistics is to distinguish sampling error from variability that may be related to another variable of interest. The outcome of the test is the probability that observed variability in the data is sampling error only. This probability is the p-value that is reported as the result of the test. If this probability is very low, then the conclusion is drawn that the variability in the data may be ascribed to variability in one or more variables.

During the past few decades, the possibilities for statistical analysis have greatly increased. There is now a large variety of different types of analysis available, some of which are simple, others more complex. The complex analyses are not necessarily better than the simple ones. A well-defined research question may be simple, and the accompanying analysis may be also. Perhaps the most important factor that determines the choice of the statistical analysis, and with that the design of the study, is that you select a test that you are comfortable with. As stated above, it is easier to adopt the design of an experiment to an existing statistical analysis then the other way around.

Different types of statistical analysis exist, depending on the variables that are included in the study. A rough two-way distinction can be made between parametric and non-parametric tests. Non-parametric tests (such as Wilcoxon, Friedman, sign test) are appropriate when the underlying dependent variable is ordinal or nominal. In eye-tracking research, ordinal dependent variables are not as common as interval or ratio variables. Nominal dependent variables, on the other hand, may occur frequently (for instance different AOIs). The distinction between an ordinal and an interval variable is not always clear. A three-point scale (e.g. cold-warm-hot) is without doubt an ordinal variable, but as more points are added to the scale, it increasingly resembles an interval variable. Nominal dependent variables are notoriously difficult to analyse. Simple statistical tests for the association between two nominal variables exist (e.g. chi-square, Fisher's exact test), but in practice the situation is usually more complicated. An overview of non-parametric tests is given in Siegel and Castellan (1988).

If the dependent variable is measured at an interval or a ratio scale, the statistical test is a parametric test. These tests rely on specific assumptions about the population from which the sample is drawn. One such assumption is that the values in the population are normally distributed, i.e. symmetrically distributed around the mean with values close to the mean being more frequent than values further away from the mean. Whenever there is evidence that the distribution of the underlying population is not normal there is a risk that the outcome of the test is unreliable. An option is to transform, using for instance a log or a square root transformation, the data so that the distribution becomes normal. The decision whether or not to transform the data may be a difficult one. There is a cost–benefit argument. The advantage is that the test results may be more reliable. The drawback is that the test results may become difficult to interpret as well as a loss of power. We lose power because, e.g. a log-transformation reduces large numbers more than small numbers, so we are less able to separate the difference between two large numbers. An alternative solution, which unfortunately is not ideal either, is to convert the measurement scale from interval/ratio to ordinal/nominal, and to do a non-parametric test. This solution is not ideal because this conversion involves loss of information, and with that loss of statistical power. We lose power if we ignore the size of the numbers and only focus on the sign (positive/negative), because we cannot distinguish between -1 and -100.

A different two-way distinction is whether there is one or several dependent variables. The collected history of eye-movement research give you access to much more than a single measure for your study. When you have multiple dependent variables, you may decide to anal-yse them separately to see which of them yields significant differences between experimental groups. In doing so, the character of your study becomes exploratory rather than confirming or rejecting hypotheses. An alternative is to 'reverse the roles' of independent and depen-dent variables, and to see which of the dependent variables best predicts group membership. Suppose, for instance, that two experimental groups were involved in a study, for instance dyslexic readers and normal readers. These two groups all read a text and several measures are obtained from their reading: first fixation durations, number of inword regressions, gaze duration, saccadic amplitudes, etc. These measures can then be used as predictors to evaluate which of them predict whether a reader was a dyslexic or a normal reader. Finally, a num-ber of multivariate statistical methods exist that may be used to see which variables 'group' together (for instance, factor analysis, principal component analysis, cluster analysis, corre-spondence analysis). This approach is exploratory rather than confirmatory. For an overview of different multivariate statistical analyses, we refer to Tabachnick and Fidell (2000).

Further factors that determine the choice of statistical analysis are the number and types of independent variables. In the following, we briefly describe a few types of analyses that are common within eye-tracking research. For each analysis, we provide a short example, and one or two references for further reading.

Analysis of variance or ANOVA is the appropriate analysis if the dependent variable is mea-sured at interval or ratio scale and there are one or more independent nominal variables (often called 'factors'). Analysis of variance may be the most common method for the analysis of experimental data. The method exist for experiments with between-subject factors, within-subject factors, or combinations of the two. As a general recom-mendation, the number of factors should be kept low, preferably not more than three. The main reason is that independent variables may interact with one another, and the number of possible interactions increases rapidly when more independent variables are added to a study. Interactions are notoriously difficult to interpret, especially those that involve more than two factors. Analysis of variance is discussed in many textbooks on statistics. An exceptionally complete handbook is Winer, Brown, and Michels (1991). There are numerous examples of eye-tracking studies in which the results were analy-sed with an analysis of variance. One example is a study by Camblin, Gordon, and Swaab (2007), who looked at the influence of two factors on eye-movement measures. These factors were word association (whether two words are easily associated with each other or not), and discourse congruency (whether a word fits in the context or not). The main question behind this investigation was whether reading processes are more strongly influenced by local context (represented by the word association factor), or by global context (represented by the discourse congruency factor). Combining ERP measurements with eye-tracking measurements, they found discourse congruency to be a stronger factor than word association. In other words, local reading processes may be overruled by global reading processes.

Logistic regression A special case of a nominal variable is a variable that takes only two outcomes (e.g. *yes–no*, *hit–miss*, *dead–alive*). A seemingly attractive solution is to convert the outcomes to proportions or percentages. This might be allowable for the description of the data, but not for the statistical test. One risk with proportions is that some participants contribute with many data points (e.g. 90 misses out of 100 trials), whereas others contribute with only few data points (e.g. 2 out of 5). If the results from these two participants were averaged, then the first proportion would be counted just as heavily as the second, which is not appropriate since the second proportion is much less reliable than the first. The solution for such dichotomous variables is to convert the proportional scale to a logarithmic scale (logit transformation) and to do the analysis on the transformed values instead. This type of analysis is called a logistic regression. An introduction to logistic regression can be found in Tabachnick and Fidell (2000). An example of a logistic regression analysis within eye-tracking research is given in Sporn et al. (2005). In that study, a number of eye-tracking variables were measured in a clinical group of schizophrenic patients and a control group. Subsequently, the results of the eye-tracking measures were used as predictors in a logistic regression analysis, to establish whether the two groups could be differentiated on the basis of the measurements.

Regression Regression is similar to analysis of variance in that there is a dependent variable measured at an interval/ratio scale. In regression, however, the factors (predictors) may be either categorical or continuous. The simplest example of regression contains one continuous dependent variable (e.g. fixation duration) and one continuous predictor (e.g. font size). A relationship between these variables implies that an increase in the predictor is associated with an increase (or a decrease) in the dependent variable. The most parsimonious representation of such a relationship is to suppose that it is linear, i.e. the change in the dependent variable is constant across the whole range of the predictor. If this is true, then the relationship between the variables can be modelled using the equation for a straight line: $Y' = b + aX$. In this equation, b is the level of Y at the lowest level of X, and a is the slope of the line, i.e. the change in Y per unit change in X. Reality may be more complex than that, however. The relationship between two variables need not be linear, and there may be more than one variable that influences the dependent variable. We recommend Cohen, Cohen, West, and Aiken (2002) as a textbook on regression.

Multilevel modelling A relatively recent development in statistical analysis is offered by so-called multilevel analysis (also known as hierarchical models, mixed models). In this type of analysis, random factors are included and parameters of the model (estimates of the contributions of the different factors) are estimated by a process of maximum likelihood estimation or variants of it. These models may be applied when the dependent variable is an interval/ratio variable, but also when the dependent variable is a nominal variable. Multilevel models have the great advantage that they are flexible. The data set does not need to be perfectly balanced, as it should be for analysis of variance. For an introduction to multilevel modelling, we refer to J. Singer and Willett (2003). An example of multilevel analysis within eye-tracking research is given by Barr (2008). The technique has been applied successfully to analyse results of studies with the visual world paradigm (p. 68), but its range of applications is far wider than that.

Loglinear analysis Loglinear analysis is a technique for analysing the relationship between nominal variables. If only two variables are involved, their relation can be represented as a two-dimensional contingency table. If there are three, the table becomes three-dimensional, and so on. In loglinear analysis, as in analysis of variance, the model for the expected cell frequencies consists of main effects and interaction effects. In a two-way table, for instance, there are two main effects, and one two-way interaction. In a three-dimensional table, there are three main effects, three two-way interactions, and one three-way interaction, and so on. The goal of the analysis is to find the most parsimonious model that produces expected cell frequencies that are not significantly different from the observed frequencies. An example of the application of loglinear analysis in eye-tracking research is given for transition matrices (p. 193). An introductory chapter on loglinear analysis can be found in Tabachnick and Fidell (2000).

3.3.4 Data modelling

The fourth stage, which is optional to many, is the modelling stage. In some cases, there is no noticeable difference between the analysis stage and the modelling stage. Many researchers settle for just finding individual significant effects and this is perfectly fine. However, once a particular domain has accumulated a number of significant predictors each targeting the same variable, then it becomes fruitful to try to integrate these predictors into a complete model. The aim of statistical modelling is to create an explicit model that can describe and predict your data, and do this as well as possible. This is important for the scientific work, because this output is something we can benchmark against, typically through some form of goodness-of-fit statistic. If we have two different models that try to describe a particular set of data, we can test both and see which model performs more accurately. We can also see whether the inferior model can be incorporated to create an even better unified model, or if it has no unique information value at all to contribute. The end result is a better understanding of what factors are involved in a particular behaviour and/or cognitive process, and how these factors interact to produce the outcome they do. Valuable outcomes from modelling include:

- Produce an explicit model that can be implemented in an application.
- Produce an explicit model that can be compared against other models to evaluate which one is better.
- Identify redundant factors that do not contribute with unique explanatory power.

Model-building is performed, not in a single, correct way, but rather by a variety of approaches. A typical rule of thumb is to achieve a good tradeoff between model complexity and explanatory power. Including many predictors that improve the model only minimally results in a very large and complex model. In that case it would be better to exclude those predictors and settle for a less powerful, but much simpler model. A simple model will be much easier to communicate and for other researchers to adopt.

Other questions, which really are beyond the scope of this book, are whether models should be built in a forward fashion, including predictors as they are identified as significant predictors, or in a backward fashion, excluding factors as they fail to improve the model. Different practices exist in different fields, and it is up to the reader to find her own way of modelling confidently.

3.3.5 Further statistical considerations

A potential problem that may undermine your conclusions is the *multiple comparisons problem* (see also the terms *family-wise error rate* or *experiment-wise error rate*). We briefly explained this before in the context of a fishing expedition, where we test many different measures and settle with whatever is significant. A significant result is a probabilistic statement about the likelihood that a given sample comes from the assumed population, or comes from the same population as another sample. If this probability is sufficiently low, we can reject our null hypothesis in exchange for our more interesting alternative hypothesis. However, this probability is only valid for a single test. If you test a hundred samples using this test, you most likely get a few significant tests even though the data are completely randomly generated with no real effect at all. In order for the hypothesis test to mean anything, the experiment and the analysis should be set up to make a single test for every research question, otherwise you are inflating the risk of a significant result where there is no true effect. There are several ways where a multiple comparisons problem could arise in your experiment:

- You do not have a single clear measure to capture your hypothesized effect, so you use several measures each tested with their own hypothesis test.

- You do not have a clear prediction about where in the trial an effect will appear, so you compute several time bins and test their significance separately.
- You test different layouts of the data, for example using time bins, then using the whole trial, then collapsing trials into larger units (*trial* → *block* → *participant*). There is a risk that you keep transforming and aggregating your data until your data becomes significant, rather than arranging the most appropriate way determined prior to the analysis.

One way to compensate for this problem, if indeed you want to investigate several measures, is to perform a Bonferroni correction (or related procedure, see e.g. S. Holm, 1979) on your significance level to compensate for the multiple comparisons. This means you lower your significance level (α) based on the number of hypothesis tests you perform. The standard Bonferroni correction is simply to calculate $\frac{\alpha}{n}$ where α is the significance level and n is the number of comparisons (hypothesis tests).

If you find effects that are only significant before the multiple-comparisons adjustment, but you still believe in them, then you can at least report them as post-hoc findings. In themselves, they are not as useful as real results, but another researcher may have a good explanation for them and proceed with her own replication of your results, if you do not do this yourself.

3.4 Auxiliary data: planning

Eye tracking is useful, fascinating, and challenging in itself, but all of these positive properties can be increased by adding further data channels. Common auxiliary data types include verbal data, reaction time data, motion tracking, galvanic skin response (GSR), and for a few years now also electroencephalography (EEG) and function magnetic resonance imaging (fMRI) data. These are added for a variety of reasons.

Verbal data, for instance, are used for methodological triangulation as an information source on cognitive processes in working memory in addition to eye tracking as information source on perceptual/attentional processes (e.g. Antes & Kristjanson, 1991; Canham & Hegarty, 2010; Charness, Reingold, Pomplun, & Stampe, 2001; Haider & Frensch, 1999; Jarodzka, Scheiter, Gerjets, & Van Gog, 2010; Lowe, 1999; Reingold, Charness, Pomplun, & Stampe, 2001; Underwood, Chapman, Brocklehurst, Underwood, & Crundall, 2003; Van Gog, Paas, & Van Merriënboer, 2005; Vogt & Magnussen, 2007. Others add verbal data to eye-movement data to study the speech processes in themselves (Tanenhaus et al., 1995; Griffin, 2004; Holsanova, 2008).

All these types of data have their own possibilities, weaknesses, and pitfalls, and none of them provide an infallible turnkey solution any more than eye tracking does. Rather, the trick is to use them in combination so that the weakness of one system is complemented by the strength of the other. This is sometimes called *methodological triangulation* and *cross-validation*.

We will now describe the possibilities of using common auxiliary data in triangulation to cross-validate eye-tracking data. Eye-tracking data, including pupil diameter data can also be used to disambiguate other data, but that is outside the scope of this book.

3.4.1 Methodological triangulation of eye movement and auxiliary data

In spite of the great opportunities eye tracking provides to a researcher, it also has its shortcomings. As we noted on page 71, eye-tracking data only tell us where on the stimulus a cognitive process operated, and possibly for how long, but not by itself *which* cognitive process is involved.

Methodological triangulation refers to the use of more than one methodological approach in investigating a research question in order to enhance confidence in the ensuing findings (Denzin, 1970). If research is founded on the use of a single research method it might suffer from limitations associated with that method or from the specific application of it. Thus, methodological triangulation offers the prospect of enhanced confidence, credibility, and persuasiveness of a research account through verifying the validity of the findings by cross-checking them with another method (Bryman, 1984). Webb, Campbell, Schwartz, and Sechrest (1966) suggested, "Once a proposition has been confirmed by two or more independent measurement processes, the uncertainty of its interpretation is greatly reduced. The most persuasive evidence comes through a triangulation of measurement processes" (p. 3). The consensus among the many reviewers of methodology, supported by empirical studies, is that it is best to rely on a wide range of complementary methods (Ericsson & Lehmann, 1996).

In psychology several methods are in use to gain data on human knowledge (for an overview see Kluwe, 1988): *probing* (i.e. interviewing a participant), *questionnaires, sorting tasks, free recall of knowledge*, as well as several behavioural measures such as *reaction times, electroencephalography, galvanic skin response, functional magnetic resonance imaging*, and *thinking aloud*. These additional data types vary both in how easy they are to record in combination with eye-movement data, the potential they have in disambiguating them, and in how well this potential is investigated.

Verbal data are easy to record and have a wide potential to disambiguate eye-tracking data, because this method allows researchers to gain insight into participants' experienced cognitive processes while inspecting a stimulus or performing a task. It has become the largest and most investigated complimentary data source to eye-tracking data, in particular in the applied fields of eye-tracking research, where participants have free and naturalistic stimuli and tasks.

3.4.2 Questionnaires and Likert scales

Both questionnaires and Likert scales can be seen as a form of elicitation where conscious answers are given by the participant to highly structured questions. The structure can be more or less rigid, where one extreme is open-ended questions (such as "How do you feel?"), and another extreme would be forced-choice questions with few alternatives ("Do you prefer option A or option B?"). The rigidity has both benefits and drawbacks. A great benefit is the ability to automatically have all the answers confined within an easily analysed answer space, for example values ranging between 1 and 7. A drawback of rigid questions is the risk of low validity due to wrong constructs or misinterpreted questions, such as participants not understanding what you are asking about or forced to provide an answer to a dimension they believe is irrelevant to them. Questionnaires may be low-tech, but they are critical to operationalizing difficult constructs. Assuming you want to find an eye-tracking measure that predicts the level of happiness of a participant, you will have no other easy access to such information because there exists no device that can measure the happiness of a participant. Fortunately, such questions are easily arranged in a questionnaire, especially if they are standardized questions used by psychologists. It is then easy to collect data about both the eye movements and the happiness of a number of participants, and then find a correlation with some measure which can then be further elaborated on and verified.

A typical psychological questionnaire often uses a Likert scale for easy analysability. Additionally, there are often many questions asking the same thing but with slightly different wording in order to reduce any effect due to particular phrasing, including some reversed questions that ask the complete opposite (with a correspondingly reversed scoring). An example in line with our above example would be the Oxford Happiness Questionnaire (Hills & Argyle, 2002).

3.4.3 Reaction time measures

Eye-tracking data offer a number of reaction time measures, for instance saccadic latency, entry time, latency of the reflex blink, eye–voice latency, and others listed in Chapter 13. Even the first fixation duration is in effect a form of latency measure. All of these are indicative of processing, such that the reaction takes longer when processing is hampered or more difficult. When latency is referred to in relation to auxiliary data in this chapter, discussions are limited to identifying cognitive processes in such a 'brain sense'. Of course, there are a multitude of complex issues to do with the latencies involved with the synchronization of machines and equipment when recording auxiliary data. Chapter 4 (p. 134) and Chapter 9 (p. 286) tackle the combinations of equipment for data recording more technically. Refer back to Chapter 2 (p. 43) to remind yourself of the latency issues involved specifically with eye-trackers.

The traditional non-eye-tracking reaction time test is a measure from onset of a task until the participant presses one of two or more buttons to mark a decision, typically between two options, for instance "yes" or "no" to the question whether a series of letters constitute a word or not. The latency of the decision is then taken as the dependent variable and used as an approximation of the ease of processing of the particular stimuli. In trials where the processing leading up to the decision is easy the participant is faster, whereas hard trials have longer latencies.

As eye tracking provides the richer spectrum of latency measures, there is often little point in adding manual reaction time tests to eye tracking, other than for pure triangulation or to compare visual and manual modalities. However, time on task-data which measures the time until a participant has finished with a stimulus or subtask is often added to the analysis of eye-movement data. This additional information comes at the cost of variable trial durations, however, which requires us to think about scaling several of the other eye-tracking measures we might think about using.

3.4.4 Galvanic skin response (GSR)

Galvanic skin response (GSR) measures the electrical conductivity of the skin using electrodes which are usually put on one or two fingers of the participant. The variation in GSR signal corresponds to the autonomic nerve response as a parameter of the sweat gland function.

When eye tracking has been supplemented by GSR, the motive has been to investigate *cognitive load* and *emotional reactions*, for instance in usability tasks (Westerman, Sutherland, Robinson, Powell, & Tuck, 2007) and social anxiety research (Wieser, Pauli, Alpers, & Mühlberger, 2009).

The GSR latency is slow, reactions appear 1–2 seconds after stimulus onset. This means that the eyes could already have left the part of the stimulus that caused the GSR effect long before the effect was registered in data. This latency is difficult to take into account, and could be one reason why there are so few combined studies.

Eye tracking offers some measures of its own that are sensitive to cognitive load and emotional variations, for instance pupil dilation (p. 391) and saccadic amplitude (p. 312). Since these eye-tracking measures react to so many cognitive states (so many c:s in the terms of Figure 3.1 on page 72), however, disambiguating them with GSR makes good sense.

3.4.5 Motion tracking

Motion trackers can be magnetic or optic, and are used to measure the movements of all (external) body parts, but not eyes. Magnetic motion trackers are sometimes optional parts of head-mounted eye-trackers. Optical motion tracking is based on infrared cameras and reflections just like eye tracking, and gives the same type of sample data stream, with comparable sampling frequency and precision, albeit 3D, for a selected number of points across the participant's body or on artefacts manipulated by the participant. Even the analysis of general movement data has similarities to fixation and saccade analysis. The obvious benefit of adding motion tracking to your study is that you will be able to measure synchronized movements of the eye, body, and objects.

The combination is not uncommon in applied research. For instance, Wurtz, Müri, and Wiesendanger (2009) investigated the eye–hand latency in violin players, as the interval from the fixation of a note until the corresponding bow reversal, and Wilmut, Wann, and Brown (2006) investigate the role of visual information for hand movements. Wengelin et al. (2009) and B. Andersson et al. (2006) describe set-ups for studying how reading of one's own emerging text coincides with keyboard writing (keylogging), and Alamargot, Chesnet, Dansac, and Ros (2006) have developed a set-up and software solution called Eye and Pen, which combines graphomotor activities with eye movements. There are also many human factors, ergonomic, and robotic applications of this combination.

3.4.6 Electroencephalography (EEG)

There are many similarities between electroencephalography (EEG) and eye tracking: sampling frequencies are in the same range, and both signals can be analysed as process measures. There are different EEG technologies (called high- and low-impedance) that require different post-processing. And with both measurement techniques, it takes some time to gather enough experience to be able to do publishable research.

EEG does not measure deep into the brain, only the surface, and there is high inter-individual variance in the thickness of the skull and scalp. High amplification is needed as the signals are often very weak. Because the noise levels are so high, many trials are needed to filter out a significant effect, and participants may find this tedious. EEG artefacts stem from alternating current but also eye blinks and saccadic and microsaccadic movements. Filters are required to remove them, and high-impedance systems may require heavier filtering.

Sampled EEG data come in waves that correspond to continuous brain activity. It is possible—with some training—to read state of arousal directly from wave plots, which is extensively done in clinical settings (hospitals). When we are excited and alert, the signal is high in frequency (Hz) and low in amplitude (μV). When we are drowsy, the activity is much slower but higher in amplitude. EEG can be analysed in the frequency domain in order to extract information about the global brain activity of the participant.

When EEG is added to eye tracking, the continuous EEG signal is seldom used. Instead analysis focuses on the EEG amplitude, direction (positive/negative), and latency of the signal with a particular scalp distribution *as a response* to external stimulus events or internal cognitive processing. This is called *event-related potentials* or ERP (Luck, 2005).

In one line of research, the purpose has been to study the neurological system itself. The *saccadic eye-movement-related potentials* (SERP) and the *eye-fixation-related potential* (EFRP) are ERP paradigms that investigate the EEG signal next to saccades and fixations. Early studies focused on the neural activity around saccades, and what that could tell us about the human visual system. Becker, Hoehne, Iwase, and Kornhuber (1972) found that around 1–3 seconds before the saccade onset, occipital and parietal posterior areas exhibit a so-called pre-motion negativity, indicative of general readiness. A pre-motor positivity can be measured 100–150 ms before the saccade onset, possibly reflecting motor programming (Jagla, Zikmund, & Kundrát, 1994). Immediately after the saccade offset, there is a strong positive response, called the Lambda response, in the posterior parietal area, and a concurrent negativity in the frontal eye fields. The shape of the Lambda response depends on the general visual background (Morton & Cobb, 1973), and is believed to correlate to the processing of new information in the visual cortex. The negativity in the frontal eye fields is probably a sign of inhibition of further saccades while the processing of information continues in the visual cortex (Jagla et al., 1994). For a recent review of research on *saccadic eye-movement-related potentials*, see Jagla, Jergelová, and Riecanský(2007).

In reading research, ERP data are used to support and strengthen interpretations made from eye-tracking data. Dambacher and Kliegl (2007) found a correlation between N400 components and fixation durations. Takeda, Sugai, and Yagi (2001) found that the EFRP in the 100–200 ms block after fixation onset decreases in a way that would reflect decline of mental concentration (i.e. carelessness) caused by visual fatigue. Using the same P200 EFRP, Simola, Holmqvist, and Lindgren (2009) show a parafoveal preview benefit for distinguishing between words and non-words in the right visual field that does not exist in the left visual field.

3.4.7 Functional magnetic resonance imaging (fMRI)

Functional magnetic resonance imaging (fMRI) measures activity throughout the whole brain, not just surface activity like EEG. The *temporal resolution* differs very much between fMRI and eye tracking. Eye tracking involves measuring how the eyes move with a temporal resolution of down to 0.5–1 ms. In contrast, fMRI involves measuring and aggregating over 1000 ms time spans. This makes it more difficult to co-analyse fMRI and ET data than EEG and ET data, where both systems have the same temporal resolution. The output from an fMRI measurement is an activation visualization of the blood oxygenation level-dependent (BOLD) signal, which in principle is identical to a heat map and the eye movement representations of Chapter 7.

Although fMRI studies very often include looking at pictorial stimuli (and/or hearing audio), the vast majority of studies that combine the two technologies only use eye tracking to control that the participant is awake, has his eyes open and looks in the general direction of the stimulus. If researchers analyse the eye-tracking data, they usually only detect saccades, and only to make sure that the eye is not moving.

As an example, Simola, Stenbacka, and Vanni (2009) measured activity in the visual cortex (V1) as participants *looked at* a central cross on the stimulus monitor and simultaneously *attended to* wedges in five concentric rings at 1.6°–10.2° from the centre. The authors showed that the enhanced activity by attention in retinotopically organized V1 directly corresponds to the locus of covert attention, and that the attended responses spread over a signicantly larger area than the sensory responses. It was important to show that the participant's gaze did not deviate systematically from the central cross, because eye movements would move the mapping of the stimulus onto the visual cortex (V1). Hence eye tracking was used.

A rare exception where saccades were actually used to align the fMRI data is Ford, Goltz, Brown, and Everling (2005). They used an antisaccade task with long intervals between saccades, which is compatible with the slow fMRI data.

3.4.8 Verbal data

This section describes the most commonly used method for knowledge elicitation in combination with eye tracking: verbal data. We use the term *verbalization* for the act of externalizing thoughts as speech and *verbal data* for the totality of data resulting from recordings of verbalization, irrespective of their form (i.e. audio or transcribed). Combined recordings of eye tracking and verbal data are made in several research areas as well as in applied usability projects. There are three major purposes to record eye-tracking data in combination with verbal data:

1. To investigate the minute relation between vision and speech over time (Holsanova, 2008).
2. For purposes of methodological triangulation, for instance to investigate working memory processes directly in addition to perceptual/attentional processes as shown by eye-tracking data (Jarodzka, Scheiter, et al., 2010; Altmann & Kamide, 2007).
3. In specific cases, eye-tracking data are recorded to help participants to elicit verbal data by a method known as "cued retrospective reporting" (J. P. Hansen, 1991; Van Gog, Paas, Van Merriënboer, & Witte, 2005).

Theoretical background: origin and idea of verbalizations as a valid data source

Initially, the easiest and most common way to gather insight into cognitive processes accompanying task performance was to interview people who are skilled performers, that is experts (Ericsson, 2006). It is questionable, however, whether experts are able to describe their thoughts, behaviours, and strategies so that it is understandable to less skilled people (Ericsson, 2006). In particular, since discrepancies have been found between reported and observed behaviour (Watson, 1913). For this reason Watson (1920) and Duncker (1945) introduced a new method of thought analysis: *thinking aloud*. This type of verbalization has been shown not to change the underlying structure of the thoughts or cognitive processes, and thus avoids the problem of reactivity, as long as the verbalizations are carefully elicited and analysed (Ericsson & Simon, 1980, 1993).

The central assumption behind the use of thinking-aloud is that "it is possible to instruct participants to verbalize their thoughts in a manner that does not alter the sequence and content of thoughts mediating the completion of a task and therefore should reflect immediately available information during thinking." (Ericsson, 2006). Those verbalizations provide data on which knowledge is currently activated and how it changes. According to Ericsson and Simon (1993) the information processing model assumes the following: (1) the verbalizable cognitions can be described as states that correspond to the contents of working memory (that is, to the information that is in the focus of attention); (2) the information vocalized is a verbal encoding of the information in the working memory. That is, only this content can be found in the data that was "on the participant's mind", respectively in the participant's attention. It is important to note that if thinking aloud is not completely free, it may interfere with task performance itself. Providing the participant with appropriate instructions is therefore crucial (p. 105).

Another crucial part in the use of verbal reports is coding (M. T. H. Chi, 2006 and page 290). The data should be coded in the context of the task. Hence, a cognitive task analysis needs to be done beforehand, so as to know the functional problem states required to be able to categorize single utterances.

Thinking aloud techniques have been successfully used in a variety of domains, like designing surveys (Sudman, Bradbrun, & Schwarz, 1996), learning second-language (A. J. F. Green, 1998), text comprehension (Ericsson, 1988; Pressley & Afflerbach, 1995), decision-making studies (Reisen, Hoffrage, & Mast, 2008), studies of text translators (O'Brien, 2006), developing computer software (R. D. Henderson, Smith, Podd, & Varela-Alvarez, 1995; Hughes & Parkes, 2003), or to investigate the relation between vision and speech (Holsanova, 2008).

This method can provide information on, for instance, the forward-strategy-use in experts (M. U. Smith & Good, 1984), or even in perceptual processes; for example it has been found that experts note more relevant features of pictures in contrast to novices (Wineburg, 1991).

It has to be noted that the method of gathering verbal data from participants is known under several other names, such as a *retrospective think-aloud* in the academic usability world (J. P. Hansen, 1991; Hyrskykari et al., 2008) and as a *post-experience eye-tracked protocol* (PEEP) in the commercial usability world (Petrie & Harrison, 2009; Ehmke & Wilson, 2007). We decompose the term verbal reports (Ericsson & Simon, 1993) into:

- Thinking aloud approaches (like concurrent reporting, retrospective reporting, and cued retrospective reporting (Van Gog, Paas, Van Merriënboer, & Witte, 2005).
- Probed reporting, like self-explanations (i.e. the participant explains a stimulus or task to himself; Renkl, 1997)
- Structured interviews.
- Free recall.
- Task-driven verbalizations (i.e. providing verbalizations according to a specific task).

Individual differences in verbal data

Already Claparède (1934) and De Groot (1946/1978) had found large differences among participants in their ability to think aloud. To give you an impression of what variation in participant verbosity can be expected, we present here frequency distributions from real data. Figure 3.8 presents data from a study, where we used cued retrospective thinking aloud (Jarodzka, Scheiter, et al., 2010). Thus, participants are very likely to vary in how much verbalization they produce. Although this situation cannot be completely avoided, it helps to train the thinking aloud and to prompt silent participants when they stop talking (see below).

Forms of verbal data

In this section, we will distinguish between different forms of verbal data according to the point in time when they have been produced: concurrently or retrospectively. Thinking aloud, self-explaining, and task-driven verbalizing are produced *during* stimulus inspection (concurrent verbalizations). Retrospective reports (i.e. reflecting what the person was thinking during stimulus inspection) can also be produced *after* stimulus inspection as well as free recall and structured interviews (retrospective verbalizations). Table 3.2 provides an overview of their properties.

Concurrent verbalizations

Thinking aloud can be produced in two points in time: concurrently or retrospectively. If the participant speaks while performing a task or inspecting a stimulus, this set-up is called *concurrent think-aloud*. Meanwhile his eye movements can be recorded. Most eye-tracker manufacturers have support for synchronized concurrent recordings of speech, but the very act of speaking may make the participant quiver or move enough that the recording of eye movements will be less precise, in particular for tower-mounted eye-trackers (p. 137). Moreover, it is very likely that participants thinking aloud perform slower (Karpf, 1973).

It has long been suspected that concurrent verbalizations alter eye movements during the task. On the one hand, psycholinguistic research in the so-called "visual world paradigm", starting in the mid 1990s (Tanenhaus et al., 1995) has thoroughly investigated the temporal relation of gaze to verbal expressions. Its main thesis, that "speech is timelocked to gaze" has been shown for single-sentence trials, again and again. However, in the task of describing complex pictures with everyday scenes, speech planning is a process in itself, which in turn requires additional time and affects eye-movement behaviour (Holsanova, 2001, 2008).

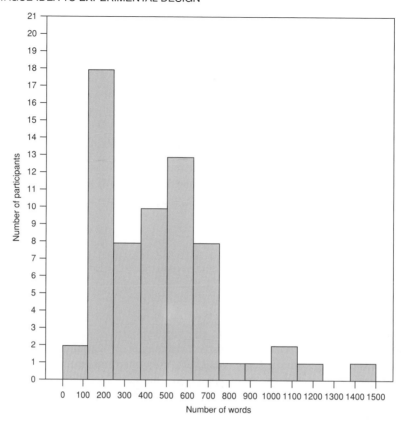

Fig. 3.8 Number of words that participants uttered during cued retrospective thinking aloud. Bin size is 100 words. Verbalization training and prompting was used in the way later described in this section. Data from Jarodzka, Scheiter, et al. (2010).

Ericsson and Simon (1993) claim that, given that thinking aloud is implemented in the manner they propose, thinking aloud should not alter task performance itself, besides slowing it down. Nevertheless, some researchers found exactly this effect: the think-aloud process takes resources from all parts of the cognitive system, and slows down not only eye movements, but the general exploration and learning processes (Nielsen, Clemmensen, & Yssing, 2002; Van Someren, Barnard, & Sandberg, 1994). Eger, Ball, Stevens, and Dodd (2007) found that fewer participants finished their online search task when thinking aloud compared to being undisturbed during the task. Davies (1995) even found that the order in which the participant performs subprocesses changes when think-aloud is required of him in a design task. The greater the cognitive load a task imposes, the more novices have problems with concurrently thinking aloud compared to experts (Van Gog, 2006).

The advantages, on the other hand, are the following. Two data sources may be recorded at one time. These data sources are very likely to be closely linked, since they have been recorded simultaneously from a single participant. Concurrent verbalization also provides the momentous perspective. This would be of particular importance in complex tasks, where cued retrospection could be expected to provide a perspective that deviates from or even ignores the momentous cognitive processes and simply becomes a post-hoc construction. This happened for B. Ryan and Haslegrave (2007) who showed videos (without gaze data) of workers in a storage room, and collected retrospectives.

Concurrent verbalization is used frequently in psycholinguistics research, where the very

Table 3.2 Overview of the different varieties of verbal reports that are combined with eye-movement data, and their properties as methods. Note: Y – yes or possible, N – no or very unlikely.

Method	Dual recording sessions necessary?	Verbal and eye-movement data synchronized?	Pre-structuring of verbal data possible?	Decreased eye-tracking data quality?	Task performance slower?	Effect on task performance?	Risk of memory loss on verbal data?	Biased verbal data?
Concurrent recording								
concurrent thinking aloud	N	Y	N	Y	Y	Y?	N	N
self-explanation	N	Y	N	Y	Y	Y	N	N
task-driven speech by describing stimulus	N	Y	N	Y	Y	Y	N	N
Retrospective recording								
retrospective reporting	Y	N	N	N	N	N	Y	Y
cued retrospective reporting	Y	N	N	N	N	N	Y	N
structured interviews	Y	N	Y	N	N	N	Y	Y
freely recalling the content of a stimulus	Y	N	N	N	N	N	Y	N

purpose is a detailed investigation of the temporal relation of visual attention to the contents of verbal data, and an investigation of the implications for speech production and reception models. Furthermore, this method is frequently used in educational psychology to investigate levels of processing involved in studying certain learning materials as well as mental overload. The suspicion that the primary task may be affected has discouraged many other applied researchers from using concurrent verbalization, however.

Besides thinking aloud, at least two more types of verbal reports exist that may be linked to eye movements: *self-explanations* and *task-driven verbalizations* (in psycholinguistics). Self-explanations are a specific variety of verbalizations which require the participant to explain the stimulus to himself. Whereas thinking aloud should not interfere with the primary task, this type of verbalization is meant to alter the task performance or the inspection of the stimulus. This method is mainly used in educational psychology, where it has been shown to enhance learning (M. T. H. Chi, De Leeuw, Chiu, & LaVancher, 1994; McNamara, 2004; Renkl, 1997). Since this kind of verbal data is recorded concurrently, it possesses similar advantages and drawbacks to the concurrent thinking-aloud method.

Task-driven verbalizations are another specific form of concurrent verbalizations. This method requires that the participant does not freely think aloud, but has a specific task in mind, like describing or recalling a stimulus. Again, this type of verbalization will change the eye-movement performance dramatically as compared to a silent stimulus inspection.

Retrospective verbalizations

The alternative to concurrent recordings is to record the thinking aloud *after* the task is performed. Separating the eye-movement recording during the primary task in time from the verbal recordings could make the study liable to loss of detail from memory as well as fabulation. The question of whether participants remember or fabulate when they explain their own eye movements was elegantly answered by J. P. Hansen (1991) who showed participants bogus recordings of someone else's eye movements. The misled participants soon detected the error, which Hansen took to indicate that they could remember their own eye movements. Participants' intact memory is further supported by Guan, Lee, Cuddihy, and Ramey (2006), who find that participants look at objects in the same order as they later (even without support from eye movement data) say that they do. Moreover, several studies have shown that *retrospective think-aloud* results in more detailed and qualitatively better verbalizations if combined with showing the participant's own eye-movement recordings compared to uncued retrospective verbalizations (J. P. Hansen, 1991; Van Gog, Paas, Van Merriënboer, & Witte, 2005). The verbalizations of the cued verbalizations were quantitatively better in terms of eliciting more information on actions done, more descriptions of how a step was performed (Van Gog, Paas, Van Merriënboer, & Witte, 2005).

This method exists in several varieties that go under names such as *cued retrospective reports* (Eger et al., 2007; J. P. Hansen, 1991; Van Gog, Paas, Van Merriënboer, & Witte, 2005), *eye-movement supported verbal retrospection* (J. P. Hansen, 1991), or *post-experience eye-tracked protocol* (Petrie & Harrison, 2009; Ball, Eger, Stevens, & Dodd, 2006), reflecting the fact that the method has been re-discovered more than once in different fields of research.

An important issue to consider is that a whole body of studies showed that cued retrospective verbalizations stimulate meta-cognitive reflection at the cost of action-related comments. Hyrskykari et al. (2008), in a test of web usability, found that cued retrospection resulted in more comments on the user's cognitive processes, while think-aloud results in more comments on user manipulation (of the software/web pages). Eger et al. (2007) found that more usability problems were identified by participants who performed cued retrospection compared to think-aloud or playback of screen without gaze data. K. L. Taylor and Dionne (2000); Kuusela and Paul (2000) found that more action and outcome statements are produced in concurrent think-aloud then in retrospective mode, which gives information about strategies and reasons for actions. J. P. Hansen (1991), in an analysis of computer interfaces, found that verbal retrospective protocols cued by an eye-movement video of the user's work are superior to retrospective protocols primed by a pure video recording. Hansen found more problem-oriented comments and more comments on manipulation in the task, when recording cued retrospection from participants that see their own eye movements compared to seeing just a video recording. Kuusela and Paul (2000) also argue that retrospective reports often only reveal those actions that led to a solution, and that attempts that led nowhere are not mentioned. Van Gog, Paas, and Van Merriënboer (2005) found that cued retrospectives result in a larger number of metacognitive comments (on knowledge, actions, and strategies of the participant), and that they elicit more information on actions done, more descriptions of how a step was performed (Van Gog, Paas, Van Merriënboer, & Witte, 2005).

The drawbacks of the retrospective method are that recordings take at least twice as long as with concurrent reporting and that the two data sources may not be as perfectly synchronized as in concurrent reporting. Moreover, if the task is too long, participants may easily forget what they have been thinking even when cued with their own eye movements. As a rule of thumb reported by researchers using this technique, recordings should not exceed ten minutes (Van Meeuwen, 2008). On the other hand, the main task performance is not disturbed by a secondary task (thinking aloud), which in turn may result in a more naturalistic task performance or stimulus inspection.

Another version of verbal data is *free recall* (e.g. Jahnke, 1965). In this, a participant simply recalls the stimulus in a free order and without cues. Free recall is used with eye tracking as an experimental condition in mental imagery studies (Johansson et al., 2006).

Another possibility of recording verbalizations is that the researcher prepares questions that she uses in *a structured interview based on gaze replays* with the participant (e.g. Pernice & Nielsen, 2009; Ehmke & Wilson, 2007). Questions should be designed as part of the experimental design and the interview should have the same structure for participants. Sometimes, however, the participant and the researcher look through the scanpath or gaze cursor playback together, simply discussing whatever strikes them as interesting, with or without prepared topics.

In usability, the joint discussion or interview is often done after the researcher previews the participant's data, before letting the participant see it, as a means of coding the scanpaths so the right questions can be asked in terms of the cognitive processes underlying the data (Pernice & Nielsen, 2009; Ehmke & Wilson, 2007). Before using this method, note that you may easily run the risk of including three severe drawbacks to your data. First, the coding of the scanpath plot is subjective. No algorithms exist as yet that would detect such patterns in real time. This means that different measurements of the same scanpath would not lead to the same questions. Thus, this measure is not *reliable*. Second, the time the participant has to wait until he can be questioned about his proceeding may easily be too long to deliver a trustworthy recall of the process. Since working memory is very limited in time, a long pause between action and recall (without memorizing) leads to forgetting the content. Since, participants are not asked to memorize their thoughts, they will not be transferred to long-term memory. This means that the measured verbalizations are not about the intended content, instead they are very likely to be made up. Under such circumstances this measure would be not *valid*. Third, if the coding of the scanpath is conducted by only one rater under time pressure depending on which experimenter is conducting the study on a certain day, the results may differ. Therefore, instructions for the coding have to be very strict and avoid subjectivity, otherwise, the measure is not *objective*. Hence, this method violates all three quality factors that a measurement must have (e.g. Lienert & Raatz, 1998).

Importance of instruction: how to elicit verbalizations from participants

Technical issues on how to record verbal data have been described in Chapter 4. Here we focus on the main challenge in providing valid verbal data, namely on how to elicit valid verbalizations from participants by the appropriate instruction. This issue is most crucial for two forms of verbalization: thinking aloud and self-explanations.

When recording verbal data and eye movements to retrieve current or remembered cognitive processes from the participant, the precise instruction to verbalize is of great importance. The instruction is done in three steps: *instruction*, *training*, and *reminding*. The three steps differ slightly depending on whether you record thinking aloud or self-explanations.

What both types of recordings have in common is that very sensitive data is recorded, namely speech without the ability to modify anything. Many people feel uncomfortable if their own voice is recorded. Even more important, telling ones own thoughts is quite intimate and requires a degree of meta-cognitive awareness and self-confidence. Thus, it is important that the participant feels secure and comfortable during recording. The training before a first recording helps to get them familiar with the situation. Moreover, it helps when as few people as possible are in the recording room, so the participant does not feel monitored.

It is important to emphasize in the instructions to think aloud to express thoughts freely and not with any specific task in mind (like evaluating the stimulus). Only such instructions minimize the effects on task performance. Note that the instructions to think aloud are general instructions, thus they are suitable for both concurrent and retrospective reporting (e.g. Ericsson & Simon, 1993).

Instruction

The instruction to *think aloud* is very important, since it tells the participant what to do. Thereby, the emphasis should be on expressing the content of working memory with as little filtering as possible. That is, effort in formulating grammatically correct sentences or meaningful content should be forgone. Only such instructions can assure that the participant is not too disturbed in his primary task performance. The following instruction has been proven to elicit the desired behaviour (Van Gog, Paas, Van Merriënboer, & Witte, 2005, based on Ericsson & Simon, 1993):

> Thinking aloud means that you should really think aloud, that is, verbalize everything that comes to mind, and not mind my presence in doing so, even when curse words come to mind for example, these should also be verbalized. Act as if you were alone, with no one listening, and just keep talking.

The instruction to *self-explain* could be as follows (adapted from Van Gog, Paas, Van Merriënboer, & Witte, 2005).

> Research has shown that learning is more effective when you self-explain the to-be-learnt content to yourself. Verbalize your self-explanations always out loud as you would talk to yourself and do not mind my presence in doing so. It is not important that the self-explanation is well formulated, even when curse words come to mind for example, these should also be verbalized. Act as if you were alone, with no one listening, and just keep talking.

Training

The training, i.e. getting acquainted with *thinking aloud* gives the participant an impression of what is meant by thinking aloud and enables him to get used to the recording situation. There are at least two common training tasks that are suitable to train thinking aloud (Ericsson & Simon, 1993):

> Please think back to the home you were living in when you were a child, and count the number of windows it had while thinking aloud, verbalising everything that comes to mind.

> Please, multiply the numbers 23 by 16 and tell me, what you are thinking during your calculation.

For both tasks, the participant should count out loud stepwise (instead of giving the result immediately) and think out loud all the while. If a participant does not manage to think aloud, the other task should be tried.

The training is a central part of *self-explanation*. Research has shown that only a successful self-explainer profits from this verbalization method. A direct intervention to foster self-explanation is to train the verbalization itself (for indirect methods see e.g. Catrambone, 1998; Renkl & Atkinson, 2003; Renkl, Stark, Gruber, & Mandl, 1998). Although, several extensive training types exist (e.g. McNamara, O'Reilly, Rowe, Boonthum, & Levinstein, 2007), we present here only a very simple version of self-explanation training (Renkl et al., 1998):

- Before the actual recording the experimenter models a self-explanation behaviour on a task that is comparable to the experimental task. The experimenter has to give hints on how to self-explain the given problem and to elicit several aspects of self-explanation (e.g. elaborating the problem given, principle-based explanations, goal-operator combinations).

- On the basis of this warm-up, hints to self-explain the rationale of the presented solution steps have to be given. The hints should focus on the subgoal of each step and the operator used to achieve it (i.e. explanation of goal–operator combinations).
- Afterwards, the participant has to self-explain on his own on another comparable task, whereby he is coached by the experimenter. The coaching procedure consists of two elements:
  * If important self-explanations are omitted, this is indicated and the participant is asked to supplement the missing explanations;
  * the experimenter answers the participant's questions concerning the self-explanations.

Prompting

Both when answering questions and when narrating freely, participants will vary in how much speech they produce (p. 102). If the participant stops verbalizing his thoughts, the experimenter has to *remind* him after 3 seconds (Van Gog, Paas, Van Merriënboer, & Witte, 2005); other researchers use even longer time spans of 15 seconds (Renkl et al., 1998) by saying: "Please try to keep talking."

The difference in time until prompting reflects what you want to elicit from the participants. If you are intereseted in working memory content, each silent second is missing data. Hence, you should prompt the participant to talk as soon as possible.

Prompting a participant may interfere with the task, in particular with eye movements, even when done neutrally (Kirk & Ashcraft, 2001), and should therefore be used very carefully in *concurrent verbalization* mode. Ericsson and Simon (1993) recommend the use of non-directive prompts such as "keep talking" if the participants fall silent, but not to intervene in any other way. In practice, many usability practitioners instead use interview-like prompts such as "what do you think it means?", which is likely to disrupt the flow of task processing and change eye movement and other behaviour (Boren & Ramey, 2000).

During *retrospective* thinking aloud, we have two different cases: if the gaze path is shown as a dynamic eye-movement visualization, then time is running on the monitor used for cueing just as much as it was during the original performance of the task. Prompting in such a case may interrupt the retrospection just as much as it interrupts concurrent thinking aloud. If the eye movements are shown as a static visualization, then there is no time running. Prompting in this case can very well be made. In the case where the participant stops verbalizing his thoughts, the experimenter has to *remind* him after three seconds by saying the same as above: "please try to keep talking." (Ericsson & Simon, 1993).

Do I really have to stick to those stiff instructions?

Sometimes studies recording verbal data reveal contradictory results. One important reason for that might be the actual use of an instruction to think aloud. In the usability world it is common to use more directed instructions to elicit verbal data. That is, participants do not simply mention what comes into their minds, but rather they are instructed to "evaluate" a material. That kind of verbalization, however, requires a lot of cognitive resources from the participant and thus is very likely to disturb the primary task and cause change to the content of the verbalizations (compare level-3-verbalizations; Ericsson & Simon, 1993).

A study by Gerjets, Kammerer, and Werner (2011) investigated this issue directly. The authors compared the verbal data of participants who either received an instruction to verbalize freely according to Ericsson and Simon (1993) or an explicit instruction to mention factors that influence their evaluation as often used in web research (e.g. Crystal & Greenberg, 2006;

Rieh, 2002; Savolainen & Kari, 2005; Tombros, Ruthven, & Jose, 2005. Results show that both groups differed significantly from each other in terms of verbal reports, eye-tracking data, and problem solving data. Obviously the natural behaviour was altered.

In the most applied eye-tracking fields, however, some practitioners do not place a high emphasis on the instruction to the participants. For instance, Pernice and Nielsen (2009, pp. 113–114) show examples of participants' awe-struck comments on the gaze cursor ("I can't believe that's my eye"). This may be an effect of poor instructions. The authors then quote a usability analyst who argues in favour of previewing the data to decide questions that participants can be asked, apparently oblivious of the danger of fabrication and biases. It is not uncommon that applied users fail to apply a sufficient methodological standard to their use of the retrospective method, and later mistakenly attribute their failures to the method rather than to their own standards. As with all scientific methods, retrospective verbal protocols also require methodological rigour.

Thus, different instructions to verbalize thoughts lead to differences in verbalizations, eye movements, behaviour, and level of disturbance of the primary task. Since, the very free instruction of Ericsson and Simon is the most examined and elaborated one, its consequences can be estimated. Whereas, if you make up your own instruction, you never know, what comes with it. Thus, we recommend to use the free instruction, in particular, since it does not disturb the primary task.

3.5 Summary

This chapter has introduced the most important parts before you proceed to record actual data. There are good reasons for spending time at the design phase of your experiment:

- Selecting how you will **approach** your research in this experiment determines the work you need to do, whether this is by an exploratory pilot, a fishing trip, a theory-driven experiment, or a paradigm-bound experiment. These approaches all have strengths and weaknesses.
- Mapping out the **logic** behind the experiment saves you the moment of despair when you realize that your study was built on false premises or a fallacious argument just as you were getting ready to write up your results.
- Selecting the correct **measures** is a decision best taken at the design stage. There has to be a clear motivation for a measure, with a theory or at least a plausible explanation linking the eye movement to the cognitive process being studied.
- The **statistics** should be prepared and tested before you record the actual data. In many cases, it is simply easier to design around a particular statistical method rather than having to learn and implement some advanced statistical analysis to cope with non-standard data.
- If required, there is always the option to **triangulate** your construct of interest using other data sources that complement the eye tracking. However, the price of this is increased complexity to your experiment.

The experimental design is perhaps the most important stage of all, and it is difficult to sum up briefly. It is all too easy to jump right in and start recording, thinking you can sort the rest later. With experience, and a couple of poor experiments, however, the lesson is learnt. A week spent properly thinking about the design saves four weeks of frustration during the analysis stage and when writing up the paper.

There are many pitfalls. For example, do the data have a distribution that is easy to work with and compatible with the statistical tests in mind? Is your selected eye-tracking measure actually measuring what you are interested in, or are there better candidates? When in doubt, record some pilot data and take it from there.

4 Data Recording

In the previous two chapters, we described the many aspects of eye-tracking systems (Chapter 2), and the importance of how to design an experiment to use in eye-tracker-based research (Chapter 3). This chapter takes us through the recording of the data.

The chapter is structured as follows:

- We begin with a hands-on summary in Section 4.1 (p. 111) to introduce the chapter.
- Section 4.2 (p. 111) discusses how to build the technical environment in which both the real data, and pilot data, are recorded.
- Section 4.3 (p. 115) covers the details of participant recruitment, and best practices when people arrive in your laboratory to take part in an eye-tracking experiment. It is important that participants feel good about the recording, not only to obtain good data and obey the laws of ethics, but also because you want participants or their friends to come back again and take part in future experiments.
- Section 4.4 (p. 116) deals with the eye camera set-up, and how to take on the challenges that some participants and environments pose to good data quality.
- Section 4.5 (p. 128) explains how to calibrate the eye-tracker on a participant.
- The instructions for the participants are important for acquiring valid data, and the most important points should be reiterated after calibration, and just before the start of recording, as Section 4.6 (p. 134) points out.
- In many cases, speech, galvanic skin response (GSR), electroencephalography (EEG), or other data sources are recorded together with eye-tracking data. As well as creating new possibilities, this also brings challenges, as described in Section 4.7 (p. 134) . This section may be regarded as optional if your sole purpose is to learn about eye tracking only.
- Debriefing (Section 4.8, p. 139) means telling the participant all he wants to know about the study. Commonly an information sheet is provided after the recording, and any additional questions are answered.
- Section 4.9 (p. 140) describes what to do once data are recorded; sorting and backing up files, as well as preliminary data analysis.
- The chapter is summarized in Section 4.10 (p. 143).

Building the recording environment and collecting data often starts before the experimental design is finalized. This is because piloting is such an important feedback mechanism to the formation of the experiment that many decisions cannot be taken before a pilot is made. When your real data are recorded, you have limited the number of possible experimental designs that you could previously choose from; the data produced relate precisely to the design you settled upon. Therefore, make certain exactly what you want to record before you record it. Carry out pilot recordings, and perform preliminary analyses of the pilot data.

Decisions made during the recording phase have a large effect on data quality, and so the researcher with the highest incentive to get good data should take part in the recordings, so she can influence the many choices made during eye camera set-up and calibration.

4.1 Hands-on advice for data recording

Recording data is the pivotal point in all eye-tracker-based research. All preparations lead to data recording, and all analyses use the data produced. Once you have started to use up your participants with a specific type of experimental set-up, you have committed to it.

- Test that any external equipment can interface with the eye-tracker correctly. Select stimulus presentation tools with care, and test them properly for timing.
- Be sure to *pilot* the technical set-up as well as instruction and data analysis properly before you bring in the real participants and start committing yourself to the recruitment and recording process.
- Treat participants so that they feel reasonably good about the task. Design the experiment so as to ensure that you get the most data and best data quality from the participants.
- Have all consent forms, rewards, and other documentation prepared and copied before participants arrive.
- Setting up the *eye camera* for a given participant is the most decisive factor for good data quality (aside from the eye-tracker itself), and requires an understanding of the principles of video-based eye tracking which can only be acquired by experience. The good thing is, this experience can be transferred to any other video-based eye-tracker.
- When he arrives, look at the participant's eyes to quickly identify any mascara, drooping eyelids, contact lenses, squint, or difficult glasses.
- Get acquainted with the degrees of freedom that you have in directing the eye camera towards the participant's eye(s), and learn how to use contrast, luminance, and focus settings to make it the best possible eye image.

4.2 Building the experiment

The preparation phase can be intense. Stimuli need to be prepared, the physical environment set up (unless the eye-tracker is fixed in a cubicle), and pilot testing needs to be run to make sure the experiment will actually work.

4.2.1 Stimulus preparation

Eye tracking is about looking at any type of stimulus, but the vast majority of all eye-tracking studies have stimuli in the form of still images, which may be simple or complex, shown successively one at a time. The order and timing of stimuli presentation is determined by the experimental design, and the stimuli are most often presented on a monitor. Images, perhaps .jpeg or .bmp files are shown one after the other according to the constraints of the design. More basic research into low-level oculomotor control and psychophysics often presents small dots or contrast patches on the screen, rather than full images. Other research fields, like psycholingustics, use images in conjunction with other presentation modes such as spoken utterances. Whichever field your research relates to, in most cases the stimuli are presented on a monitor with a fixed or controlled physical relation to the eye camera, and on- and offsets of stimuli are controlled by you and your stimuli presentation software. In some cases, eye tracking is used even though any visual stimuli are of no or peripheral interest. For example, tracking the eyes while presenting a narrative in a pitch-black room (Johansson et al., 2006), or while stimulating the frontal eye fields with *trans-cranial magnetic stimulation* (Neggers et al., 2007). Perhaps the most demanding stimuli preparation occurs when you use the real world as the recording environment with real objects as stimuli, as this involves physically constructing the stimuli, placing or moving them between trials, or post-hoc segmenting the recordings into actual trials. All these stimuli types have benefits and drawbacks that need to be considered by the researcher. An alternative to real-world stimuli is to trade some realism for better stimuli control. This would be the case for eye tracking in virtual environments, such as car simulators, where the world is like an interactive video.

Animations and videos are usually shown on monitors, and represent a step up in realism compared to still-image viewing, but add extra requirements on your technical set-up due to the dynamics. In particular, *synchronization* becomes critical. Be sure to check the following synchronization issues in your system:

- The timing between your stimulus program and the recording software of the eye-tracker: does the start of a new stimulus picture co-occur in time with the corresponding trial mark in the eye-tracking data?
- Are there cumulative synchronization errors between your stimulus program and the presentation of videos, due to variable frame rates caused by other processes competing for the CPU? If the trials are terminated immediately after video playback, does the same video consistently produce the same trial lengths?
- What is the timing between your stimulus program and other recording systems, such as EEG, GSR, and sound recordings?
- Do you assume a particular and fixed frame rate? Is the 24 fps video really 24 fps, or rather 23.976 fps (NTSC)?

In complex set-ups with many stimulus presentation forms and several recordings, synchronization issues often become difficult to solve, and you risk losing control over the important temporal dimensions, and end up with no or false results, as in Figure 2.22 on p. 46. Furthermore, videos (i.e. moving stimuli) are problematic due to their interaction with current oculomotor event detection processes, which may give you invalid data (p. 168).

However, in some research settings which use the real world as the stimulus, like real car driving, your participant looks at real-life traffic that you cannot control. Pedestrians come and go to their own liking, not according to your experimental plan. You simply have to take what you get. If you record from two people in a collaborative or face-to-face setting, you have the same lack of control. Participants may or may not say or do what you hope they will. In these cases, it is extra important to pilot your stimuli and your task, to make certain that you are likely to naturally encounter the behaviour that you want to measure.

If you are preparing a monitor-based experiment, there are a number of commercial stimuli programs that you can use: e.g. E-prime, Presentation, MatLab with Psychophysics Toolbox, PsyScope, as well as a number of dedicated slideshow presenters and experiment programs that have been developed in labs or by manufacturers. The commercial programs allow for more advanced experiments, and also for interfacing with additional soft- and hardware, such as audio, GSR (galvanic skin response), and EEG (electroencephalography), as well as mouse devices, keyboards, and button boxes. There are, however, important considerations when selecting what solution you want to use to present your stimuli.

Programming environments MatLab in conjunction with Psychophysics Toolbox (Brainard, 1997; Pelli, 1997; Kleiner, Brainard, & Pelli, 2007) and Python with PsychoPy (Peirce, 2007), are extremely versatile, but the learning thresholds keep some users away. Additionally, a programming approach often takes more time to implement and consequently it is usually only preferred if no ready-made tool can present the stimuli as desired. Some programming software may require you to manage licence numbers, licence servers, or hardware keys (dongles), which may cause problems if you often change stimulus computers and relocate your set-up. However, if you have the ambition to perform many experiments in the future, it will very likely pay off to incrementally implement your stimulus presentation needs in a cross-platform, open source programming environment. This will gradually reduce the time spent coding each experiment as you recycle a lot of code. Open source solutions means it is easy to share code with students and colleagues, as well as replicate others' set-ups. Coding skills are crucial in a laboratory working with large amounts of quantitative data, and having students or laboratory assistants work with modifying coded experiments could be a good learning opportunity for what may become future PhD students.

Professional stimuli presentation software Commercial programs, such as E-prime, Presentation, and PsyScope, provide a fairly high flexibility, significantly lower learning thresholds, and are quick to program using the graphical user interface. There is a large user community which means you can often get help to implement more advanced routines, and simpler experiments already have user-contributed templates. On the negative side, you are limited to the capabilities provided for you by the software developers, and you do not have access to the underlying code. Synchronization with the eye-tracker may be an issue, and there is also the question of handling licences and hardware keys. This is typically the most common option, as it offers a good balance between simplicity and capability.

Eye-tracker manufacturer software The quality of software varies between manufacturers. Overall, the programs are easy to integrate with the hardware as the companies use it themselves in demonstrating their equipment. No single manufacturer software supports all kinds of experiments, and manufacturer software is usually very limited, often just catering for their main customer segment. For instance, one may lack support for using the web as a stimulus, another may lack support for gaze-contingent research. There is no general advice as the softwares vary greatly, but always examine these programs sceptically for bugs, latencies, and odd data processing procedures.

Non-experiment programs Programs used for presentations such as Powerpoint, Impress, and Open Office Presentation should not be used for stimuli presentation if you care about latencies. They may be a quick fix to a slideshow experiment, but if you depend on correct timings, you run the risk of getting results you cannot rely on and, consequently, not be able to publish.

Real life On the positive side, using the real world will, naturally, have a high generalizability to real-world behaviour since the study is more natural. On the negative side, you get poor or no control over random events and noise inherent in a complex and real environment. Also, any synchronization with eye-tracking equipment will often be manual and as such you will not have clear-cut trial starts and stops. Consider a consumer approaching a target product shelf: when does the trial actually start? Will it be when the user is already in front of the shelf, possibly missing any pre-views of the shelf the consumer has had, or should it be as soon as the shelf is remotely visible from a large distance in the scene camera. Will the gaze cursor be meaningful from a large distance where you cannot make out what precise products the consumer is looking at?

All stimulus presentation software should be tested as part of building the recording environment. Do not accept them at face value.

4.2.2 Physically building the recording environment

Some experiments are simple enough so that you just use a permanent set-up, typically consisting of eye-tracker, recording computer(s) with appropriate software, monitor, keyboard, and mouse, possibly speakers, microphone, and video camera. In other cases, you have to build the environment from scratch; for instance if you are recording on paper newspapers with a head-mounted system and magnetic head-tracking, or if you are combining a virtual reality environment with eye tracking. Building the environment is the physical correspondent to programming the stimulus presentation.

With a static monocular eye-tracker and a stimulus monitor, set up the two so that the recorded eye is placed in the middle of the imagined volume extending from the monitor. In such an eye-centred set-up, you minimize the risk that saccades in the two horizontal extremes of the monitor will be different, although such placement effects should already be controlled for in the design by counterbalancing the stimuli positions.

Be careful with lighting conditions (p. 17), so that you do not have additional infrared reflections or poor contrast in the eye image. Be careful to have a stable environment to avoid environmental noise in your data (p. 35).

If you are using a system with magnetic headtracking, it needs to be set up separately—in a process that measures the geometry of the scene. Also beware of magnetic disturbances near the recording area, such as fans, elevators, and computer equipment of various kinds.

Similarly, magnetic systems such as TMS and fMRI may cause interference, as the magnetic field causes induction in the eye-tracker electronics. Therefore, most researchers working with video-based systems and TMS or fMRI prefer to use remote or even long-range systems.

4.2.3 Pilot testing the experiment

Pilot testing the experiment is essential. Always pilot! Everything will improve, in particular your stress level during real data collection. There are a multitude of reasons why you should pilot your experiment:

- You find out what cables are missing in the eye-tracker and stimulus set-up.
- You will be able to see if your proposed stimuli and instructions do not elicit the behaviour that you want to measure and quantify, so you can get to change them well before the real recording.
- You practise handling of participants and equipment for this particular experiment.
- You check the geometry of the recording environment, and that you can calibrate and record data in all gaze directions required by your experiment.
- You will find out whether the software that you thought would work in fact does not.
- You can ask your pilot participants how well they understood your task instructions.
- You will see whether the proper data files are generated by the eye-tracking and stimulus software and that these contain the data you will be using.
- You can run a pilot analysis on the pilot data to see that the selected dependent variables and your method of analysis really work.
- Running a quick pilot or dummy recording at the beginning of each day that you will be recording will help you discover if your set-up has been tampered with; perhaps somebody borrowed a cable or some other critical part and forgot to return it or reconnect it properly?

After piloting, alter your experiment so that it does what you want it to do, and then reiterate the pilot. When you are happy with your pilot study, you can start recruiting the real participants.

4.3 Participant recruitment and ethics

When booking a participant for your study, allow time for him to ask questions. Prepare what you will answer when the participants ask questions, which they will. The most common question tends to be "What is the purpose of your study?". Have a good cover story, or tell them that they will get to know afterwards. Prepare a list so that you can offer to send participants the general results, your publications, etc. Other difficult questions that sometimes come up are "Is this testing my intellectual abilities?" and "Can I do anything wrong?"

Decide beforehand who will be in the room during the experiment. In some studies, participants will feel more comfortable if they are left alone with their task.

When he arrives, welcome the participant and introduce him to the equipment and to the people working with the experiment. Be social to him. At the same time, be certain to look at his eyes. Look for things that may mess up your recording: mascara, downward pointing eyelashes, certain types of glasses, and contact lenses. Is the participant squinting? The sooner you know about such problems, the better you can plan what to do. This is particularly true if you are on a tight recording schedule.

Also, remember that the second a participant shows up for your experiment, his thoughts are occupied mostly with non-laboratory ideas; home-work assignments, evening schedules, romantic plans and other pressing business. Different participants will be in different states of mind, and they will associate your instructions with slightly different things depending on their reference frame of the world and of themselves. Similarly, their physiological states will differ. Some have come running directly from a class, their minds working at full capacity with all newly learned ideas, and others have come directly from home, still not wide awake. These differences will contribute to the heterogeneity of the participant sample and may add variance to data, which may detrimentally influence your later statistical analysis.

One thing the participants *do* have in common is that they are all located in your laboratory for testing, and this you do have control over. You should give them a chance to settle and assume a similar state of mind. Allow the people coming directly from class to sit down and gather their thoughts, and allow the people coming straight from home to take a minute to wake up and think about why they are here. Let the laboratory setting work its magic and frame the procedure for each participant in the same way as you take them into the experiment room and give them their instructions. Keeping these things constant makes it more likely your instructions will be interpreted similarly across participants, and this will help you to get a more homogeneous sample.

If your study allows it, showing the eye camera image to the participant as part of setting it up may help the participant to cooperate better and move about less. If your participant is a child, showing and explaining what you are doing is particularly important, since a child is more likely to move his eye out of the eye camera view. When you do work close to the participant, such as adjusting the equipment, tell him in advance exactly what you are going to do, so you do not startle them. Be sure to tell the participant that it is OK to stop the experiment at any time. You do not want your participant to silently suffer through the second half of your experiment.

4.3.1 Ethics toward participants

Ethics towards participants are comprised of two elements: 1) The law, which varies across regions in the world. 2) The researcher's common sense, empathy, and desire to have a good relationship with the participant pool.

In many parts of the world, experiments on children, clinical populations, or participants that are likely to experience some degree of psychological stress due to the task, require the experimenter to apply to a regional board of ethics before running the study. The ethical board will then decide whether the study follows the local law, and whether the scientific purpose of the study outweighs the hardships and/or sufferings of the participants. You may think that participants do not suffer very much from taking part in an eye-tracking study, but participants with clinical diagnoses, such as dyslexia, can feel bad about doing a reading study in a highly technical laboratory, in particular if the participant is young and has already been subjected to excessive testing.

Ethics fundamentally means that the participant should have a good feeling about having participated in your study. This is in your own interest, because your participant will tell his friends about your experiment and the laboratory in which it took place. Not only will you increase the chances that your participant will come back therefore, you potentially gain new participants for future studies also. If you have treated your participants well, and if they are interested in your study, they may even recruit their friends for you! If you get them to be really interested, after a few years, one of your former participants may suddenly be your student. All in all, you should treat your participants well.

Many ethics-related issues are dealt with in the 'consent form', a written statement that the researcher may use the data collected from the participant, and that the participant considers himself fully informed about the purpose of the study and the consequences for himself of signing off the rights to the data. Laws may require consent forms to be signed *before* data recording, but the objectives of the study sometimes require this to be done *after* the recording (so that the participant is not aware of the purpose of the study during the recording). This can be solved by preparing two consent forms: one which is more general in its experiment description, and a second post-experiment consent form which fully explains the experiment and gives the participant the option to have the recorded data destroyed if no consent is given.

4.4 Eye camera set-up

Now we are ready to put the participant into one of the eye-trackers described in Chapter 2. This section describes how to adjust the eye camera view so as to get data of high quality. Eye camera set-up is of great importance to the quality of your data, and largely decides whether you can use them in analysis, and for what measures. Knowing your eye video and the algorithms that calculate gaze position from it allows you to get better data from a larger spectrum of participants, more quickly and with less anxiety.

Some manufacturers have hidden the eye camera set-up in automatic processes, giving an appearance of increased usability and simplicity (Figure 4.1(b)), but at the same time with-holding control over the data recording from the user of the system. The result in terms of data quality may be acceptable in a large number of cases, but some loss of quality will go unnoticed, or be difficult to understand and alleviate. Experienced users of these mostly re-mote systems will with time learn to move or tilt a whole system (camera unit and monitor) to set up an optimal eye-camera angle, behaving in accordance with the advice we give be-low, but without the feedback that a full eye-image can provide. Most eye-tracking recording software shows one or another image of the participant's eye, however. Figures 4.1(a) and (c) are examples from the ASL MobileEye, and the SR EyeLink respectively. In this section, we will use examples from SMI and EyeLink systems, because the video image can be very clearly seen with their systems, but the presentation and majority of advice in this section are valid for all video-based pupil–corneal reflection systems. We will use reading data to show the effect on data quality, because the lines of text provide a good reference point against which to compare data.

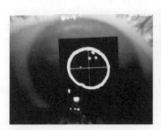 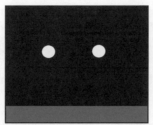 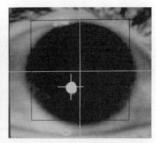

(a) The ASL MobileEye eye image (b) The Tobii Studio eye image (c) The EyeLink 1000 eye image

Fig. 4.1 The eye images of three video-based pupil-corneal-reflection eye-tracking systems. To the left ASL MobileEye eye image, in which the highlighted ring indicates the circumference of the pupil. In the middle, Tobii Studio in which the eye image is hidden, and to the right the EyeLink eye image, with pupil and corneal reflections clearly marked by colour and cross-hairs.

The Marketer: Alchemist, Magician, Sorcerer and Medicine Man

Is marketing an art or a science? Perhaps marketing is more like

sorcery. Think of a sorcerer collecting ingredients from different sources

and mixing them into a potion, accompanied with the magical effect of a

flash of light and the illusion to follow. To some extent this fits with

Culliton's vision of a marketer as a 'mixer of ingredients'. Of course

Fig. 4.2 Example of good quality data in raw format, recorded with a tower-mounted eye-tracker at 1250 Hz. The figure shows raw gaze samples; one dot per sample. Fixations are seen as blobs of many dots in a small area. Saccades are strings of dots; the more sparsely the dots are placed, the faster the saccade.

Errors can arise in the eye (feature) detection and gaze estimation algorithms at the heart of the eye-tracker due to *covering* of the pupil or corneal reflection, *confusion* between the pupil or corneal reflection and a number of other optic entities, *distortion* of the image, or because of *loss* either of the pupil or corneal reflection by the camera and its supporting software. A number of causes behind these problematic conditions are summarized in Table 4.1.

In order to get high-quality data such as that shown in Figure 4.2, you should see to it that the eye camera records the eye from slightly below the eye with regard to the direction the participant has when facing the stimulus area. If your eye camera is too low, it will be difficult to calibrate and record in the upper corners of the calibration area because the corneal reflection is more easily occluded by the lower eyelid. If the camera angle is too high, the upper eyelid will often cover some participants' pupils when looking at the bottom corners, and calibration will be difficult or faulty. Figure 4.3 shows how camera positions, the participant, and the mirror should be moved to achieve a better image. When you are moving cameras or mirrors close to your participant's eyes, take care always to talk to him about what you are doing, so that he is prepared and you do not startle him. Remember that by participating, he puts trust in you. Of course, you must be careful not to hurt him or scratch his glasses.

The participant and cameras should be placed in a position so that the eye camera shows a good image of the eye for each corner of the calibration area. This involves directing cameras and/or mirrors as well as raising or lowering the participant's chair, or the table with eye-

Table 4.1 Summary of optic conditions that may endanger data quality. For instance, both pupil and corneal reflection may be covered; the pupil foremost by droopy eyelids, and the reflection by laughter, or more specifically, the accompanied narrowing or closure of the eye. Confusion refers to cases when other objects are mistaken for the whole or part of the pupil or corneal reflection. Optic distortion can be caused by, for instance, bifocal glasses, while extreme gaze angles may cause loss of the corneal reflection.

	Pupil	**Reflection**
Covering	Droopy eyelids	Laughter
Confusion	Mascara	Retinal
	Glasses	Glasses
	Ambient infrared light	Contact lenses
	Retinal reflection	Sunlight
	Specks and dirt	Lamps
		Other infrared light sources
		Wet eye
Distortion	Bifocal glasses	
Loss	Head movement	Extreme gaze angles

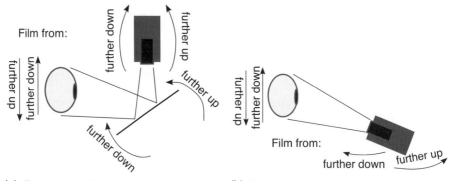

(a) Tower-mounted and some head-mounted systems

(b) Remote systems and some head-mounted systems

Fig. 4.3 How to move the eye camera, the mirror, or the participant, so as to get a camera angle from further up or further below.

tracker and stimulus monitor. If you are using a head-mounted system, camera set-up often involves positioning and directing a whole construction of mirror and cameras. If you are using a remote eye-tracker or a head-restraining static system, remember that participants tend to sit very attentively during camera set-up and calibration, but may slide down during the actual recording, so your camera angle changes or you have to move mirrors or camera during recording (or it is done automatically), which may cause an offset in data.

A pupil–corneal reflection system calculates the participant's gaze direction on the basis of the relative position of the pupil and the corneal reflection centres. When calculating the centre of the pupil, it is important that the eye camera sees the entire pupil in all gaze directions. Two examples of good eye images can be seen in Figure 4.4. Partial occlusion of the pupil causes a movement of the calculated centre point, and thus a movement in the data coordinates, although no real eye movement has been made. In fact, even very small movements of the calculated pupil centre can cause considerable movement in the coordinate files. The identified corneal reflection may also move artificially, jumping to other reflections

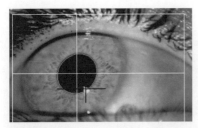 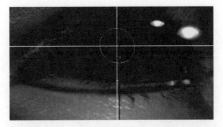

(a) Both pupil and corneal reflection are uniquely identified with white and dark cross-hairs, respectively.

(b) The large white blobs in the right-hand picture are infrared reflections in the participant's glasses, but they do not interfere with the gaze estimation algorithm.

Fig. 4.4 Eyes with good eye camera set-up, filming from below. Both eye images are from head-mounted systems.

in the eye video, most commonly just under or on top of the upper eyelid. This movement of the calculated corneal reflection causes large and very fast, but entirely false, movements in the data samples, which we call *optic artefacts* in Chapter 2.

Ocular dominance

If your participant is squinting or if there is reason to believe that one eye is better than the other, see to it that you select the so-called *dominant* eye. Ocular dominance can be determined using a number of different tests; one simple test for this is the 'Miles test' (Miles, 1929). Here, the participant extends both arms and brings both hands together to create a small opening while looking at an object with both eyes simultaneously. The observer then alternately closes the left and the right eye to determine which eye is really viewing the object. That is the eye that should be measured. Around two thirds of the population have a right eye dominance and men are more commonly right dominant (Eser, Durrie, Schwendeman, & Stahl, 2008).

If you are recording monocularly and you notice that you have to change the camera to the other eye, for instance recording a left eye after a series of right eyes, you may need to take care that the position of the left eye relative to the monitor will be the same as that of the previously recorded right eyes (if your experiment demands control over this). If not, the result may be small variations in fixation and saccade data in the outskirts of the monitor. The best solution is to control for this in the experimental design, so horizontal stimuli positions are counterbalanced.

4.4.1 Mascara

Mascara is considered a serious problem for data quality. This may be less of an issue for a bright-pupil system, as the pupil is bright but the mascara dark (see Applied Science Laboratories, 2011), but mascara also blocks filming through sparse eyelashes, making it not completely unproblematic for bright-pupil systems. Therefore, regardless of eye-tracking system, always tell your participants beforehand not to wear mascara. Do not tell them not to wear make-up, because some participants think that mascara does not qualify as make-up. If the mascara is left on, only expect to make a good recording on participants with large, open eyes and upward eyelashes. This is because in a dark-pupil system, the software that identifies the pupil is confused by the other large dark area in the immediate vicinity of the pupil, and may lock onto the mascara rather than the pupil. This is detrimental to subsequent calibration, as well as to the recording. A make-up removal kit should therefore be an indispensible piece of

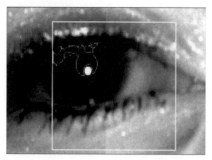 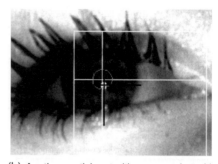

(a) Participant with drooping eyelid and downward eyelashes. A thick, dark brush of lashes melds with the pupil and makes it impossible for the recording software to identify the pupil.

(b) Another participant with mascara, but with upward-pointing lashes; in this case the mascara is easy to exclude, and lashes like these seldom occlude the pupil.

Fig. 4.5 Mascara interferes with pupil detection.

equipment in all serious eye-tracking laboratories. If you ask your participant to remove the mascara, watch out for any remaining mascara blobs that often have a round pupil-like form which can be mistaken for a pupil and later cause offsets in your data.

Some recording software can exclude portions of the eye video from the eye feature detection process, which allows quality recordings without asking participants to remove mascara. In Figure 4.5, only the parts of the eye video that are inside the white rectangle are analysed for pupil and corneal reflection. This works relatively well in the majority of cases, provided the lashes point upwards and the head is fixed so the eye does not move relative to the eye image (as for a fixed contact system with chin rest). Moreover, software programs often give the user the option to reject pupil-like objects that are too small or too large, such that mascara blobs with extreme sizes can be discarded automatically.

The right side of Figure 4.6 shows a raw, unfiltered plot of data samples from a participant for whom we had a good eye video in all gaze directions. It shows one pixel for each sample, of which there are 1250 per second. Where samples cluster to blobs, the eye has been still in a fixation. Where samples trace a line, the eye has moved quickly in a saccade. The vertical pairs of lines are blinks; the eyelid going down and then up again. All else is noise of various kinds. It can been seen that we have fixations and saccades almost right on the word for each line. The left side of Figure 4.6 shows data from a participant with mascara and downward eyelashes. The data plot is largely OK all the way to line eight, which is the gaze direction at which the mascara aligns with the pupil in the eye video. Data for the lower five lines consist of useless optic artefacts.

4.4.2 Droopy eyelids and downward eyelashes

The problem with droopy eyelids grows with the age of your participants, but it is also a matter of individual variation. Droopy eyelids are a major problem in eye-tracking research even if there is no mascara, because the eyelids, or the eyelashes, cover the pupil in the lower gaze directions (Figures 4.7 and 4.8). In your data, you will see very large downward offsets, because a pupil partially occluded from above has a lower mass centre and resulting data will be at an artificially lower vertical position. At a certain gaze angle, the pupil is completely covered, and you will then have complete data loss in the lower part of the screen/visual field. Notice that pupil occludance may not appear dangerous during calibration, when the participant is more tense and focused, and the eyes are more open. It is when he gets into

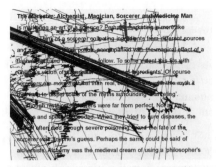

(a) Data from participant wearing mascara and having slightly downward eyelashes. Data plotted in the upper half of the stimulus image shows data recorded when the eye was open and all of the pupil seen. Below this is the data where the pupil is covered by lashes with mascara.

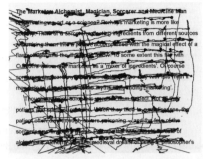

(b) Good eye-tracking data. Vertical lines are blinks. Some noise can be seen in the upper left corner and the bottom line. However, all lines of text have accurate and precise data samples on top of them, that the event detection algorithms can make use of.

Fig. 4.6 The effects of mascara on slightly downward eyelashes.

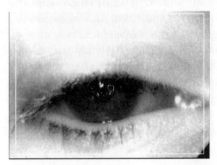

(a) A thick brush of lashes covers the pupil and make it impossible for the recording software to identify either pupil, or corneal reflection.

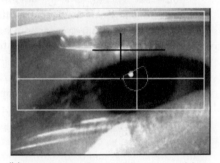

(b) In this drooping eyelid, on a participant with glasses, the eye-tracker locks onto a false corneal reflection on the eyelid, because the real corneal reflection is partially occluded underneath lashes. Also notice the partial pupil occlusion. Gaze data from this eye video will have considerable data loss, a very large offset, and many optic artefacts.

Fig. 4.7 Participant with drooping eyelid and downward eyelashes.

the task and relaxes that the eye closes and you get an offset. In fact, you may get better data quality if you calibrate the bottom calibration points with a relaxed participant, who closes his eyes a little, because that is what the eye will look like when you record your participant looking in that direction. However, that is a gamble and the correct solution is to redo the set-up to handle the drooping eyelids or the eyelashes.

There are at least four possible solutions for droopy eyelids and downwards eyelashes:

1. If possible, move the camera or the mirrors to film the eyes from even further below.
2. Ask the participant to use an eyelash curler to turn the eyelashes upwards. This instrument should be desinfected between participants.
3. Is the participant tired? Ask him to return at another date and time that is more appropriate.

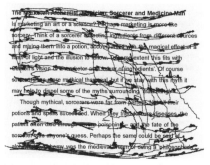

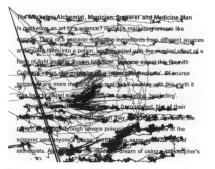

(a) Mild effects. The bottom five lines have a one-line offset, and the two last lines are smeared together into one thick data line.

(b) Strong effect. Note the offsets and optic artefacts in the bottom four lines, and the centre. The data in the upper paragraph are fairly good, since the eye is open while the participant is looking there.

Fig. 4.8 Example of the effect in reading data of droopy eyelids.

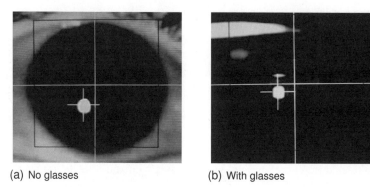

(a) No glasses   (b) With glasses

Fig. 4.9 Effect of glasses on one and the same participant. Note in (b) the extra reflection just above the corneal reflection, the darker image with lower contrast, and the large reflection in the upper left corner.

4. As a final resort, use some sticking plaster to fixate the participants upper eyelid. This works well for most elderly participants, but may not be comfortable for some participants.

4.4.3   Shadows and infrared reflections in glasses

Glasses make eye tracking more difficult in several ways. First, glasses, or possibly the surface treatments of the glasses, may make the eye image darker, reducing the contrast between pupil and iris, which may decrease accuracy and precision in a dark-pupil system. Access to contrast and brightness settings in the eye camera is useful to remedy this. Second, the light from the corneal reflection can be reflected back to the eye and give a second, but fainter corneal reflection higher up in the eye image (compare the eye images in Figure 4.9). Third, the shadows from the brim may confuse the pupil detection in dark-pupil systems. All these three effects are seen in Figure 4.10.

Another major problem is infrared reflections in the glasses themselves. If the infrared reflection is on top of the pupil or near the corneal reflection in any of the gaze directions—ask your participant to look around—your calibration or your data recording will be jeopardized. This problem is particularly large if the participant wears old, scratched glasses, or glasses

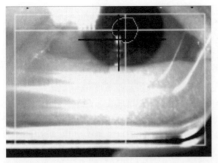

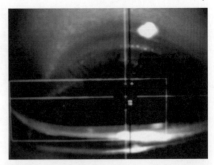

(a) Eye with shadow from glasses, and an infrared reflection high above the eye. Dark areas could confound the pupil detection but have been excluded from detection.

(b) Eye with multiple infrared reflections and refractions from glasses, both above and below the pupil. Were the eye to move, the pupil might be covered.

Fig. 4.10 Shadows and reflections in glasses.

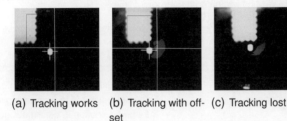

(a) Tracking works   (b) Tracking with off-   (c) Tracking lost
set

Fig. 4.11 Reflection in glasses covering more and more of pupil and finally making tracking impossible.

that have been treated to reflect sunlight, while glasses with anti-reflection treatment tend to elicit much fewer reflections. The solution is to move the eye camera angle so these reflections appear far from the pupil and corneal reflection (see Figure 4.11). It may take a while to find a view on the eye without interfering reflections, in particular with tower-mounted eye-trackers, but then these systems usually have good tracking throughout the experiment as the participant is fixed. For remote eye-trackers you are usually limited to changing the filming angle and then hoping that the participant does not switch to a disadvantageous position during the experiment.

Some people wear small glasses with thick designer frames. This may cause a dark shadow on part of the eye, which can interfere with both pupil and corneal reflection. Again the solution is to move the camera position and angle until an optimal viewing angle is found.

Some glasses are more difficult than others, in particular if they are so dark that the contrast in the eye video is too low, very small so the frame comes too close to the eye, or because they are very scratched and create many infrared reflections. A frame too close to the eye is problematic because it may occlude pupil or corneal reflection in certain eye positions, or the frame itself may be mistaken for a pupil or a corneal reflection if it is dark or reflective. If your eye-tracker allows you to change the luminance (and contrast) of the eye image, do that. Another solution, used by some eye-tracking researchers, is to have a set of their own eye-tracker-friendly glasses of different strengths that they lend to participants with problematic glasses.

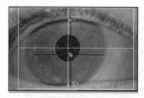 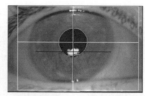 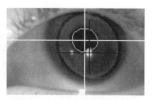

(a) No air bubbles at the point of the corneal reflection. (b) The effect of air bubbles on the corneal reflection. (c) Hard contact lens; no air bubbles, but if the border of the lens passes over the corneal reflection, a similar offset will occur.

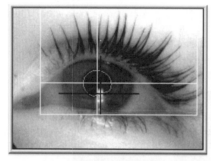 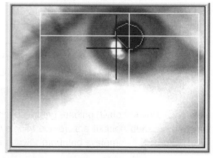

(d) Focused camera. Two corneal reflections; cross-hair on the upper one. (e) Unfocused camera. Several corneal reflections merged into one, so tracking is stable, but the pupil detection is deformed, giving a small offset.

Fig. 4.12 *Soft contact lenses* in (a), (b), (d), and (e): Reduce focus on camera to avoid multiple corneal reflections. The *hard contact lens* in (c) does not generate bubbles.

4.4.4 Bi-focal glasses

Bi-focal glasses introduce a border in the midst of the eye video that makes calibration difficult and recording close to impossible. Ask your participant to wear other glasses.

4.4.5 Contact lenses

Soft contact lenses cause only one problem in eye tracking, but it is a major problem, and it is not uncommon. For some people, because of a less than perfect fit between lens and eyeball, small air bubbles gather underneath the contact lens. When the infrared illumination is reflected in such a collection of small air bubbles, the light is split up into a number of reflections (Figures 4.12(b) and 4.12(d)). As the eye moves, the bubbles shift. Your eye-tracker will randomly select any of these reflections as the corneal reflection, and jump between them. This results in erroneous data samples and apparently very fast movements of the eye (Figure 4.13), known as optic artefacts. When this occurs it can be devastating for your data quality. You cannot always see the bubbles while setting up and calibrating a participant; they may appear in the midst of data collection, ruining your recording session.

Fortunately the solution is mostly very easy. If your participant wears soft contact lenses, which you should ask them about or can even see in the eye image, always reduce the focus of the eye camera somewhat. This way the many small bubbles will merge into one larger corneal reflection. Your data will sometimes be slightly less accurate, because the larger corneal reflection pushes the pupil slightly to the side. Nevertheless, an unfocused recording is much, much better than if you had continued with full focus and a split corneal reflection.

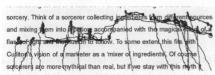

(a) Participant reading one line of text.

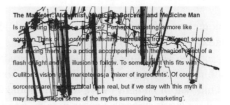

(b) Participant reading two lines of text.

Fig. 4.13 Offsets and optic artefacts, due to contact lenses causing a split corneal reflection. The length of the false movement lines corresponds to the distance in the eye video between the two corneal reflections. As Figure 5.14 on page 163 shows, velocities in these artefactual movements is far beyond that of saccades.

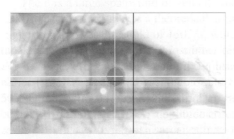

(a) Full sunlight. Low contrast and high luminance; pupil is identified but corneal reflection is not.

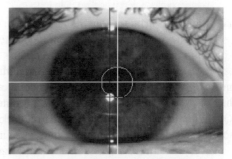

(b) Indoors with only artificial illumination.

Fig. 4.14 Same participant wearing a head-mounted eye-tracker.

This will work in all cases, except the most extreme and rare ones, when the corneal reflection splits into a multitude of points that can cover up to a quarter of the iris.

Hard contact lenses are formed to fit the eyeball much tighter, and appear to gather no air bubbles, and data can be recorded at full eye camera focus. Hard contact lenses are very clearly seen in the eye camera image, as in Figure 4.12(c). Only if the border of the hard lens moves across the corneal reflection, which can occur often for some participants, will data quality suffer.

4.4.6 Direct sunlight and other infrared sources

Direct sunlight contains much infrared light, enough to outshine the infrared illumination many times over. The result is typically complete and immediate data loss (compare Figure 4.14). This can be particularly difficult during car driving, especially when the sun is close to the horizon, shining directly onto the eyeball. One of the authors was once in a car-driving project where we drove along the Scanian coast with a western sun shining through a sparse forest. The resulting rapid alternations between sun and shadow yielded equally rapid alterations between data capture and data loss. Such data, of course, are useless. In cars, one option is to attach an infrared filter film to the windows, but a more common option is to simply record on a cloudy day. The SmartEye systems that are specifically designed for use in cars select a part of the infrared frequency spectrum in which the sun has a lower effect on the eye-tracker camera, compared to the normally used infrared frequency.

Static systems can also be affected by sunlight, for instance through a window. Good shades or no windows at all are therefore recommended in an eye-tracking laboratory.

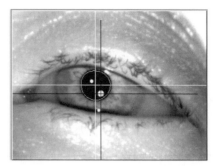

(a) A hot incandescent bulb gives a second reflection in the cornea, and the corneal reflection cross-hair has locked onto it.

(b) The fast-moving fourth Purkinje reflection in the upper left quarter of the pupil.

Fig. 4.15 Additional reflections.

A video-based motion capture system illuminates the scene to be measured with several infrared lamps, which could seriously compete with the infrared diode of the eye-tracker. We have on several occasions tested head-mounted systems with motion capture systems such as Qualisys. This combination has always worked. Obviously the shorter distance from the eye to the eye-tracker infrared diode more than compensates for its weaker luminousity.

In fact, some ceiling-mounted indoor lights can be more harming to eye tracking than motion trackers as measured by the intensity of the corneal reflection that they give rise to. In Figure 4.15(a), an incandescent light from the ceiling caused an additional corneal reflection, which is similar to the double reflection of the contact lenses, but only now it is permanent. If we were to calibrate on such an eye image, the danger is that some of the calibration points are calibrated with the correct reflection, and other on the false reflection, as in Figure 4.15(a). Terrible offsets result from such a calibration. Solutions include turning off the light, or using a lamp that does not emit infrared light,[14] and if that is not possible, use recording software settings to select properties such as reflection perimeter and distance to pupil centre to tell the eye-tracker which reflection to use.

4.4.7 The fourth Purkinje reflection

You may sometimes see an additional reflection inside the pupil, as in Figure 4.15(b). It moves very quickly when the participant moves his eyes, but as soon as it reaches the border of the pupil, it disappears. It is produced at the back of the lens, and can therefore only be seen through the pupil. This reflection is used by dual-Purkinje eye-trackers, and is the reason they are so precise and have such a small tracking range. It may on rare occasions—for only a few samples—interfere with the corneal reflection and undermine data, but it is the weaker one and will not overly displace the cross-hair from the corneal reflection, as long as the eye camera is focused. If the camera is out of focus, this reflection may be much bigger and undermine the calculation of the pupil area.

4.4.8 Wet eyes due to tears or allergic reactions

When the participant's eye is wet, the corneal reflection splits up into several reflections, similar to the split corneal reflection in a contact lens. This may happen due to allergic reactions in the pollen season, or if you instruct the participant to try not to blink. The latter case makes

---

[14] You can check any lighting source for infrared by covering the eye-tracker's infrared source and pointing the camera at the light—if the system picks it up you know it emits infrared light.

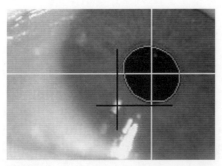
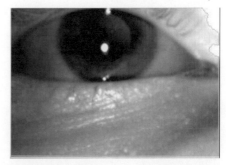

(a) Allergic reaction resulting in a wet eye and multiple corneal reflections. The identification cross is on a false reflection.

(b) Infrared reflections in the retina giving a semi-bright pupil.

Fig. 4.16 Reflections in tears and retina.

them gaze until their eyes are dry and then the eye compensates with more tear fluid. The distance between reflections is often larger in this case, so the problem cannot be solved by decreasing eye camera focus. However, it mainly appears when gaze is in the far upper corners, as in Figure 4.16(a), and can mostly be solved during manual calibration with little or no data loss.

4.4.9 The retinal reflection (bright-pupil condition)

On rare occasions in dark-pupil systems, you may happen to have the infrared illumination almost co-axial with the line of sight, and then see the reflection in the retina. Unless you are using a bright-pupil system, you do not want this, because it makes pupil identification difficult or impossible, as in Figure 4.16(b). This condition can be solved by moving illumination and the mirror.

4.4.10 Mirror orientation and dirty mirrors

Wrong mirror orientation is a very uncommon problem, but one which may occur—it did in our laboratory. During the preparations for a large study (310 participants in six days using four tower-mounted systems), we were cleaning the mirrors of the systems, and happened to put one of them upside down. Now, the mirror that is part of many eye trackers, is covered on one side by a thin layer that reflects infrared light but lets through visual light. It is usually difficult to place the mirror upside down, but when it happens, by accident, in the hurry of the last preparations, the infrared light is spread into four corneal reflections along the vertical axis, as in Figure 4.17(a). The diagnosis was difficult, but once the problem was found, the solution was easy.

Specks on mirrors may give rise to weak reflections in the eye image that reduce the contrast and increase noise levels, as shown in Figure 4.17(b). The solution is simple: clean the mirror.

The examples above should be ample proof of the importance of the user being able to see the eye video and influence its quality. Hiding the eye video from the user, and relying on automatic set-up of the eye video, is a current trend in manufacturer development. It is an understandable ambition to attempt to make this part of data recording more easy, but if this automatization is not properly done, it can make eye camera set-up and recordings more difficult, give data of a poorer quality, and leave the user with fewer clues on how to improve data quality.

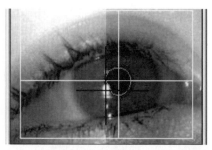 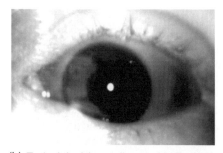

(a) Four corneal reflections along the vertical axis, as a result of an infrared-reflecting mirror turned upside down.

(b) To the left of the pupil, a weak reflection is visible, equal in size to the pupil, that reduces the contrast and will increase noise levels in recordings. Clean the mirror from fingerprints and specks.

Fig. 4.17 Mirror reflections and lowered contrast due to a dirty mirror.

The entire eye camera set-up and positioning of the participant should take no more than a minute or two once you start to gather experience.

4.5 Calibration

Individual calibration of each participant is necessary for a variety of reasons. For instance, the eyeball radius varies by up to 10% between grown-ups, and it may also have different shapes. Glasses alter the size of the eye in the eye video image. These variations change the geometrical values underpinning the calculation of gaze direction (Hammoud, 2008).

If you are using a head-mounted system out of the laboratory, see to it that the level of ambient infrared light is as low and stable as possible. If you calibrate in an area with a lot of infrared light, and then record in a darker area, the contrast between pupil and iris may change and result in poorer data, unless the camera compensates and the system dynamically resets the contrast thresholds. For maximal data quality, always calibrate in the same luminance conditions as you will have during data record, and minimize luminance variation in the trials (see Chapter 2).

4.5.1 Points

Calibration is typically made on a 2D area which has a number of predefined calibration points: 2, 5, 9, 13, and 16 are common numbers. Calibration points should cover the area where the relevant stimuli will be presented, whether it is a monitor, a scene video from a head-mounted system, or even just a part of a screen. Using the pupil and corneal reflection positions recorded in calibration points with known coordinates, the recording software can calculate a function to estimate any given location on the stimulus, given the extracted pupil and corneal reflection positions. Systems with just one or even no calibration points are being developed. By calibrating the system on just a few calibration targets, the system can then fit a function that allows it to interpolate between all intermediate positions and also extrapolate to positions outside the calibration area. It should be noted that accuracy is better within or close to the calibration targets and the stimuli should preferably be appearing within the area encompassed by the calibration points.

Points should be small and visually salient, so that participants gaze at them as exactly as possible during calibration. Any misalignment of gaze towards the actual calibration point will introduce a corresponding offset in your data. Some laboratories use high-frequency Gabor patches that are only visible when participants look straight at them. Animated calibration targets seem to work better than static ones, as participants gaze at them as long as they are animated rather than looking around for the next target. Having the participant mouse-click on very small points rather than just looking at them may increase accuracy even further. For small children, it can be an advantage to exchange the standard point for objects that are fun or somewhat familiar to them: a yellow sun, a blue star, etc.

The position of points differs substantially between systems that give data files and those that only give gaze-overlaid video output, such as the head-mounted systems. For data files, the calibration points should be put on the stimulus surface (i.e. most commonly the computer monitor on which the experimental stimulus is displayed). For gaze-overlaid data, the calibration points should be in the coordinate system of the scene video camera. When calibrating the scene video of a head-mounted system, a laser pointer is commonly used to project an actual target overlapping the calibration coordinates determined from the scene camera. Alternatively, it is possible to position the scene camera at an exact position where known physical targets will coincide with the calibration targets of the system.

4.5.2 Geometry

There are a number of geometry settings that the calibration routine needs access to: the size (and position) of the calibration screen in pixels and/or millimetres, the precise position of the calibration points, and the distance from the eye to the monitor. These values can be set manually with some eye-tracking systems, but are automatically estimated or measured in some of the remote systems.

Monitor distance affects data quality in corners, and what really matters is how much of the visual field is covered. Unless the participant has difficulties accommodating, there is little benefit in presenting on a 24 inch screen at a position chosen so that is covers a visual angle equivalent to a 17 inch monitor at a shorter distance. You have to find the proper compromise between the position when the corneal reflection is lost in top corners, when the pupil is covered with eyelashes at the bottom corners, and between the distance and height of the monitor in the overall set-up. Even with a very good set-up, some participants' eyes will nevertheless cause problems in bottom and top corners.

4.5.3 The calibration procedure

Always test the quality of your eye video before calibrating. Let the participant look at the corners of the calibration area and watch whether the eye video looks good with a stable pupil and corneal reflection in all corners. Then you can calibrate.

The participant looks through all calibration points, and at each point the eye-tracker software samples a few hundred milliseconds of data. The participant in Figure 4.18 looks at nine different points. Notice how the spatial relation between pupil and corneal reflection differs in the different gaze directions. It is of vital importance for the quality of your data that the full and correct pupil and corneal reflections are selected at every single calibration point. An eye video set-up with the images in Figure 4.18 would give a successful calibration and good quality data.

The progress through the points, as well as acknowledgement that the sampled data are valid, can be done *manually* either by the operator or by the participant, or *automatically* by the recording software. The current trend among manufacturers is to provide automatic calibration as their default. Tests that the authors have carried out with close to 60 participants in each of the three conditions (i.e. operator controlled, participant controlled, auto-

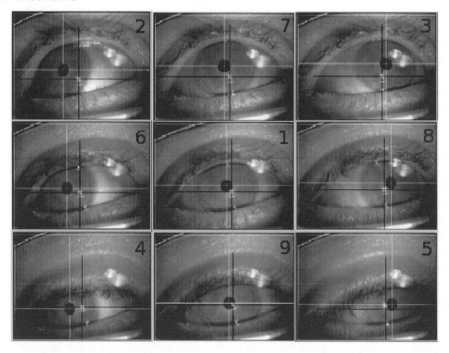

Fig. 4.18 Participant (with glasses) looking at the nine points of a calibration screen in the order given by the numbers 1 to 9. The bright reflections are always out of the way for successful detection of pupil and corneal reflections, although close in calibration point 3.

matic) showed that data quality (precision and accuracy) is superior for *participant-controlled* progress and acknowledgement of calibration points (Holmqvist, Nyström, & Andersson, 2011). In other words, participants know best themselves when they are looking at a point, and the researcher can hand over the calibration process with confidence.

Irrespective of calibration method, the participant must cooperate in looking at the calibration points, and they virtually always do. Exceptions may include children or animals who lose their interest in the calibration procedure after a few points. Patients who have difficulty keeping their eyes still, e.g. due to congenital nystagmus (common with albinos), are also difficult to calibrate.

You may sometimes miscalibrate participants simply because they happen to look in the wrong direction while you or the eye-tracker acknowledges one of the points. Sometimes, a participant tends to fixate the calibration points for a very short time, not knowing that you need a second or so to verify the image in the eye video and press the acknowledgement button. Other participants may make involuntary so-called square wave jerks during calibration (see Figure 5.30), giving an offset because the participant looked away slightly from the calibration point just at the moment that point was confirmed in the calibration procedure. To reduce the danger of such errors, always instruct your participants to keep their gaze fixed in the centre of each calibration point until it disappears, and watch out for participants from groups that are known to have a higher rate of square wave jerks (p. 407).

4.5.4 Corner point difficulties and solutions

Many systems allow you to watch the eye camera image while calibrating, so you can see that the eye is still, that it is looking in the right direction, and that corneal reflection and

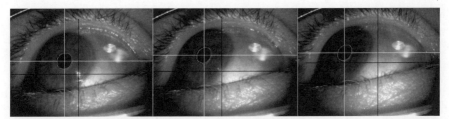

Fig. 4.19 More and more extreme gaze directions towards the upper left calibration corner. The first eye is OK, the second is dubious, and the third will give a considerable offset in data, as in Figure 4.20.

pupil are correctly identified, as in Figure 4.18. The most difficult calibration points are the corners. *Bottom corners* are problematic if your participant has downward eyelashes partially or completely covering the pupil, when looking down at the bottom corners. In that case, there are three things that you can do:

1. Ask the participant to open his/her eye. This will temporarily keep the eyelid or lashes from blocking the eye feature detection and lets you proceed with the calibration. But during recording, when your participant is fully occupied with the task and no longer thinks about holding the eye open, you will get optic artefacts, offsets, and data loss at that bottom corner. This may be a viable option if the problem only concerns the corners of the screen and the interesting parts of the stimuli are mainly located in the centre.

2. Acknowledge calibration of that point even if half the pupil is covered. This is gambling that your participant's pupil will also be half-covered during recording. Your data will have a smaller offset compared to the corners in case one, but the poorer precision and accuracy will remain, and will likely contain optic artefacts. If you are planning to do area of interest-based analysis this may be OK, but fixation and saccade measures will be affected.

3. Go back and set up the eye camera to film from further below, or ask the participant to curl the eyelashes. This takes more time, but it is the only guarantee of good data. With a remote, try tilting the camera or moving it closer or further from the participant to change the angle.

The *top corners* are usually easier, but they have a problem of their own, illustrated by the eye images in Figure 4.19 and the resulting data in Figure 4.20. When the corneal reflection moves across the border of the iris, it changes position and form. If you calibrate with a corneal reflection outside of the iris, then you will later have a considerable offset for data samples in that corner. There are of course large individual differences between participants as to the gaze direction at which this corneal reflection leaves the iris. For some participants with a narrow eye opening, the corneal reflection is instead covered by the lower eyelid. In any case, there are three things you can do to remedy this situation:

1. The quick solution is—if your recording software allows it—to move the calibration point further in, and ask your participant to look at the new position, hopefully thus moving the corneal reflection back into the iris. This solution will give precise and fairly accurate data when recording, especially if the task normally does not require the participants to look at extreme angles but rather in the centre of the screen.

2. You could also move your eye camera and/or infrared illumination so as to film the eye from further up. This takes more time, and you also run the risk of creating problems at the bottom corners if you change the camera angle too much.

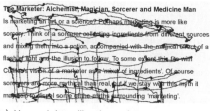 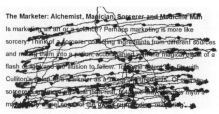

(a) Upper right calibration point   (b) Upper left calibration point

Fig. 4.20 Offsets—poor accuracy—resulting from calibrating participants whose corneal reflection had left the iris, as in Figure 4.19. In 4.20(a), the upper right calibration corner was problematic. In 4.20(b), the upper left calibration corner. These errors are easy to spot in a highly structured design and task, such as in reading, whereas in other tasks it will be much more difficult to identify these offsets.

3. The most proper solution is to position the stimulus (monitor) so that both top and bottom corners are OK for the large majority of participants. This you have to do when building the recording environment and setting up the geometry of your experiment. A greater distance from the participant to the monitor will lower the maximum visual angles required and alleviate these problem, but it will also lower the difference in angles between different areas of interest and lower the accuracy and precision.

4.5.5 Calibration validation

It is important to never take a calibration at face value. A participant may have shifted his eyes just as you or the system captured the eye as representative for that particular calibration marker. The simplest solution is, right after the calibration, to show an image containing the calibration markers and ask the participant to look at the markers while you verify them visually on the control computer.

Some systems provide a numeric accuracy value of the average deviation between markers and gaze position. This accuracy value should be reported when you submit your article or report, but in the past this has been unusual. High-end systems exhibit values around 0.2°, whereas a maximum average deviation of 0.5° should be demanded for most studies. An average deviation of 1.0° would be unacceptable for instance for reading research investigating preview benefits and word landing positions, and some remotes produce 1.5° or larger average offset. If you use this number, be sure to relate the reported visual degree value to your particular stimuli display: how much off can the data be before your analysis suffers? Recalibrate until the validation values is below your required accuracy. Only then start the data recording.

It is important to keep in mind the difference between the estimated accuracy and the real accuracy. Even if you perform a validation, the validation points will also suffer from a random or systematic error. A realistic goal would be to have the offsets for the calibration/validation targets as small and random, i.e. offset equally in all directions, as practically possible. For studies that require very high accuracy, there exist correction methods that can be used immediately subsequent to calibration. For instance, Santini, Redner, Iovin, and Rucci (2007) describe a method in which raw data samples are shown on top of the calibration points, and a joystick is used to alter the underlying transformation matrix so that data are right above the points.

Although precision is just as important to validate as accuracy, in practice precision validation is very uncommon. An exception is Santini et al. (2007).

4.5.6 Binocular and head-tracking calibration

There are two special cases in which additional calibration work is necessary: binocular calibration, and calibration using head-tracking based eye-trackers.

Liversedge, White, et al. (2006) recommend a separate calibration for each eye when using (true) binocular recording and you are interested in investigating the disparity between the eyes. Calibrating both eyes at once may give an erroneous (absolute) disparity value, because the calibration routine believes that both eyes are directed towards the calibration point, when in fact one eye may be off. Other researchers, for instance Nuthmann and Kliegl (2009) argue that making separate calibrations of each eye is ecologically invalid, and report disparity measures even after simultaneous binocular calibration. Clearly, the relative disparity, and changes in disparity, will still be correctly measured.

When using head-tracking systems, additional calibration of the combined measurement system is typically necessary, but we refer to manufacturer manuals for details.

4.5.7 Calibration tricks with head-mounted systems

This section presents four calibration tricks that can be used on versatile head-mounted video-overlay eye-trackers to improve their performance. This concerns eye-trackers mounted on and moving with the participant, but otherwise working on the same eye-tracking principles described in this book.

Since calibration for such a system really only concerns calibration points in the scene video—the physical calibration points are only there to make the participant look at what corresponds to the right point in the video—it is possible for the participant to turn his/her head just as much as they want. This can be used in cramped places with partially unfortunate lighting conditions, such as sunlight, where there only is a single good physical target available. Choose one single physical calibration point so that the eye video looks good when the participant is looking in that direction. Then, for each calibration point, turn the participant's head so that the single physical calibration point is aligned with the calibration point in the video. If the participant continues to look at the physical point, he will in effect look in the correct directions for calibration, and the gaze-overlaid video data will be fine.

Another trick is to make a head-mounted system into an eye-tracker that yields a data file with absolute coordinates for an easier analysis. To do this, lock the head-mounted eye-tracker onto something, so it does not move relative to the stimulus monitor. You would probably have to build some construction. If successful, the eye video coordinates of your eye-tracker will be possible to use as coordinates in the stimulus monitor, and you can use the data file for fixation analysis, area of interest analysis, etc., which is currently not possible when your participant is moving around. There may be cases when such an approach is the easier option, e.g. in very specific environments when your standard remote or tower-mounted eye tracking will not fit, such as in a vehicle.

Yet another trick is to tilt the calibration area, if your system only supports a single stimulus area or plane. Suppose you are studying a car driver's gaze to interior controls on the dashboard, and also want to get high quality data for the outside traffic. If you calibrate all points outside the car, you will have a considerable parallax error (p. 60) for gazes inside the car. If you calibrate inside the car, you will have parallax error for outside targets. However, the calibration plane does not have to be orthogonal to the line of sight. Put the lower calibration points on the dashboard, and the upper points 10 metres in front of the car, to get a (more or less) parallax-free precision both on the dashboard and on the outside of the car.

A final tweak to get good data is when you have already calibrated, but notice that the gaze cursor is systematically offset in one direction or another due to movement of the head-band or the helmet, then it is possible to ask the participant to keep the eyes still at a particular position and then gently shift the scene camera or the entire system so that the offset disappears. This will allow you to fine-tune your calibration without re-doing the complete calibration, which may be an option in the field. Always do a validation test after this adjustment so you can determine later, during post-processing when you are looking at the recorded data, whether to include this data or not.

4.6 Instructions and start of recording

The last thing you should do before recording is to instruct your participants about the task. Be precise, and use exactly the same instructions for all participants. A written instruction is usually more similar between participants than a verbal instruction. If your participants have different conceptions of the task, they are very likely to behave differently. Task instruction has a very strong influence on eye-movement behaviour, as elegantly shown by Buswell (1935, p. 136ff) and Yarbus (1967, p. 174ff), and later largely replicated by Lipps and Pelz (2004) and DeAngelus and Pelz (2009). Note that when recording participant speech, additional specific instructions may be necessary.

If a computer program shows your stimuli, have that program start and stop your recording, as well as synchronizing it with changes in the stimulus display. Starting and stopping manually requires some amount of post-recording cutting of the data files. Synchronizing change of stimulus manually gives errors anywhere from 500 ms up to many minutes (if the operators are distracted). Sometimes manual start of recording is necessary, however, for instance, for field recordings in the real world.

Manipulating the eye camera set-up during recording can be necessary when the eye slowly disappears from the eye video, usually as a consequence of a head-mounted eye-tracker slipping or the participant slumping together slightly when relaxing. It will always disturb the participant, however, and often introduces measurement error. Some eye-tracking systems have built-in tools for quick recalibrating, which can be used in a pause between trials. On some older systems, recalibration was required often, such as once per line of read text. Newer systems with stable tracking can be left running for a long time without recalibrating or drift correction. However, if you know your system has drift issues, i.e. when the offset increases over time, then it is important to plan for frequent drift corrections between trials or blocks.

During recording, keep your eye on the eye video, and preferably keep a record of what happens: is the data good in the entire visual field? Is there a downward offset in the upper left corner? Is there a split corneal reflection problem? Is the data stable, or are there many optic artefacts? Taking such quality notes will be important for later interpretation of the data. Some of the problems can be remedied after recording, but some should be taken care of during recording. You can improve the eye video during recording: changing the focus of the camera and altering the threshold for pupil identification typically alters you data very little. But do not change the camera angle towards the eye, or the position of the infrared illumination. Such alterations will give you a permanent offset in your data, unless followed by immediate recalibration.

4.7 Auxiliary data: recording

This section covers the concurrent recording of auxiliary data along with eye movements and therefore may be regarded as optional for those solely concerned with learning the techniques of eye-movement recording. If you record only eye-movement data, you can skip to p. 139, but as we noted on pp. 95–108, there are many reasons why you may want to combine eye-movement data with other types of recordings. Here we will describe how to make combined recordings in three different types of technical set-ups:

Non-interfering set-ups *Reaction time tests* and *galvanic skin response* (GSR) are both technically simple and do not interfere with the eye-tracker in the sense that they do not cause reflections in the eye movements, large head movements, or other large sources of error.

Interfering set-ups *Motion tracking, EEG/ERP*, and *fMRI* are technically and methodologically challenging, and may interfere with the eye-tracker (or the eye-tracker may interfere with the auxiliary hardware). For example, a contact-based eye-tracker will generate noise if the EEG electrodes touch the eye-tracker or if the eye-tracker generates much electromagnetic noise.

Verbal elicitations *Verbal data* may interfere with the eye-tracker, or vice versa, and may require additional instructions in order to acquire a high enough data quality (pp. 105–106), but is such a common auxiliary data source that it warrants its own section.

4.7.1   Non-interfering set-ups

Reaction time tests are often measured using a so-called *button-box* with a limited number of buttons, and giving the participant the instruction to click the correct button—right for yes, and left for no, for instance—as soon as they know the answer to the question. Using a third-party stimulus and synchronization software, reaction time latency measurements are easy to combine with eye tracking. Unless the click causes vibrations in the eye-tracker (p. 35), there is no interference between reaction time tests and eye tracking. Some manufacturers (e.g. SR Research) provide software for reactions time tests to be incorporated into the design of an experiment simply using the existing keyboard, but note that button boxes have better temporal characteristics, and other software specifically designed for the kinds of reaction time tests used in studies on attention can easily be used in conjunction with eye tracking.

Galvanic skin response (GSR) measures the electrical conductivity of the skin using electrodes which are usually put on one or two fingers of the participant. The variation in GSR signal corresponds to the autonomic nerve response as a parameter of the sweat gland function. Most GSR systems can be run at the same sampling frequency as eye-trackers, but stimulus presentation and synchronization may have to be dealt with using third-party software. There is no mechanical or electromagnetic interference between the GSR and eye-tracking systems.

4.7.2   Interfering set-ups

Eye-trackers that work for participants inside the intense magnetic field of the fMRI tunnel have been sold for quite some time, but the market is small, and the benefit of eye tracking to fMRI (or vice versa) is still unclear to many users.

An eye-tracker that works in a strong magnetic field must be built differently from the eye-trackers we saw in Chapter 2. All electronics must be at a far enough distance from the magnet, so fMRI-compatible eye-trackers use long-range cameras and mirrors close to the participant, as in Figure 4.21.

Initially, eye-movement recording in combination with *EEG* was done using an EOG (electro-oculography) system. EEG sensors and EOG sensors are the same, only placed differently. As eye movements and blinks give rise to problematic artefacts in EEG data, many current-day EEG systems include EOG sensors. The EOG data can then be used to filter the

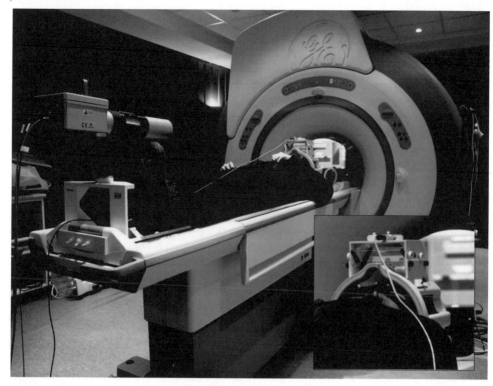

Fig. 4.21 Long-range eye-tracker for use in fMRI environment. The participant has two mirrors above his face: one mirror for the eye camera to film through, the other for projecting the stimulus image. Image used with kind permission from SMI GmbH.

eye movements and blink signals in the EEG data (T.-P. Jung et al., 2000). Even now, EOG data is used to remove the movement and blink artefacts from the EEG signal, using what is known as the *surrogate multiple source eye correction* (P. Berg & Scherg, 1994). Here, a number of reference eye movements are recorded before the actual experimental data. a PCA (principle component analysis) reveals the artefact topographies, and the waveforms from these can be modelled in the experimental data so that overcorrection is avoided. After subtraction of the artefact waveforms, the EEG data will be cleaned from oculomotoric artefacts.

In later years, EEG recordings were also combined with video-based eye-movement recordings. Figure 4.22 shows how a tower-mounted high-precision eye-tracker and a remote eye-tracker are used in combination with EEG. In neither of the two studies where these combinations were used could we detect electromagnetic interference between the two systems, not even in the tower-mounted eye-tracker where the electronics are really close. We did see some mechanical interference in the tower-mounted eye-tracker, however (Simola, Holmqvist, & Lindgren, 2009). Leaning a forehead covered with EEG sensors against the head stabilizer of the tower-mounted eye-tracker was easy for some participants, but it was difficult for some to keep still. The eye-tracker tended to lose data as participants changed position and the eye moved out of camera view, but EEG data appeared not to be affected, either from eye-tracking equipment or TFT monitors. CRT monitors may have to be shielded.

The EEG system should be mounted and calibrated on the participant first, as it will always take longer than the eye-tracker set-up and calibration.

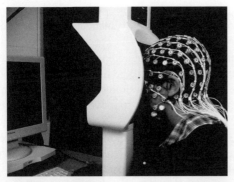 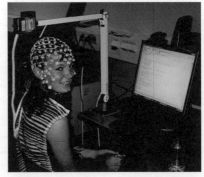

(a) When the EEG net is in close contact with the head-stabilizing part of a tower-mounted eye-tracker, data in both systems are sensitive to slippage: the eye may move outside of the camera image as the participant attempts to find a comfortable position. The foremost sensors on the cap or net may slip on the forehead. For participants who can remain still, data is excellent, however. The 128-channel HydroCel EGI Geodesic SensorNet and the SMI 240 Hz HiSpeed eye-tracker.

(b) With a remote eye-tracker, there is no contact between the two systems. The participant is free to move her head, and there is less physical interference. Remotes invariably give a poorer data quality than tower-mounted systems, however. The 128-channel HydroCel EGI Geodesic SensorNet and the SMI RED IV 50 Hz remote eye-tracker.

Fig. 4.22 EEG and tower-mounted versus remote eye tracking.

Motion trackers exist both as magnetic and optic varieties, but optic ones are more common and versatile. Since they also operate with infrared light and reflections, optic motion trackers could potentially disturb the eye-tracker, or in odd circumstances the other way around, but in our experience this rarely happens. Directing the motion tracker cameras differently and turning down the light intensity of their lamps may remedy interference. Many motion trackers run at the same range of sampling frequencies as eye-trackers.

4.7.3 Verbal data

Verbal data can be recorded *concurrently* during eye-tracking recording or *retrospectively*, after eye-tracking recording (pp. 101–105). The point in time of recording the verbal data may influence the quality of the eye-tracking data dependent on the *type of eye-tracker*, as we will see in the following. Thus, before deciding when to record the verbal data, you have to consider which type of eye-tracker you have and what kind of cutbacks you are willing to accept in the quality of your eye-tracking data. If you decide to record the verbal data retrospectively, the verbal data should be cued by a replay of the participant's eye-tracking data to stimulate the participant's memory of their thoughts (compare Van Gog, Paas, & Van Merriënboer, 2005). Consequently, you have to consider *how to present* these eye-tracking data to the participant. Irrespective of when you record the verbal data, the crucial issue is how you *instruct* your participants to provide unbiased verbalizations (p. 105).

Task interference and tracking robustness

When recording verbalizations *concurrently*, make sure that the participant is able to speak freely. Remote, tower-mounted, and head-mounted eye-trackers interfere differently with the speech movements of the participant, as will be stressed in this section. Having participants talk while being eye-tracked also introduces a somewhat poorer quality in the eye-movement data, in the form of increased noise levels, optic artefacts, or inaccuracies, simply because participants move more when they speak, and the various head movement compensations can not always keep up.

When recording with a *remote* eye-tracking system (without adding a forehead rest), the influence of speech movements on eye-tracking data quality will be moderate. For instance, fast head movements may not be compensated for, and the physiology around the eye may change as speech muscles move. The freedom of the participant to move their head is likely to give better concurrent speech quality, however.

When using a *head-mounted* system (or a remote system with a forehead rest), concurrent verbalizations do not disturb the eye movement recordings as much. In this case, an additional microphone needs to be used, which will be attached to the participant.

A *tower-mounted* high-end system does restrict head movements, but care must be taken not to restrict jaw movements during concurrent speech; such precautions may however jeopardize eye-movement data quality instead. Retrospective verbalizations will provide the best eye-tracking data.

When recording *retrospective* verbalizations, the major technological challenge is to minimize the delay from the end of recording eye-movement data until recording of retrospective verbalizations is started. A longer delay means poorer quality of verbal data, as the participant's memory quickly deteriorates. The bottleneck is the possibility of showing the eye-movement data very quickly to the participant, and start sound recording fast. Different manufacturers offer varying support for this. Some software allows for a direct and quick replay of recorded eye movements. Others require the researcher to export the recorded eye-movement data from the recording software and then import these data to the analysis software before they can be shown. Another important technological feature for retrospective verbalizations is the ability to replay the recordings full-screen, so that the participant is not distracted by the user interface of an eye-tracking data analysis software. Further potentially important technological features include being able to display the participant's eye movements with transparent dots and scanpaths, so that important parts of the display are not occluded.

Note that participants may not only speak about their own eye-movement data, but may very well point to them, using deictic references like "there" and "it" towards the indicated item. With frequent pointing comes a need to record video along with sound, and to transcribe pointing activities.

How to display the eye-movement data when recording cued retrospective verbalizations

When recording verbal data retrospectively, the aim is to elicit thoughts as close as possible to the actual thoughts during the experiment. This leads to better results—in terms of less forgetting and less fabricating—when participants' verbalizations are cued (Van Someren et al., 1994).

Participants' eye-movement data may be shown to him either as *static* visualizations (showing a longer sequence at once), or *dynamic* visualizations (momentous). It is likely—although not proven—that these two types of eye movement visualizations elicit different verbal data from the participant, since they deliver different types of information. We would argue that each visualization has its own advantages depending on the task participants have to accomplish during the experiment and your research question, but academic research into this method is lacking.

Static visualizations of eye movements give an overview over a longer span of time, typically the entire trial (webpage, learning instruction, or sentence to be translated). The temporal order of a short scanpath can be shown by order numbers of the fixations. For longer sequences, the temporal extension during which the scanpath is visible may be interactively altered to reveal the order. Having an overview can be expected to prime the participant to comment on relations between inspecting different areas, like why there are a lot of saccades between two areas, but not between others, or explaining the inspection of areas with lots of fixations. However, it is very likely that the order of inspection will be neglected, and that only areas that were intensively inspected are mentioned.

A dynamic visualization of eye movements instead shows the momentous dynamics of visual behaviour, with no overview at all. The real-time perspective of the dynamic eye-movement visualization is likely to trigger participant comments on the instant decisions, hesitation, and considerations, but it is also more demanding for the participant. Since the participant has no overview of his gaze behaviour over the whole inspection, it is very un-likely that he will comment on larger attention shifts in space over time. Since dynamic eye-movement visualization is also quite fast, reducing the playback speed may be necessary to allow the participant time to reflect on what he had been thinking during the task (Kammerer, Bråten, Gerjets, & Strømsø, 2010). However, slowing down the recording is not always ap-propriate. For stimuli that depict dynamic content a slowed speed would change the features of the stimulus itself. Another possibility is to reiterate the dynamic eye-movement visual-ization several times to give the participant several chances (Jarodzka, Scheiter, et al., 2010). This possibility, however, is difficult in terms of analysis later on. For instance, what if a par-ticipant, who viewed the eye-movement visualization several times, makes a more detailed description of the stimulus than another participant who viewed his eye-movement visual-ization only once? In such cases, at least time on task has to be added as covariate into the analyses. A third possibility is to enable a self-paced, participant-governed eye movement visualization; this might help the participant even more to deal with the complexity of the presented data (Van Gog, Paas, Van Merriënboer, & Witte, 2005). Again, very different du-rations of inspecting eye-movement visualizations may however occur. Moreover, it is likely that not all participants are equally able to estimate their need to adapt the eye-movement vi-sualization. This in turn would result in diverse quality of verbal data. A final concern would be if dynamic visualizations put social pressure on the participant to produce more, as more events unfold in the visualization, yet the participant has nothing to contribute. Then this social pressure may result in a participant confabulating to escape the pressure.

How to elicit verbalizations from participants

When recording verbal data as thinking aloud the precise instruction to the participants is of great importance (p. 105). The instruction for the participant is done in three steps: *instruct-ing*, *training*, and *reminding*. It is important that the participant feels comfortable during recording. Training before the actual recording helps the participant become familiar with the situation and task. Moreover, it helps when as few people as possible are in the recording room, so the participant does not feel monitored. In case the participant stops verbalizing his thoughts, the experimenter has to gently *remind* him to go on.

4.8 Debriefing

After all data collection is done, debrief the participant. It may be a good idea to start by asking the participant if he can guess what the study was about. You might do this to see if the actual purpose of the study is (too) transparent. Then, tell the participant what the study was really all about. This is particularly important if the experiment was based on deception or the nature of the experiment is likely to influence the participant's belief in his abilities, such as a reading test (see e.g., D. Sharpe & Faye, 2009 for a discussion about debriefing). As part of debriefing, you should also ask them to sign your written informed consent document, unless this was done before the data recording. Inform the participant that his recorded data

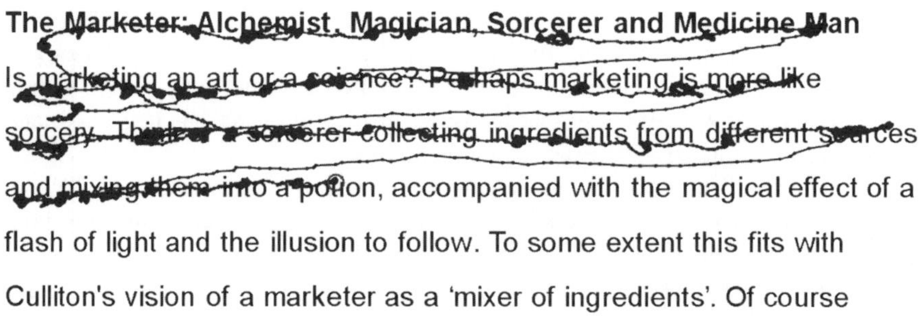

The Marketer: Alchemist, Magician, Sorcerer and Medicine Man

Is marketing an art or a science? Perhaps marketing is more like

sorcery. Think of a sorcerer collecting ingredients from different sources

and mixing them into a potion, accompanied with the magical effect of a

flash of light and the illusion to follow. To some extent this fits with

Culliton's vision of a marketer as a 'mixer of ingredients'. Of course

Fig. 4.23 Good data quality. Raw samples (1250 Hz), showing fixations as blobs and saccades as lines.

will be anonymized and that he can withdraw data at any point. Make sure to underline that the participant is welcome to get in touch anytime, with any questions he may have. He might not want his data to be used in the overall analysis of the study, and if this is the case ethical principles dictate that this request must be respected. Also during debriefing, see to it that your participant has your contact information. In practice, previous participants almost never get in contact with us, but they should be able to if they wish.

If possible, procure an inconvenience allowance for participants, but beware of tax regulations and complex administration. Some tax legislations force experimenters to formally hire their participants above a certain reward level. This is important to check before you start giving out money. Finally, ask the participants not to reveal the purpose of the study, should they bump into someone they know, who might be your participant the next day, and who should not know about its purpose.

If you have done everything right, your participant will leave feeling at ease, happy with having contributed to research.

4.9   Preparations for data analysis

After the data recording is finished, backup and classification of data proceeds. We now have a set of files containing data that will be pre-processed and then analysed.

4.9.1   Data quality

As we pointed out on page 87, the first thing to do after data are backed up is to investigate data quality. Data quality can to some extent be measured by recording participant fixations on a collection of points just before, during, and after recording, and then calculating precision and accuracy values in each point. Usually, however, data quality is estimated by visual inspection of scanpath visualizations, of which many have been shown in this chapter, and velocity over time graphs, which we introduced on page 48, and which will be much used in the next chapter.

When exhibited as a scanpath, good data quality looks as in Figure 4.23. When we recently recorded reading data from 310 participants—of which one is shown in Figure 4.23—around 90% of the data have this quality. Fixations are more or less right on the word (so we can make area of interest analysis), and the precision is good enough for the fixation and saccade algorithms. The figure shows raw samples, because disturbances are more clearly seen—event detection smoothens scanpaths considerably, as we will soon see.

In some portions of your data, quality may be lower. A participant can have good data for some trials or parts of trials, and horrible data elsewhere. Data quality can also vary across the stimulus, being excellent in one part and awful in another. Whether the problem is an offset, low precision, optic artefacts, or complete data loss in one portion of the field of view, it matters, because the nature of your data quality determines its suitability for different subsequent analyses. For instance, the corner offset in Figure 4.20 does not prevent you from making a calculation of fixation durations, but area-of-interest order data based on word-position regions would be invalid. Therefore, it is useful to make data quality notes during recordings when you can see in real time what is going on— and use those notes to sort your data files to different analyses. Later, confirm uncertain judgments by inspecting raw scanpath and velocity-over-time plots. Some data files you will simply have to throw away, for some you can possibly do partial analysis—like the top half of the monitor when you had a drooping eyelid participant; maybe you can only calculate fixation durations for some recordings. Just remember that if you use data with poor quality for a dependent variable that it is not suited for, you will end up presenting false results in your papers.

How much of the data can you expect to have to throw away? In our experience, around 2–5% of the data from a population of average non-pre-screened Europeans needs to be dismissed due to participant-specific tracking difficulties. However, this number varies significantly: Schnipke and Todd (2000), Mullin, Anderson, Smallwood, Jackson, and Katsavras (2001) and Pernice and Nielsen (2009) report data losses of 20–60% of participants/trials, and Burmester and Mast (2010) excluded 12 out of 32 participants due to calibration (7) and tracking issues (5). The amount of data loss can be related to several factors such as the experience of the experimenter, the quality and flexibility (possibility of changing set-up of camera and mirrors) of the hardware, the complexity of the experiment, the calibration procedure, and how well the recording environment is controlled. Also, when combining EEG nets and tower-mounted systems, the data loss may increase to almost 1/3 of the data (Simola, Holmqvist, & Lindgren, 2009). Using an eye-tracker outdoors, near sunlight, and in cars may lead to a considerable data loss due to ambient lighting conditions. Y. Wang et al. (2010) lost data from 32% of the participants in field car driving, for instance. However, these data losses should also be seen in a wider perspective, for at least two reasons. Screening participants beforehand so only those with no glasses, no lenses, wide-open eyes, not too bright iris, and upward lashes, are invited as participants, can give a 100% tracking robustness, but it should also be noted that this may involve recruiting a subset of the population that may not be representative. Additionally, reading about data loss in an article paper must not necessarily mean there were technological difficulties, but that the researchers were very picky about their quality criteria and rather removed data than include overly noisy or invalid data.

There is no standard criterion for *how* to select the data to discard, however. Criteria used in literature include, for instance, the percentage of zero values in the raw data samples, a high offset (poor accuracy) value during validation, a high number of events with a velocity above $800°/s$, and an average fixation velocity above $15°/s$ (indicative of low precision). For an example of accuracy and data loss criteria, see Komogortsev, Gobert, Jayarathna, Koh, and Gowda (2010).

4.9.2 Analysis software for eye-tracking data

Analysis softwares naturally lag behind the research front. The ones that exist sometimes leave the researcher no other option than to program the analysis herself. Historically, analysis software have moved through three levels of sophistication.

- The simplest (and oldest) ones can import one data file (that is one participant) at a time, and include a calculation of fixations (using some algorithm), the possibility of drawing areas of interest on stimulus images, and a few visualizations—typically a scanpath or a proportion of gaze to different areas of interest—but only for one participant at a

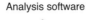

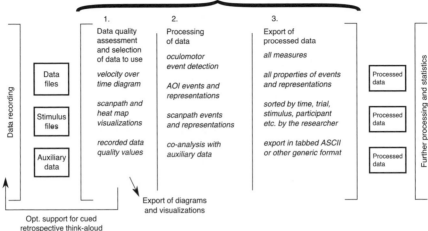

Fig. 4.24 An analysis software takes data files resulting from recording for an experiment. The three stages 1–3 correspond to a typical workflow in research, with italicized terms for visualizations, tools, and export possibilities. After data analysis, further processing and statistics take part in other, dedicated software.

time. Randomization of stimulus images is not resolved. Up until around 2000, this is what most researchers had to work with, unless they programmed analysis themselves.

- The middle level software is more integrated with recording and stimulus presentation programs. It can import a large number of stimulus images that have been used in an experiment, and resolve randomization. It exports a few (4–30) types of tables with data for several participants or several images at once. It is still more oriented towards visualizations than to export of structured data, however. These softwares first appeared in the early 2000s.

- The highest level of software is tightly integrated with recording and stimulus presentation software. The software allows for analysis of data from varying technical set-ups. It allows the user not only a choice between several fixation algorithms, but also powerful area of interest, scanpath, and attention map analyses. It allows the user to group participants, stimuli, and areas of interest according to the experimental design, supports the workflow suggested in this book, including the formatted export of a vast number (50–200) of research-relevant dependent variables into formats that can easily be processed further in a statistics package such as SPSS.

Figure 4.24 shows what three components you should expect in a commercial analysis software. First, tools for assessing the data quality and selecting which data has good enough quality to use. Second, several eye-tracking-specific processing tools, corresponding to Chapter 5–9, should be represented. Third, the export of structured data from the processing tools to statistical software is of great importance.

When we have interviewed them, the developers of analysis software have mentioned two different strategies. Some only provide the most basic output in stage 3 of Figure 4.24, arguing that researchers will be so inventive that new measures will appear all the time and seldom be reused, and that each user should implement any further analyses themselves. Others try to define and implement a set of often recurring analyses that many users can benefit from, which is a much larger undertaking.

	Time	Type	Set	R Raw X [px]	R Dia X [px]		
				R Raw Y [px]	R Dia '		
▼ 📁 Fp1							
📄 fp1_20030405.idf	20529264944	MSG	0	Mpg File: C:\Program Files\SMI			
📄 fp1_20060401.idf	20772109812	MSG	1	# Message: lunch.bmp			
📄 fp1_20061021.idf	20772114110	SMP	1	185.99	41.40	49.68	50.58
📄 fp1_20070331.idf	20772134064	SMP	1	185.32	41.61	50.38	50.53
▼ 📁 Info_and_questions	20772154167	SMP	1	184.67	41.76	49.65	50.54
📄 1_info.mat	20772173852	SMP	1	184.60	41.19	49.75	49.60
📄 1_svar1.mat	20772193838	SMP	1	185.44	35.74	49.62	50.64
📄 1_svar2.mat	20772213743	SMP	1	185.08	36.56	50.49	50.58
📄 1_svar3.mat	20772233878	SMP	1	184.82	36.70	49.71	50.57
📄 1_svar4.mat	20772253904	SMP	1	184.67	36.70	49.73	50.56
📄 1_svar5.mat	20772273651	SMP	1	184.60	36.81	49.65	50.57
📄 wminfo_1.mat	20772281453	MSG	1	# Message: Audiofile: 20070430:			
▶ 📁 Fp2	20772293593	SMP	1	184.39	36.89	50.53	50.58
▶ 📁 Fp3	20772313630	SMP	1	184.21	36.92	50.69	50.57
▶ 📁 Fp4	20772333425	SMP	1	183.96	37.16	49.66	49.55
	20772353814	SMP	1	183.87	37.16	49.72	49.63
	20772373312	SMP	1	183.67	37.27	49.75	49.54

(a) Data files.   (b) Inside each eye-movement data file.

Fig. 4.25 Typical data after data recording is completed, but before analysis is started. Data often reflect the experimental design. In this case (a) shows four binary eye-movement files (`*.idf`) for each participant because there were four conditions, and several auxiliary Matlab (`*.mat`) files with data from questionnaires taken during the trials. Correspondingly, (b) shows that inside each eye-movement file, we find the data for raw samples, one for each line, time stamps, x and y coordinates in the stimulus for the right eye, horizontal and vertical pupil dilation, and on some lines, the onset of stimuli (`lunch.bmp`) and audio recordings.

This book covers the analysis options present in the most advanced types of existing analysis software. Many established eye-tracking laboratories do program their own analyses, however, either because the current software solution for their system is not ideal, not cutting edge, or they do not trust its output. Also, the particular analysis that the researcher wants may not be supported by the software. MatLab seems to be the dominating choice of programming environment for eye-tracking labs, but the freely available programming language Python and the open-source statistical language R are quickly increasing in number of users. Code can easily be shared among laboratories, and some code is made publicly available on the Internet. One absolute requirement for continuing with custom-made analyses is the ability to export into neutral file formats accessible by all software, such as tabbed ascii (.tsv). These files, with eye-tracking data, will look something like Figure 4.25.

When co-analysing eye movements with other data (p. 286), researchers typically use one analysis tool for each type of data, and then do an additional joint analysis in MatLab, R, or other software packages.

4.10 Summary

This chapter has discussed all the potential pitfalls you may encounter during data recording. Additionally, you should now know enough to be able to troubleshoot accuracy and precision problems, and be able to handle participants with more challenging eyes.

Some key insights include:

- Selecting the appropriate stimulus presentation solution for your experiment, knowing the benefits and drawbacks of each.
- Several degrees of freedom are available in most eye-trackers to reposition the system or angle it differently to overcome mascara problems and reflections in glasses.

- Simple tricks can be very effective, such as slightly defocusing the camera if the participant wears contact lenses, or simply having a make-up removal kit in the laboratory to be able to ask participants to remove mascara.
- Participant ethics is important, not only because you have to follow the rules, but because happy participants come back for more experiments, and may help recruit their friends as well.
- If needed, there is the option to record with auxiliary data sources, although these may be more or less disrupting or interfering with your eye-tracking set-up. EEG is challenging to include, but button-box reaction time tests are very unproblematic.

This and the plan you designed for your experiment are the raw material for your data analysis.

Recording high-quality eye-tracking data is a skill that must be learnt through training. Poor data quality can never be remedied by later data processing and statistical analysis, just like a good quality of your data can never compensate for an inadequate experimental design.

Part II

Detecting Events and Building Representations

So far we have dealt with hardware and all the pragmatic issues involved with designing an eye-tracking experiment and recording eye-tracking data. In Part II of this book we explain Events and Representations; Part II thus provides detailed coverage of what you actually do with eye-tracking data once it has been recorded. This includes algorithmic parsing of raw sample data into fixations and saccades, and how eye-tracking data can be gathered together to form meaningful representations, such as attention maps.

5 Estimating Oculomotor Events from Raw Data Samples

In this chapter, we will present the algorithms responsible for calculating *fixations*, *saccades*, *smooth pursuits*, and other events directly from the raw data samples. This chapter is organized as follows.

- In Section 5.1 (p. 148) we introduce the illusively simple calculation of fixations and saccades, illustrated by manufacturers' analysis software.
- Section 5.2 (p. 150) introduces what the algorithms have to work on; namely position, velocity, and acceleration data. We classify the events to be detected and the algorithms that do it.
- In Section 5.3 (p. 153) we provide a condensed list of hands-on advice for the beginning user of an event detection algorithm.
- Current algorithms are far from perfect. In Section 5.4 (p. 154), the major challenges are listed. The selection of settings is given particular emphasis. Read this if you want to know in detail what the algorithms may do with your data.
- If you are interested in the algorithms themselves and the design issues and computational reasons behind them, read Section 5.5 (p. 171).
- Section 5.6 (p. 175) focuses on data recorded onto gaze-overlaid video, for which manual segmentation of fixation duration and other events is often the only option.
- Blink events (Section 5.7, p. 176) are easily detected, but smooth pursuit is not (Section 5.8, p. 175).
- Noise and artefacts (Section 5.9, p. 181) are not even considered events, but there are good reasons for algorithms to detect such periods, and for us as researchers to decide how to treat them.
- There are detection algorithms also for some of the lesser known events, for instance microsaccades and square-wave jerks (Section 5.10, p. 182).
- The chapter is summarized in Section 5.11 (p. 185) by listing the events that can be detected and the values of which we carry with us for further analysis.

Very often, the first step in data analysis is the calculation of *events* such as fixations and saccades, with all their parameters. Indeed, the fixation and saccade values exported by the algorithms of this chapter are of great importance. They are heavily used in research in themselves, as well as in a multitude of combinations with other ways to measure and visualize eye-tracking data. Sometimes, it is even thought to be impossible to analyse eye-tracking data without this calculation. This is wrong, however. In many cases, fixation and saccade analysis is *not* a prerequisite to data analysis. For instance, heat map visualizations and the dwell time measure (p. 386) and scanpath length (p. 319) can all be calculated on raw unprocessed data just as well. Only raw data, but not fixations, can be taken as input when the analysis is tightly connected to running sample time, as with proportion over time curves (p. 197).

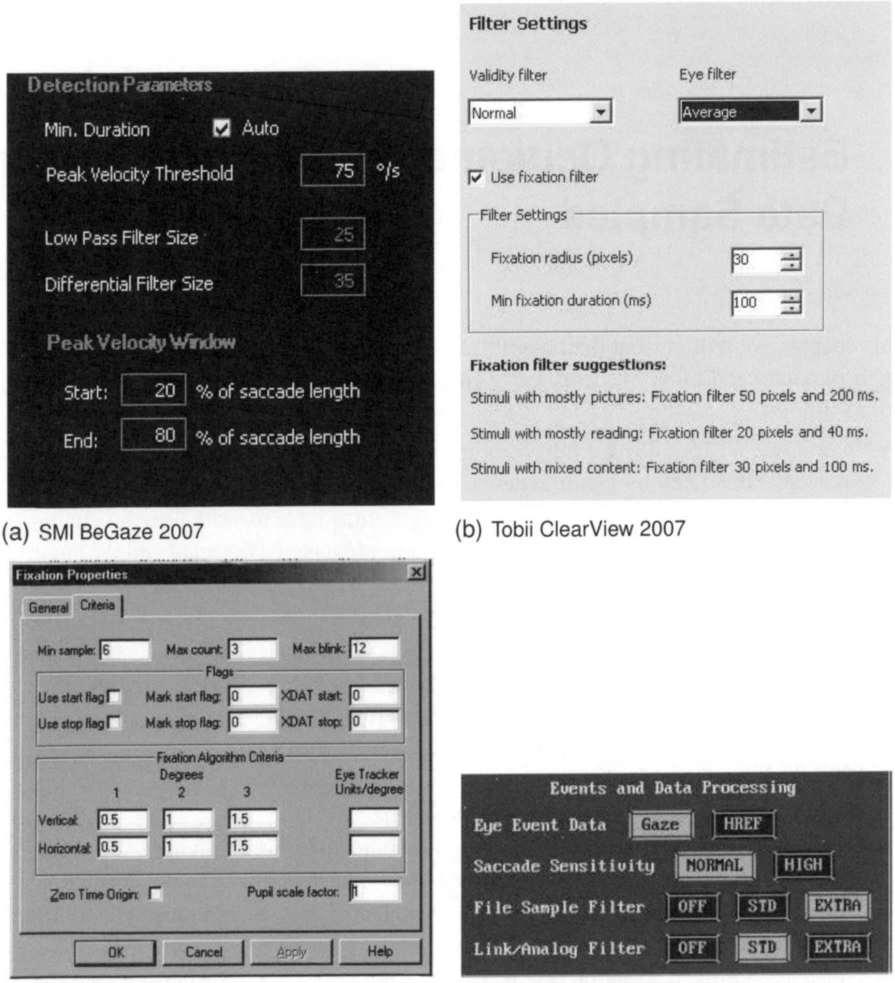

Detection Parameters

Min. Duration ☑ Auto

Peak Velocity Threshold [75] °/s

Low Pass Filter Size [25]

Differential Filter Size [35]

Peak Velocity Window

Start: [20] % of saccade length

End: [80] % of saccade length

(a) SMI BeGaze 2007

Filter Settings

Validity filter   Eye filter

[Normal ▼]   [Average ▼]

☑ Use fixation filter

Filter Settings

Fixation radius (pixels)   [30 ⇕]

Min fixation duration (ms)   [100 ⇕]

Fixation filter suggestions:

Stimuli with mostly pictures: Fixation filter 50 pixels and 200 ms.

Stimuli with mostly reading: Fixation filter 20 pixels and 40 ms.

Stimuli with mixed content: Fixation filter 30 pixels and 100 ms.

(b) Tobii ClearView 2007

Fixation Properties   ✕

| General | Criteria |

Min sample: [6]   Max count: [3]   Max blink: [12]

Flags

Use start flag ☐   Mark start flag: [0]   XDAT start: [0]

Use stop flag ☐   Mark stop flag: [0]   XDAT stop: [0]

Fixation Algorithm Criteria

	Degrees			Eye Tracker Units/degree
	1	2	3	
Vertical:	0.5	1	1.5	
Horizontal:	0.5	1	1.5	

Zero Time Origin: ☐   Pupil scale factor: [1]

[OK]   [Cancel]   [Apply]   [Help]

(c) ASL Eyenal 2004

Events and Data Processing

Eye Event Data   [Gaze] [HREF]

Saccade Sensitivity [NORMAL] [HIGH]

File Sample Filter   [OFF] [STD] [EXTRA]

Link/Analog Filter   [OFF] [STD] [EXTRA]

(d) SR EyeLink 2007

Fig. 5.1 Settings dialogues for fixation analysis in three analysis packages and one recording software from commercial eye-tracking manufacturers.

5.1 The setting dialogues and the output

In theory, the event detection algorithm takes raw, possibly filtered data samples and tries to detect events within them. The most reported of such events are fixations and saccades. It sounds simple and something that could be done automatically, and that we should not really have to bother thinking about, and indeed software engineers have made it illusively simple to use fixation algorithms. All you have to do is to accept the pre-set values in a dialogue like those in Figure 5.1, and click OK.

In reality, however, these setting dialogues provoke many questions: What does minimal time or minimum fixation duration actually mean? What is a fixation radius, and how does it relate to monitor resolution, measured in pixels? And what is peak velocity threshold? When is a normal saccade-detection sensitivity better than a high sensitivity; should not high sensitivity always be better? And what do all the ASL Eyenal parameters mean? How sensible are the suggestions given in the Tobii dialogue? Why should there be different settings for different kinds of stimuli: are fixations more stable in reading than in picture viewing when

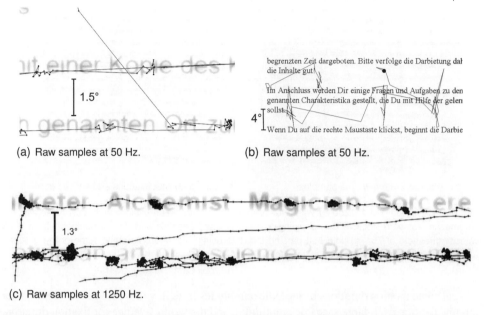

(a) Raw samples at 50 Hz.

(b) Raw samples at 50 Hz.

(c) Raw samples at 1250 Hz.

Fig. 5.2 Enlarged views of raw samples plotted against the stimulus background. Note how close samples are to one another in the 1250 Hz recording compared to the 50 Hz data, in particular during long saccades. Also note the low precision in (b) recording compared to (a) and (c).

such recordings are taken on the same eye-tracker? Is there a danger that my data is too noisy to do a fixation analysis, or does filtering automatically fix this? Does it matter what settings I choose? The purpose of this chapter is to give a better understanding of how event detection works, and provide insights into how to approach a settings dialogue such as the ones in Figure 5.1.

Figure 5.2 shows the *input*, the raw data samples, from three different eye-trackers. The raw data constitute the data that you get from your eye-tracker after recording. When plotting raw data against the background of the stimulus, each data sample is a little dot. During a saccade, when the eye is moving quickly, the distance between dots is large. During fixations, the dots aggregate to form one large blob from many dots. How closely the raw sample dots are positioned is directly related to the sampling frequency of your eye-tracker. How smooth the raw data appear is a direct consequence of the precision of the eye-tracker. Both these system properties are crucial to how the fixation and saccade algorithms are designed, and largely decide what a given algorithm can deliver.

In Figure 5.2(c), a full stimulus display is shown with an overlaid raw data plot. Fixation blobs and thinner saccadic lines are clearly seen. Vertical lines are blinks in progress. At the bottom and to the left, there is some high-velocity noise, probably caused by a dual corneal reflection; either a split corneal reflection, or one real and one falsely detected. Overall, this is the type of data you should expect from your eye-tracker. Figure 5.3(b) shows fixations and saccades calculated from the same raw data, using manufacturer software and default settings. Fixations are now seen as circles with a diameter indicating the duration, and abstracted straight lines for saccades. During the fixation analysis, blinks and artefacts were filtered off. In total, the fixation scanpath looks much cleaner than the raw data plot. Nevertheless, there is something deeply wrong with the scanpath of fixations and saccades. A lot of fixations that we can clearly see in the raw data plot are gone. There are two fixations on the word "Magician" in the first line, for instance, that have simply disappeared after event detection. Each line has lost one or more fixations. If you were to export this fixation and saccade data,

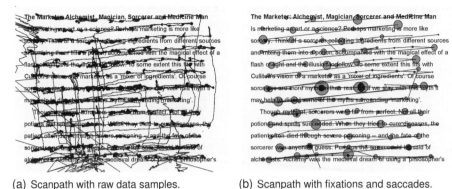

(a) Scanpath with raw data samples.   (b) Scanpath with fixations and saccades.

Fig. 5.3 Data recorded at 1250 Hz with a tower-mounted eye-tracker. Fixations were calculated with the commercial software BeGaze 2.1, applying a velocity-based analysis and default settings with a peak velocity threshold of $75°/s$. Note that parsing the data using this algorithm omits some of the grouped samples of 'blobs' which from manual inspection seem to be valid fixations.

and calculate fixation durations or saccadic amplitudes from it, you would get erroneous data: too few fixations, too large saccadic amplitudes, and the wrong average for fixation duration. You would use corrupted data, and the results you present in your report or journal paper may not be valid.

5.2 Principles and algorithms for event detection

Before we start addressing event detection in more detail, let us stop for a moment and reflect over what an event is. For example, should we always look for blobs in the raw gaze plots when we want to find a fixation, or can the fixation event be defined by other criteria?

The only raw material all algorithms have to work with is the stream of data samples recorded by the eye-tracker. In this stream of data samples, there are sometimes portions that exhibit a prototypical behaviour signifying that an *oculomotor event* has been recorded. For example, the saccade event is loosely defined as a period when the eye 'moves fast', and the fixation event where the eye 'is rather still'. The goal of *event detection* is to, according to a set of rules, robustly extract such events from the stream of data samples. Most often, this is done automatically by applying a detection algorithm to the gaze data, but it can also be done manually using subjective judgements.

Event terms such as 'fixation' are used both for the events algorithmically or manually detected in the data stream, and the oculomotor events of the eye that were recorded. In reality, perfect matches between the fixations detected by an algorithm and moments of stillness of the eye are very rare. To make matters worse, the term fixation is sometimes also used for the period during which the fixated entity is cognitively processed by the participant. The oculomotor, the algorithmically detected, and the cognitive 'fixations' largely overlap, but are not the same. When reading, for instance, it is considered proven that a word can be processed parafoveally prior to being fixated (Rayner, 1998). It is in fact easy to decouple the fixation position from the position where attention is located and processing takes place, if the task and stimuli are simple (Posner, 1980).

Furthermore, there are 'eye-in-head' fixations when the eye is still in its socket, irrespective of whether the head moves or not, and 'eye-on-stimulus' fixations when the eye is fixated on a target but possibly moving inside the head to compensate for head and body motion. Only when the head is immobile relative to the stimulus are they identical.

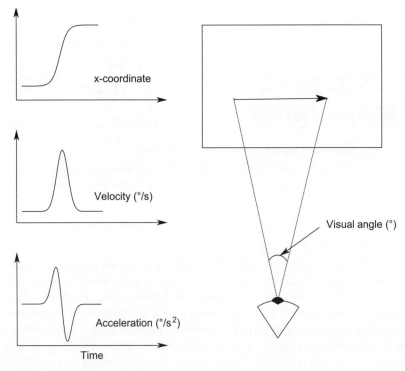

Fig. 5.4 Idealized gaze position, velocity, and acceleration profile over time showing one saccade in-between the end of a fixation (to the left of the saccade) and the beginning of a new fixation (to the right of the saccade).

The term 'fixation' in this chapter refers to an event in the data file that has been detected by an algorithm or subjectively by a person. 'Fixation' in this chapter does *not* refer to the cognitive event during which the fixated entity is processed by the participant (for a discussion about the relationship between fixation and cognitive processing, see page 377).

Event detection algorithms make use of three data streams from the recording and subsequent calculations: Gaze position (x, y), gaze velocity (in $°/s$) and gaze acceleration (in $°/s^2$). Besides pupil size which is sometimes used to detect blinks, that is all there is. Figure 5.4 illustrates such data from an idealized saccade[15] represented by the vector to the right in the figure. Velocity is calculated using the distance between two data samples (first derivative of gaze position), while acceleration is estimated from three consecutive samples (second derivative of gaze position).[16] Wyatt (1998) proposes the use of jerk (the third derivative of gaze position) to identify saccades, but it is noisy and fairly impractical in software implementations. As we saw in Chapter 2, filtering can significantly influence the data, in particular velocity and acceleration profiles. In the remainder of this chapter, we assume that filtering has already been done, but acknowledge that the results of event detection are tightly coupled to both the precision of the eye-tracker and the filters applied to the recorded gaze positions, as well as used in velocity and acceleration calculations.

There are some general principles many algorithms use to detect specific events:

1. Fixations are predominantly detected by a maximum allowed *dispersion* or *velocity* criterion. In the former case, temporally adjacent samples must be located within a

---

[15] Saccade taking the shortest path between two fixation positions.

[16] See page 48 for details about these calculations.

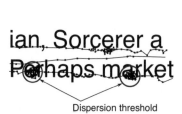

Dispersion threshold

(a) Data samples must reside within the circle for a minimum amount of time to be a fixation.

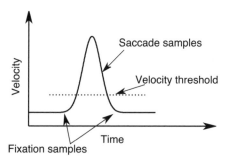

(b) Velocity samples below the threshold belong to fixations and the samples above the threshold belong to saccades.

Fig. 5.5 Fixation identification by maximum allowed (a) *dispersion* and (b) *velocity*.

spatially limited region (typically 0.5–2.0°) for a minimum duration (anywhere from 50–250 ms in the literature) whereas in the latter case, fixations are identified as contiguous portions of the gaze data where gaze velocity does not exceed a predefined threshold (about 10–50°/s) . These scenarios are depicted in Figure 5.5(a) and 5.5(b).

2. Saccades are commonly identified as periods where the eyes 'move fast', and are in practice defined by velocity or acceleration thresholds; everything above the thresholds are saccades (as in Figure 5.5(b)). Saccade detection thresholds vary significantly, but are usually in the range 30–100°/s (velocity) and 4000–8000°/s^2 (acceleration).

3. Smooth pursuit identification does not exist in any current commercial implementation, and it is currently an open research problem to develop a robust and generic algorithm for such a purpose. The few algorithms that do exist mostly use information about the velocity (typically less than 30–40°/s) and direction of smooth pursuit eye movement.

4. Blinks are often identified as $(x = 0, y = 0)$ coordinates or when the pupil diameter is zero, indicative of a closed eyelid. Note, however, that a careful investigation of blink parameters requires us to measure eyelid movement, and this information is only crudely (if at all) related to the coordinates from your eye-tracker.

5. An artefact is a rather ill-defined 'event', but can for example occur when data samples report high velocity movement that physically cannot derive from real movement of the eye. Typically, such parts of the eye-movement data are identified and removed during initial analysis (e.g. the filtering stage), and sometimes even online during recording. More generally, artefacts can be considered as consecutive data samples that do not conform to any known eye-movement event. If the percentage of such 'unknown' data samples is high, this may be an indication that the data is of poor quality and should not be used in further analysis. It can also indicate that the algorithm is not appropriate to use on your recorded data.

6. While the above events, in particular fixation and saccade events, will be of main focus in this chapter, other events indeed exist and algorithms have been developed to detect them. For *nystagmus*, for instance, Juhola (1988) presents an adaptive digital recursive filter capable of detecting all maxima and minima in a sequence of alterations. The *square-wave jerk* (p. 183) is another event that occurs frequently in healthy participants' eye movements. Then there are fixational eye-movement drifts, microsaccades, and tremor, for which a few algorithms exist (the one by Engbert & Kliegl, 2003 for microsaccade detection, for instance). Nyström and Holmqvist (2010) proposed an al-

gorithm to quantify movements known as *glissades*, a type of wobbling eye movement at the end of saccades.

The existing algorithms do not detect all event types; in fact they rarely detect more than one. The common *identification by dispersion threshold algorithm*[17] (I-DT) detects fixations only and does not separate between remaining events. Other algorithms detect only saccadic portions of the data. Overall, the existing methods can be divided into three broad groups:

Dispersion- (and duration-) based *fixation detection algorithms* using positional information, and the related clustering algorithms using Principle 1. By making alterations to the dispersion criterion, several varieties have developed: Salvucci and Goldberg (2000) test five different dispersion-based algorithms, and Urruty, Lew, Ihadaddene, and Simovici (2007) have developed a completely new algorithm based on projection clustering. Santella and DeCarlo (2004) developed a mean shift clustering algorithm that could be used for fixation detection. This group of algorithms is common in commercial implementations, such as Gazetracker, ASL Eyenal, faceLab, and SMI BeGaze, and are not uncommon in research papers. Typically, dispersion-based algorithms are used for data collected with a low-speed eye-tracker.

Velocity and acceleration algorithms using Principles 1 or 2, (mostly) use velocity and/or acceleration data to calculate events. Software packages by Tobii, SMI, and SR Research (EyeLink) include detection algorithms based on such principles, although their details are quite different. This class of algorithms typically requires data collected at higher sampling rates (say > 200 Hz).

Manual detection of events where a number of experienced eye-tracking researchers subjectively parse data samples into events. This is a method to find fixations, but it is not an algorithm. Many researchers trust only manual detection, in particular when data are collected with head-mounted eye-trackers without head tracking.

5.3   Hands-on advice for event detection

If you need to analyse your data with a fixation or saccade detection algorithm, and care about the validity of the output, what should you do? Some general recommendations are:

- Perhaps most importantly, plot your fixations next to your raw data, as in Figure 5.3, and examine what the algorithm does at different settings.
- Examine the distributions of events in your measure at different settings (look at the histograms), before you decide which setting to use.
- Make parallel analyses with several settings, and see how this affects your results; see M. J. Green (2006) who does this.
- Recommendations for algorithmic settings depend on factors such as the eye-tracker used for data collection, individual traits such as fixation stability, and the particular circumstances during calibration and recording (see pp. 154–161 for a detailed discussion).
- If you want to compare your results to previous literature, use similar algorithms and settings. Unfortunately, however, not all researchers report the settings they use.
- Fixations with unreasonably low durations often result from the current algorithms. Remove them if they significantly influence your results, or use a better algorithm.

[17]Refers in this book to the implementation described in Salvucci and Goldberg (2000).

- Beware of smooth pursuit or movement that looks like smooth pursuit in your data file. This is likely to be part of your data if you use animated stimuli or a head-mounted eye-tracker. Current algorithms have been designed to analyse only data recorded from static stimuli.

- Dispersion based algorithms are not suited to analyse data collected with higher sampling frequencies (> 200 Hz). If you have access to velocity-based algorithms, they are more likely to produce a good output.

- Using velocity and acceleration data, make sure that you understand how the filters used to generate the data affect detection. For example, lowpass filtering smooths out velocity peaks and thus effects where the peak threshold intersects with the velocity curves.

- Some researchers use measures that require data samples as input, but only from fixations. The fixation detection algorithms can then be used to 'clean' the data from all other events prior to using the measure.

- Beware that some implementations divide events (such as a fixation) that cross a trial border into two parts. This may lead to artificially low first fixation durations for trials; one option is to exclude such partial events from the analysis.

- In you article, always report the algorithm and the detection parameters you have used.

- Clearly define the events you use in your article. For example, do 'fixations' refer to implicitly detected inter-saccadic intervals or explicitly detected oculomotor periods of stillness?

5.4   Challenging issues in event detection

There are a range of issues that influence the results of event detection. As we saw in Figure 5.1, some of them are possible to control in the settings dialogue boxes in commercial software, while others may require post-processing or new algorithmic solutions. The validity of your results depends on how you deal with these issues.

5.4.1   Choosing parameter settings

Given a set of raw data samples, parameter settings are used to identify a specific event or to separate different types of events from each other. Therefore, they largely define the properties of a detected event. While the settings mostly serve to distinguish between event types, they are also commonly used by researchers to exclude data that are unreasonable with respect to what is known about the physiological limitations of eye movements, or with regard to the experimental design. With the important choice of parameter settings in mind, what are the proper values to choose for the settings in event detection algorithms, and how are they motivated?

Recommendations, arguments, and practices

Some manufacturers have provided their customers with recommendations for fixation analysis settings, but how well founded is such advice? In the Tobii Clearview settings dialogue (p. 148), the recommended lower fixation duration threshold of 40 ms for reading studies compared to 200 ms in picture viewing probably reflects the observation that fixations are typically shorter during reading than during picture viewing (p. 377). But what if the researcher has participants making 165 ms fixations during picture viewing? Should she then just lose those fixations from later statistical calculations, as Figure 5.3 exemplifies? And what about the 50 pixel radius suggestion for picture viewing, compared to 20 pixels for reading? Are fixations more stable during reading than while viewing images? If the participant makes two fixations close to one another during reading, the fixation analysis would give two fixations. But if the same person makes two fixations at the same close distance during picture viewing, should the fixation analysis produce just one long fixation?

The ASL Eyenal Manual (2001) offers the following motivation for their thresholds (defaults are 1° and 100 ms): "Specifically, there is research documenting the minimum latency of saccades in response to visual stimuli (thus suggesting a minimum fixation duration) and data defining the maximum amplitude of involuntary eye movements during the fixation (thus establishing maximum fixation boundaries)". Involuntary eye movements such as drift and microsaccades indeed make up part of the movements inside a fixation, but the imprecision in the specific eye-tracker and the specific measurement may be much larger than 1°.

Also, dispersion can be calculated in a number of different ways. Blignaut and Beelders (2009) present the following varieties of dispersion:

1. The maximum horizontal and vertical distance covered by the gaze positions in a fixation, $((\max(x) - \min(x)) + (\max(y) - \min(y)))/2 \leq$ threshold (Salvucci & Goldberg, 2000).

2. The distance between points in the fixation that are the furthest apart (Salvucci & Goldberg, 2000).

3. The distance between any two successive points, which is an estimate of the eye velocity (Shic, Scassellati, & Chawarska, 2008).

4. The distance between points and the centre of the fixation, i.e. the radius (Camilli, Terenzi, & Nocera, 2008).

5. The average or the standard deviation of the distances of all points from the centre of a fixation (Anliker, 1976; Applied Science Laboratories, 2001).

ASL Eyenal uses the standard deviation as dispersion measure and sets it to 1° as default, but for many of the other implementations, it is unclear what dispersion is. Surprisingly many softwares ask for dispersion thresholds in pixels instead of visual degrees. SMI's BeGaze 2.1 software uses 100 pixels as default. To make sense of this value, the experimenter first needs to convert them to degrees of visual angle, taking into account the viewing distance as well as the size and resolution of the screen (p. 24), and also understand which calculation of dispersion is used in the particular implementation they have at hand.

The dispersion setting is closely connected to the imprecision of the recorded data, and some implementations attempt to compensate for such noise. For instance, the ASL Eyenal dispersion algorithm for 50 Hz data requires three data samples to be outside of the dispersion radius for the fixation to end, not just one. Allowing single data samples to deviate is an insurance against low precision in the data; what we saw in Figure 5.2(b). In a way, this can be seen as a temporal increase of the dispersion threshold to allow one or two deviating fixation samples to pass unnoticed. In contrast, the I-DT ends the fixation as soon as the dispersion criteria are violated, which makes it more sensitive to noise, possibly requiring a higher dispersion setting.

Researchers have not paid too much attention to the dispersion setting, but Rötting (2001) reviews studies with dispersion settings ranging from 0.5°–2° of visual angle. Blignaut and Beelders (2009) and Blignaut (2009) argue that the optimal dispersion setting is 1° (for the radius dispersion measure), but relies heavily on the dispersion measure used.

The minimal fixation duration setting has been a long-standing discussion among researchers, however. Inhoff and Radach (1998) write that they themselves mostly use a cutoff point for fixation duration of 50 ms, but that many of their reading research colleagues use cutoff points ranging from 70–100 ms (but do not state which algorithms they use). Rötting

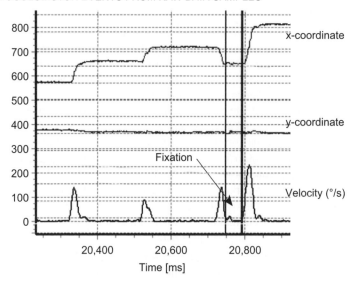

Fig. 5.6 A <45 ms fixation; following a regressive saccade during reading (Data from our example reading set). Excluding the glissade (the little bump in the velocity curve), the fixation duration becomes even shorter; about 30 ms. Data recorded at 1250 Hz with a tower-mounted system.

(2001) summarizes a number of studies, mainly in human factors, that use dispersion algorithms and duration settings ranging from 60–120 ms. At the other end of the scale, Granka, Hembrooke, Gay, and Feusner (2008) use a 200 ms duration setting. Manor and Gordon (2003) notice that 200 ms has become the de facto standard in clinical studies, originally derived from a 1962 study of eye movements in reading. Engmann et al. (2009) used no cutoff at all, but found that only 3.9% of the fixations in their study had a duration of less than 100 ms. Is this divergence in settings a problem for researchers who want to compare their results against someone else's?

Perhaps we could decide duration setting on the basis of what is known about how short fixations can be. However, there seems to be no concensus on how common even shorter fixations really are. They do exist, that is clear, as shown by the fixation in Figure 5.6, which measures exactly 45 ms when including the smaller velocity peak after the main saccade. If we exclude the glissade duration, the true fixation is around 30 ms in duration.

As we will see on page 377, information intake may be closed for the entire duration of such short fixations, but is this a good reason to exclude them? Rötting (2001) seems to argue that we should, while others use cutoffs without specifying the motivation. But the short fixations are still real oculomotor events, even if intake is closed. The fixation blob in the raw data files represents an oculomotor event, and it is our task to measure it as best we can, and distinguish it from other short periods of stillness that can be found in the data. The question of intake is very important, but should not be built into the event-detecting algorithms.

The EyeLink velocity algorithm allows for 'low', 'medium', or 'high' saccade sensitivity, although the settings dialogue in Figure 5.1(d) shows only 'normal and high'. Medium sensitivity corresponds to a velocity threshold of $30°/s$ and an acceleration threshold of $8000°/s^2$, while the high sensitivity uses $22°/s$ and $4000°/s^2$. The algorithm assumes that a given sample of raw data is part of a saccade in progress, if at least one of the velocity and the acceleration values is above the respective threshold. This is sensible when detecting saccades online. It is safer to use two criteria than only one, as there is only one chance to get it right. For the same reason, the settings for the EyeLink algorithm are chosen *before* recording the data. The EyeLink manual of 2007 recommends the more sensitive setting for oculomotor research, and the medium setting for cognitive and reading research (compare the recommendations in Figure 5.1(b)), arguing that "The larger threshold also reduces the number of microsaccades detected, decreasing the number of short fixations (less than 100 ms in duration) in the data" and noting that "Some short fixations (2% to 3% of total fixations) can be expected, and most researchers simply discard these". Not everyone discards the short fixations, however. Velichkovsky, Dornhöfer, Pannasch, and Unema (2000) not only take them seriously, but name them 'express fixations', after finding that they make up 7% of the total number of fixations given by their EyeLink system in a car simulator task. However, do poor data, noise, microsaccades, smooth pursuit, and a too low velocity threshold—below the precision level of the system—lie behind these frequent 'express fixations', rather than actual oculomotor behaviour?

There is a large spanwidth of velocity threshold settings among researchers. Duchowski (2007, pp. 149–152) makes a theoretical argument about the settings for velocity algorithms, suggesting a lower threshold of $130°/s$, which "should effectively detect saccades of amplitudes roughly larger than $3°$". Most other researchers use lower velocity threshold settings. For instance, Smeets and Hooge (2003) used a velocity threshold of $75°/s$ when studying rather large saccades, and Inchingolo and Spanio (1985) compare the settings $10°/s$ and $50°/s$. Beintema, Van Loon, and Van Den Berg (2005) chose the very low setting of $20°/s$, but added a minimal saccade amplitude criterion of $1°$, and a minimal duration between saccades of 30 ms to distinguish saccades from noise.

While the dispersion setting may be difficult to motivate, the choice of thresholds for velocity algorithms could be made in relation to the purpose of your study: what size of saccades do you want to detect, how much noise is there in the recorded fixations, and where is the line between the velocities of the fastest saccades you want and the slowest movement due to artefacts you have? The precise settings inside these spans could be selected from visual inspection of some typical samples in your data, using a plot of velocity and position, such as Figure 5.7. The following paragraph summarizes issues related to the saccade velocity threshold:

- **Saccade velocity threshold** The major setting. How small are the saccades you need to detect? Detection of small saccades requires a lower threshold. How much noise is there in the fixations? A lot of noise requires a higher threshold. Settings in the literature typically range from $20–130°/s$, as discussed above.

In fact, the problem with undetected fixations seen in Figure 5.3 was that the default saccade velocity threshold ($75°/s$) was set too high. This means that short saccades and their two surrounding fixations are grouped as one single fixation. We can see four such short saccades in Figure 5.7, three of which move with a velocity below $50°/s$. An appropriate setting for this data is rather $30–40°/s$.

Although the saccade velocity threshold is the most commonly used, there are three additional thresholds for velocity and acceleration based algorithms:

- **Saccade on- and offset velocity** Deciding when a saccade starts and stops, and is always equal or lower than the saccade velocity threshold. For high-quality recordings, a setting of $10–15°/s$ is often used but there is no consensus on how such thresholds should be set.
- **Maximum velocity threshold** A little-used artefact-removal threshold. The fast-moving artefactual movements from split and false corneal reflections, mascara, and droopy eyelids are above the interval $750–1000°/s$, which can be considered as a physical limitation on how fast the eye can move. Not many algorithms use an upper velocity

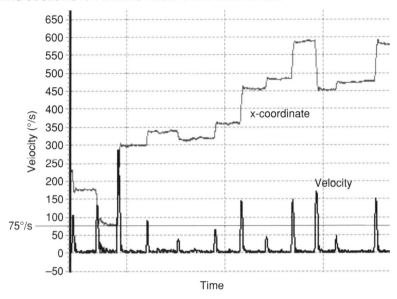

Fig. 5.7 Gaze velocity (black) and gaze x-coordinate (grey) for reading data. The vertical scale is in $°/s$ and pixels, respectively. The horizontal scale is samples (time). $75°/s$ is marked by a line, which is clearly too high for many of the saccades. 1250 Hz data from a tower-mounted system.

threshold, but Duchowski (2007) makes a theoretical argument suggesting $750°/s$ as a suitable threshold.

- **Saccade acceleration threshold** Used in the EyeLink algorithm to allow for quick detection of saccades online. An acceleration threshold can also be useful for distinguishing saccades from periods of smooth pursuit; quick pursuit velocity can be larger than slow (small) saccade velocity, but saccades always have larger accelerations (Behrens & Weiss, 1992).

The EyeLink software allows for *post-recording filtering* of the fixation and saccades resulting from the online saccade algorithm. The filter takes minimal fixation duration and minimal saccadic amplitude as settings. Defaults thresholds are 50 ms and 1°. Subsequent fixations that are shorter and closer than the threshold settings stipulate are merged into one fixation. Remedying noisy recordings post-hoc seems to be the major function of this tool. It introduces two new settings, however, making it a total of four settings for the algorithms deciding what fixations and saccades should remain for data analysis. Overall, the many heuristic elements of the EyeLink online saccade algorithm appear to be difficult to overview for the average user, which is perhaps why the settings dialogue primarily provides the summary settings of 'medium' or 'high' saccade sensitivity (Figure 5.1(d)).

Effects of settings

It has long been known that fixation and saccade output is very sensitive to the choice of algorithm settings (Karsh & Breitenbach, 1983, e.g.). Using 60 Hz data and a dispersion-based algorithm, Shic, Scassellati, and Chawarska (2008) show that the effect of parameter changes on mean fixation duration is a linear function of parameters, with a considerable slope. As our reading data (p. 5) in Figure 5.8 show, the effect is that all basic fixation measures are heavily altered when using the common dispersion-based I-DT algorithm. Both the dispersion and the duration settings may give rise to artificially significant differences that may change the result of a study completely. For instance, the average fixation duration at setting

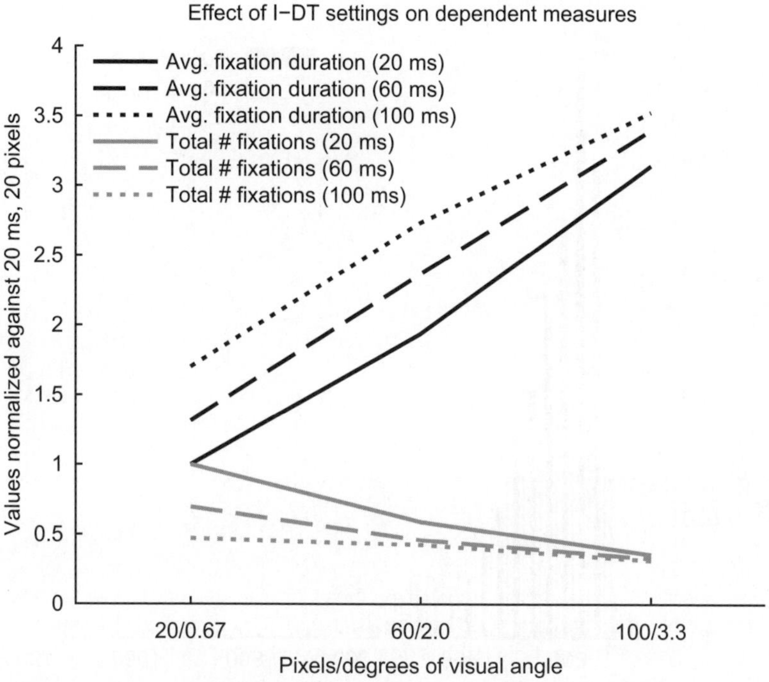

Effect of I−DT settings on dependent measures

Fig. 5.8 How fixation measures differ with different dispersion diameters and duration settings in a commercial implementation of the I-DT algorithm (1250 Hz reading data from page 5). The slope is similar to that from 50 Hz data in Shic, Scassellati, and Chawarska (2008).

60 ms and 60 pixels differs significantly from the average fixation duration at 100 ms and 60 pixels (two-sided t-test with 36490 fixations each, $t(36489) = 3.07$, $p < 0.01$). The same thing happens if you change the dispersion from 60 pixels to 100 pixels while keeping the duration at 100 ms ($t(26950) = 3.22$, $p < 0.01$).

Fixation durations will not only differ in their averages—a change in dispersion and duration thresholds also alters the distribution, as shown in Figure 5.9. A change from a 100 ms 60 pixel setting to a 100 ms 100 pixel setting dramatically decreases the number of 'fixations' around the 200 ms duration, and increases the number of 'fixations' with durations around 400–600 ms. Such a change in distribution affects averages but also the variance of the data, which in turn affects all your variance-based significance tests (t-tests and ANOVAs, for instance). Even this small examination of the I-DT algorithm clearly shows that dispersion and duration settings should be chosen with the utmost care.

These effects are not unique for dispersion-based algorithms, but are also present in algorithms using velocity data. Figure 5.10 shows how basic saccade and fixation measures are affected by parameter changes in the SMI velocity algorithm; at a $90°/s$ setting, for example, the average fixation is 2.5 times as long as it is at the $30°/s$ setting ($t(14340) = 2.85$, $p < 0.01$). Shic, Scassellati, and Chawarska (2008) found similar variation when changing the saccade velocity setting from $18°/s$ to $81°/s$. It is clear that the choice of setting can be *the* determining factor to the success or failure of an eye-tracking study. Although otherwise similar, studies using different settings of the peak saccadic velocity are not directly comparable. It is important to notice that the basic measures in Figure 5.10 are the foundation that many other dependent measures in eye-tracking research are built upon. Virtually all dependent measures will alter their values when this setting is changed.

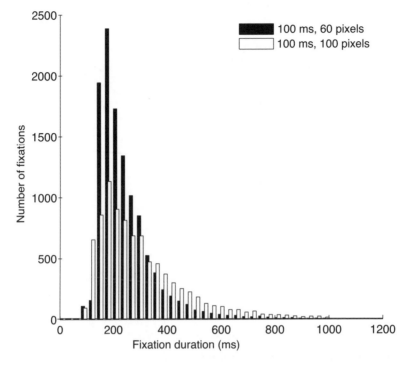

Fig. 5.9 Distribution of fixation durations for two dispersion settings of the I-DT algorithm (data source described on page 5).

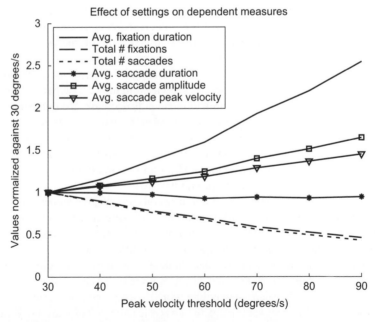

Fig. 5.10 How important dependent variables change with the setting of saccade velocity threshold in the SMI velocity algorithm (a commercial implementation of Smeets & Hooge, 2003). Reading data recorded at 1250 Hz and described on page 5.

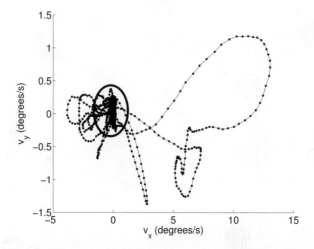

Fig. 5.11 Control ellipse for saccade detection where samples outside the ellipse—where the eye velocity is large—are saccade candidates. One and a half seconds of data collected at 1250 Hz with a tower-mounted system during reading.

Data driven threshold

It is well known that the noise levels in eye-tracking data can change across individuals, tasks, trials, and even within trials, so why should we choose a setting subjectively and stick with it throughout the entire analysis? This particular question has led researchers to develop algorithms that let the data itself assist in how to set the thresholds. Tole and Young (1981) suggested locally adapting the acceleration threshold used to detect saccades to compensate for varying noise levels they observed in the data. Similarly, Behrens, MacKeben, and Schröder-Preikschat (2010) proposed a saccade detection algorithm where an adaptive, momentary acceleration threshold was calculated based on the preceding 200 samples (for data acquired at 1000 Hz). A related algorithm is described by Marple-Horvat, Gilbey, and Hollands (1996), who use a "double-window" technique where two temporal windows on each side of the current velocity sample are subtracted, and a saccade is detected only if the difference between the average value within each window exceeds a certain threshold. Niemenlehto (2009) based the resilience against varying noise for saccade detection on a constant false alarm technique.

Assuming the noise is constant over a trial, one can estimate the noise level over the whole trial, and then use this estimate to set the thresholds. For fixational eye movements, the dominant principle for microsaccade detection is based on the algorithm proposed by Engbert and Kliegl (2003), who first estimate the velocity noise in x and y-dimensions separately, and then set the thresholds as multiples of the estimated variance in the noise; all samples outside the control ellipse formed by such thresholds are saccade candidates, as Figure 5.11 illustrates. Since the dynamics of microsaccades are similar to normal saccades, the same principle can be used to find appropriate saccade detection thresholds. Similar strategies for choosing saccade detection thresholds have been employed in other recent work (Nyström & Holmqvist, 2010; Van Der Lans, Wedel, & Pieters, 2010).

5.4.2   Noise, artefacts, and data quality

Noise can derive from the oculomotor system, the eye-tracker, or the environment, and adds unwanted variation to the acquired data. Artefacts can be seen as a special type of noise,

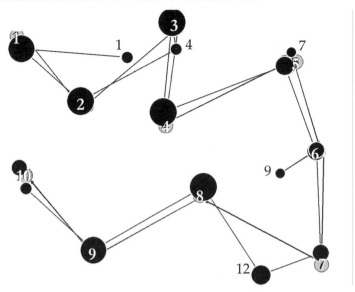

Fig. 5.12 False fixations with black numbers 1, 4, 7, 9, and 12 result from imprecision (p. 33) in data. This means that raw data differ so much from sample-to-sample even within a single fixation that some of the samples end up outside of the dispersion radius, and will be segmented into minute fixations of their own. Recorded at 50 Hz on the remote system on a blue-eyed participant with contact lenses, and analysed using a dispersion-based algorithm with manufacturer standard settings. The task was to look at the centre of each white number in increasing order. Dark filled circles represent detected 'fixations'.

but are typically larger and easier to distinguish from known eye-movement characteristics. Data quality is a more imprecise term, but is related to accuracy, precision, percentage of data loss, perhaps in addition to a subjective rating from the person responsible for the recording. Having access to all these quality indicators gives you an idea of whether the recorded data are useful for further analysis, or should be discarded.

It is generally easier to detect events in recordings with high data quality. Figure 5.8 showed results from data with high quality in the sense that the calibration was judged as good and no problems were reported by the operator during the recording. Unfortunately, not all recorded data have the same high quality, and the algorithms need to deal with the imperfections too. In fact, data quality is an important factor to consider when using the algorithms, which can erroneously interpret various recording imperfections as actual eye-movement events.

In dispersion-based algorithms, high noise levels can make a sample that rightfully belongs to a fixation move outside of the dispersion radius, end the fixation, and trigger a new one. Figure 5.12 shows how a number of such false 'fixations' are created from stray samples in the vicinity of the real fixations. Some varieties of dispersion algorithms attempt to address this problem by temporarily allowing a few samples to exceed the maximum dispersion threshold without ending the fixation (such as ASL Eyenal). High velocity artefactual eye movements will also be assumed to be saccades with intermediate fixations, but the 'fixations' will now be deleted because they are too short.

The velocity algorithms are also best suited for high quality data. High velocity artefacts and imprecision are major obstacles; if the imprecision inside a fixation has a velocity above the velocity threshold used, it gives rise to false 'saccades', effectively ending the fixation. The velocity threshold can be superseded many times, giving a whole array of unrealistically short 'fixations'. Figure 5.13 shows how this happens during the first and fifth fixations.

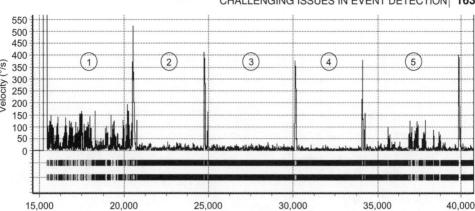

Fig. 5.13 Variable precision. Data acquired for oculomotor fixations 1–5 are noisy (imprecise) when the participant looks at the top of the stimulus (first and fifth fixations) and precise at the bottom (second to fourth fixation). Recorded with a remote system at 250 Hz and analysed with a velocity-based algorithm with a threshold of 75°/s.

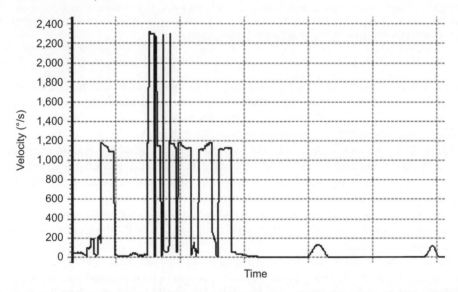

Fig. 5.14 Saccadic velocity plot showing the effect of having multiple competing corneal reflections (eye image in Figure 4.13). High-speed artefacts to the left, and slower reading saccades on the right. Recorded at 1250 Hz a tower-mounted system, participant with contact lenses.

With both dispersion- and velocity-based algorithms, the effect of imprecision can to some extent be alleviated by raising the threshold setting. With a larger dispersion radius, or a higher velocity threshold, sample-to-sample motion can be quicker without endangering the consistency of fixations. This remedy comes at a price, however. For instance, raising the velocity threshold of Figure 5.13 above the peaks of this imprecision will make it so high that many real saccades will not be identified. When a saccade is not identified, the two surrounding fixations are reported as one single 'fixation', with a duration that equals the sum of the two real fixations and the intermediate saccade.

Figure 5.14 shows high-speed *optic artefacts*: false eye movements with velocities well over 1000°/s and virtually infinite acceleration. Such velocities appear for instance when the

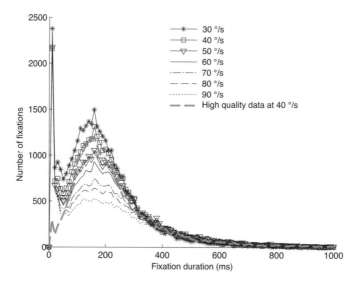

Fig. 5.15 13 readers with very poor recording quality (mascara, contact lenses, drooping eyelids, etc). The SMI velocity algorithm in BeGaze 2.1 with different peak (saccade) velocity threshold settings. 10 readers with very high data quality at setting 40°/s for comparison.

corneal reflection moves instantly from one position to another, as in Figures 4.12(d) and 4.13 on page 124. The two 'bumps' further right are real saccades, included for comparison. In the reading data used for examples here, 0.4–0.9% (depending on settings) of the saccades had a velocity higher than 800°/s. In corresponding data with low quality, 4–9% of the saccades had such high velocities.[18] Obviously, the poor data quality caused this tenfold increase, by having the algorithm identify as saccades various false 'saccadic' movements like the ones in Figure 5.14. As a comparison, the return sweeps, when readers switch from one line to the next, across the entire monitor, a distance about 25° of visual angle, had an average peak velocity of 440°/s. In between the false high speed 'saccades' of the artefactual data, the SMI velocity algorithm finds false 1 ms 'fixations', as it attempts to fill the almost non-existent period between two false 'saccades'.

In fact, when running data with poor quality through the SMI velocity algorithm of BeGaze 2.1, it identifies a huge number of false 'fixations' with durations shorter than 40 ms, as clearly shown in the histogram of Figure 5.15. Similar 'blips' of very short 'fixations' in the related I-VT algorithm were reported by Salvucci and Goldberg (2000). In both cases, the lack in many velocity-based algorithms of a temporal criterion for fixation duration could be one part of the problem. The other part is the lack of an upper velocity threshold that could eliminate high-speed artefacts with intermediate 1-sample false 'fixations'. For very high quality data, the number of unreasonably short 'fixations' is much smaller (dotted comparison line), but they still exist. For durations above ∼80 ms, the distribution is very similar. This suggests that with an improved algorithm, a good portion of the poor quality data could in fact be used, at least for some types of analyses.

5.4.3 Glissades

Interestingly enough, the very high quality data in Figure 5.15 *also* exhibit a small proportion of 1 ms 'fixations'. In the high quality data, the unreasonably short fixations are not found

---

[18] Analysis was made using the SMI velocity algorithm of BeGaze 2.1 with a threshold of 40°/s

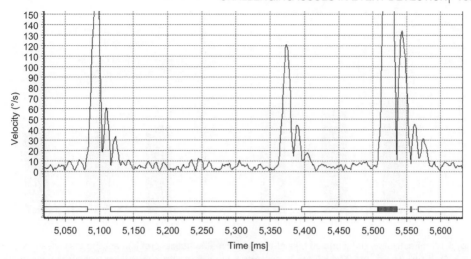

Fig. 5.16 Saccades with multiple velocity peaks and false 1 ms fixations between them. Recorded at 1250 Hz with a tower-mounted system. Fixations (white lines), saccades (grey lines), and undetected events (gaps in between) according to SMI BeGaze 2.1 are indicated at the bottom of the graph.

amongst noise, but when the algorithm faces a main saccade ending with smaller velocity peaks, knows as *glissades* (see definition on page 183), as in Figure 5.16. The saccade of this participant does not stop at the intended fixation goal, but continues beyond it, and then back again, but too far, and thus wobbles back and forth for a while, before it comes to a standstill and the fixation can start. The velocity peaks in these very strong glissadic movements are well beyond the normal velocity threshold (here $40°/s$), and therefore the SMI velocity algorithm finds, not a fixation right after the saccade ending, but essentially a new 'saccade'. Therefore, two of the saccades in Figure 5.16 are not recognized as saccades at all. The third saccade *is* recognized, but only its first velocity peak. We see false 1–10 ms 'fixations' between the peaks inside the second and the third saccades. Glissades of this extreme size are not uncommon in data that we have recorded from reading, mathematical problem solving, and many other tasks. Between 20–40% of all saccades end with a glissade, but almost no saccades start with this type of movement (Nyström & Holmqvist, 2010).

Some algorithms treat glissades like just another type of noise. Stampe (1993) describes glissades as noise that "includes ringing or overshoot artefacts following saccades, which can confuse the saccade detector into extending the saccades into the next fixation". Similarly, Duchowski (2007) describes filters that are optimized for idealized saccades (without glissades), thus smoothening out the glissades before the fixation algorithm gets the velocity data. The EyeLink parser seems to assign glissades to fixations, as shown in Figure 5.18. However, from this figure it remains unclear whether the EyeLink algorithm at times generates very short fixations as a result of poor glissade treatment, or whether it is robust enough to avoid that. The manual tends to point in the former direction: "Post-processing or data cleanup may be needed to prepare data during analysis. For example, short fixations may need to be discarded or merged with adjacent fixations, or artefacts around blinks may have to be eliminated" (SR Research, 2007). However, whether the short fixations are due to glissades remains to be investigated.

First fixation duration values are *extremely* sensitive to these short 'fixations' in data, because when a participant makes a saccade into an area of interest, the saccade very often ends with a glissade, and the SMI velocity algorithm often outputs a false 'fixation' before the glissade, and also before the real fixation. Therefore, during analysis, forgetting to remove short

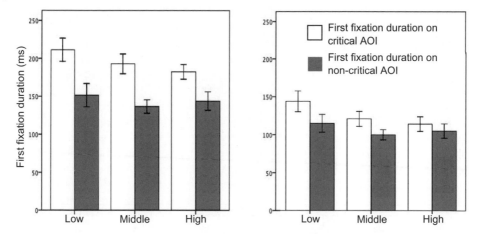

Fig. 5.17 First fixation durations on critical areas in a mathematical problem solving task (described on page 5). 'Low', 'High', and 'Middle' are three groups of participants with varying levels of mathematical competences. Fixations were detected using the SMI velocity algorithm and a 40°/s threshold. The same data is presented both left and right, but to the right the data include the small 'fixations'. Why such a huge difference on first fixations? After a saccade into an area, the very short 'fixation' that the SMI velocity algorithm finds between the saccade and the following glissade is taken as the first fixation, since it precedes the real fixation. Note that the very short 'fixations' not only make the averages much lower, they also introduce noise that conceals significant effects.

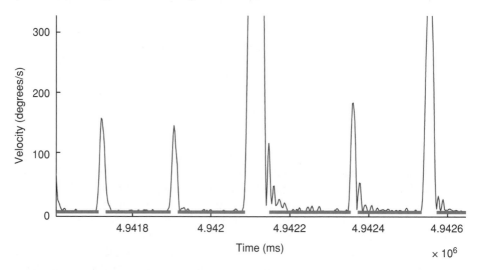

Fig. 5.18 Event detection with the EyeLink parser for reading data ('Normal' sensitivity). Data were collected with the head-mounted system at 500 Hz. Thick lines at the bottom of the graph indicate where 'fixations' have been detected. Note how glissadic movements are systematically assigned to the following fixation and how parts of the saccades are also attributed to fixations.

'fixations' before calculating first fixation duration values means using lots of unreasonably short 'fixations', and getting averages that are lower, as in Figure 5.17.

Glissades have until recently been treated unsystematically and differently across algorithms and even within the same algorithm, sometimes being attributed to saccades, other times to fixations. Some researchers express the need to exclude them completely from further analysis. Gilchrist and Harvey (2006) require the velocity to remain below 30°/s for at least five samples (20 ms) to count as a fixation, which "excludes the interval of ocular instability just after the saccade", and argue that this leads to a more accurate calculation also of fixation location, although fixation durations may be shorter than typically reported, as the glissade is assigned to the saccade. Investigating post-saccadic drift, Collewijn et al. (1988) considered the eye velocity during a 100 ms period after a saccade, but arguing that "This period started 20 ms after the end of each saccade in order to avoid contamination by the dynamic overshoot frequently associated with a saccade".

The prevalence of glissades appears to vary across eye-trackers, being more common, larger, shorter, and heavily curved in DPI-systems compared to video-based, while they are eradicated or transformed to post-saccadic drift in coil-based eye-trackers (Deubel & Bridgeman, 1995; Frens & Van Der Geest, 2002). Glissades can be observed in data collected with any video-based high-speed eye-tracker with good precision. In low-speed, remote systems, they may be more difficult to see, since the average glissade duration is only slightly larger than 20 ms (one sample in a 50 Hz eye-tracker) (Nyström & Holmqvist, 2010).

Positioned in between saccades and the following fixation, the question is which to assign the glissade to. The fact that perceptual visual intake appears to be closed during glissades (McConkie & Loschky, 2002), as well as the fact that glissades follow the same main sequence relationships as saccades (p. 318) tells us that they are predominantly saccadic in nature. As glissade-detecting algorithms become more available, we can surely expect to see more studies using this event.

5.4.4 Sampling frequency

There is a tendency for dispersion-based algorithms to be used for data collected at a low sampling frequency, such as 50 Hz, and velocity algorithms for data collected at higher sampling frequencies (say > 200 Hz), but there are also exceptions. The Tobii Fixation filter is a velocity-based algorithm for fixation detection in data as slow as 30 and 50 Hz, for instance.

Dispersion-based algorithms end a 'fixation' as soon as the raw samples cross the border defined by the dispersion radius. In high-speed data, this border can be crossed just about anytime. The two 'saccades' identified by the I-DT algorithm in Figure 5.19, indicated by black lines, start a bit into a real saccade, and two thirds into a real fixation, respectively. This is clearly incorrect, and reflects the fact that the dispersion algorithm is only aware of centre points and dispersion, but only indirectly velocity and acceleration. Take the 'fixation' in Figure 5.19 that starts in the middle of the first real saccade. I-DT starts calculating the centre point of the new 'fixation' here, even though the eye is in full motion and some distance away from its landing point in the real fixation. Once the eye has reached the real fixation, data samples are close to the dispersion radius border, as most of the distance was spanned by the saccade. This means that even very small movements inside the real fixation make I-DT think the dispersion border has been crossed. In Figure 5.19, this happens at time 8360 ms, deep inside the real fixation. After a minimal 'saccade', the I-DT starts a new 'fixation', with its new centre point and dispersion, which happen to be chosen generously enough to accommodate the next real saccade inside the 'fixation'.

Dispersion-based algorithms have a large problem with their imprecise estimate of individual saccade and fixation durations. The same miscalculation of fixation onsets occurs at all sampling frequencies, but for the lowest sampling frequencies, this is not as big a problem since the sampling frequency by itself is the major limiting factor.

Velocity-based saccade detection algorithms are better suited for use with a wide spectrum of sampling frequencies. With suitable filtering when velocity data is calculated, it is quite possible to get clear velocity peaks even for 50 Hz data, as shown for instance in Figure 5.20. The reason it is uncommon to use velocity algorithms for low-speed data is that velocity, and in particular acceleration, can be calculated only crudely when the sampling frequency is low.

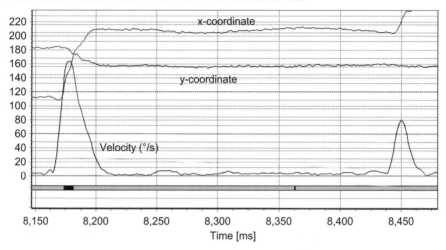

Fig. 5.19 Note how the dispersion algorithm reduces the duration of saccades, and even inserts false 'saccades' in the midst of a fixation in this reading data recorded at 1250 Hz with a tower-mounted system. Grey lines depict the x- and y-coordinates in the coordinate system of the scene video. The dark line is eye velocity. The bottom bar indicates 'fixations' (light) and 'saccades' (darker) according to the I-DT algorithm with 100 ms and 80 pixels settings.

If our task is to detect saccades correctly rather than to measure them with high precision, all we need is a fair estimate of peak velocity, and this we can get even at 50 Hz.

In conclusion, while dispersion-based algorithms do not produce valid event data for higher sampling frequencies, the velocity algorithms have good potential for the entire spectrum of sampling frequencies. The use of acceleration is only suitable for data acquired with high-speed systems, however.

5.4.5 Smooth pursuit

An increasing number of studies use stimuli and experimental set-ups that induce the participant to make smooth pursuit movements, for instance by using animated or video stimuli, or taking the participant out with a head-mounted eye-tracker to make simultaneous head and eye movements. Many of these studies use data recorded at low sampling frequencies, and dispersion algorithms are used to calculate fixations.

Figure 5.20 shows data from a participant walking past a shelf in the supermarket (experiment 3 on page 5). He walks, turns his head, and moves his eyes simultaneously. When applying the I-DT algorithm to the data in this figure, three fairly correct saccades are indeed found, but also four or five false ones. The impact on variables such as fixation duration or saccade rate is therefore disastrous. Such event data cannot be used. Interestingly, the velocity peaks of this 50 Hz data seem to better estimate where the saccades are located, posing the question of whether a velocity-based algorithm would have been a better choice (which finds some support in Munn, Stefano, & Pelz, 2008).

Velocity algorithms typically assign smooth pursuit data into the same category as fixations. Itti (2006), using video data, applies a velocity algorithm to remove all saccades, arguing that the remaining mixture of fixation and smooth pursuit data can be seen as a 'visual intake' category. Depending on the purpose of the study, such a mixed category could be sound or not. Itti wanted to compare all visual intake to that predicted by his algorithm, but made no duration statistics on the data. In most commercial software packages, this is indeed also the best case scenario of how smooth pursuit is handled; in the Tobii Fixation filter im-

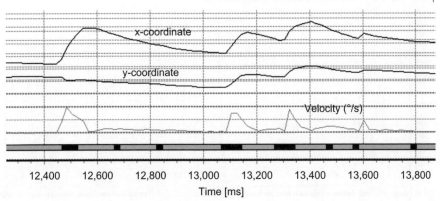

Fig. 5.20 Eye movement data from a head-mounted eye-tracker at 50 Hz on a participant walking past a shelf in a supermarket. Dark lines are the x- and y-coordinates in the coordinate system of the scene video. The grey line is eye velocity. Bottom bar indicates fixations (light grey) and saccades (dark grey) according to the I-DT algorithm with 80 ms and 80 pixels settings.

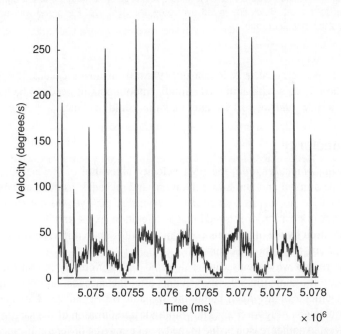

Fig. 5.21 Event detection with the EyeLink parser for smooth pursuit data ('Normal' sensitivity). Data were collected at 500 Hz with the head-mounted system from a person viewing a pendulum movement. The lines at the bottom of the graph indicate where 'fixations' have been detected. Notice how fixation and smooth pursuit are merged into the same category.

plementation, the 'visual intake' category is still labelled 'fixations', and users with smooth pursuit data may be misled into making various statistics on the duration and prevalence of these 'fixations'. This is also the current status for parsers of high-speed data from EyeLink and SMI. Figure 5.21 illustrates how the EyeLink parser treats smooth pursuit data from a person following a pendulum movement on a computer screen.

The worst case scenario, Figure 5.20 is an example of this, is that smooth pursuit eye movement causes an algorithm to output events that are clearly not present. Using velocity thresholds only, it may be hard to separate fast smooth pursuit, which can reach velocities

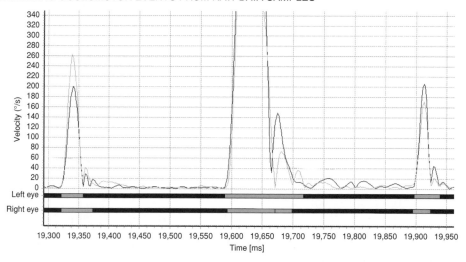

Fig. 5.22 Reading near the borders of a flat monitor: Velocities of saccade far to the right, return sweep, and saccade far to the left. Black line is left eye; grey line right eye. Recorded with a tower-mounted system at 500 Hz in binocular mode.

of 100°/s (C. H. Meyer, Lasker, & Robinson, 1985), from slow saccades. If we want correct fixation and saccade data with animated stimuli, smooth pursuit needs to be identified as an event in its own right, and we will see later how this could be done.

5.4.6 Binocularity

When processing *binocular data*, the SMI velocity algorithm of BeGaze 2.1 finds differences in both the number and duration of fixations and saccades, as indicated by Figure 5.22. This should come as no surprise, since it is known that the eyes do not move in complete synchrony, either in position or in speed and acceleration (p. 24 and 449). Nevertheless, the hard thresholds used by the algorithms could make even subtle differences in eye movement between the left and the right eye count.

Part of the reason why events can be detected very differently is that the two eyes do not make exactly the same glissadic movements after the saccade, and sometimes only one of the eye velocities reaches down below the saccadic offset threshold, examplified by the right (grey curve) eye in Figure 5.22. The amplitude and duration of the saccade then differs between the eyes. Another reason is due to the two eyes having different distances to the right and left part of the monitor. Figure 5.22 shows first a saccade in the far right of the monitor (at around 19,350 ms), then a return sweep (at about 19,650 ms), and finally a reading saccade at the far left of the monitor (at around 19,900 ms). At the right-hand side of the monitor, the right-eye saccades have a larger amplitude and the fixation durations are shorter than for the left eye. Conversely, on the left side of the monitor, the fixations of the left eye will be shorter, and its saccadic amplitudes longer than in the right side of the monitor (compare Figure 2.4 on page 24). This is not really a problem of the algorithm, but rather questions whether we should continue to record monocularly, and accept only the saccades and fixations of the one eye that we happen to select.

Since the majority of eye-tracking research is monocular, velocity algorithms have mostly been applied to monocular data. The I-DT algorithm appears not be used in any real binocular research, probably as it is too imprecise in itself. Binocular event detection algorithms using the covariance between the eyes have been developed (Van Der Lans et al., 2010).

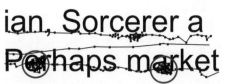

Fig. 5.23 The I-DT detection criteria: gaze must reside within a limited spatial region for a specified minimum duration. Two fixations clearly fulfil the spatial dispersion criterion, but what about the more dispersed blob on Sorcerer? Is that one fixation or two? In the end, your settings will decide.

5.5 Algorithmic definitions

5.5.1 Dispersion-based algorithms

Dispersion-based algorithms are the most common type of event-detection algorithms, and are implemented in many commercial analysis software packages. They have mostly been used for low-speed data, and have long been considered the prime choice when analysing 50 Hz data. In short, dispersion algorithms detect only fixations and collect all other events to a common category. They identify fixations by finding data samples that are close enough to one another for a specified minimal period of time. They do not make any use of velocity or acceleration information to calculate the precise on- or offsets of fixation. Related cluster algorithms are presented by Urruty et al. (2007), Santella and DeCarlo (2004), and Goldberg and Schryver (1995b). The most used and also best of the dispersion algorithms is, according to Salvucci and Goldberg (2000), the *identification by dispersion threshold* (I-DT) algorithm; they tested six fixation algorithms with respect not only to accuracy and robustness, but also ease of implementation and speed. There are a number of commercial implementations of dispersion-based algorithms, for example by ASL, and SMI.

The pseudo-code for the I-DT algorithm is:

```
I-DT. Input: (raw data samples, dispersion threshold, duration threshold)

   1. While there are still data samples

       (a) Initialize window over first samples to cover duration threshold
       (b) While dispersion <= threshold, add samples to window
       (c) Note a fixation at the centroid of window samples
       (d) Remove window points from samples
```

Dispersion is defined as $d = [\max(x) - \min(x)] + [\max(y) - \min(y)]$, where (x,y) represent the samples inside the window. The dispersion algorithms combine a temporal window (duration threshold) with a spatial requirement (the dispersion threshold). For instance, the temporal threshold may be 100 ms, and the dispersion threshold $1°$ of visual angle. This would then mean that only when the data samples stay within a $1°$ diameter for at least 100 ms is that sequence of data samples considered a fixation. This principle is illustrated in Figure 5.23. The I-DT algorithm has a number of cousins who all use a temporal threshold, but calculate the spatial dispersion criterion somewhat differently (Blignaut, 2009; Shic, Scassellati, & Chawarska, 2008; Salvucci & Goldberg, 2000). Moreover, the algorithmic variations have different ways to deal with noise, as we have pointed out above.

5.5.2 Velocity and acceleration algorithms

Fixation detection algorithms

As for dispersion algorithms, *fixation velocity algorithms* use a duration criterion, but instead combine it with a stillness criterion based on eye velocity. The eye velocity is seldom at the

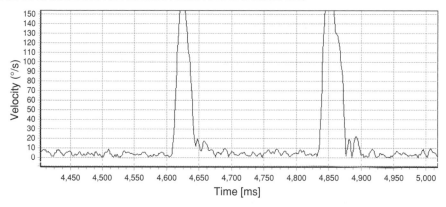

Fig. 5.24 Velocity chart for three fixations and two saccades, recorded at 1250 Hz with a tower-mounted system. Velocity calculated with BeGaze 2.1.

absolute zero level, because of micro-movements in the eye and eye-tracker-related noise. Therefore users of this algorithm must decide an upper velocity threshold for fixations. Figure 5.24 shows a velocity over time chart for three fixations and two intermediate saccades. The velocity during fixations in this reading data has its peaks at 6–10°/s. The shortest saccades typically have velocity peaks of about 30–40°/s. Rötting (2001) summarizes settings for the velocity threshold used for this type of fixation analysis in five quoted studies: $< 16°/s$, $< 20°/s$, $< 6.58°/s$, $< 50°/s$, $< 37.7°/s$. The two last settings most likely reflect a considerable noise in the eye-tracking systems used in the quoted studies, and definitely run the risk of categorizing some short saccades as parts of fixations. Thresholds could also vary since the velocity samples have undergone different types of lowpass filtering prior to detection; little filtering requires higher thresholds.

This type of algorithm also requires an additional minimal duration threshold for fixations, which can be set to anything between 60 and 120 ms, according to Röttings review, also see pages 155–156 for an extended discussion. The algorithm thus finds fixations as periods longer than a minimal duration, during which the eye velocity is below a maximum velocity threshold.

Even though the 'fixation radius' and 'Min fixation duration' settings in Figure 5.1(b) on page 148 invite the user to believe that it is a dispersion-based algorithm, the Tobii ClearView fixation algorithm is in principle similar to the I-VT algorithm by Salvucci and Goldberg (2000); the 'fixation radius' setting refers to the maximum distance between two consecutive samples in pixels. Fixations comprise consecutive samples whose distances are shorter than the 'fixation radius' over a period longer than the minimum fixation duration. Note, however, that according to Blignaut and Beelders (2009) classification of dispersion metrics on page 155, the Tobii Clearview algorithm could well fit the under the umbrella of dispersion-based algorithms.

Saccade detection algorithms

A velocity-based saccade detection algorithm focuses on identifying the saccadic velocity peaks. Motion above a velocity threshold, for instance $75°/s$, is assumed to be a saccade. In order to differentiate real saccades from artefacts, which can also be fast movements, there are usually additional constraints on saccades, such as a clear speed peak near the middle of the saccade (Smeets & Hooge, 2003), or that the peak saccade velocity cannot be higher than a certain threshold (Nyström & Holmqvist, 2010). What is not identified as a saccade is typically assumed to be a fixation. Surprisingly, very few, if any, algorithms have used the fact that saccades follow what is known as the *main sequence* to exclude 'non-typical' saccades (i.e. eye movements have a typical path from which deviating saccades are obvious).

Velocity-based algorithms have been implemented by many researchers themselves, but are also available in some commercial analysis software. One such implementation can be found in the commercial software BeGaze 2.1 by SMI. It has been used in this book to illustrate strengths and weaknesses of current centre algorithms. The SMI velocity algorithm is a more elaborate version of the I-VT algorithm of Bahill, Brockenbrough, and Troost (1981) and Salvucci and Goldberg (2000), and also very similar to the algorithms tested by Inchingolo and Spanio (1985), and possibly stemming back to the algorithms by Boyce from 1965 and 1967 as referred to in Ditchburn (1973).

The particular implementation of the SMI velocity algorithm we have used in many examples above is based on the algorithm described and used by Smeets and Hooge (2003). This paper spells out the algorithm in detail, because the authors thought that researchers should be specific about their algorithms. In fact, few other papers provide such detail, so when one SMI employee a little later made a literature search for saccade detection algorithms being used in research papers, that particular version came to be the algorithm SMI implemented in their BeGaze software.

The SMI velocity algorithm is a two-pass algorithm, i.e. it looks through the complete data stream twice. The first time to calculate velocities and *detect saccades*, and the second time to find saccadic onsets and offsets. The following is the pseudo-code.

```
SMI velocity algorithm. Input: (raw data samples, velocity threshold,
saccade peak location threshold)

  1. For all samples:

      (a) Calculate angular velocities
      (b) Detect peaks in eye velocity
      (c) Calculate fixation velocity threshold

  2. For all velocity peaks:

      (a) Collect all data samples to the left of the peak, but only until the velocity
          is so slow that the sample must be part of a fixation (the fixation velocity
          threshold).
      (b) Collect all data samples to the right of the peak, but only until the
          velocity is so slow that the sample must be part of a fixation.
      (c) Detect a saccade from the collected data samples only if the
          velocity peak of the saccade is located within the central
          part of the saccade. Otherwise it is discarded.
      (d) Detect blinks as periods where only zero data ((x,y) = (0,0)) are found
          between two saccades.
      (e) Fixations are everything that are not saccades or blinks.
```

In other words, this algorithm finds the velocity peaks that rise above the threshold, and accepts these as saccade candidates. Originating at the saccadic peak, the algorithm then walks down the slopes on both sides (see Figure 5.24). The calculated fixation velocity threshold tells the algorithm when the speed is so low (the eye is so still) as to stop counting this as a saccade, but rather as a fixation. The SMI implementation of this algorithm takes it that the saccade on- and offsets are when the saccade velocity is three standard deviations higher than the average velocity of fixations, as calculated from the beginning of the stream of data samples. For the two saccades in Figure 5.24, the onset velocities are $12.56°/s$ and $10.95°/s$, and the offset velocities $13.98°/s$ and $15.83°/s$, somewhat higher than the average fixation noise of $6–10°/s$. As a very simple check that the saccade velocity profile seems valid, only

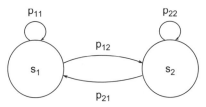

Fig. 5.25 A finite state machine with two states: one representing fixations and one saccades.

saccade candidates that have velocity peaks in the central portion (default are 20%–80% of saccade length) of the saccade are finally accepted. Finally, fixations are detected implicitly as everything that is not saccades, blinks, or undefined events.

Velocity algorithms are better to use with high sampling frequencies, since saccades are short (in the area of 20–50 ms) and you need many samples in each slope (10–25 ms) to calculate velocities correctly in the critical slope ends. A 200 Hz recording gives 2–5 samples per slope (depending on the size of the saccade), which should be considered an absolute minimal sampling frequency for accurate saccade duration calculations (p. 29). If the algorithm is used just for *detecting* the saccade, rather than *measuring* it, then a sampling frequency as low as 50 Hz can be sufficient. For saccadic detection, it is enough to have one velocity sample above the peak threshold, which means two data samples at a large enough spatial distance between them, which you find in 50 Hz data.

The 'Tobii fixation filter' developed by Olsson (2007) is used with low speed data using a 'double-window technique' (similar to the one proposed by Marple-Horvat et al., 1996). First, the algorithm uses two sliding windows on opposite sides of the current velocity sample and finds the average velocity within each such window. These averages are subtracted, and only if the difference exceeds a threshold, a saccade is detected. To prevent two fixations from being identified too closely in space and time, another set of thresholds is used to control for fixation proximity.

An increasingly popular event detection algorithm was presented by Engbert and Kliegl (2003). It was originally developed to detect microsaccades, but works equally well for saccade detection. To detect saccades, the algorithm searches for velocity samples exceeding a threshold, which is calculated based on a median estimation of the eye velocity during a trial. Thus, it adapts the threshold over different trials and participants. Horizontal (v_x) and vertical (v_y) velocity components are treated separately by the algorithm.

Hidden Markov Models (HMM) use a probabilistic model to classify data samples into saccades and fixations based on velocity information. The I-HMM model described by Salvucci and Goldberg (2000) uses two states, S_1 and S_2, each representing the velocity distribution of either fixation samples or saccade samples (see Figure 5.25). Each state is associated with transition probabilities, which estimate the likelihood of the next sample belonging to a fixation or saccade, given the status of the current sample. Typically, consecutive samples have a high probability of belonging to the same type of eye movement, giving small inter-state transition probabilities, $\{p_{12}, p_{21}\}$. The two-state I-HMM model reported by Salvucci and Goldberg (2000) needs eight parameters, which can be estimated from similar sample data. Besides two transition parameters for each state, the model needs to know the observation probabilities in the form of velocity distributions (means and standard deviations). Given the model parameters and a sequence of gaze positions to be classified, dynamic programming such as the Viterbi algorithm can be use to map gaze positions to states (fixation or saccades) in a way that maximizes the probability of a correct assignment according to the model. Finally, neighbouring samples are collapsed into fixation and saccades based on e.g., majority decisions.

Extending the two-state approach, Rothkopf and Pelz (2004) proposed a four-state HMM to analyse data collected using head-mounted eye-trackers. The two additional states represented data from smooth pursuits and vestibular ocular reflexes (VOR).

The I-HMM is, according to Salvucci and Goldberg (2000), accurate and robust, and it is possible to adapt by re-estimating the parameters. In comparison with other dispersion-based methods, it is more complex, however, and requires more parameters to be set (or estimated). Algorithms based on HMMs are uncommon and cannot be found in any commercial software.

Velocity in combination with acceleration

Information about eye acceleration is particularity useful when distinguishing saccades from smooth pursuit. Velocity by itself is not sufficient since the slowest saccade velocity can be slower than the fastest smooth pursuit movement (Behrens & Weiss, 1992). Acceleration is therefore used in high speed data for detecting saccade on- and offsets, where the eye acceleration reaches its maximum value.

A widely used velocity- and acceleration-based saccade detection algorithm was developed by SR Research and thus primarily applied to eye-tracking data acquired with EyeLink-systems, but it is not the only algorithm using acceleration data (see Tole & Young, 1981; Behrens & Weiss, 1992). The algorithm developed by SR Research is perhaps the most heuristic of the different algorithms, with several settings and a number of pragmatic assumptions built in. This may stem from its fundamental difference compared to previously described algorithms: it is primarily designed to detect saccades *online* using the position and movement of the eyes, which is (and must be) reflected in its design. This difference gives the EyeLink parser some advantages. First, only the detected events have to be stored on the recording computer, not raw data samples. This saves a substantial amount of space. Second, and maybe most importantly, it allows for gaze-contingent research where stimuli can be manipulated online in synchrony with the eye-movement events. On the other hand, an online algorithm does not have access to all data samples in a trial before detection, and thus needs to make its decisions based only on data recorded before the currently available sample. Moreover, it has only one chance to get this right, whereas a multipass algorithm has the chance to correct initial mistakes.

In the EyeLink algorithm, saccade on- and offsets are detected by comparing the instantaneous velocity and acceleration against user defined thresholds. To make the algorithm more robust, detection is triggered when either velocity or acceleration become higher/lower than their respective thresholds for a predefined number of samples. Besides saccades, the Eye-Link parser detects blinks and fixations; blinks are identified when the pupil size is very small, or cannot be found at all in the camera image of the eye; fixations are everything that is not saccades or blinks.

5.6 Manual coding of events

Manual coding means that a person subjectively decides, for example, when the gaze position is still enough to be a fixation or moves fast enough to be a saccade. An example of coding instructions and procedures is given in C. M. Harris, Hainline, Abramov, Lemerise, and Camenzuli (1988). While it is very time consuming, manual coding may sometimes be the only real option, as in the case where data is available only as gaze-overlaid videos or when data are recorded from dynamic stimuli. Compared to algorithmic detection, manual coding has the advantage of being able to utilize the powerful pattern matching ability that humans have, but also the weakness of human subjectivity and inconsistency.

To identify fixation durations from video, you need to look through it frame by frame,[19] and notice when the gaze overlay cursor is still and when it moves. Stillness is typically defined as the gaze cursor remaining on the same position (usually an object) in the scene, even if the head is moving, rather than stillness in the head.

Fixation duration coding from gaze-overlaid videos is not very common, and when it is done, the method is rarely published. For instance, Tatler, Gilchrist, and Land (2005) recorded the eye video image onto the gaze-overlaid video, and thus could see the movement in the *eye video* while watching the gaze cursor move when coding for fixations. According to Benjamin Tatler,[20] the movement in the eye video is a much more reliable indicator of fixation and saccade events than the gaze cursor, especially as the scene video looks a bit blurred during saccades and head movements.

Munn et al. (2008) tested three coders, with on average 300 hours of coding experience. They were given the instruction to code the gaze-overlaid 30 Hz video for fixation start- and end-frames. They used a 200 ms fixation duration criterion. Coding a 100 second period of data took 80 minutes on average. One data period was from a participant walking around in an office environment, and the other from an animated film. The authors compared the coded fixations to fixations produced by a velocity-based type of algorithm, also taking 30 Hz data, with the addition of an extra fixation duration criterion of 200 ms. Results show that the human coders agreed with each other slightly more often than with the algorithm, but this could be due to the low sampling frequency of the eye-tracker. For head-mounted systems with a higher sampling frequency, we should expect a better performance on the part of the algorithm. In conclusion, Munn et al. (2008) found that the algorithm they tested was quite robust in finding fixations (or rather non-saccadic portions of data), and that the algorithm could be used as a preliminary parser that reduces the effort of manual coders to find potential fixations.

Methods for dwell time coding are described on pages 227–229. In dwell time coding, the coded values are the total gaze durations on objects in the scene, irrespective of whether that gaze is composed by fixations, saccades, or smooth pursuit.

5.7 Blink detection

Blink detection is an important component of an event detection algorithm, both since blinks are related to cognitive functions (p. 410 and Fogarty & Stern, 1989), and because they need to be separated from other types of events such as fixations and saccades. Moreover, blinks are often considered to be artefacts in both eye-tracking and EEG data, and inaccurate detection causes these undesired data to be included in the subsequent analysis. For example, the EyeLink manual advises the user that "it is also useful to eliminate any short (less than 120 millisecond duration) fixations that precede or follow a blink. These may be artificial or be corrupted by the blink" (SR Research, 2007). Together these reasons motivate why most eye-trackers report information about blinks, even though they are not movements of the eye, but rather movements of the eyelid.

There are a number of methods to detect and measure blinks, for example by analysing the eye video directly (Grauman, Betke, Gips, & Bradski, 2001; Moriyama et al., 2002), by identifying large vertical EOG potentials (Abel, Troost, & Dell'Osso, 1983), by monitoring markers attached to the upper and lower eyelids (Collewijn, Van Der Steen, & Steinman,

[19]If you record eye movement data at 50 Hz on a video with 25 interlaced frames per second, you can go through the video field by field to see *all* data samples during coding. Not all video viewers allow this, however.
[20]Personal communication, October 21, 2009.

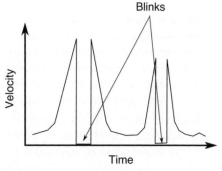

Blinks

Velocity

Time

(a) Two blinks seen as pairs of artefactual down- (b) Two blinks in a velocity plot.
ward saccades with intermediate loss of data.

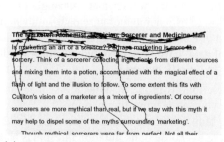

Fig. 5.26 Typical appearance of blinks when they appear in data collected with tower-mounted high-
-speed eye-trackers.

1985), or simply by manual counting of blinks (J. R. Taylor et al., 1999; Epelboim & Suppes,
2001). The focus of this section, however, is blink detection with data from modern video-
based eye-trackers that output at least time stamped (x, y) coordinates and pupil size.

Blinks are detected as the eyelid descends downward to eventually cover the entire eyeball. On its way down, it covers increasingly more of the pupil, making the calculated pupil
centre move downward, and with it the data samples, as though there was a rapid downward
saccade. When the eyeball is completely covered, both the pupil and the corneal reflection
cannot be tracked any more. Consequently, the eye-tracker reports neither data samples nor
pupil size, and instead typically outputs zeros (0). When the eyelid re-opens a corresponding
upward-moving saccade-like movement is produced, and actual eye tracking can continue.
Figure 5.26 illustrates the typical appearance of (a) data samples and (b) velocity during two
blinks recorded with a high-speed tower-mounted eye-tracker.

There are surprisingly few published articles dedicated to blink detection, and the ones
that exist can mainly be found in the data analysis sections of the paper. Indeed, most blink
detection algorithms consider pupil size and gaze coordinates, often also with a required
minimum duration. Bonifacci, Ricciardelli, Lugli, and Pellicano (2008), for example, define
blinks as sudden losses of the position signal for more than 96 ms, and Van Orden, Jung, and
Makeig (2000) use a pupil diameter threshold in combination with an 83.3 ms minimum duration requirement. Using both pupil and gaze coordinate information, Geng, Ruff, and Driver
(2009) required a loss of pupil data for at least 50 ms in combination with eye movement
of at least 13° of visual angle. Similarly, Brouwer, Van Ee, and Schwarzbach (2005) defined
blinks simply as "those samples during which no eye position was recorded". Karatekin, Marcus, and White (2007) used one of three criteria, defined as followed: "(a) the pupil diameter
falling below 1.86 mm or above 5.96 mm, (b) the horizontal or vertical positions of the eye
falling outside the limits of the screen, or (c) the diameter of the pupil changing by more than
0.74 mm over 16.7 ms."

Several researchers do not use their own software, but rely on blink detection algorithms
implemented by manufacturers. Examples are:

- SMI's analysis software package BeGaze 2.3 detects blinks when "zero data is embedded in 2 saccade events" (SMI, 2007), i.e. exactly what is depicted in Figure 5.26. Note
  that this makes the algorithms depend critically on how saccades are defined.
- The EyeLink parser describes blink detection as follows in the manual: "Blinks are
  defined by a period of missing pupil surrounded by a period of artefactual saccade

caused by the sweep of the eyelids across the pupil." (SR Research, 2007).

- Tobii Studio's (version 2.1.12) help function hints to the user that "A couple of gaze data with validity code 4 on both eyes followed by a number of gaze data with validity code 0 on both eyes are usually a sure sign of a blink". According to the help function, the validity code 0 means that all 'relevant data' have been recorded, whereas validity code 4 indicates that data is missing or is "definitely incorrect".

A common denominator for the algorithmic descriptions in the manufacturers' manuals is that sufficient detail to implement the algorithm yourself is typically missing.

Although visual intake is suppressed during blinks, it is not clear for how long (p. 324). Therefore, it seems suboptimal in the general case to choose blink duration thresholds based on what is known about blink suppression.

Data from eyelid trackers show that closing the eyelid is generally faster than opening it (p. 325). This allows us to define at least four duration measures: closing time, closed time, reopening time, and blink duration. The baseline is the position of the eyelid before closing. As we have seen in the eye camera set-up section, eyelids can be more or less droopy in the baseline state, and a droopy eye will have a smaller amplitude during blinks. There are several alternative measures of blinks. For instance, blink closure duration was defined by Morris (1984) as the time from when the lid is half closed and going down, until it is at the same position but heading upward. Lobb and Stern (1986) introduced a whole range of measures, such as time between blink initiation and incursion of the lid on the pupil, duration of lid over the pupil, duration between lid over pupil and full closure, and how long the lid remained closed.

Note that an eye-tracker typically does not measure the movement of the eyelid, and therefore cannot provide detailed information about individual blinks. However, it may give a good idea of how much of the pupil is covered. For instance, closing time could refer to the time it takes the eyelid to traverse the pupil on its way down. Sometimes there is no need to know the precise dynamics of a blink, as long as it can be detected and *blink rate* can be calculated.

5.8 Smooth pursuit detection

Smooth pursuit is the slow motion of the eye as it follows something moving. There is a common belief that smooth pursuit can *only* occur when there is a target to follow, but some studies contradict this. It appears that participants can follow the mental percept of an imagined or offset stimulus for at least a few seconds (Whittaker & Eaholtz, 1982; De'Sperati & Santandrea, 2005). So, for instance, if the participant controls a moving object, the eye can pursue it smoothly even in total darkness (Gauthier & Hofferer, 1976).

Smooth pursuit can be studied in its own right, indirectly revealing properties of the neural systems that underly it. Alternatively, the effect on smooth pursuit of drugs, alcohol, and a variety of disorders can be a reason to use smooth pursuit measures. For instance, Trillenberg, Lencer, and Heide (2004) review a large number of eye-tracking studies with a focus on smooth pursuit, and conclude that "eye movements provide an important tool to measure pharmacological effects in patients and unravel genetic traits in psychiatric disease". Similarly, the large review by O'Driscoll and Callahan (2008) indicates that smooth pursuit impairment is robust in schizophrenia.

Figure 5.27 shows the *x*-coordinate, velocity and acceleration of a person's gaze when trying to follow a pendulum movement—a task that requires smooth pursuit movements. As the figure illustrates, smooth pursuit is characterized by periods with more or less constant velocities accompanied by what is known as 'catch-up saccades'. These are employed when

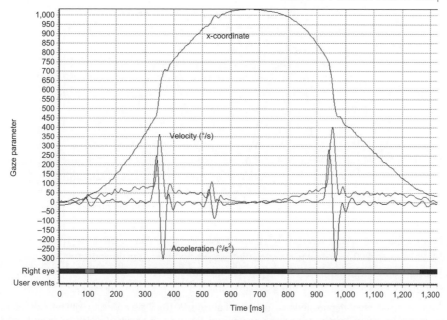

Fig. 5.27 Gaze following a pendulum movement. Recorded with the SMI HiSpeed 1250 Hz. 'Fixations' (black) and 'saccades' (grey) as detected with the SMI velocity algorithm in BeGaze 2.1 are shown at the bottom of the graph.

the gaze position lags behind the target it follows, and therefore temporarily needs to increase velocity to catch up with the target. Besides catch-up saccades, another two types of saccades can interrupt smooth pursuit: *back-up saccades* (in the direction opposite target motion which reposition the eyes on the target when eye position was ahead of the target) and *leading saccades* (anticipatory saccades of any amplitude over 1°). Square-wave jerks can also occur during smooth pursuit (Black, 1984). Fixations interrupt smooth pursuit when it is very slow, at least from the viewpoint of the detection algorithm, which ignores whether or not the smooth pursuit brainware continues to move the eyes.

In the medical research community, data on smooth pursuit is typically calculated in relation to a moving object (dot) that the participant looks at. To estimate how accurately the participant can follow a target dot as it moves, the ratio (*gain*) or distance (*phase*) between target velocity and eye velocity over time can be calculated. There is then no need to *detect* the smooth pursuit first; calculations can be made directly from the raw data stream. However, it may be necessary to remove saccades (including catch-up saccades) and interpolate saccadic gaps to obtain accurate values (Ebisawa, Minamitani, Mori, & Takase, 1988).

Applied researchers use more complex video stimuli, as well as head-mounted eye-trackers without head tracking, and get data where smooth pursuit is mixed with fixations and saccades. Using the current dispersion or saccade velocity algorithms to calculate fixation duration, saccadic amplitude or the percentage of smooth pursuit is of little use here, but can be directly misleading, as we saw earlier in this chapter. For such applications, a general smooth pursuit detection algorithm is needed.

As previously described, some algorithms co-classify fixations and smooth pursuits into a general 'intake' category, like the fixation velocity algorithms used by Itti (2005) as well as the Tobii Fixation Algorithm and the EyeLink parser, which report these combined events as fixations only. Such 'fixations' may not be comparable with fixations recorded from still images.

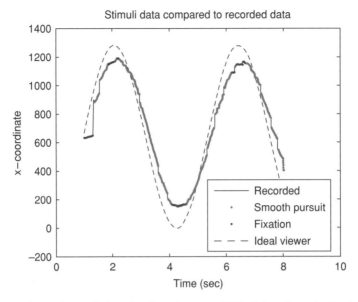

Fig. 5.28 Result of smooth pursuit detection (from Larsson, 2010). Data collected with a tower-mounted system at 500 Hz from a participant looking at a sinusoidal target (the path of which is marked as 'ideal viewer').

Smooth pursuit detection is much less investigated than fixation or saccade detection. Nevertheless, a number of methods have been proposed. Sauter, Martin, Di Renzo, and Vomscheid (1991) developed a technique based on Kalman filtering, which tries to model and predict eye velocity online based on previous velocity samples. If the predicted velocity is significantly different from the observed velocity according to a χ^2-test, a saccade is detected. Otherwise, it is a smooth pursuit movement or a fixation. Komogortsev and Khan (2007) extended this approach by detecting a fixation when the predicted eye velocity was $< 0.5°/s$ for at least 100 ms. Smooth pursuit was defined as everything that was not a saccade or a fixation, and where the predicted eye velocity did not exceed $140°/s$.

A different approach was used by Agustin (2010), who in an initial step separated saccades from fixation and smooth pursuit with simple velocity thresholding, and then separated fixations from smooth pursuit by looking at the direction of movement over a limited time window; smooth pursuit was detected only when the standard deviation of the movement directions was below a certain threshold. Since fast smooth pursuit velocity can exceed the velocity of slow saccades, Larsson (2010) used the algorithm by Engbert and Kliegl (2003) adapted to the acceleration domain to separate the quickly accelerating saccades from fixations and smooth pursuit. Smooth pursuit was separated from fixations by statistically testing the uniformity in distribution of sample-to-sample vectors around the unit circle. Only portions of the data where the hypothesis of uniformity was rejected by a Rayleigh test were accepted as smooth pursuit. Finally, a dispersion-based threshold was used to find fixations. Remaining data comprised undefined events. Figure 5.28 shows the result of applying the algorithm by Larsson (2010) to data collected from a participant looking at a sinusoidal target.

Analysing smooth pursuit in monkeys, Ferrera (2000) presented an algorithmic method drawing on eye velocity. Assuming that saccades have already been removed from data, it is implemented as follows. A moving window of 100 ms is applied to velocity samples, for each stop comparing whether the data in the current 100 ms window differs significantly from the data in the previous 100 ms window. Ferrera then uses the calculated significance values to make an ROC (receiver operating characteristic) curve along the eye-velocity curve.

When the ROC curve reaches 0.95, onset of smooth pursuit is assumed to have taken place. This appears to be a fairly precise calculation of onset, and it is based on eye velocity only. Ferrera's major argument for using a velocity- rather than an acceleration-based algorithm is that acceleration is a noisier measure, being a second derivative. Smooth pursuit offset is the inverse of onset. In theory, therefore, Ferrera's method could be used to calculate the offset by simply exchanging the positions of the two windows.

D. J. Berg, Boehnke, Marino, Munoz, and Itti (2009) used principal component analysis (PCA) to classify raw eye-movement data within a temporal window. A small ratio of the explained variances (minimum divided by maximum) for each of the two principal components was interpreted as a saccade. Raw data samples with a ratio near zero but with insufficient velocity to be considered as a saccade were taken as smooth pursuit samples.

5.9 Detection of noise and artefacts

There are good arguments to discard imprecise data entirely. But in order to know how much noise there can be in a recording before we delete it, we need to quantify the amount of data which is overly noisy. Detecting which sections of the data are too poor to be used is important, in particular if manufacturers use lower quality eye cameras in the systems they sell.

There are many different types of noise detection. First, there is the *system inherent noise* that is related to the precision of your eye-tracker. In high-end systems, this type of noise is low enough to allow the measurements of fixational eye movements, whereas this is not possible for lower end systems. System inherent noise can be hard to separate from real eye movements under normal conditions, and is reduced by filters rather than detected and removed.

Second, there are the high velocity *optic artefacts*—very quick jumps in eye-movement data—that do not originate from actual eye movements, but derive from situations where the eye-tracker temporarily fails to correctly track the pupil and/or the corneal reflection. As a result, movements that violate known eye-movement dynamics can appear in the data. Fortunately, most artefacts with high velocities can be removed by excluding data samples with velocities and accelerations that exceed the theoretical values for how fast human eyes can move; in 1250 Hz data, Nyström and Holmqvist (2010) use upper thresholds of $1000°/s$ and $100000°/s^2$ for this purpose.

Data loss, when the eye-tracker cannot report a value of how the eye moves, can also be seen as noise. Typically, lost samples are indicated in the data files, which makes it simple to calculate and report. Depending on your research question, blinks are sometimes included in this category.

Event detection algorithms are typically designed under the assumption that there is relatively little imprecision and few artefacts in the data, and in particular that the level of imprecision is even throughout the recording. In some cases, as in Figure 5.13, precision varies over time. Assuming we have a velocity-based algorithm, there are three options for how to deal with this variation:

1. Let the velocity threshold adapt to the local precision level in the data, as proposed by Tole and Young (1981); Niemenlehto (2009). When precision is high, lower the threshold, when it is low, increase the threshold. This makes the best possible use of data, but since fixations are defined by different criteria due to the varying noise levels, they may not be comparable with each other.

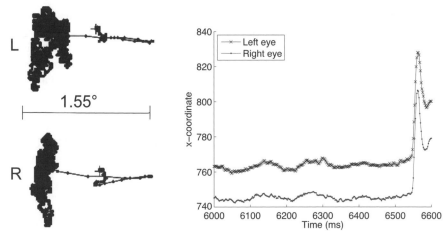

(a) Scanpaths with raw data samples. Long fixation to the left, and microsaccade with immediate backward moving 'overshoot' or 'microglissade'. Left eye above, and right eye below.

(b) The same microsaccade as in (a) shown as a position-over-time plot.

Fig. 5.29 A large microsaccade recorded binocularly at 500 Hz in pupil-only mode, with a video-based tower-mounted eye-tracker and a participant staring at a very small point.

2. Use a fixed, low threshold throughout all data. This will give proper fixations in the high-precision sections of data, but a plethora of unreasonably short fixations and saccades in the low-precision section.

3. Use a fixed, high threshold throughout all data. Noise would be ignored, but also many small saccades.

In summary, noise can be detected as artefacts, data loss, and blinks. The proportion of this type of noise can (and should) be reported in your study. Physiological and system generated noise is more difficult to detect, and is usually reduced by filtering.

5.10   Detection of other events

A number of other patterns occur in eye-tracking data, that could be parsed into events.

Fixational eye movements consist of microsaccades, drifts, and tremor. Of these three types of micro-movements, microsaccades, as illustrated in Figure 5.29, are the most investigated. They can be detected by the algorithm of Engbert and Kliegl (2003). From a ballistic point of view, microsaccades can be regarded as smaller versions of normal saccades, possibly ending with larger overshoots (Møller, Laursen, Tygesen, & Sjølie, 2002).

In short, the algorithm estimates the standard deviation $\sigma_{x,y}$ of the velocity

$$\sigma_{x,y} = \left\langle v_{x,y}^2 \right\rangle - \left\langle v_{x,y} \right\rangle^2 \tag{5.1}$$

in x- and y-dimensions with a median estimator $\langle \cdot \rangle$ to alleviate the influence of noise. Then, velocity samples above a threshold $\lambda \sigma_{x,y}, \lambda \geq 1$ are potential microsaccade samples. Several researchers use the fact that microsaccades occur in both eyes simultaneously, and therefore only accept those that have a minimum overlap in time between the left and the right eye (Engbert & Mergenthaler, 2006; Otero-Millan, Troncoso, Macknik, Serrano-Pedraza, &

Martinez-Conde, 2008). Hafed and Clark (2002) detected microsaccades as movements of size $0.12°-1°$ with a velocity $> 8°/s$, whereas Martinez-Conde, Macknik, and Hubel (2000) used $0.05°-1°$ and $> 3°/s$. Møller et al. (2002) accepted fixational movements as micro-saccades only if their velocities and accelerations exceeded $5°/s$ and $2500°/s^2$, respectively.

Given the microsaccades, inter-microsaccadic intervals (IMSIs) can easily be calculated as periods between the microsaccades (Engbert & Mergenthaler, 2006).

The term **glissade** was coined by Weber and Daroff (1972) to describe a slow, drift-like movement without latency that "corrected dysconjugate refixations". In other words, the glissade was seen as a post-saccadic movement intended to realign the eyes before steady fixation. Bahill, Clark, and Stark (1975a) propose that glissadic overshoot last 30–500 ms, and are therefore different from dynamic overshoot, which they argue last only for 10–30 ms.

Later, glissades were hypothesized to be errors in the measurements, not something to be detected as an event in its own right. For instance, Deubel and Bridgeman (1995) explain the observed "post-saccadic movement" as a form of inertia in the eye lens during saccade retardation, that makes it go further than the eyeball tissue, which then pulls then lens back again. This movement of the lens (but not the eye) would cause what is essentially a mea-surement error in the data, which would be especially grave for the Dual-Purkinje eye-tracker which relies on the fourth Purkinje reflection at the back of the lens. The video-based pupil and corneal reflection systems are much less sensitive to such swinging of the lens, assum-ing that this is the explanation, but yet the authors of this book see the many large glissadic movements very clearly in our data from all our video-based eye-trackers, including high-end systems from SMI and SR Research.

For simplicity, Nyström and Holmqvist (2010) suggested naming all types of high-velocity over- and undershoots that occur directly after a main saccade glissades, and this is also the terminology used in this book. According to this definition, glissades could be seen as ocular 'wobbling' that sometimes occurs at the end of main saccades (for an example see Figure 10.28 on page 338), and it thus differs from the slow post-saccadic drift that may go on for the entirety of the next fixation.

In current detection algorithms, glissades are mostly assigned either to the fixation (e.g. the EyeLink parser), or to the saccade (for instance Gilchrist & Harvey, 2006). Nyström and Holmqvist (2010) detected glissades separately as movement peaks that exceed a velocity threshold within 40 ms after the offset of a saccade. According to Nyström and Holmqvist's definition, the onset of a glissade equals the offset of the preceding saccade, whereas the glissade is terminated when reaching the first local velocity minimum after the last glissadic movement peak. Using this definition of glissades they found an average glissade duration of 24 ms in reading and scene perception, but glissades between 10–50 ms were common.

The **square-wave jerk** is an involuntary, conjugate saccadic intrusion that takes the eye off the visual target, and then back again (Leigh & Zee, 2006, p. 164). Its typical motion pat-tern can be seen in Figure 5.30. Square-wave jerks mostly consist of pairs of small saccades $(0.5-5°)$ in opposite directions, separated by a normal or slightly longer (200–400 ms) sac-cadic latency. Around 10% of square-wave jerks are biphasic, which means that they return with saccadic overshoots, and must be followed by a third, corrective return saccade. Orig-inally called 'Gegenrücke', and sometimes 'saccadic intrusions' (into fixations), they were first termed square-wave jerks by R. Jung and Komhuber (1964). They can derive from both physiological and pathological sources (Abadi & Gowen, 2004). In normal participants, they can occur at a rate of 0.3 Hz or more (Leigh & Zee, 2006, p. 164).

Research papers used a variety of detection techniques, including amplitude and velocity criteria (Abadi & Gowen, 2004). Fahey et al. (2008) used a detection algorithm that searched for a pair of saccades in opposite directions, separated by a 60–900 ms period of stillness. Sac-cades were detected using a velocity threshold of $10°/s$. Moreover, Fahey et al. classified the

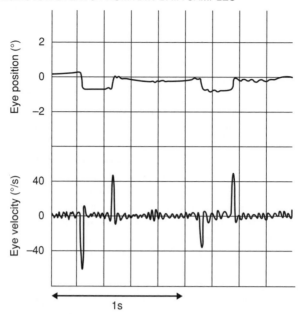

Fig. 5.30 Position and velocity pattern of two square-wave jerks. Recorded from an 11-year old boy fixating a target, using a video-based 120 Hz eye-tracker with magnetic head-tracking. Reprinted from *Pediatric Neurology*, *38*(1),Michael S. Salman, James A. Sharpe, Linda Lillakas, and Martin J. Steinbach, Square Wave Jerks in Children and Adolescents, Copyright (2008), with permission from Elsevier.

square-wave jerks into micro ($< 0.5°$), and macro ($0.5–3°$) events. Using a similar strategy, Feldon and Langston (1977) detected square-wave jerks as pairs of opposing microsaccades separated in time with at most 750 ms.

If the intrusive movement lacks the intersaccadic interval present in square-wave jerks, and saccades appear 'back-to-back', it is most likely due to *ocular flutter* (horizontal movements shown in Figure 5.31) or *opsoclonus* (movements in all directions) (Leigh & Zee, 2006, p. 165). Unlike square-wave jerks, these types of movements seem to appear mainly in participants with saccadic abnormalities.

Undefined events Some portions of data may simply not be possible to assign to any known category, either because the algorithm is not designed to identify this particular type of event, or because the portion of data does not fit according to any known prototypical pattern. Typically, this is what is left after every known event has been detected, and is sometimes categorized together with noise and artefacts.

Notice that the physical appearance of glissades, small saccades, microsaccades, and the beginning/end of a square-wave jerk can be very similar, and therefore the same algorithm could successfully detect all three types of eye movements. In the end it is up to the researcher to decide which event has been detected, and its functional role. Sometimes terms are used interchangeably; Abadi and Gowen (2004), for example, make no terminological difference between dynamic overshoots (i.e. glissades) and microsaccades, and Hafed and Clark (2002) equate square-wave jerks with a "pair of back-to-back opposing microsaccades".

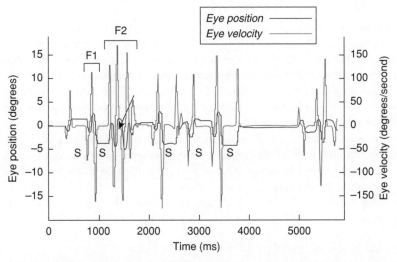

Fig. 5.31 Square-wave jerks (S) mixed with ocular flutter (F1, F2). Reproduced from *Brain*, *131*(4), Michael C. Fahey, Phillip D. Cremer, Swee T. Aw, Lynette Millist, Michael J. Todd, Owen B. White, Michael Halmagyi, Louise A. Corben, Veronica Collins, Andrew J. Churchyard, Kim Tan, Lionel Kowal, and Martin B. Delatycki, Vestibular, saccadic and fixation abnormalities in genetically confirmed Friedreich ataxia, Copyright (2008) with permission from Oxford University Press.

5.11 Summary: oculomotor events in eye-movement data

From this chapter, we can conclude that a comprehensive oculomotor event detection algorithm should deliver the following data, correctly calculated, to be used directly or in further analysis:

- **Velocity-** and **acceleration** values calculated from the raw data coordinate samples, via a filtering that does not undermine the detection of any of the events.
- **Fixation** events, each having values for at least position, dispersion, onset, and duration. Inside fixations, we find the fixational eye-movement events, divided into:
  * **microsaccades**, with at least amplitude, duration, and velocity values
  * **drifts**
  * **inter-microsaccadic intervals**
- **Saccade** events, each having values for at least starting position, landing position, amplitude, starting time, duration, peak velocity, and peak acceleration.
- **Smooth pursuit** events, with values for ... well, there is no consensus on how smooth pursuit events should be represented. Within smooth pursuit, we find the event triple:
  * **catch-up saccade**
  * **back-up saccade**
  * **leading saccade**
- **Blink** events, with values for at least *starting time* and *duration*.
- **Glissade** events, with at least the same values as a saccadic event.
- **Square-wave jerk** with at least *amplitude* and *starting position* and *duration*.

None of the algorithms described in this chapter detect and measure all events reliably. They all have settings that are not easy to grasp for the beginning eye-tracking researcher, but which have profound effects on the results produced. Most worryingly, the algorithms treat the raw samples so differently that basic measures such as fixation duration and saccade amplitude will be difficult to compare between algorithms using the same data. The majority of eye-tracking researchers appear to have faith in the algorithms provided by manufacturers, and manufacturers mostly support this faith when they hide the algorithm properties in settings dialogues that are difficult to see through, and when not simultaneously showing raw data and detection results in the same scanpath or velocity graph.

The dominating dispersion algorithm I-DT delivers fixations with a distribution (shown in Figure 5.9) which simply does not look credible, independent of setting. It is imprecise in its calculation of fixation onset and duration, and presents little more, yet bothering the user with the two settings and their unclear interaction. The single setting of a velocity algorithm is easy to relate to the velocity diagrams: just by looking at a few portions of data you can estimate the proper threshold value. Also, the fixation duration distribution of the various velocity algorithms looks more like a representation of a real distribution. For data with a high sampling frequency, the velocity algorithms are the only realistic choice. In the near future, however, we are likely to see improved algorithms for all these events.

6 Areas of Interest

In the previous chapter, we explained how to process data samples into events such as fixations, saccades, and smooth pursuits (Chapter 5). This chapter defines and discusses areas of interests (AOIs) as a tool for the further analysis of eye-movement data. In simple terms, AOIs define regions in the stimulus that the researcher is interested in gathering data about: did the participant look where expected, and what were the properties of their eye movements in the area looked at? But more importantly, AOIs allow further events to be defined and detected: *dwells, transitions,* and *AOI hits*; these will be introduced in this chapter. In addition, segmenting stimulus space with AOIs allows us to transform and simplify the recorded data into representations such as *strings, transition matrices,* and *proportion over time graphs.*

Using AOIs in data analysis requires a number of issues to be addressed:

- First, we emphasise the important relationship between your hypothesis and what can be done in an AOI editor (Section 6.1, p. 188).
- In Section 6.2 (p. 188), we provide condensed hands-on advice for work with AOIs.
- We then define the three basic AOI events in Section 6.3 (p. 189): *AOI hits, dwells,* and *transitions.* We also define three related events: *returns, first skips,* and *total skips.*
- Five major representations of eye-movement data, based on the subdivision of space using AOIs, are described in Section 6.4 (p. 192): *AOI strings, dwell maps, transition matrices, Markov models,* and *proportion over time graphs.* Many of these come with several varieties.
- Section 6.5 (p. 206) describes the properties and usage of several types of AOIs: dynamic, distributed, gridded, and fuzzy AOIs, just to mention a few.
- It is commonly believed that AOIs are very simple to use. However, there are a number of challenging issues concerning the usage and analysis of AOIs that are discussed in Section 6.6 (p. 216). For example, can we use AOIs that are arbitrarily small, or is there a minimal allowed size?
- Finally, the summary in Section 6.7 (p. 229) draws together the most used AOI events and representations that will follow us through the remainder of the book.

Since AOIs have been repeatedly re-invented by different researchers, and because software developers want to contrast their products with those from other manufacturers, there is no standard terminology for AOI measures, and some of the measures are referred to by up to seven different names. Sometimes the same name is used about different measures (like 'gaze duration' which can be either 'dwell time' or 'total dwell time'). Even the AOIs themselves are known under different names, such as 'ROIs' (regions of interests), 'IAs' (interest areas), and 'Zones'. We use 'AOI' because it appears to be the most established term in eye-tracking research. The unclear naming situation causes unnecessary confusion in many research papers, and a one goal of this chapter is to propose a standardized and more logical vocabulary.

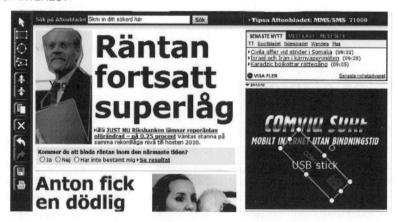

Fig. 6.1 Two AOIs drawn on a stimulus background (a webpage); one a polygon (named 'Yngves') and the other a rectangle (named 'USB stick'). The AOI editor is seen on the left as a number of tool buttons. AOI editors today give the user lots of freedom to position and edit the AOIs.

6.1   The AOI editor and your hypothesis

AOI events are defined *in relation to entities in the stimulus*. In this, they contrast with fixations and saccades which are calculated on the basis of data alone; the event detection algorithms of the previous chapter know nothing about the stimulus content.

AOIs are created using a tool for spatial segmentation sometimes called 'the AOI editor' or similar. AOI editors are usually supplied in the analysis software for the eye-tracker. AOIs are always drawn against the background of the stimulus. Figure 6.1 shows an AOI editor with two AOIs drawn on top of a stimulus.

The precise segmentation of the stimulus is crucial to your analysis, and will be discussed in detail on pages 216–224. Remember that the AOIs you draw are *part of your hypothesis*, because they decide which areas in space dwell and transition data should be calculated against. This has two important consequences:

- If you alter your AOIs, you alter your hypothesis.
- If you draw your AOIs after data recording, while inspecting the data, you are forming post-hoc hypotheses.

The freedom of AOI editors allowing you to alter AOIs however you like and at anytime, must therefore be used with great care in order not to undermine the validity of the study.

6.2   Hands-on advice for using AOIs

Before you apply AOIs to your stimuli, consider the following:

- There are many measures that use the events and representations of this chapter, and each and every one of them is very sensitive to how you divide your stimulus into AOIs.
- Let your *research hypothesis decide* what AOIs you put on the stimulus. If you edit or move your AOIs, you alter your hypothesis.
- Each AOI should cover an area with homogeneous semantics, and the semantics should be founded in the rationale behind your experimental design.
- If you are free to design your stimulus, do not put objects so close together that you cannot have a margin between AOIs.

- Overlapping AOIs should not be used unless the hypothesis and stimulus demand it, and then the calculation of first fixations, dwells, and transitions must be reconsidered.
- Do not distribute a single AOI over many areas of your stimulus, unless there is a clear link between the semantics in those areas, your research hypothesis, and the measures you employ.
- When using transition measures, report what is known as 'whitespace' (parts of the stimulus not covered by any AOIs) as a proportion over the whole stimulus. Define how transitions are calculated with regard to whitespace.
- Be aware of measures that are scaling dependent with respect to, e.g. the size or the content of an AOI. However, this must be motivated by the semantics of the stimulus, and the baseline probability of looking towards each area.
- The *minimal AOI size* is limited by the precision and accuracy (pp. 33–41) of your recorded data.
- Avoid arbitrary AOI positioning; ensure your AOIs are as precise as possible in relation to the important elements of the stimulus. For complex real-life stimuli, use an external method (such as expert ratings) to decide if your division of stimulus space is suitable.
- Manually coding dwells and transitions from gaze-overlaid videos is not intractable for limited sections of data.
- Inaccurate data (offsets) can be repaired, but this should not be done unless you know exactly what calculations to make and the consequences for your data.

6.3 The basic AOI events

AOI hits, dwells, and transitions are events in the same sense as fixations and saccades, but to be calculated they require AOIs that connect the data to stimulus space. AOI hits, dwells, and transitions are events used in a very large number of measures; from basic ones like *dwell time* to complex ones like *entropy* and the *string edit measure*. They are used in virtually all branches of eye-tracking research, from human factors to reading.

The following subsections introduce AOI hits, dwells, and transition, and discuss how they should be calculated. We then present the *return*, and the two *skip* events, derived from the basic AOI events.

6.3.1 The AOI hit

The most primitive AOI event is the *AOI hit*, which states for a raw sample or a fixation that its coordinate value is inside the AOI. The sample-based AOI hit underlies all raw AOI measures, including those based on fairly complex representations like proportion over time graphs. In the right side of Figure 6.2, dark portions of the line along the path of samples indicate AOI hits on one of the two AOIs, while where the line is grey, no AOI hit has taken place. Sometimes an AOI is not considered to have been hit until it has been looked upon during a minimum amount of time, reflecting the minimum time it takes to cognitively process the information therein.

The fixation-based AOI hit is important in many of the counting measures with AOIs. Figure 6.2 also shows (on the left side) fixations that directly correspond to the raw data in the graph of the right side.

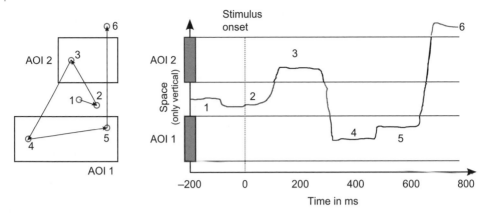

Fig. 6.2 Principle for the trials in which AOI data are calculated: stimulus space is divided into two AOIs, shown on the left side, with fixations from 1 to 6. Trial time is divided by a stimulus onset (at time 0), shown by a dashed line. The space–time diagram on the right side uses black lines to indicate the idealized path of raw data samples over the AOIs, corresponding to the fixations on the left side.

6.3.2 The dwell

The second AOI event is *the dwell*—often known as 'gaze' in reading and 'glance' in human factors (P. Green, 2002)—which is defined as one visit in an AOI, from entry to exit. Figure 6.2 (right) shows the raw data samples included within an AOI as black segments, and those samples outside AOIs as grey segments; a whole black segment equals a dwell. The dwell has its own duration, starting point, ending point, dispersion etc., as it is in several ways similar to a fixation, but a much larger entity both in space and time.

Dwell data represent sample data at a coarser level. If you only know that there is a dwell in the AOI, it can refer to any of the data samples; or in other words, you have lost information about the precise positions of samples. In return, you can categorize the AOI, giving its spatial extension a name that has a meaning to your experiment.

6.3.3 The transition

Another well-known event is *the transition*, also known as 'gaze shift', which is the movement from one AOI to another. For instance, any eye movement between text and graphics in a study of textbook reading counts as a transition. The notation for a transition between AOIs I and E is `IE`, in typewriter font. When AOIs have names with multiple letters, such as AOI RF and AOI LF, the transition is written `RF LF`. The predominant exception in the usage of the term transition comes from reading research, where researchers typically do not describe the movement from one word to the next as a transition but as a forward saccade.

Transitions are similar to saccades; they traverse spatial locations, they could have some sort of duration, an amplitude, and latency measures could be built from them. But transitions can be larger entities than just one saccade, since the transition can move from one AOI to another via fixations in parts not covered by AOIs (Figure 6.3). Indeed, any intermediate portion of the raw data sample in between AOI visits may be counted as part of the transition—the grey segments of the line in Figure 6.3. Note the two dubious cases, however: the term transition is usually reserved for the change in gaze allocation between one AOI and another, rather than exit and re-entry to the same AOI. Also, is it correct to characterize a movement as a transition even between two AOIs when several fixations have been made along the way?

A saccade within an AOI is not and should not be called a transition. Sometimes you may

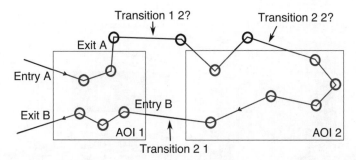

Fig. 6.3 Two AOIs 1 and 2. There is clearly a transition 2 1, but should the movements marked as transitions 1 2 and 2 2 count as transitions? Transition 2 1 is an entry and a return to AOI 1.

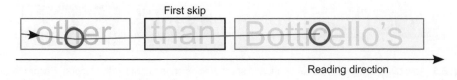

Fig. 6.4 An AOI (word) first-skipped: a later word was looked at without first looking at the skipped AOI.

see "within-AOI transitions" in transition matrices and other measures, but they confuse both the concept and the statistics. They are and should be called "within-AOI saccades".

Studying text–image integration, Stolk and Brok (1999) differentiate between *one-way* and *two-way transitions*. One-way transitions occur when a text has been finished and the graphics is then read, but there is no connected return. Two-way transitions back and forth between the two modalities were taken as indications of actual integration.

Obviously, the particular division of the stimulus space into AOIs is crucial to all transition calculations, and may in fact determine whether a result will be significant or not. It is therefore of the utmost importance to motivate the choice of AOIs based on hypothesis, task, and stimulus, before making the transition calculations to be presented as results.

6.3.4 The return

The *return*, also known as 'revisit', is a transition to an AOI already visited, examplified in Figure 6.3, but the event exists in a version without predefined AOIs also. In research on radiology, it has been operationalized as the event when the eye strays further than 2.5° of visual angle—the approximate area of acute foveal vision—from the centre of any previous fixation and then comes back within that circle.

6.3.5 The AOI first skip

The *AOI first skip* event assumes that the AOIs are ordered, as in reading, and that more or less all AOIs are looked through. An AOI (that is, the word) is taken to be first-skipped if the eye of the reader lands on a later AOI (word) before landing on the word itself, as illustrated in Figure 6.4. The first-skip status of the AOI is not changed if the reader immediately regresses back to it. It was still skipped first, and will remain so.

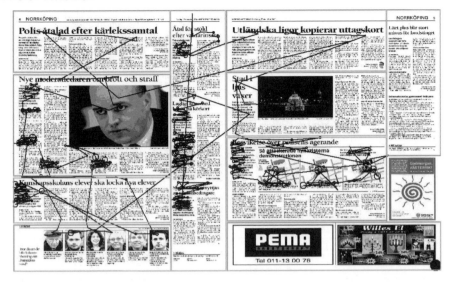

Fig. 6.5 Advertisements at the bottom right and short articles on the right totally skipped. Recorded with a 50 Hz head-mounted eye-tracker with head tracking.

6.3.6 The AOI total skip

The *total skip* status is given to an AOI that a participant does not look at for the entirety of a trial. While the AOI first skip is a dedicated reading event, the AOI total skip is a very general event, since it does not presuppose conventionalized order. For instance, in newspaper reading, an AOI total skip occurs for those AOIs (for instance advertisements) that were never looked at. Figure 6.5 shows an example of data where some parts of the newspaper spread have been totally skipped.

Figure 6.5 also illustrates that skipping may be too coarse a measure for semantic AOIs with a large coverage. Even the non-skipped AOIs are not very much read, which we can quantify with the more flexible reading depth measure (p. 390).

6.4 AOI-based representations of data

There are five AOI-based representations of eye-movement data that many measures make use of. The first is the dwell map, a gridded AOI with dwell time in the cells. Then there are the AOI strings, the most used sequence representation. The third is the transition matrix, which tells us how frequent transitions were between any combination of AOIs in our stimulus. The fourth are the Markov models, the probabilistic variety of the empirical transition matrices. The last are the proportion-over-time graphs and the other AOI over time representations.

6.4.1 Dwell maps

A *dwell map* is simply a list of all AOIs with dwell time (p. 386), as illustrated in Figure 6.6. If gridded AOIs (p. 212) are used, the dwell map can be superimposed onto the stimulus, with the dwell time value filled into each cell in the grid. Although calculated from dwell time data in the gridded AOIs, this simple representation can also be seen as a downsampled heat map, as will be evident in the next chapter, and is of great value in several position dispersion and similarity measures.

0.9	4.0	2.3	2.2	0.1	0.2	
1.4	1.4	4.5	9.4	9.8	3.3	1.3
0.8	0.4	1.0	10.8	11.8	2.4	0.5
0.4	0.9	1.7	2.9	2.4	0.8	0.1
	0.2	0.3	0.9	1.5	0.7	0.1
	0.2			0.2	0.8	
						0.3
						0.1

(a) Dwell map: a gridded AOI with dwell time filled into cells.

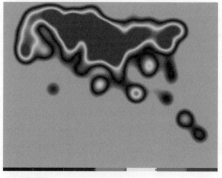

(b) Heat map of the same data.

Fig. 6.6 Dwell map versus heat map for the same data produced by BeGaze 2.4. The dwell map shows dwell times in seconds.

6.4.2 The AOI strings

The *AOI string* is a sequence of either fixation-based AOI hits or dwells in the order of occurrence. There are at least three different varieties:

1. In the string MMTCCHGM, each letter is a *fixation in an AOI* with the name of the letter. Each fixation is included, so we have cases of repetition in the string.
2. A *compressed* string consist of *dwells only*, which means that repetitions are removed when sequences of fixations within the same AOI are collapsed into a single dwell, to give MTCHGM.
3. A string with *first entries* only lists a dwell on the first entry into the AOI. This means that each AOI appears in strings only once, as in MTCHG, and that the maximal string length equals the number of AOIs in the stimulus.

We will write AOI strings as MTCHG when all AOIs have single letters as names, and as A6 C5 F0 I1 J1 K2 I3 or 1 3 4 in all other cases.

There are three applications of the fixation- and dwell-based AOI strings, according to Privitera (2006), each corresponding to a different timescale:

Full history analysis Using the string edit measure for calculating *scanpath similarity* (see p. 348).

Short history analysis Calculating *transition similarity*—a Markov model of transition matrices (p. 193).

No history analysis Calculating *locus similarity* as defined by the number of AOIs shared by both strings, independent of order, and as such could be a coarse pairwise position similarity measure (p. 370).

6.4.3 Transition matrices

A *transition matrix* is a full catalogue of all AOI sequences of length ℓ equal to the dimensionality of the matrix. A fictitious two-dimensional transition matrix is shown in Table 6.1, which shows the transitions between different parts of a machine control panel that the operator looks at. In this transition matrix, the AOIs are listed in rows and columns, and the number in each cell indicates how many times gaze has shifted from one AOI to another. For instance, after the operator looked at the left side (LS) of the dashboard, he often moved his gaze to the left front (LF) part (77 times) and only rarely to the right front (RF) part (3 times).

Table 6.1 A length-2 transition diagram from a fictitious human factors study. The movement direction Left Side to Left Front (LS LF) has scored the largest number of transitions. Dots indicate structural zeros, illegitimate cells representing saccades inside AOIs.

		To						
		LS	LF	RF	RS	I	E	O
	Left Side (LS)	.	77	3	0	17	0	1
	Left Front (LF)	18	.	14	1	56	2	9
	Right Front (RF)	1	52	.	15	16	1	14
From	Right Side (RS)	0	7	35	.	13	15	30
	Instruments (I)	3	54	2	1	.	4	37
	Engine (E)	0	9	0	3	27	.	61
	Other (O)	2	60	2	5	27	4	.

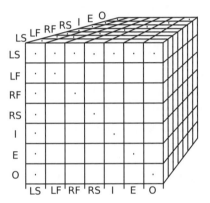

Fig. 6.7 Visualization of a 3D transition matrix for studying the frequency of AOI strings of length 3. Dots again mark structural zeros. The empty cells fill with the number of specific sequences of length three.

Note that the matrix ignores saccades within the same AOI, which is why the values on the diagonal of the table are all so-called structural zeros—they can never be larger than zero. Structural zeros are fundamentally and statistically different from cells that contain sampling zeros, such as transitions from left side (LS) to right side (RS), which were not observed during the study, but could have been. It is important that the software producing values for transition matrix cells clearly distinguishes between the many structural and the many real zeros. Note that some older software replace structural zeros with the number of within-AOI saccades.

Transition matrices can easily be extended to encompass longer sequences. For studying the prevalence of sequences of length 3, a three-dimensional (3D) transition matrix is formed. Continuing with the same fictitious example, Figure 6.7 shows the principle of a 3D transition matrix. Each cell corresponds to, not a transition, but a subsequence such as RS RF LF, a substring of the total AOI string produced by a participant.

There are three complications we need to observe when entering the higher dimensions. First, occurrences of strings shorter than 3 are counted twice or more. For instance, given the AOI string I RS RF LF I LF RF of one participant, the one and same RF LF transition of length and dimensionality 2 appears once in the two length-3 subsequences RS RF LF and once in RF LF I. This means that values in transition matrix cells cannot be straightforwardly compared between dimensions. Second, in the 3D transition matrix, there are structural zeros not only along the central diagonal, but also on the sides and along the corners. This is because any cell that represents an immediate repetition, such as RF RF LF or IEE, but not IEI, is disqualified. The number of remaining valid cell values (N) in a transition matrix from n AOIs and with a dimensionality of ℓ is described in Equation (6.1). The authors have verified this calculation in computer simulations with n ranging from 2 to 12 and ℓ from 3 to 8.

$$N = n(n-1)^{\ell-1} \tag{6.1}$$

The third methodological issue with transition matrices for longer strings is that the number of cells grows exponentially with string length ℓ. Unless enormous amounts of data are recorded, the vast majority of these cells will be empty, and many others will have low values. Not only do these empty cells make it more difficult to achieve statistical power, the zero-inflated data also contorts the statistical distribution. As explained in detail on pages 339–346, this exponential growth and the resulting sparseness of transition matrices as the sequence length increases can be dealt with in very different ways. First, by using probabilistic methods such as Markov chains, which convert the transition frequencies to probabilities and ignore probabilities at or close to zero. Alternatively, one can count only a limited number of the most frequent transitions, the 20 most frequent, for instance. Third, categorizing sequences (cells in the matrix) into a few meaningful groups is also a way of dealing with exponential growth.

The usefulness of transition matrices for strings longer than 2 can be disputed. For instance, C. M. Harris (1993) and Pieters, Rosbergen, and Wedel (1999) found no effects in higher-order Markov models, concluding that free-viewing is a reversible first-order Markov process. Using a 3D transition matrix to study scanpath sequences of multiple lengths in an air traffic control weather station, Ahlstrom and Friedman-Berg (2006) found that the most common sequences across all participants were single transitions of length 2, but very few longer sequences in the data were common over all participants. This means that a first-order Markov model—essentially a 2D transition diagram—governs the scanpath in these situations. In fact, we have found no studies reporting longer sequences than four AOIs even though, in theory, there are situations where longer sequences would be interesting to study.

It is usually taken for granted that a transition matrix is always a 'change of position' matrix, in that it counts transitions between AOI positions. However, Ponsoda et al. (1995) developed a *change of direction matrix*, based on their segmentation of saccadic direction in Figure 10.2(c) on page 302. They argue that a full 8×8 transition matrix would be inappropriate due to high standard errors in matrix cells when small data sets are used, and proceed with a 2×2 matrix, using only horizontal and vertical directions.

Usage of transition matrices

Transition matrices are flexible representations that have been used in many research fields. In human factors, Itoh, Hansen, and Nielsen (1998) constructed a model of ship navigation using a transition matrix in combination with dwell time analysis. Moray and Rotenberg (1989) found that instruments were fixated more frequently after a plant failure, but that dwell times were unchanged, and that operators tend to deal with multiple disturbances sequentially. Morrison, Marshall, Kelly, and Moore (1997) used a transition matrix to investigate whether different decision strategies can be visible in transition matrix results from interactions with military decision support displays.

Cook, Wiebe, and Carter (2008) investigated learning from displays with multiple representations of osmotic cell transportation. They showed that low prior knowledge students transitioned more frequently between macroscopic and molecular representations, interpreting this as evidence of a higher difficulty in coordinating the representations. The 'eye movement matrix' of Hyönä, Lorch Jr, and Rinck (2003) uses sentences as AOIs, and is one of the methods for studying global text reading. The likely but hypothetical examples given by

Hyönä et al. show that they can be useful in the study of inconsistent texts. Lastly, Holmqvist, Holsanova, Barthelson, and Lundqvist (2003) used transition matrices to compare internet newspapers.

The relation between dwell time and the number of transitions

S. R. Ellis and Stark (1986) point to the possibility that by chance alone, there are *more transitions between AOIs with a higher dwell time*, simply because the gaze is more often there. It is clear, however, that this correlation between dwell time and number of transitions is more likely with some stimuli and tasks than with others. In newspaper reading, for instance, the number of transitions a participant makes between two texts that he has read for 2 minutes each cannot be 24 times higher than the number of transitions between texts that he has read for 5 seconds each. The texts are separate and unrelated units, and there is no need to look back and forth between them to solve the task of understanding the news. But in human factors studies, in particular surveillance tasks where participants look at radar or instruments in a cockpit that all play a part in the task, it is much more likely that dwell time influences the number of transitions, simply because such tasks require many integrative transitions.

S. R. Ellis and Stark formally differentiate between three cases with different base probability of transitions:

Random Each AOI has the same dwell time, which is interpreted as the same probability of being fixated. The expectation is that transitions will be equal between all pairs of AOIs. This could possibly occur during task-free viewing of random scenes.

Stratified random All AOIs have different dwell times. The probability of transitions from/to an AOI is proportional to its dwell time. This is the case with the human factors task where information from all AOIs contributes to solving a single task.

Statistically dependent As in our newspaper example, the probabilities for transitions cannot be calculated from the dwell times in the AOIs. Such a situation can be modelled by a Markov chain with states for the AOIs and their dwell time, and transition probabilities for the transition frequences.

6.4.4 Markov models

Markov models are related to transitions matrices, but there are important differences. First of all, while a transition matrix is only a descriptive summary representation of collected data, the exact same numbers in the cells of a Markov model are assumed to be *the probabilities* for each transition. That is, the highest transition probability in a Markov model indicates the most probable sequence of two or more AOIs. In other words, Markov models can be used to examine the stochastic processes underlying observed transition sequences, and to explore the goodness of fit of a predicted model. Another difference between Markov models and transition diagrams is that Markov models can include the dwell time between transitions in the probability model.

Markov models exist at several levels, known as orders, which directly correspond to the dimensionality of transition matrices. The zero-order Markov model would be the dwell map for the set of AOIs. The first-order Markov model corresponds to the standard 2D transition matrix, that is, probabilities of movements between the cells of the zero-order Markov model. The second-order Markov models describe the probabilities of all triple-AOI sequences, i.e. all strings with a length of three AOIs. Higher-order Markov models can model even longer sequences of AOIs. In practice, however, Markov models higher than second order (three AOIs) are hardly ever used.

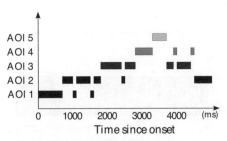

(a) AOI sequence chart with five AOIs and data from one participant.

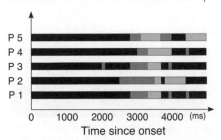

(b) Scarf plots from fictitious five participants and the same five AOIs as in Figure (a). Participant 1 here has the same data as shown in Figure (a).

Fig. 6.8 Sequence chart and scarf plot.

Markov models have been used for very basic research on scanpath planning. For instance, recording data from airline pilots, S. R. Ellis and Stark (1986) compared statistically the empirical transition matrix to a first-order Markov model derived from zero-order probabilities (dwell times), noting the model fits the data better at the first-order level than if only comparing dwell times. C. M. Harris (1993) reanalysed the data from Buswell (1935), finding that they are readily modelled by a so-called stationary, reversible first-order Markov model. This result, replicated by Gordon and Moser (2007), Epelboim and Suppes (2001), and Pieters et al. (1999), can be interpreted as showing that the probability of fixating an object depends significantly on the object of the immediately preceding fixation, but not on the objects fixated further back in the scanpath.

Hidden Markov models include hidden states that may correspond to theoretical entities. Studying consumer brand awareness, Van Der Lans, Pieters, and Wedel (2008) use a model with two states, "localization" and "identification".

6.4.5   AOIs over time

There are many *AOI over time* representations, the best known of which are the *proportion over time graphs*. They represent time more accurately than transitions (p. 205). AOI over time representations use a time line which starts usually some time before the introduced and measured effect and stops at a point in time where the effect is likely to have dissipated. By observing and analysing the changes in the attended AOIs, the presence and actual parameters of the effect in question can be measured.

Each measure that can give values over successive points or windows in time along the sampled eye-movement data can produce value-over-time graphs. Figures 6.8 and 6.9 show how this is done with the binary measure AOI hit. Figure 6.8(a) shows an AOI *sequence chart* (also 'order versus time diagram') with five AOIs and data from one participant. The sequence chart shows the order and duration of dwells to each AOI. This participant starts looking at AOI 1, and then looks at AOI 2. After two short returns to AOI 1, the participant continues to AOI 3 and so on.

In Figure 6.8(b) we have collapsed the sequence charts of each participant to one line, and thus formed a *scarf plot*. The *scarf plot* is a condensed version of the AOI sequence chart, where the AOIs of each participant have been placed on a single line, so as to form what looks like a scarf, as in Figure 6.8(b), where each colour in the scarf refers to a unique AOI. With multiple participants, scarf plots allow visual comparisons over several participants.

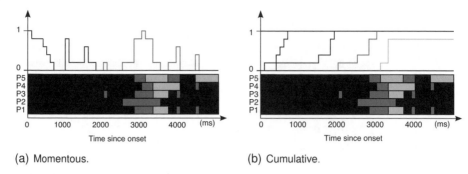

(a) Momentous.   (b) Cumulative.

Fig. 6.9 Illustration of how momentous and cumulative proportion over time graphs are calculated from scarf plot data. Bottom: Scarf plots for five participants. Top: The proportion over time graphs for two of the five AOIs.

Whereas the scarf plot is excellent for visualizing the AOI behaviour of a particular individual, it is less apt for identifying a particular AOI trend that is present, but scattered in many participants. For this case, it is appropriate to make a line graph showing the proportion of participants gazing at a particular AOI at a given point in time. Figure 6.9 plots the data from Figure 6.8 as proportion values over time.

Sampling frequency of data in the fictitious example in Figure 6.9(a) is however very low, only 10 Hz, and the number of participants in actual research is much larger than five. This makes the actual proportion over time graphs much smoother than the ones shown here, but the principle is exactly the same. Additional smoothing typically improves visual interpretation of the graph.

Proportion over time graphs have two varieties. The *momentous proportion over time graph* shows the differences in gaze behaviour for *one moment at a time*. It is very simple to calculate as the average over a scarf plot, as illustrated by Figure 6.9(a). An AOI having a large area under the curve in a momentous proportion over time graph also has a high average *dwell time*, and vice versa. This is because the proportion of samples that fall within an AOI during a time window will sum up to the total amount of dwell over all participants in the same time window.

For studies where it is important what proportion of participants have *so far seen* an AOI, the *cumulative proportion over time* diagrams can be a good tool. For each AOI, if it has been seen by a participant, then that AOI is marked as seen for the rest of that participant's data. The cumulative proportion over time graphs provide for latency measures closely related to the *entry time measure* (p. 437), expressing what percentage of participants have entered an AOI over time. What is known as 'hazard curves' and 'survival probability analysis' (S. N. Yang & McConkie, 2001; Hirose, Kennedy, & Tatler, 2010) plot the probability over time that an AOI will survive in the sense of not being hit by any fixations. As such, they are the mathematical inverse of cumulative graphs.

Proportion over time graphs were originally used with *fixed trial durations*. This means that exactly the same participants contribute at the beginning as in the end. When recording data with *variable trial durations*, this means that more participants contribute in the beginning of the graph than towards the end. In cases where the experimental design requires trials to be of different lengths for different participants, we need to choose either:

- For each raw data sample, count the number of participants that look at each AOI, relative to the total number of participants at the onset of the trial. Curves will generally decline as participants finish with trials and drop off.
- Count the proportion of participants, relative to the remaining number of participants

who look at each AOI at the point in time of that raw data sample. Data for each AOI will always sum to close to 100%, and curves will not decline, but they are based on a declining subset of participants.

A word of caution: these proportion-over-time graph only tells us *that* a proportion of participants look at, or have looked at, the AOI, not *what* proportion looks there. Participants may take turns.

The time-locking hypothesis, and the order and duration of the processes

Before we can enter into a discussion on the many varieties of AOIs over time, we need to ask what they can be used for. In what is now known as the visual world paradigm of psycholinguistics, a hypothesis soon emerged that points out that eye movements appear to be *time-locked* to the linguistic and cognitive processes being studied (Tanenhaus et al., 1995; Eberhard, Spivey-Knowlton, Sedivy, & Tanenhaus, 1995; A. S. Meyer, Sleiderink, & Levelt, 1998). Time-locked means that the development of a proportion over time graph coincides with the development of the linguistic processes of the task.

As an example, Allopenna, Magnuson, and Tanenhaus (1998) investigated the lexical activation of words in competition with cohort words and rhyming words. For instance, "beaker" will compete with words which begin with the same sound, such as "beetle", and also words which rhyme, such as "speaker". Allopenna et al. wanted to test competing computational models of lexical activation, but the precise theoretical applications are not important here. The important issue is that the models made predictions in terms of the activation of each word over time. These activation curves could be plotted against time, and compared to proportion over time curves from eye-tracking data both visually and statistically. So, to get proportion over time curves, Allopenna et al. set up an experiment with stimuli as in Figure 6.10(a). Participants were given instructions such as "Look at the cross. Pick up the beaker. Now put it above the square". The hypothesis is that about 200 ms after the sound "beaker" starts, the participants gazes will move to the most likely objects; namely those two that start with the "bee..." sound. After a few more milliseconds, the pronunciation of "beaker" has reached the "..ker" sound, and then gazes on the cohort "beetle" will drop. After data were recorded, the proportion over time curve in Figure 6.10(b) was calculated.

The recorded proportion over time curve turned out to be almost identical to the predicted activation curve of the model, which illustrates how the development of the proportion over time graphs can be time-locked to associated linguistic processes. If this result were to be a general principle of eye movement coupling to linguistic and cognitive processes, one that holds for a variety of tasks, proportion over time graphs would be a valuable tool for investigating many aspects of both language and general cognition.

Before we start to examine this approach more generally, there are some things we need to consider. First of all, the time-locking hypothesis is a close relative of the eye–mind hypothesis of page 378, claiming that processing of words during reading goes on for exactly as long as the duration of fixations, which is now known to be not fully correct. Moreover, in psycholinguistic research, where these graphs originate, participants always hear speech, the same speech, developing at the same speed for all participants. When psycholinguists use proportion over time curves and exploit the time-lock between linguistic processes and eye-movement processes, they use speech that is synchronized with particular moments in the trial, to guarantee that all participants are presented the same speech at the same time. If we were to use proportion over time curves for studies where no speech synchronization occurs, we may get very variable and noisy graphs as the eye-movement effects belonging to specific linguistic and cognitive processes are spread out over the trial instead of occurring at a distinct moment for all participants, resulting in a flatter curve with no obviously distin-

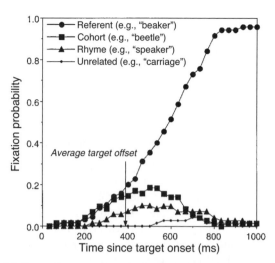

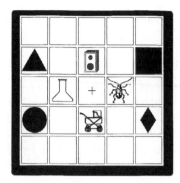

(a) Stimuli used while participant heard sentences such as "Pick up the beaker".

(b) Proportion over time graph from onset of target (e.g. "beaker"). The curve is almost identical to the predictions of the lexical activation model TRACE. Because they are so similar, we only show the data.

Fig. 6.10 An example of proportion over time graphs that could be time-locked to linguistic processes. Figures are reprinted from Allopenna et al. (1998) with kind permission from Elsevier Limited.

guishable peak. This risk increases if we cannot guarantee that the processing starts almost immediately when we present the synchronized part of the stimuli. In psycholinguistic research, proportion over time curves only stretch over fairly short time periods, from around 1 s (Allopenna et al., 1998) up to around 2.4 s (R. Andersson, Henderson, & Ferreira, 2011) . In our example above, Allopenna et al. (1998) analyse data over a single up to a few seconds. What if we were to give participants tasks that range over 10 or 20 seconds with only an initial synchronization? Would we be able to see any common gaze pattern between different participants after more than the first second?

Lexical activation processes are not only fast, they are also very automated with little or no conscious deliberation involved. If we have a much more complex task, such as mathematical problem solving, is it not a risk that individual participants will each have their own pace and carry out the task using their own particular strategy? If so, if we calculate the averages taken at specific times over *all* participants, these averages will not reflect that some people are only at stage x_1 at time t_1 while others are at stage x_2. At any given time we will therefore have averages collapsed across participants at different stages, and the proportion over time graph will be very hard to interpret.

Taken from our mathematical problem solving task (p. 5), the proportion over time graphs in Figures 6.11 and 6.12 use data at 1250 Hz, and show the first 20,000 samples, or about 16 seconds. Participants were shown a mathematical task, the 'input AOI' in written text for 5 seconds, and then four alternatives for solutions appear, while the input remains. The graphs start at the onset of the four alternatives. Participants were either students of mathematics ($n = 21$) or students in the humanities ($n = 24$). The five curves do not sum up to 1 (i.e. 100%) because the AOIs cover only a portion of the monitor, and blinks cause further non-AOI time.

Visual inspection of proportion over time graphs produced from longer trials provides a valuable tool for explorative analysis of eye-movement data. It can be seen that at the onset of the four alternatives (time 0 in the graphs), no participants were looking at anything else

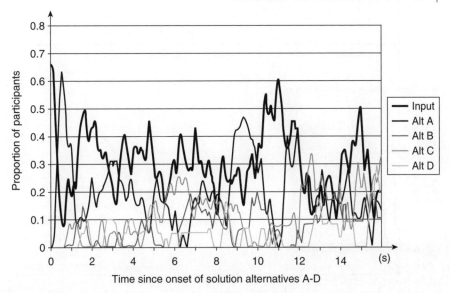

Fig. 6.11 Proportion over time graph of how *humanities* students look at the AOIs in one mathematical task. The AOI 'Alt A' is the correct alternative. The graphs have been smoothened by an averaging filter of 200 samples (160 ms).

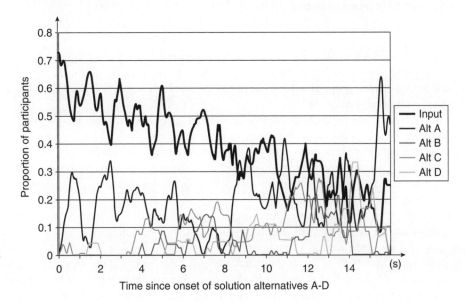

Fig. 6.12 Proportion over time graph of how *mathematics* students look at the AOIs in one mathematical task.

except the input AOI. At the onset, virtually all humanities students jump directly to the A alternative, while the mathematics students remain longer at the input with only few looks at the A alternative. This difference in visual behaviour between the groups could be interpreted as evidence of two different strategies to solve the task: the mathematicians appear to try to derive the solution from the input, while the humanities students seek help to understand the task by looking at the possible solutions. Granted, the mathematicians also look at the A al-

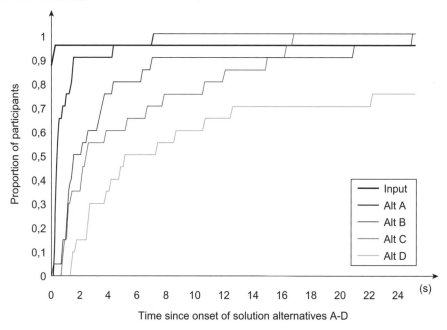

Fig. 6.13 Cumulative proportion over time graph of how humanities students look at the AOIs. Same data as in Figure 6.11, but not smoothened.

ternative, but to a much smaller degree (peak at 0.3 compared to 0.6 for looking at Alternative A). At this point we would like to have a way to calculate the periods in time during which the difference between proportion levels is significant, and when it is not. Such methods are only just being developed (p. 440).

It is much less clear in this example that participants in either group are in sync with one another in their process of comparing the input with the alternatives. There are some pulses of 1.8 second duration for both groups, but they would need to be substantiated by another analysis. Clearly, there is more variation and noise in the proportion over time graphs over longer periods of data where there is not speech to synchronize, because of variation in the precise timing between participants.

The cumulative proportion over time graphs are much easier to interpret over longer recordings than are the momentous graphs. Figure 6.14 shows a cumulative proportion over time graph for the same data as in Figure 6.12. It can immediately be seen that after about 2 seconds, more than 90% of the mathematics students have looked at the alternative A, but only about a third have looked at the second alternative. We can also see that while after about 3.5 seconds all mathematics students have seen the alternative A, the other three alternatives are seen only by 70–86% of them. Some 14% of them appear to have considered the A solution to be so obviously right that they did not even bother to look at any of the others. In contrast, the humanities students much earlier have much higher 'so far seen' proportions on the incorrect answers (Figure 6.14), in particular during the 2–10 second period after onset.

The time until 50% of the participants have seen an AOI—the T50 latency measure on page 438—can be read directly from cumulative proportion over time graphs. For the humanities students, T50 is 0.4 s for Alt 1, and 1.5 s, 2.4 s, and 5.2 s for the other alternatives. For the mathematics students, T50 latencies are much higher.

If we combine what we see in the momentous and the cumulative proportion graphs, we see plenty of evidence that the humanities students immediately go to the alternatives to seek

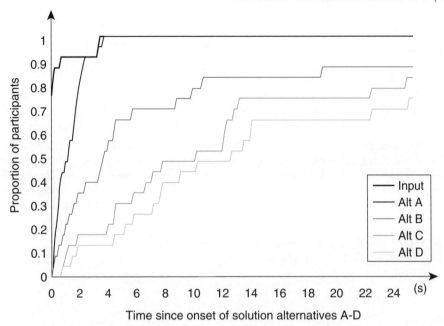

Fig. 6.14 Cumulative proportion over time graph of how mathematics students look at the AOIs. Same data as in Figure 6.12, but not smoothened.

clues for the solutions, while the mathematicians to a higher degree adopt a strategy of first thinking thoroughly about the input, and then directly selecting the correct alternative, not bothering about the incorrect ones.

Proportion of seen AOIs over time

Suppose that we were interested in finding out how many AOIs a single participant has seen over time. Figure 6.15(a) shows a graph of such data for a single participant. This participant progresses steadily through the AOIs, and after 3500 ms all AOIs have been seen. When using more participants, we can either stack each such participant graph on top of the others, to make a three-dimensional graph (not shown), or we can collapse the participant dimension by averaging their data. We would then arrive at a graph like Figure 6.15(b), in which one (fictitious) group of participants progresses through the AOIs much more rapidly than the other.

Both types of graphs in Figure 6.15 are cumulative, that is they sum up the number seen so far. Momentous graphs of seen AOIs over time are measures of dispersion, in that they show how spread out versus focused participants are over time. They differentiate from the spatial dispersion measures on pages 359–370 in that the underlying AOIs can be semantic units. A hypothetical measure based on these graphs would therefore reflect semantic dispersion, and would be particularly appropriate when using dynamic or distributed AOIs for which semantics can be very different from spatial extension. Note that the probability of a middle value in Figure 6.16 is always higher than the probability of a high or low value, and that if the number of participants is fewer than the number of AOIs, the graph can never reach the value 1.

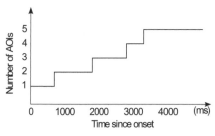

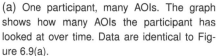

(a) One participant, many AOIs. The graph shows how many AOIs the participant has looked at over time. Data are identical to Figure 6.9(a).

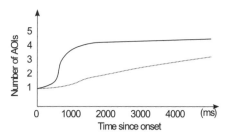

(b) Many participants, many AOIs. The two graphs show how many AOIs participants have so far seen over time. The dashed line shows a group that explores the AOIs more slowly, while the black line shows a group that quickly examines all AOIs.

Fig. 6.15 Cumulative graphs of how many AOIs have been seen over time.

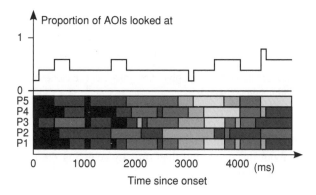

Fig. 6.16 The proportion of AOIs looked at by five participants is shown at the top, based on data in the five scarf plots below. At around 3000 ms, all participants look at the same AOI, so the proportion sinks to 20%. At around 4700 ms, they look at four different AOIs, and the proportion value is 80%. The same fictitious data as in Figure 6.9.

Proportion of transition sequences over transition time

The proportion of transition sequences over transition time is a useful representation if there are large differences in dwell time across participants, and you want to measure the development of transitions over time, accepting a shift between participants' data, in opposition to a strict time-locking hypothesis. For instance, in our example with momentous proportion over time graphs in Figures 6.11 and 6.12, participants' differing dwell times on AOIs may blur the pulse effects from being seen in the graph. When using transition time, the duration of dwells are ignored, and we can see sharper results.

To form the representation, align the lists of transitions for each participant, so you have everyone's first transition next to everyone else's first transition, and so on. Then simply count the number of transitions of each type at each time. In Table 6.2(a), AB means 'from AOI A to AOI B'. 100% of the first transitions were from AOI A to AOI B, and 75% of the second transitions went back to AOI A again. The measure can easily be developed for use with longer sequences of transitions. Table 6.2(b) shows how sequences of three consecutive AOIs are distributed across the participants and over transition time.

The transition over transition time data could be drawn in the same way as a normal

Table 6.2 Proportion of transition sequences over transition time. In (a), single transitions, in (b) double transitions. Out of four participants, we calculate for each transition in the order the proportion of each type of data.

(a) Single transitions

	1st	2nd	3rd	4th
Part1	AB	BA	AC	CD
Part2	AB	BA	AB	BC
Part3	AB	BC	CA	AD
Part4	AB	BA	AB	BC

(b) Double transitions

	1st	2nd	3rd	4th
Part1	-	ABA	BAC	ACD
Part2	-	ABA	BAB	ABC
Part3	-	ABC	BCA	CAD
Part4	-	ABA	BAB	ABC

Table 6.3 Types of time usage with measures, and whether it involves downsampling or a shift in time relative to the original sample time.

	Downsampling	Shift in time
Momentous/cumulative	*No*	*No*
Binned time	*Yes*	*No*
Left-, or rightward alignment	*No*	*Yes*
Event based time	*Yes*	*Yes*

proportion over time graph, although with discrete time. Since there are a total of 20 different two-AOI transitions with five AOIs, and 80 three-AOI transitions triples, the graph could be rather crowded, but in practice, only a few of the transitions and transition sequences actually appear in data.

In an explorative study, Goldberg, Stimson, Lewenstein, Scott, and Wichansky (2002) used a simpler version of the transitions over transition time diagram, which they call *navigation pattern*, on several tasks on a web portal page. Their study indicates that headers in a portlet were not usually visited before the body, by finding either the Header-Body-Customize or Header-Customize order of AOIs, in all cases but one.

6.4.6   Time and order

Time runs from the start of trial and onwards, at a sampling frequency decided by the specific eye-tracker. This basic, original time in the recordings is used for duration calculations in many eye-movement measures, including momentous and cumulative proportion over time graphs. In this section, we will look at three other organizations of time which are important for AOI events but also for the oculomotor event fixations, saccades, and smooth pursuit: binned time, left- and rightward alignment, and event based time. Each of these either downsample or shift data in time, as summarized in Table 6.3.

Binned time and ordinal positions

When data consist of fixations, dwells, transitions, or other events with variable duration, rather than raw data samples, we no longer have one point per time sample and cannot plot measure values over true time. One solution is then to use binned time and ordinal positions. We will use the example in Figure 6.17(a), which shows numbered fixations of two participants P1 and P2 laid out in true recording time. This is how we usually think about time.

Measuring how fixation durations develop over time requires grouping the fixations in bins of for instance 500 ms. Then all fixations starting during 1–500 ms after onset are grouped into a first bin, while saccades launched during the next bin 501–1000 ms are a second group etc. Figure 6.17(b) presents the same data from P1 and P2 as binned average fixation durations. Binning means downsampling time, cutting it up in larger chunks, so this calculation comes at a loss of information, namely about precise start and end of fixations. Binning does not introduce a shift in time, however. Each bin in (b) represents a period of time from the original data in (a), which is the same for each participant.

The precise bin size is in effect an arbitrary setting that should be chosen as part of the experimental design or in relation to the data analysis, for example to ensure statistical independence between samples in successive bins. In literature, 500–1000 ms are commonly seen bin sizes. Occasionally, time bins may be much larger. For instance, Knoblich, Ohlsson, and Raney (2001) divided their trials into thirds: first, middle, and last bin.

In Figure 6.17(c), fixation durations are ordered by the fixation number; we compare the fixation durations between P1 and P2 for fixation number 6, for instance, regardless of the fact that the P2 fixation number 6 occurs much earlier than the P1 number 6 fixation.

Using ordinal positions to define the flow of time in measures has two consequences: first, time is *downsampled* into larger and variable chunks, in effect using fixation number as chronometric units, by which we lose information. Second, data are *displaced* between the two participants, so that although fixation 6 of one participant coincides with fixation 4 in true time, the comparison always uses fixation 6 of both participants, which is also a reduction in information. Whether this is desirable or not should be decided by the rationale of the experiment at hand, and in particular the expectations on the temporal flow of perceptual and cognitive processes, that is how much time they take, and in what order they occur, compared to fixations made.

The most common events that use chronometric units in measures are fixations, saccades, dwells, and transitions. Examples of such measures are the unique AOIs (p. 343), entry time (p. 437), and the ambient versus focal distinction (p. 266).

Leftward versus rightward alignment

When trials have different lengths, examining what happens just after onset of a stimulus event requires a *leftward alignment of trials*. Examining what happens just before the end of trials requires a *rightward alignment*. Figure 6.18 illustrates left versus right alignment for two participants with trials of different lengths. Aligning data does not downsample it any more than is already the case, but it shifts data in time between participants/conditions. In the example in Figure 6.19, Glaholt and Reingold (2009) calculate proportion over time curves with rightward alignment in a decision task between two images with variable trial duration. The two curves are calculated for a long time period of backward time, towards the decision.

6.5 Types of AOIs

The most basic type of AOI outlines a region in the stimulus that encapsulates what is 'interesting' from the perspective of your experimental design, and is used to quantify whether and how much someone looked at this particular region. Most of the time, the AOI is a single, static, and content-less region with well-defined borders. However, as we will see in this section, there are many varieties of the basic AOI type, and some of them violate one or many of these basic properties.

6.5.1 Whitespace

The areas of the stimulus *not* covered by AOIs can be referred to as *whitespace*. Whitespace has usually been regarded as wholly unproblematic: after all, if there is nothing there, why

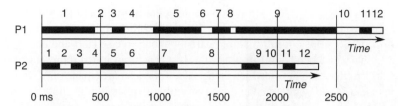

(a) Participants 1 and 2, with numbered fixations laid out in real time. For P1, executing 12 fixations takes 2.87 seconds, for P2 it takes 2.33 seconds.

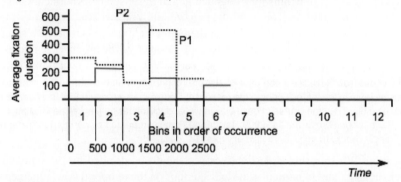

(b) Bins of size 500 ms have been applied to the two data in (a). For each bin, the graph shows the average fixation durations for fixations starting in the bin. Each bin represents a period of time in the original data in (a), which is the same for each participant.

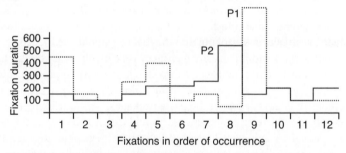

(c) Duration of fixations in the order of occurrence. Ordering data by events, such as fixations, efficiently shifts the original recording time. For instance, here we compare fixation number 6 of both participants, when in real time P1 produces his sixth fixation more than 400 ms later than P2.

Fig. 6.17 Real time data (a), binned time data (b), and data ordered by events (c). Three very different views of the same data.

Leftward	ACABCD AACB
Rightward	ACABCD AACB

Fig. 6.18 Leftward and rightward alignment of AOI strings over time. Leftward alignment is for studying behaviour just after onsets, and rightward alignment behaviour before offsets.

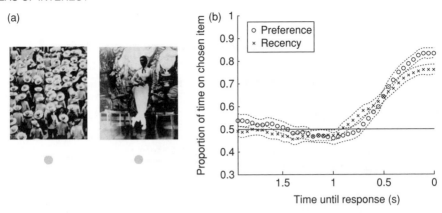

Fig. 6.19 (a) Two items in a decision task. When the decision is made, the user looks at a grey dot below the item he chose. (b) 'Gaze likelihood curves' plot the proportion of time spent on the chosen item, for each 50 ms time bin in the interval prior to the response. Dotted lines represent 95% confidence intervals about each time bin. The time course of gaze bias in visual decision tasks, Mackenzie G. Glaholt, Eyal M. Reingold, *Visual Cognition*, © Jan 11, 2009, Taylor and Francis, reprinted by permission of the publisher (Taylor & Francis Group, http://www.informaworld.com).

would anyone look at it? And if participants look there, why not just put in another AOI for the whitespace? Indeed, in most tasks participants will not look at whitespace, because the experimental task is set up to direct them to the objects selected as AOIs.

However, in longer experiments which require problem solving, looking at whitespace may indicate a mental process, afterthought, or perhaps mental imagery while solving the task, or simple indifference over a task which the participant was expected to do correctly. Moreover, as soon as we take eye tracking into the real world, outside the lab, the whitespace area becomes much larger, and affects the measures very much, in particular the order and transition measures. For instance, consider an eye-tracking study of product selection in the supermarket. Perhaps the researcher wants to do an AOI analysis only of the pasta shelves, but the participant looks only at very few of the pasta packages, before walking away over to the vegetable area (whitespace) for a few minutes. Should this movement count as a transition between the last AOI the participant looked at before the vegetable area and the first AOI looked at when returning? The percentage of whitespace is virtually never reported, but for many measures, in particular transition measures, it should be, so researchers can relate the reported results to it.

6.5.2 Planes

Planes are super-AOIs that exist in studies with multiple frames of reference, commonly due to combined eye and head tracking (supplied only by a few manufacturers). Technically, a plane is a two-dimensional surface in a three-dimensional space. A measurement procedure at the set-up ensures that the recording software knows exactly where each plane is located. The measurement system also knows the position and direction of the participant's head. This allows for online detection of AOI hits, in addition to saving data files with coordinates in each plane.

The keyboard and monitor depicted in Figure 6.20 are two planes, the picture behind is the third. Control rooms and aircraft cockpits are other examples of experimental settings that may require division of the stimulus space into a number of different planes. Some eye-tracker systems produce data where planes do not share coordinate systems, but each plane has its

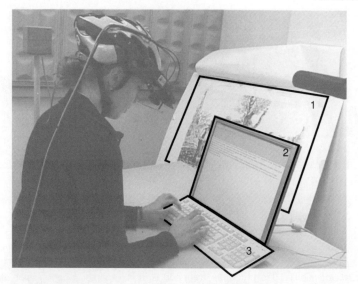

Fig. 6.20 Three 3D planes, numbered 1 for stimulus, 2 for monitor, and 3 for keyboard, in a study of reading while writing. Each plane is a super-AOI that can contain its own AOIs. The recording software knows where the planes and the participants head are, and can calculated AOI hits online.

own coordinate system (SMI head-mounted systems with Polhemus head-tracking, for instance), while others may have the same global coordinate system across planes (SmartEye). Also, planes need not be parallel, but can have any direction. A plane may contain many AOIs. Each AOI of course resides in one plane only, and all of the AOIs of that plane use the same coordinate system. Nevertheless, most of the AOI measures are applicable to planes as well. It makes perfect sense, for instance, to analyse dwell time on the monitor plane, or transition matrices between different planes in an air traffic controller's working space.

6.5.3 Dynamic AOIs

If your stimulus consists of animated stimuli or videos, the objects that you try to cover with normal, static AOIs will move away from under the AOI. You then need to use *dynamic AOIs*. These have recently been introduced in commercial software, and move in sync, following the underlying object. However, in current implementations, they require of the user not only specification of the AOI shape, size, and position, but also of how the AOI moves and changes form over time (Papenmeier & Huff, 2010). Figure 6.21 illustrates how a movie of a flying butterfly is tracked by a dynamic AOI throughout a short clip from a video sequence.

In the implementation of dynamic AOIs available in one of the commercial software packages, manual adjustments of AOI shape are required only for certain key frames, then the software automatically estimates the shape in the intermediate frames. This makes it easy to create AOIs following objects that move with constant direction and speed, whereas objects that move in a non-linear fashion require more manual work. Dynamic AOIs created this way are perhaps of most practical use when there are relatively few objects of interest in a stimulus, which is common to all participants.

Once the dynamic AOIs are in place it will be possible to use all AOI measures with the data. When dynamic AOIs overlap, however, a difficult prioritization is necessary (p. 221). Dynamic AOIs were first available in commercial analysis software in 2008, and have thus not yet been much used in research.

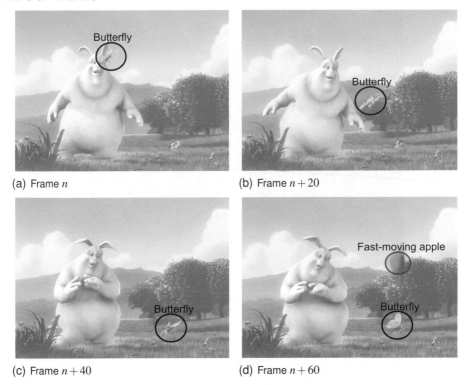

(a) Frame n (b) Frame $n+20$

(c) Frame $n+40$ (d) Frame $n+60$

Fig. 6.21 Four frames of a film with 20 frames (833 ms) between them. A circular dynamic AOI tracks the flying butterfly, and the last frame also introduces another dynamic AOI to track the falling apple. Reproduced here with permission from the Blender foundation `www.bigbuckbunny.org`.

6.5.4 Distributed AOIs

The four instances of the man in Figure 6.22 are really only one single individual in four different locations according to narrative time when the picture is described. If we want to treat them as one in the statistical analysis, it can be seen as appropriate to use one single *distributed* AOI to cover all four instances of the man.

Holsanova (2008) notes that when participants describe Figure 6.22 and use phrases such as "it looks like early spring", there is no single, well-delimited item in the picture that corresponds to the concept "early spring". Spatially, the spring is spread out in all sorts of objects that provide evidence for the season (the dandelions, the birds in the tree, and the garden work). Distributed, non-connected AOIs are needed whenever the stimulus has semantics that are not spatially precise. "Early spring" is one such example, but also, "crucial information areas for solving mathematical tasks", as in Figure 6.23. Similarly, Morrison et al. (1997) collected several different and distinct areas into three categories: "situation awareness regions", "explanation-based reasoning regions", and "recognition-primed decision regions". Their analysis is based on this categorization rather than on the included physical regions. In fact, in experiments that have non-manipulated, natural stimuli, it is very common to have *a number of different AOI divisions* each pertaining to its own specific semantic level and subsequent analysis.

When using distributed AOIs, it is important to consider the interpretation of the measures used. The distributed AOI in Figure 6.23 seems semantically inconsistent with respect to first fixation durations, for instance, which can be expected to be lower for the ρ and θ parts of the AOI than for the $(\rho cos\theta, \rho sin\theta)$ part, simply because the latter is more complex to

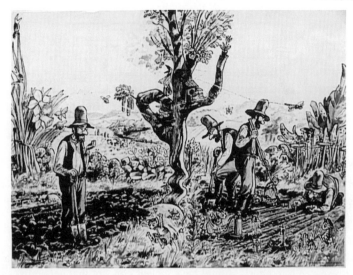

Fig. 6.22 Complex stimulus picture used by Holsanova (2008), Johansson, Holsanova, and Holmqvist (2005) and others. Reprinted from Nordqvist (1990), with kind permission from the author.

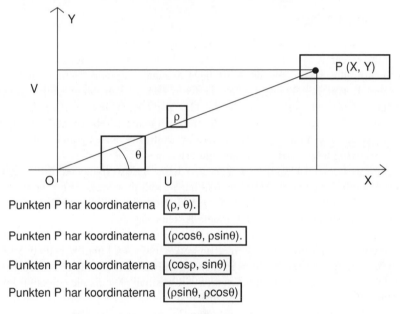

Punkten P har koordinaterna (ρ, θ).

Punkten P har koordinaterna $(\rho\cos\theta, \rho\sin\theta)$.

Punkten P har koordinaterna $(\cos\rho, \sin\theta)$

Punkten P har koordinaterna $(\rho\sin\theta, \rho\cos\theta)$

Fig. 6.23 A distributed AOI indicating crucial mathematical information as selected by experts. All seven AOIs are treated as one single AOI, only distributed in space.

understand. With a distributed AOI, we treat the first fixation in any of the seven part AOIs as the first fixation in the distributed AOI. If we compare first fixation durations between two groups, and the participants in one group look at the ρ first, while the participants in the other group look at $(\rho\cos\theta, \rho\sin\theta)$ first, then these durations will be different just because they land on areas where one requires deeper processing than the other. Moreover, ρ is closer to the centre of the display, where fixation is normally directed at the start of a trial, therefore any measure of latency to reach the AOI will obviously be contaminated because it is distributed

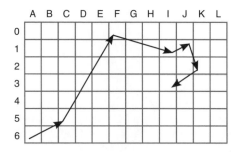

Fig. 6.24 Scanpath over gridded AOIs. A string representing this scanpath would be A6 C5 F0 I1 J1 K2 I3. On pages 273–278 and 348–353, such string representations will be used to quantify the similarity between scanpaths.

in space.

A distributed AOI should therefore have consistent semantics across all part AOIs. For instance, your research hypothesis should have a clear concept that generalizes over the different part AOIs, such as "crucial information", that can be motivated in relation to the dependent measures that you employ.

6.5.5 Gridded AOIs

The 'I' in AOI stands for interest. If we take the viewpoint that AOIs should be defined in relation to the research hypothesis, AOIs almost always coincide with the natural semantic units of the stimulus scene. But do AOIs have to match semantic entities in the picture? Goldberg and Kotval (1999) differentiate between *content-dependent analyses*, where the AOIs are linked to meaningful units in the stimulus, and *content-independent analyses*, which simply place a grid across the stimulus and let each cell in the grid be an AOI, see Figure 6.24. The fact that semantics of the stimulus are divided arbitrarily makes gridded AOIs unsuitable for directly studying *what* participants are interested in.

As we saw earlier (p. 192), gridded AOIs also define the dwell map representation of data. In fact, using a grid for creating AOIs and making a dwell time analysis for them, results in a crude version of an attention map (heat map) made from the same data. The larger the cells (AOIs), the cruder the approximation. For details, see Chapter 7.

Gridded AOIs found their way into eye-tracking research very early. In his seminal work on picture viewing, Buswell (1935) divided an image into a 4×4 matrix, and added a number representing the percentage of fixations in each AOI. Gridded AOIs can be useful for studying *how* participants scan the overall stimulus area, irrespective of semantic content (Goldberg & Kotval, 1999; Brandt & Stark, 1997). In particular, the string edit measures use the gridded AOIs representations, of the kind exemplified in Figure 6.24.

However, an inherent problem of gridded AOIs is how to choose the number of cells. Different cell sizes could yield very different results (Foulsham, 2008, p. 72). To avoid arbitrariness, studies using gridded AOIs in the analysis should employ several different cell sizes for the AOIs and show the same effect for each, which Pomplun, Ritter, and Velichkovsky (1996) do.

6.5.6 Fuzzy AOIs

All AOIs in use today have sharp borders. This means that a data sample or fixation is located either inside ('hit') or outside ('miss') the AOI. A fixation located directly outside the AOI border is therefore considered a 'miss' just as much as another fixation much further away.

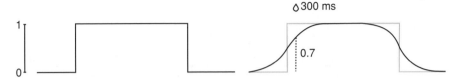

Fig. 6.25 AOIs can be seen as a function with infinitely sharp edges that defines the probability of 'hit' (left). If the edges are softened, we would have fuzzy AOIs (right), for which fixations share their duration with two bordering AOIs in proportion to the probability of being a hit, so that for instance a 300 ms fixation at height 0.7 adds 210 ms to the AOI and 90 ms to its neighbour.

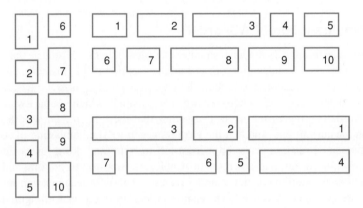

Fig. 6.26 The three most common conventionalized AOI orders, without which concepts like 'first skip' and 'regressions' would not be possible.

This motivates having AOIs with 'soft' or 'fuzzy' borders that, instead of a binary hit/miss decision, register partials hits. Figure 6.25 shows the principle for AOIs with soft borders. In a fuzzy AOI, the uncertainty of whether a fixation falls on the correct side or not is turned into a probability measure that assigns part of the fixation to one AOI and the other part to the neighbouring AOI or whitespace. In the case of duration, for instance, if the 300 ms fixation falls at a location where the probability of a hit is 0.7, the AOI is assigned a value of 210 ms $(300 \cdot 0.7)$. The level of fuzziness can be varied, for instance to correspond to the degree of imprecision and inaccuracy in your data, such that data with poorer quality have increasingly less sharp borders.

An alternative implementation of fuzzy AOIs is to append a Gaussian function around each fixation, and distribute the fixation duration to AOIs according to the volume covering each AOI (Buscher, Cutrell, & Morris, 2009). This approach emphasizes the other reason for smudging AOI borders; visual uptake may be distributed over a wide area, and this should be reflected in the measure values.

Although fuzzy AOIs are applicable to both dwell time and transition measures, the concept of fuzzy AOIs or the alternative of using a Gaussian attention deployment has not been thoroughly investigated in the literature, and validity experiments are needed to be able to confidently use fuzzy AOIs. For example, does attention constituted by a longer peripheral fixation equal a spot-on fixation, if they both result in the same weighted (as per above) dwell time?

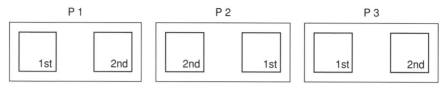

Fig. 6.27 Three participants and the same stimulus, with two AOIs. Participants have later answered questions about what is their first and second choice of the two items shown in the AOIs. The hypothesis wants to compare entry and dwell times (AOI measures) for first versus second choice AOIs. This require same-position AOI to have different identities for different participants.

6.5.7 Stimulus-inherent AOI orders

Mostly, AOIs in a stimulus do not have an inherent order to them that tells us that one of them is the first, another the second, and so on. The great exception is the conventionalized reading order that has made the reading researchers define a large number of AOI measures that make little sense for other stimuli, like "between-word regression", which is a backward movement to another word. The regression in itself assumes that there is an AOI with a lower order number than the current one, and that the gaze moves to it. The numbering of AOIs follows the conventionalized reading order, be it from-left-to-right, and down (as in European languages), from-right-to-left, and down (as in Arabic), or from-top-to-bottom, and to the next right column (as in traditional Chinese and Japanese). These three are examplified in Figure 6.26. There are also other lesser known reading orders. In traditional Mongolian, words go from-top-to-bottom, and to the next left column, whilst in the ancient Boustrophedon system words follow a zig-zag-pattern, with alternating reading directions for every other line.

Few other stimuli than text, if any, have a conventionalized order of AOIs. Rather, a common research question is to investigate whether a particular type of stimulus has a conventionalized scanning pattern or not. Of course, a participant's reading order may be reflected in the order he looks at other objects other than text. For instance, Lam, Chau, and Wong (2007) show that participants scanning thumbnails on commercial web pages do so in an order reflecting their dominant reading direction.

6.5.8 Participant-specific AOI identities

AOI identities are not always independent of the participants looking at them. For instance, we may have a stimulus picture with two toys that the child participants are also asked to rate after the recording was made. Now we want to have an AOI that is "the best-liked toy", i.e. for each child that toy which was rated the highest. This AOI will cover different toys for different children, as in Figure 6.27. A similar situation appears if you have an internet study with different articles and ads, and you want to let the interests of the participants decide the identity of the AOI. To the extent that they handle *individual AOI identities*, modern analysis software solves this by letting the user name AOIs differently for different participants; the name then decides the AOI's identity during analysis. The analysis in Glaholt and Reingold (2009), exemplified on page 208 assigns AOI identity based on participants' choice between two AOIs; i.e. 'chosen' versus 'non-chosen'.

6.5.9 AOI identities across stimuli

The identity of an AOI can be just as much decided from the experimental design as it can from participant actions. In both cases, this overrides the basic definition of AOI by it spatial extension. For instance, in a study where stimuli are always a face and a cellular phone (we

Image 1   Image 2   Image 3

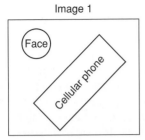 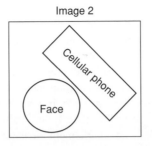 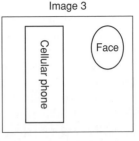

Fig. 6.28 Three stimulus images with a face and a cellular phone AOI in each. Although each face looks different, has a different size and position in the image, from the perspective of our experimental design we can view them as a single AOI concept of faces instantiated in three trials.

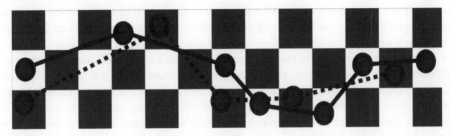

Fig. 6.29 These two scanpaths appear very similar when visualized in space, and many spatial similarity measures would give a high similarity score, but note that one participant scans only white areas, and the other only grey areas.

may be in the advertisement field now), but always different faces of different sizes at different positions, as in Figure 6.28. In her experimental design and result summary, our hypothetical researcher nevertheless considers all these different AOI as identical, and presents a single average entry time and dwell time value for the face AOI.

Letting a single AOI concept from the experimental design cover a number of AOIs from different stimulus images is then a way to increase generalizability and overall validity of the study, because if our researcher finds that entry times are significantly lower and dwell times higher for the cellular phone than for the face, then she can support that from a wide variety of combinations of sizes and positions. Again, software handle AOI identities across stimulus images by letting the name of an AOI decide its identity.

6.5.10 AOIs in the feature domain

AOIs can be defined in space and in terms of *features*, which take into account selected aspects of the content in the AOI. Feature analysis provides an important addition to all measures, increasing their usefulness manyfold by replacing space with a quantification of the semantics in the stimulus. As a simple example of how a feature space analysis works, Figure 6.29 shows two scanpaths over the same checkered stimulus. At first glance, the scanpaths are very similar: their spatial extension and form coincide very well, and would score high on many similarity measures. Looking more closely, however, you will find that one of the scanpaths hits only white and the other one only grey areas. If the grey–white difference is important in our study, the two scanpaths are not at all similar. In order to have measures that capture feature similarity, rather than spatial similarity, we should analyse data in a space spanned by the grey and white and not by the spatial x and y dimensions.

In Figure 6.29, the features are very simple, clearcut, and regular. It is not difficult to set up two distributed AOIs G and W that cover all grey and white in the stimulus. We can then represent one scanpath with the AOI dwell string WWWWWWW and the other with GGGGG, which are obviously very different, irrespective of which method for scanpath comparison we use. We thus make a string analysis in the feature domain rather than in the spatial domain.

The grey and white areas have only two colour values, but the feature values of the AOIs may also be continuously variable. For instance, in a supermarket study, all products that a participant would look at have values for price, brand, carbohydrate content, etc, that serve equally well as a feature space that can complement the natural one. Instead of measuring, for instance, the saccadic amplitude in pixels or degrees of visual angle between successive fixations, we can now measure amplitudes along the scanpath in price or carbohydrate content: a saccade from pasta AOI number 1 to pasta AOI number 7 can have an amplitude of €–3.6 , calculated as price of AOI 7 minus price of AOI 1, or for that matter +1.6% of carbohydrates. The average of the absolute saccadic amplitudes of one participant may be €0.18 , which would indicate that every new pasta he looks at deviates very little in price from the previous pasta.

Feature-space analysis quantifies the semantics of the stimulus and replaces space with that quantification. As a consequence, the unit of the measure values are changed: instead of centimetres and visual degrees, we measure distances in colour or in price or in carbohydratic content.

As long as the objects carrying the feature have sharp edges, a feature-based analysis can be implemented with AOIs, and comparisons made using for instance semantic distances within a substitution matrix (p. 276). In real-life mammography images, however, there are no clear-cut borders where AOIs can be laid. Dempere-Marco et al. (2006) therefore used five previously developed *visual feature detectors* for mosaic attenuation, nodules, reticulation, ground glass, and bronchiectatis, which are theoretically important for understanding the search behaviour of radiologists. A visual feature detector is a small algorithm that takes a piece of the stimulus image and returns a value; as though saying for instance "this patch has 0.7 in mosaic attenuation, so the fixation should be given that value." Using five feature detectors, a fixation f_i that lands in a mammography image can thus be attributed a five-dimensional $(ma_i, n_i, r_i, gg_i, b_i)$ vector, where each dimension gets its value from a feature detector (ma for 'mosaic attenuation' etc.). Dempere-Marco et al. made all analyses in that five-dimensional feature space rather than in the two-dimensional spatial space.

More generally, Dempere-Marco, Hu, and Yang (2011) propose that a feature-based data analysis can be made in two steps:

1. Select a feature domain with dimensions such as price and carbohydratic content or the five-dimenional features of X-ray images. Feature domain selection crucially includes a mapping function from spatial positions in the stimulus images to feature values, which is trivial for the pasta case (feature value for price is read from the price tag), but less obvious for radiology studies.

2. Impose a measure on the feature domain. Dempere-Marco et al. focus on pairwise position similarity, but nothing prevents us from using any other of the many measures where space can be substituted for a feature domain, including the vast majority of measures in Chapters 10 and 11.

6.6   Challenging issues with AOIs

The precise location and shape of an AOI needs to be decided in close relation with the hypothesis, the composition of the stimulus, the quality of the recorded data, and the method of analysis.

6.6.1 Choosing and positioning AOIs

How do you decide how your stimulus should be divided into AOIs? It is your hypothesis that decides what your AOIs should be, and there is therefore no point in using more AOIs than required by the hypothesis. This is easy for many simple constructed stimuli, but difficult for natural and cluttered scenes.

Semantic composition of stimuli

In many experimental settings, the stimuli are so constructed that the assignment of AOIs to parts of the stimulus is very straightforward; often there is a set number of objects and nothing else, except whitespace. The only issue then is how large to make the margins. With pure reading stimuli, individual morphemes, words, or sentences can each be given an AOI. Also, for many stimuli which were not originally conceived for use in eye-tracking experiments, but are nevertheless man made, AOIs can often easily be assigned to segments. For instance, an ad on a web page makes an obvious AOI, as well as shelf space for particular product brands in the supermarket. Such man-made pre-divided stimuli are *largely* unproblematic.

Properties of visual intake and recognition may complicate the AOI division however. If your stimulus is so simple, and your AOIs so close that your participants are able to take in one AOI in peripheral vision while looking at the other, it is dubious to contrast dwell times from the two areas and argue that visual intake is larger from one AOI than the other. Fortunately, the visual phenomenon known as 'crowding' (which originates from work by Loomis, 1978) tells us that, as peripheral information becomes more cluttered, it is very difficult to distinguish between different elements away from the current point of fixation. Therefore, for complex displays, AOIs which are close to each other may not cause a problem because crowding restricts focus to the fovea. In fact, in many studies, peripheral detection is manipulated by crowding the target with additional letters and characters.

If instead you use a naturalistic complex picture, like the stimulus image in Figure 6.22, where there is very much natural crowding, what is the proper division? Should the man to the left be represented by one AOI only, or should we make one AOI for his face, one for the soil he holds in his left hand, and one for the shovel? We could continue, and enclose each minimal semantic element within an AOI; one for each spider, butterfly, and the bird in the tree. However, we have to draw the line somewhere (literally!); every blade of grass and leaf on the tree should not be given AOI status. As pointed out earlier in this chapter, your hypothesis should guide your AOI divisions so that they are sensible and can provide answers to the empirical questions you are asking.

The stimulus can be divided into AOIs on several levels, according to your hypothesis. In Holsanova (2008, 2001), a crucial question was how speakers coordinated the spoken name "Pettson" with looking at the man, during free spoken descriptions of the picture. Then, each portion of the image in which the man is present should be given its own AOI, but with the same reference label. In another type of analysis, the transitions between the face, the hand with the soil, and the shovel were of main interest (as they may signify a sudden deeper understanding of the picture thematics). This requires an AOI analysis at a finer level of semantic composition.

Who should decide AOI positioning?

The exact positioning of AOIs is crucial, because it can determine whether you reveal a significant effect or not. However, who should make this important decision, and on what grounds? Usually, the researcher herself decides where to position the AOIs. This is an option when interesting regions in the stimulus are easy to separate from each other, and there is no uncertainty of whether they qualify as AOIs, preferably using an unambiguous and exhaustive list of criteria, but otherwise it may open up for various degrees of subjectivity. Therefore we will discuss the following alternatives:

- Using *experts* to define the AOIs. This can be done before recording, but it is manual with the risk of being subjective. Nevertheless, using human experts improves the semantic link between your stimuli and their respective AOIs. To this extent the degree of objectivity may be greater than if you position AOIs yourself.
- Using *scene stimulus*-generated AOIs. Here, the positioning is algorithmic, and therefore more objective. The scene properties themselves plus algorithms define the areas.
- Using *attention maps* to define the AOIs. This is post hoc, but it is at least done by algorithms, although threshold settings are arbitrary. No semantics involved.
- Using *clustering algorithms*. Again post hoc, but also again algorithmic with arbitrary threshold settings. No semantics involved.

Expert-defined AOIs The manually defined AOI can be made somewhat more objective by having experts define it. Experts can be expected to have a very detailed knowledge of the semantics in the stimulus. When given the task to decide which are the most important areas in the stimulus for solving the task, mathematics professors selected AOIs as shown in Figure 6.23 above. Expert judgements of AOIs can be used in a variety of stimuli: air traffic control interfaces, nuclear plant control rooms, art, architectural facades, and medical education videos are just some examples. For mathematical stimuli, it is relatively difficult to point out which are the most important semantically coherent AOIs even for an expert, since mathematical problem solving is a process that uses many if not all parts in combination. It is easier for air traffic controller environments where the scene has been designed with clear functional distinctions between areas, and probably even in medical education videos, where one or two small areas on a patient's body can be decisive for a diagnosis.

Stimulus-generated AOIs The scene stimulus itself can be used to create AOIs. Mossfeldt and Tillander (2005) present several attempts to automatically identify AOIs using edge detection and colour segmentation. They conclude that using image processing to automatically find AOIs is very dependent on the specific stimulus. Edge detection may not work adequately for natural images (photographs), and colour will not always be an effective method of segregating the stimulus. Constructed images such as text, logos, and illustrations have clearer edges however, and also more uniform colour. Therefore these classes of stimuli are better suited for image processing segmentation of AOIs. When the stimulus is not an image per se, but a computer generated display perhaps, it is sometimes much easier to have the computer render the AOIs directly from the stimulus. For instance, when studying reading of long texts (hundreds or thousands of words), a lot of time can be saved if the stimulus software can be made to produce the many AOIs directly from the stimulus. You just take your formatted text, paste it into a window, and it can be processed to a stimulus image with AOIs for each item in the text, such as words, inter-punctuation, sentences and in some cases even graphics. Not only does it save time, but it also adds precision, since each AOI is positioned at the same height as the others, with the same margins. Figure 6.30 shows AOIs generated by such a system. The same approach is possible for some non-reading scene stimuli also, namely those where the stimulus software handles the objects of the scene and can automatically attribute AOIs to them. In an animated game, for instance, you may make a log of all the sizes and positions of the automated AOIs, and then use that log

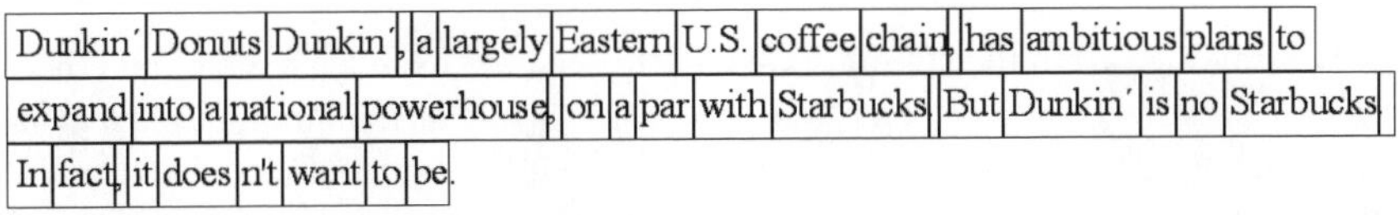

Dunkin'	Donuts	Dunkin',	a	largely	Eastern	U.S.	coffee	chain	has	ambitious	plans	to
expand	into	a	national	powerhouse,	on	a	par	with	Starbucks.	But	Dunkin'	is	no	Starbucks.
In	fact,	it	does	n't	want	to	be.

Fig. 6.30 Stimulus-generated AOIs for a short text.

to calculate AOI hits after recording or even online (Papenmeier & Huff, 2010; Holmberg, 2007). This could be the case for animations of various kinds and possibly for internet pages.

Attention maps for AOIs The attention maps described in Chapter 7 offer an alternative way to define AOIs by cutting off the top of the attention map, and letting the flat region(s) generated by the cut define the AOIs. As an alternative to cutting peaks in attention maps, Hooge and Camps (2009) hand-coded AOIs from heat map visualizations by manually drawing them at a specified colour (height in the attentional landscape, p. 233). This is an approximate, relatively objective, and not too time consuming method of obtaining AOIs that correspond to clusters. Page 248 provides more detail on the use of attention maps for AOI definitions.

Clustering for AOIs Clustering algorithms are used to divide an initial set of data samples or fixations into subsets that are similar in some sense, most often in term of spatial proximity. The strategies behind clustering differ somewhat between methods. A number of algorithms look only at the spatial proximity of the data points, such as Goldberg and Schryver (1995a), who present a clustering algorithm for finding fixation-like spatial clusters. Random samples are chosen for clusters, and iteratively the closest neighbour sample to each cluster is added to the cluster, resulting in what is known as a minimal spanning tree. Another related approach is the mean shift algorithm by Santella and DeCarlo (2004), which iteratively shifts points to higher-density areas in order to reach local maxima. However, the most common method by far to cluster data points is the k-means algorithm. It is related to Lloyds and the Linde-Buzo-Gray algorithms (Linde, Buzo, & Gray, 1980) used in vector quantization, and is straightforward to implement. In its basic form, it divides the image space into voronoi partitions based on the cluster centres. The user must define the number (k) of clusters to be found, and results may vary by each new run. Also, it does not provide actual AOIs, but only shows which points group well together; a convex hull could then be used to produce the AOIs from these points. A convex hull describes a selected set of raw samples or fixations by a minimal area that covers all points, as in Figure 6.31. This example illustrates that while it could perhaps be possible to use cluster-based AOI generation for image stimuli, it is considerably more difficult to find natural clusters when groups of raw samples are close to one another, as in the case of the text. In fact, these cluster-based AOIs have completely lost the connection to the natural semantics of the display, for both text and image. Using these AOIs for dwell time or transition analysis without substantive manual post-editing of AOIs may yield meaningless results, and manual editing would nullify the time saved by the algorithm. From a statistical point of view, using clustering techniques to create AOIs may violate assumptions of independence. The same points that are used to create an AOI are also used to calculate its contents. The result may be inflated values for AOIs that are large, positioned in relatively free areas and consequently capture more stray raw data samples. These values will be inflated compared to smaller AOIs located at areas with high competition from other AOIs, which will not capture stray raw data samples to the same degree.

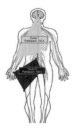
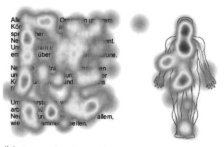

(a) Convex hulls around recorded fixations define AOIs as a result of clustering. Proportion
of participants looking at each cluster are reported.

(b) Proportion-based heat map visualization on
the same data.

Fig. 6.31 Clustered AOIs versus heat maps in the Tobii Studio analysis software. Hand-drawing AOIs around heat map centres may be less arbitrary and not take much longer.

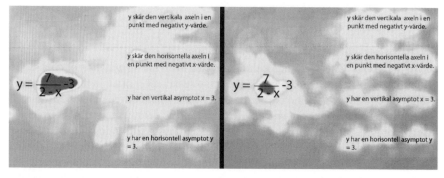

Fig. 6.32 Heat map visualizations of 21 students of mathematics (left) and 24 students of humanities (right) solving the same task. Same settings for kernel width and colour mapping in both heat maps.

Can we modify AOIs post hoc?

Ideally, your choices over precise levels of composition and divisions are matters which should be decided when developing your experimental design. But what if you prefer to record the data first, then look at the attention maps or scanpaths, before deciding where to put your AOIs?

For instance, Figure 6.32 shows the heat map visualizations of mathematics and human-ities students when solving the same mathematical problem. The researchers are interested in finding which information the mathematics students use that the humanities students do not. Suppose that at the onset of the project, the researchers did not have a clear idea which parts they should choose for candidate AOIs. The heat maps show that the semantic item "-3" could provide the crucial difference, so it would be tempting to choose a fine-grained AOI analysis, and in particular put an AOI over "-3" and test the dwell time difference be-tween mathematics and humanities students for that AOI. In doing this, we abandon the ideal of constructing the hypothesis before the data recording, and in effect enter into a semi-explorative research mode. This is not necessarily a bad thing: experiments often gain from being re-conceptualized on the path from original design to presentation of results. We must remember, though, that whenever a researcher alters AOIs to adapt better to her data, she is also altering her hypothesis and the whole story behind her study. This does not conform to proper empirical practice.[21]

In reality, however, it is not uncommon that researchers do not position AOIs until early in the data analysis stage, long after they designed the hypothesis. Even if the hypothesis is very clear about the general position of AOIs, it is often inexact, if the stimulus is particularly complex for instance. For stimuli with small spatial distances between semantic units, it is advisable to get into the habit of drawing the AOI positions in the analysis software *before* data recording. Some post-hoc refinement of AOI positioning may be necessary afterwards, but at least you do not run the experiment blind to its analysis, and the important AOI-related data will be captured *with respect to your hypothesis*. This is particularly important if there is a substantial gap between the initial design stage and the analysis stage, during which many participants are recorded and important details about the study may be forgotten.

6.6.2   Overlapping AOIs

In general, AOIs should not overlap at any single level of composition, because of the danger that single AOI hits and transitions will be counted twice, rendering your statistics difficult if not impossible to interpret. Most statistical tests assume that the data are independent—such double occurrences invalidate this assumption. Counting twice also inflates the data from overlapping AOIs compared to non-overlapping ones.

Nevertheless, there are cases when AOIs indeed overlap. Figure 6.33 shows four such situations. In Figure 6.33(a), there are two distinct levels of composition. The smaller sub-AOIs are completely engulfed by the larger AOIs within which they reside. This would be the case if the stimulus were two documents with sections of text and images inside them. Here, counting dwell time on both levels is appropriate, because the larger documents are semantic owners of the smaller ones. In these cases, we can then just subtract the AOI dwell time of the 'important information' AOI from the 'other information' AOI to get a corrected dwell time for the latter. Transition counting is not as obvious. For instance, does a saccade from the small area into its larger owner area count as a transition from one AOI to the other, or only as a movement inside an AOI? It makes most sense if transitions are counted only at each level of composition separately.

Figure 6.33(b) shows the unfortunate case when two static AOIs overlap partially. Should a dwell in the overlap area be counted as belonging to neither, one, or both the AOIs? Deciding which saccades should count as transitions is even worse. If one AOI covers the other, being in front of it, then it would be clear that any data in the overlap area only belongs to the frontmost AOI. But what if the stimulus image consists of two semi-transparent and partially overlapping objects, as is often the case in advertisements and graphic design? How to quantify AOI measures for studies with such material must be decided depending on the particular experimental design.

Figure 6.33(c) represents an AOI from a drop-down program menu overlapping the underlying taskbar AOI. As it is not transparent, the menu dwell time is not shared with the taskbar AOI, and the saccades between them should be counted as actual transitions. However, the menu AOI has a limited duration which is decided by the clicks of the participant.

---

[21]The danger becomes apparent when we realize that the precise position of the AOI over the "-3" in Figure 6.32 could decide whether the researchers obtain a significant result. If the dwell time comparison between mathematics and humanities students yields a p-value of 0.074, it might be enough to move the border of this AOI just a little to be able to creep below the magic boundary of 0.05. Under pressure to produce results, a weak researcher might be tempted to argue to herself that there is really no objective and precise spatial border between the "-3" and the larger quotient that is more correct than any other spatial border next to it. If so, she may say, what harm is there then in moving the AOI border a pixel or two? That small distance is far below the precision and accuracy of the eye-tracker, anyway.

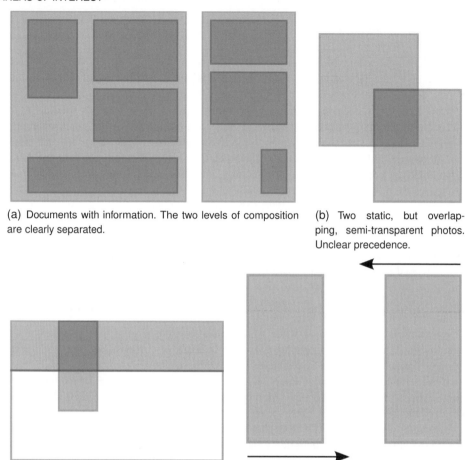

(a) Documents with information. The two levels of composition are clearly separated.

(b) Two static, but overlapping, semi-transparent photos. Unclear precedence.

(c) Menu selection overlap in computer software. The menu suddenly appears and disappears.

(d) Two people walking past each other. Dynamic overlap.

Fig. 6.33 Four different ways that AOIs can overlap.

The case in Figure 6.33(d) shows two dynamic AOIs moving towards an overlap situation. They could be two people walking towards each other, or, in a car-driving study, a pedestrian and a cyclist crossing the junction ahead. Such dynamic AOIs could occur at different depth planes according to the field of view of the observer. Is a hit on the pedestrian also a hit on the cyclist when they overlap? Should only the AOI closest to the driver be hit? This could easily be calculated if the scene is a 3D model, but it becomes more difficult if it is a real traffic scene, or just a video recording, and the AOIs are at different distances in depth. But even if we could calculate which the closest object is, seen from a visual intake perspective, how can we be certain that only one and not both objects are perceived and processed? The foremost object may not cover the more distant one completely, then, we have an overlap of AOIs that could allow both to be perceived. Even small children can easily recognize two objects in an overlap situation (Ghent, 1956), given time, but as Duncan (1984) shows, participants still tend to allocate attention only to *one* object at a time when looking at two objects which overlap.

There are at least five ways to deal with the potential problem of getting more than 100% of total dwell time in these dynamic overlaps. None of them is perfect.

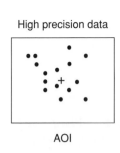

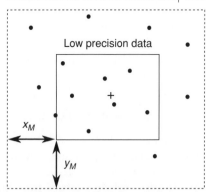

• Data samples

+ Fixation location

High precision data

AOI

Low precision data

x_M

y_M

Fig. 6.34 Additional margins (x_M, y_M) have to be added to an AOI when the precision is low, otherwise some samples will miss the AOI resulting in, for example, shorter average and total dwell times. In this example, all data samples belong to the same fixation, which is located in the middle of the AOI.

1. Accept it, and modify the statistical tests. This alternative assumes that participants fully perceive both AOIs.
2. Simply divide the dwell time of each AOI by the total sum in all AOIs. This forces the excess to be spread equally onto all AOIs, whether they overlap or not.
3. While recording data, create an overlap duration matrix, which for each pair of dynamic AOIs tells us for how long that pair overlapped. Then take the excess dwell time (the part above 100%), and let each pair of AOIs pay for that excess in proportion to their share of the total overlap duration in the matrix. This is more fair to overlap per se, but ignores whether the AOIs have actually been looked at.
4. Calculate the distances between a data sample landing in the overlapping area and the AOI centres. Then assign the sample to the nearest AOI.
5. In an overlap situation, if we have a dwell on two transparent AOIs, we give each of them one half of the dwell time.

Alternative 5 has the advantage that none of the AOIs that were neither overlapping nor looked at need to contribute to the reduction in dwell time caused by normalization. From a visual intake perspective, we could argue that from eye tracking alone, we do not know which of the two transparent objects has been attended, nor how much attention has been allocated, so the equal distribution of dwell time is a fair probabilistic estimation. For transitions, we should only count saccades that move between the two AOIs at the time when the AOIs do not overlap.

6.6.3 Deciding the size of an AOI

The accuracy achieved in your measurements (pp. 41–43) is the major factor that decides the smallest element that can be given an AOI. In theory, it would be possible to use AOIs as small as 0.5° for participants and systems that give a high accuracy after calibration. In practice, however, this is rarely applicable since imprecision of the eye-tracker (pp. 33–41) requires additional margins to enclose all data samples, as illustrated in Figure 6.34. Taking both accuracy and precision into account, the practical minimal size of an AOI can be expected to be around 1–1.5° for high-end eye-trackers, because this is the size of the fovea and the best eye-trackers have the precision to accommodate such as size. Consequently, this is also a minimum margin to be added around objects of interest in your stimuli.

If your AOIs are smaller than the precision in your data, the results that you get from the AOI analysis will have shorter dwell times and a massive amounts of entries and transitions, invalidating your results. Inaccuracy instead causes dwell time and transitions to be assigned to other AOIs than the correct one. In gaze interaction with low-cost eye-trackers, it is common practice to lowpass the data and this way make is possible to select small menu items, even though the precision is typically poor.

6.6.4 Data samples or fixations and saccades?

In the previous chapter, we have discussed both data samples and fixation-based data at length. Which should we use together with AOIs? Data samples are closer to the real eye movements, as they are not influenced by your fixation algorithm and its settings, but data samples also include artefacts from blinks and varying optic conditions during recording. Moreover, dwells could be dispersed throughout an AOI whereas fixations are typically evaluated solely based on their centre locations and durations. Taken together, this makes dwells and fixations different from each other in a number of aspects.

The dwell is comprised of all samples from entry to exit, regardless of whether they originate from a fixation or not. All samples belonging to a fixation, however, do not necessarily have to reside in the AOI, as long as the central location of the fixation does. In Figure 6.34, for instance, the fixation duration assigned to the AOI is the same regardless of whether the data have high or low precision (15 samples). However, both average and total dwell time calculated from the data samples differ significantly between the two cases.

When several consecutive fixations and data samples reside in the same AOI, total dwell time is per definition longer than the sum of fixation durations, and you can expect them to differ by about 20%. When investigating general viewing behaviour, it does not really matter which you use as long as you are systematic. However, if you are investigating a specific claim in the literature you should be aware of how duration has been previously calculated.

Some AOI hit and dwell-based measures require the use of data samples, like the proportion over time graphs. Running them through an event detection algorithm, as noted in one of the hands-on points on page 153, is then one possibility to exclude everything but, e.g. fixations, and then use data samples only from within the detected fixations.

For the *transition* event, artefacts from using data samples may be much larger, since a saccade may cross an AOI or be split by an intervening fixation, depending on the algorithmic definitions you choose.

6.6.5 Dealing with inaccurate data

Offsets in the data are major concerns for any AOI analysis, whether caused by *drift*[22] in the eye-tracker, droopy eyelids, a miscalibration in one corner, or something else. Before running an AOI analysis, always check whether data from any of your participants exhibits systematic offsets in parts of the image. You may have recorded 80 participants, for instance, and for 18 of them, data coordinates may be slightly shifted up or down, so that for a specific AOI, a large portion of the samples that rightfully belong to that AOI are in fact allocated to a neighbouring AOI. In reading studies, for instance, dwell times for one line of text may have been shifted to the line above or below it. The effect in your data analysis may be large enough to render another statistical result than the true one, and profoundly undermine the validity of your study. There are four ways to deal with this problem:

1. Before recording, when you construct your stimulus and your AOIs, be sure to add *a margin* to your AOIs, so that small offsets can be captured in the margin. Select margin

---

[22]System-inherent drift in the eye-tracking equipment causes increased inaccuracies and is not the same as drift of the eye during prolonged fixations.

sizes based on the expected precision and accuracy levels with your particular eye-tracker and participants. In some cases, competing AOIs are so close that you have no space for margins, as in Figure 6.1 on page 188; or there may be just a little space in between AOIs, as in Figure 6.30 on page 219. You need to be aware of this because it can lead to both false positives and false negatives in your statistics.

2. After data have been collected, consult the data quality ratings you made during recordings, or scanpath visualizations, and *remove participants with offset data or with high imprecision* from further analysis. You may have to record further data to compensate for the loss.

3. On a participant-by-participant basis, *move the AOIs* so they cover the correct data rather than the correct portion of the stimulus image, as in Figure 6.35(a). This takes time, and is difficult to do correctly, unless your stimulus material is text.

4. On a participant-by-participant basis, *shift the data* back so the offset is neutralized and data again covers the correct part of the image, where the AOI is, as in 6.35(b). The option to manually move fixations is currently implemented only in EyeLink software,[23] but automated "drift correction" and "offset repair" algorithms have been developed for reading data, for instance the iDict software by Hyrskykari (2006).

Alternatives 1 and 2 are the only fully satisfactory solutions, although alternative 2 adds a somewhat larger level of insecurity about your results. The two data repair alternatives are equivalent, but it is important to remember that such shifts of data or AOIs should be made only if it is *obvious* from scanpath visualizations how the repair should be made. For some stimuli, like text or newspaper reading, the scanpaths are so systematic in their alignment to the stimulus that any offset is immediately visible, and its size and direction easily calculable. For general scene images with a varying content, it is often much more difficult to correctly estimate the needed offset repair.

The problem with correcting data is of course that while increasing your chances of getting the right result, it also undermines the credibility of your conclusions, whether it is called "offset compensation" or "post-recording drift correction". If the reader of your paper knows that your data were not of sufficient quality to yield a significant result without corrupting them, then he will be in doubt about whether to believe what you report. Sometimes data corrections may increase the validity of your results, but we have no guarantee (other than the integrity of the researcher) that data were not shifted to make a non-significant result significant. Also, what about other measures; is saccadic amplitude affected when fixations are moved, for instance? The only sure solution is to remove data so poor that the resulting values for measures are not reliable.

6.6.6 Normalizing AOI measures to size, position, and content

When comparing AOI measures such as number of fixations and dwell time between AOIs (rather than between participants), you may sometimes feel that it would be fairer to the data to scale—or normalize—the dwell time value to the area, position, or content of the AOI.

---

[23] A pragmatic aspect of the EyeLink software/algorithms is the possibility of "performing drift correction on fixations" (SR Research, 2007, p. 25) by simply grabbing any fixation or group of fixations and pulling it to a new position. It is unclear from the manual whether saccadic amplitudes and velocities also change during these data editing operations, or only fixation positions. A tip is given that a whole line of fixations can be aligned to have the same vertical value while retaining their horizontal value; this is useful in reading research. The EyeLink manual states that when batch-moving fixations like this, more than a 30 pixel movement is not acceptable; however, for those users who want to move fixations more than this, the 30 pixel setting can easily be changed.

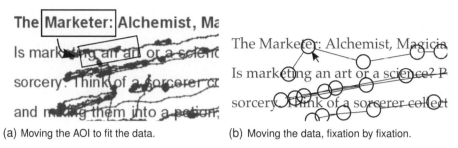

(a) Moving the AOI to fit the data.　　　(b) Moving the data, fixation by fixation.

Fig. 6.35 Correcting offsets by moving (a) AOIs or (b) fixations.

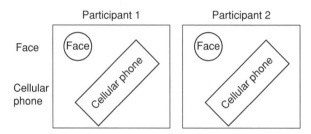

Fig. 6.36 The same stimulus image, two participants and two AOIs. Normalization is only motivated when comparing between AOIs, not when comparing between participants.

For instance, Altmann and Kamide (2007) explicitly refrained from reporting statistical comparisons of the proportion of fixations between AOIs because of differences in their relative size.

Scaling is not necessary if you are only comparing between participants who looked at the same images (Figures 6.36), as the AOIs are kept constant across the comparison. However, when comparing between AOIs within one stimulus image, or between the same AOIs in different stimuli, sizes and positions differ across the comparison.

Note that the scaling factor—or function—is not easy to find. Scaling can be motivated for three different reasons, of which only one is easy to use.

Size If gaze can be expected to be *equally distributed* across the monitor—uncommon due to central bias—and two AOIs in your stimulus have *quite different sizes*, but only *small or unknown semantic differences* between them, we can then expect that gaze will be equally distributed across the stimulus, so that larger stimuli will have more data samples just because of their size. For instance, in their analysis of social stimuli, Birmingham, Bischof, and Kingstone (2009) normalize for AOI sizes by dividing proportion values by AOI area, and report large differences compared to non-scaled proportion values, in particular for the eye and head regions of people in social scenes. Using photographs of parks, Nordh (2010) also found that dwell time positively correlates with size, so that scaling by area is motivated. The reading depth measure for newspaper items on page 390 is one solution for scaling dwell time by AOI area.

Position If your stimulus is so constructed that there is one central AOI and four AOIs in the corners, you can expect that the central AOI will receive more attention simply because of the *central-bias effect* (Tatler, 2007). You may then need to scale down dwell time values on the central AOI, but it is currently unclear exactly what function to use for this.

Content Two AOIs may have very different contents, so that *in one case the task requires more dwell time* than in the other. An obvious example would be two AOIs of the same size but containing different length text within them. The longer text would invariably have a higher dwell time, but not because it was more difficult to process. Two pictures with different content (number of faces, for instance) may also have different require-ments of gaze behaviour that can be taken as a baseline and used for normalization. In this case, scale by the unit causing the difference; for instance number or words or number of faces.

6.6.7   AOIs in gaze-overlaid videos

If data were recorded onto gaze-overlaid video only, as is typically the case with head-mounted eye-trackers without head tracking, the AOI hits must be coded manually, which may or may not be very time consuming. Once data have been coded, however, the same AOI measure may be used for gaze-overlaid data as for coordinate data. To be able to use AOI-based statistics is often reason enough to spend many weeks coding hours of video data. We will discuss current possibilities and some future directions.

Researchers are still lacking quick and robust methods for analysing gaze-overlaid scene video from head-mounted eye-trackers with no head tracking. Each of the methods below has serious limitations: they are either very slow, or they allow only for a small number of AOIs in a very limited space. Assume that in your study, you want to record eye movements from one hundred participants buying their groceries, and that they all go through the same supermarket. Such a study can be operationalized and conducted, but will have at least one thousand AOIs that you would want to code for. The ideal system would let me code AOIs using only *one* of the 100 video files, and then the computer would do the rest of the work for me. And, of course, the same coding method should also work for car-driving studies where all participants drive the same route.

The coding methods here give dwell times, that is dwell start, stop, and order of dwells. Such a coding renders possible the majority of measures defined for AOIs, that is the dwell- and transition-based measures, but not those that involve fixations. Fixations can be coded either from the gaze-overlaid video, (p. 175) or if contamination by smooth pursuit is accept-able, by using a velocity-based algorithm on gaze coordinates (Chapter 5).

Frame-by-frame coding from video Use a video player that allows you to play the gaze-overlaid video one frame at a time. When the overlaid gaze marker has reached an AOI, you start counting the number of frames until it leaves the AOI again. Such a procedure gives you the dwell time measure, in the unit of frame time. The AOI in itself is only implicit (absolute in stimulus coordinates, dynamic in head coordinates), since the coding is done on the basis of the actual semantic area rather than a geometric representation put on top of it. You can have as many AOIs as you want. This is a very general, but quite time-consuming method that has been used in studies of supermarket decision making (Vikström, 2006), newspaper reading (Garcia & Stark, 1988), cricket batsmen (Land & McLeod, 2000), gestures and face-to-face interaction (Gullberg & Holmqvist, 1999, 2006), and many other applied studies where it has been the only possible option.

Inter-coder reliability is virtually never reported, probably because the frame-by-frame coding method is considered very precise. If the study requires only limited sequences of the video to be analysed, such as the few minutes before a particular shelf in a supermarket, rather than the entire 30 minutes of shopping, it is fairly achievable to use such manual frame-by-frame coding. However, head-tracking or marker-based systems should be considered as a time-saving alternative, whenever possible.

Simulating gaze movement by hand motion Connect a graphic tablet to your computer, and draw the AOIs on a paper that you put over the tablet. Try to make the layout of the AOIs similar to that of the actual stimulus. For example, if you are studying an air traffic control station, and the communication radio used is to the right of the radar monitor in the scene, then put the radio AOI to the right of the radar AOI. Have the computer program learn where the areas are on the tablet, so when you hold the tablet pencil over an AOI, the computer program logs the time it stays there. If you hold the pencil over the radio AOI for five seconds, you get a 5 second dwell time mark in the data file. When the tablet and the computer are all set up, you play back the video at half speed, look at where the gaze marker goes, and move the tablet pencil to the corresponding AOIs on the tablet. A system like this was developed in the late 1990s at Halden research station in Norway, which Hauland (2002) used when coding 56 hours of analogue gaze-overlaid video data recorded from air traffic controllers. Hauland had a student do the same for inter-coder reliability (which was moderate at 70–75%). This is a fairly fast form of data coding, running at half recording speed, but it does not allow for more AOIs than there is room for on a tablet. Neither can you have more AOIs than it is possible to learn the positions of; at most 15 or so. This method of coding fits rather static stimuli, like control boards in aeroplanes, nuclear plants, and air traffic control operating rooms.

Dynamic AOIs in head-mounted videos As with any dynamic stimulus, dynamic AOIs can be used to code data from head-mounted videos. Put the dynamic AOIs on top of the areas in the gaze-overlaid scene video that you want for AOIs, and adjust for form, size, and motion changes. Since these AOIs are in the same coordinate system, again that of the scene video, as the coordinates in the data files, you can use the normal AOI inclusion algorithm to calculate the measures. This is a useful method if your participants make few and slow head movements, and if there are not too many AOIs in the scene. For car-driving studies, with AOIs for rear mirrors and internal controls, it works particularly well. For studies of consumers in supermarkets, the AOIs are too many, and the head movements too fast.

Computer vision solutions Use computer vision algorithms to calculate what parts of the video frames should be made into AOIs. If the contrast, patterns, and colour vary a lot between the different areas and the background, you stand a fair chance of succeeding. An extreme case to exemplify this would be if you are measuring how much students look out of a bright window compared to at the blackboard. Since the calculated AOIs will have the same coordinate system as the data file, namely that of the scene video, the calculated AOIs will fit the gaze data coordinates just as well as if we had shown the video on a monitor. Motion blur and other imperfections in the scene video can easily make the project difficult, and if the stimulus has only small visual differences between AOIs, it is not the way to go. An alternative solution involves markers. For instance, a simple and computationally tractable version of this is to attach black and white, or for that matter infrared markers with specific patterns onto the stimulus, and let the computer vision algorithm use the markers as corners of a coordinate system (essentially a plane) in which AOI can be defined. Marker-based systems typically have drawbacks, in particular a limited operative range. Markers may additionally look odd in many environments and distract natural viewing behaviour in a way that may make your study difficult to publish. An alternative could be to place the marker in the scene video—rather than on the stimulus—and have the software learn the image statistics around the marker and build a model from that.

Head tracking Knowing the position and direction of the participant's head in the measure environment gives the same result as using markers: within a certain range, coordinate systems can be defined in the measure space, and AOIs set up in them. Head tracking has mostly been magnetic, requires a certain knowledge to calibrate and set-up, but can be combined with high-speed head-mounted eye-trackers.

6.7 Summary: events and representations from AOIs

A large number of events in, and representations of, eye-movement data are built upon what we call *areas of interest* (AOIs). They are regions in the stimulus that are interesting with respect to the experimental design, and are used to quantify whether and how much participants looked at the particular regions. There are different types of AOIs, and using them comes with a number of challenges.

Basic AOI events are calculated from raw data samples or events over AOIs:

- **AOI hit** with at least information about the fixation or raw data sample.
- **Dwell** events with at least AOI name, starting time and duration values, and information about the number of fixations.
- **Transition** events with at least starting time and duration, and names of exit and entry AOIs.

Each such event has its own values. A dwell, for instance, has a duration and a starting point. These values will later appear as measures, and as parts of measures. The following derived AOI events are often seen in the literature:

- **The return** event with information about the AOI name and the time.
- **The first skip** with AOI name and time.
- **The total skip** with AOI name.

Representations of eye-tracking data that draw on AOI division are:

- **The AOI string** A sequence of fixations or dwells in AOIs, such as MMTCCHGM, where each letter is a fixation in an AOI, and the order corresponds to the sequence in which the AOIs are looked at.
- **The dwell-map** The visualization of a gridded AOI in which each cell is given the value of the average or summed dwell time for data in it. As we will see in the next chapter, this representation of data is essentially a down-sampled attention map. Not only dwell time is used, gridded AOIs can be filled with a variety of measures that give rise to visualizations of *how early* different parts of the image have been looked at, for instance.
- **The transition matrix** A two- or higher-dimensional catalogue of the number of transitions or transition sequences of each kind.
- **The Markov model** A probabilistic model describing or modelling the data in a transition matrix.
- **The proportion over time graphs** An important representation for studying processes over time, with many varieties, including **sequence chart, scarf plot, cumulative proportion graph**, and **proportion of transition sequences over time**.

In the remainder of the book, we will very often refer to AOI events and representations defined in this chapter.

AOIs can be productively combined with fixation- and saccade measures to produce a range of other measures which take both aspects into account; for instance first fixation in an AOI, saccadic amplitude within an AOI, or total dwell time. In addition, AOIs allow for substitution of the spatial dimensions with feature dimensions derived from the position. Remember, however, that the values in all these events and representations, as well as the validity of your conclusions, depend crucially on how you segment space with AOIs.

7 Attention Maps—Scientific Tools or Fancy Visualizations?

In the previous two chapters we have explained how to use data samples to estimate oculomotor events (Chapter 5) and how to divide stimulus space into areas of interests (AOIs) to detect further events and define complex representations (Chapter 6). In this chapter, we introduce a representation of eye-tracking data called *attention maps*, which is very often visualized in the form of a *heat map*, but which also has mathematical forms that can be used for quantitative testing.

Although it does not represent attention per se but the spatial distribution of eye-movement data, we consider the term 'attention map' an appropriate homage to the two papers that first introduced them as a general representation form for eye-tracking data: Pomplun et al. (1996) ('Attentional landscape') and Wooding, Mugglestone, Purdy, and Gale (2002) ('Fixation map').

This chapter is organized as follows:

- Section 7.1 (p. 231) introduces the settings dialogue you face when using a number of common commercial software packages.
- In Section 7.2 (p. 233), general principles and terminology of attention maps are described.
- How should we use attention maps? In Section 7.3 (p. 238), we provide hands-on advice to people who want to use attention maps.
- Section 7.4 (p. 239) presents issues and challenges that one should be aware of when using attention maps.
- Attention maps have so far almost exclusively been used to visualize eye-tracking data. Section 7.5 (p. 248) lists applications of attention maps that go beyond visualization.
- The summary Section 7.6 (p. 252) repeats the major methodological issues surrounding attention maps, and reiterates the two representations that the dispersion and similarity measures in Chapter 11 make use of.

Heat maps provide quick, very intuitive, and in some cases objective visual representations of eye-tracking data that naive users and even children can immediately grasp a meaning from. Their intuitiveness has made heat map visualizations very popular in parts of the applied and scientific eye-tracking community, and they are now available in all major analysis softwares for eye-tracking data.

7.1 Heat map settings dialogues

When a researcher wants to generate heat maps from recorded data, but not implement the software for doing it, she is faced with software developed by the eye-tracker manufacturer or by independent companies. It is remarkably easy; just click a button and you will immediately see the defaulted heat map visualization. Typically, regions with many fixations or data samples are highlighted with warm colours (red) and regions where few or no people looked

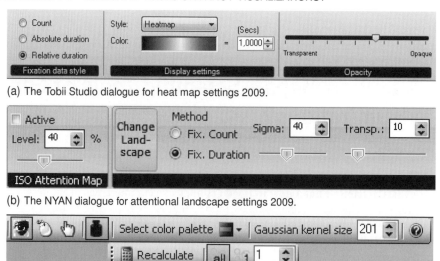

(a) The Tobii Studio dialogue for heat map settings 2009.

(b) The NYAN dialogue for attentional landscape settings 2009.

(c) The OGAMA 2.5 dialogue for attention map module 2009. The eye icon corresponds to 'use gaze data for attention maps', and the weight icon 'weight fixation by length'. The two icons in between are related to visualization of mouse data.

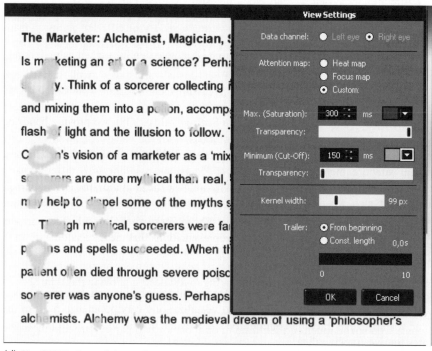

(d) The SMI BeGaze dialogue for attention map settings on top of heat map visualization 2009.

Fig. 7.1 Examples of settings dialogues for attention maps.

are marked with a colder (blue) colour. In the software, there are settings that allow you to vary the appearance of the visualization, and Figures 7.1(a) to 7.1(d) show dialogue boxes from four softwares: Tobii studio, NYAN, OGAMA (Vosskuhler, Nordmeier, Kuchinke, & Jacobs, 2008), and SMI BeGaze.

While the heat maps themselves look very simple and intuitive, it is not always obvious what settings to use in the dialogue boxes. For instance, what is 'Kernel width', what does the size of that kernel have to do with the visualization produced? Is 'Sigma' the same, or something wholly different? What does it mean that a certain colour equals the time of 1 second? What are 'Fixation data styles', and why is it necessary to choose between them? Can the user accept the default settings, whatever they are, or is it a better approach to move the values up and down until the heat map looks good? Is there such a thing as correct settings at all?

7.2 Principles and terminology

To understand what the settings in the dialogue boxes are, and why they produce the results they do, we have to understand how attention maps are generated. Two seemingly different but closely related principles have been used to achieve this: gridded AOIs and topological (Gaussian) landscapes.

The gridded AOIs (p. 212) divide space into a set of rectangular AOI cells. When filled with dwell time values, the gridded AOI becomes a dwell map. Although the dwell map as such does not qualify as an attention map visualization, it would if the numbers were converted into colour or intensity.

Gridded AOIs are versatile tools for generating a variety of different attention maps and interesting visualizations to them. To make a *dwell map*, for instance, for each cell (each AOI) in the grid, the total dwell time (p. 389) is calculated, and this value determines the colour of that cell. Figure 7.2 shows such a heat visualization of a dwell map constructed from data recorded from newspaper readers. There are clear hot-spots stretching over several of the cells, indicating lots of gaze at that area. There are also parts that are much cooler (less looked at).

While it is most common to fill the cells (AOIs) with the values for dwell time or number of fixations, gridded AOIs offer several other possibilities to build attention maps. For instance, if we were interested in a map that shows on average *how early* different parts of a scene have been visited, an *entry time map*, we could use the AOI-measure *entry time* (p. 437) as the height of each of the cells in the grid. The map would then show red where participants look early on average, and blue where they arrive late in the trial.

We could also fill the AOI cells with the measure *proportion of participants* (p. 419): for each cell in the grid, the proportion of participants having fixated that cell is calculated. 15% in the cool areas, and perhaps 97.5% in the hottest peak. Heat maps produced by the Eye-tools company, a commercial player using eye tracking to test design, provide this type of heat map (Hernandez, 2007). It has to be properly understood, however: a 'proportion-of-participants map' shows what areas have been looked at by how large a proportion of the participants, but participants who spend much of their time in only one or two parts of the stimuli will make a very small contribution to the map compared to participants who visit many grid cells with only a few fixations in each.

Despite their versatility, gridded AOIs have not become the dominating principle for visualizing heat maps. In fact, none of the settings in Figure 7.1 refer to gridded AOIs. Instead of a grid with sharp borders between cells, smoother, 'landscape-like' representations have become more prominent.

As Figure 7.3(b) illustrates, a heat map looks just as flat as fixations plotted on your stimulus, but the underlying attention map represents a smooth landscape with hills and valleys. An attention map landscape is successively built from the sequence of fixations or raw data, simply by putting a basic form at each point in space where the fixation or raw data sample is

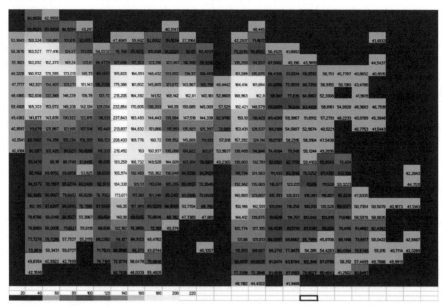

Fig. 7.2 Gridded AOI heat map. 40 readers of a tabloid newspaper; all participants and all 20 folds. Numbers in grid cells are total dwell time values. Recorded using a head-mounted eye-tracker with Polhemus head tracking at 50 Hz.

located. Various basic forms are being used: Pomplun et al. (1996) and Wooding et al. (2002) use mathematical constructs called Gaussian functions, while most manufacturer implementations use cone-formed constructs which approximate the top of a Gaussian function. Given that a sufficient number of forms have been dropped on your stimulus, the final maps will look more or less the same, even though the shape of the basic construct varies somewhat (a consequence of the central limit theorem).

For gridded AOI representations, heat map visualizations can easily be made by choosing what colour is attributed to what height values, but borders between cells will be sharp. In the landscape-like representation, smooth colouring is possible. First, we must recognize that in the commercial software, the altitude in an attention map is mostly time, in which case the altitude unit is milliseconds (ms). For example, the location of a fixation can be assigned an altitude value of its duration, say 325 ms, which decides how high the attention map will be in this point. In Figure 7.4, a single fixation hill is shown from the side, with two thresholds on the right side. Suppose we set the lower threshold to 150 ms and blue, and the upper to 300 ms and red. Then, for all altitudes from 150 to 300 ms, the attention map is coloured with hues ranging from blue to red. Using SMI's software package BeGaze 2.2 with similar settings, Figure 7.1(d) illustrates what this can look like. The resulting heat map has hot-spot areas with very distinct borders, because all the areas where the attention map is lower than 150 ms have been made transparent. In the interval between 150 and 300 ms, the colour intensifies, but above 300 ms, the colour remains constant.

Colour (in a heat map), luminance, and transparency (used in Koivunen, Kukkonen, Lahtinen, Rantala, & Sharmin, 2004) can all be mapped to the altitude in the attention map. For instance, with luminance mapping, low altitudes become dark and high become whatever the original picture was at that position. Figure 7.5(b) shows this type of mapping, which we call a *luminance map*. Yet another possibility would be to map the altitude to an image's contrast, to have an image which is sharp and in focus at high altitudes and increasingly more blurred

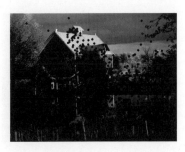

(a) Image with fixations

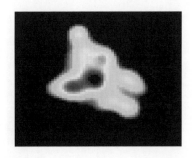

(b) Heat map

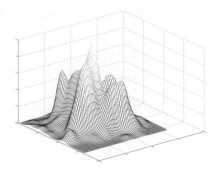

(c) Attention map

Fig. 7.3 Three different ways to visualize the same eye-tracking data. The fixations are recorded from 12 people viewing the image for five seconds.

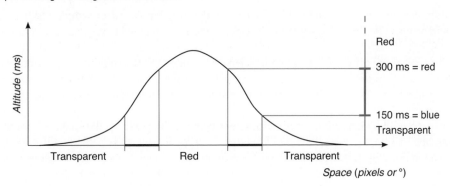

Fig. 7.4 A single Gaussian seen from the side at a point where a 325 ms fixation has landed. The figure shows how a gradual colour dimension is mapped onto altitude so as to generate a 2D heat map visualization.

as we move down the hills into the areas not looked at. Such techniques are explored, e.g. by Geisler and Perry (1998) and Nyström (2008) for the purpose of improved video compression.

There are basically four parameters that decide what your Gaussian attention map will look like. One decides the *mapping from colour to altitude*, another controls the *width of the basic construct*, a third gives you an option to build the attention map with or without taking

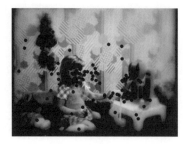

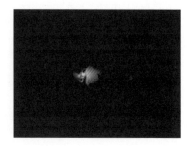

(a) Fixations on stimulus

(b) Luminance map; low altitude (few fixations) is made dark.

Fig. 7.5 In a luminance map, the altitude of the attention map decides the *luminance* of the visualization.

Table 7.1 Attention map settings in four analysis software packages; versions as of 2009. Fillings are as yet restricted to fixation duration and number of fixations.

	SMI BeGaze	Tobii Studio	NYAN	OGAMA
Colour mapping	Saturation, and minimum cutoff	colour = time	n/a	Colour palette
Width	Kernel width	n/a	Sigma	Gaussian kernel size
Filling	n/a	Fixation data style	Method	Yes
Does it use both fixations and raw samples?	Fixations are always used for images, raw samples always for video.	Yes	Fixations are always used.	Fixations are always used.

fixation *duration* into account, and a fourth decides whether raw data samples or fixations should be used. In Table 7.1, some of these parameters are mapped to the dialogue settings in Figure 7.1.

So what is the difference between gridded dwell maps and the smoother representations? In a way, they represent the same data, only at different spatial scales; gridded dwell maps can be considered mathematically a sub-sampled smooth attention map after being interpolated to its original size by a nearest neighbour method. Conversely, if we convolve a gridded dwell map with a Gaussian kernel of sufficient width, it will take on the shape of a smooth landscape.

The major reason that the smoother form of attention maps have come to dominate over gridded AOIs is probably that they are more pleasing to look at. Although being aesthetically pleasing is a seemingly superficial reason, the advent of smooth-looking heat maps helped to radically expand the eye-tracker market in favour of the manufacturer who could first deliver them as part of their software.[24] Another reason could be that the gridded dwell maps provide only a coarse representation of the original data, since fixations or raw data samples are quantized to the grid elements, and thus contain less information about the original data than do Gaussian based attention maps. A less explored reason is that attention maps built from a

[24] Qualitative interviews that the authors have made with salespeople and applied practitioners clearly show the craze for heat maps in the mid 2000s. Several salespeople report on customers asking only for the ability to produce heat maps before ordering. Applied practitioners have told us how they have tried to sell quantitive AOI analysis to customers in the advertisement and web business, but that their customers returned their analysis and asked for heat maps.

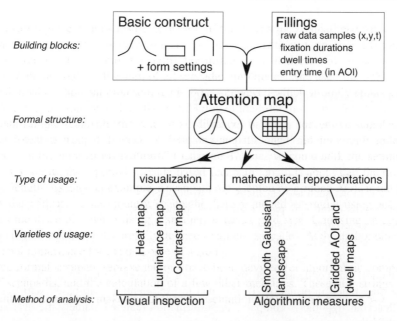

Fig. 7.6 Attention maps are created using a *basic construct*, often (but not always) a Gaussian function, and a *filling* into the construct. The filling can be number of fixations, fixation durations, dwell time, or any other AOI measure. The resulting *attention map* is a smooth landscape or a gridded AOI partition of space, that can be *visualized* in a number of ways (heat maps being the best known), or used in *measures* of e.g. position dispersion and similarity.

Gaussian function can be analysed with a suite of powerful mathematical tools; however, in principle this is also true of gridded AOIs.

Figure 7.6 summarizes this introduction to the representations we call attention maps. It shows that attention maps:

- Consist of two different, but related, representations: the smooth *Gaussian landscapes*, and the hard-edge *gridded AOIs*.
- Are built from a variety of *basic constructs*, including the basic Gaussian function, the grid cell and the various cylinder-like constructs that manufacturer implementations make use of. One such construct is placed or 'dropped' at the position of each fixation or raw data sample. This is not the case for gridded AOIs however, where a grid is simply used to divide up stimulus-space, rather than 'dropping' constructs at specific positions.
- Have *settings* that pertain to the basic constructs rather than to the full and finished map itself. When changing construct settings such as number of cells (in a gridded AOI), 'Kernel width' (of a cylinder or cone) or 'sigma' (of a Gaussian function), the full map only changes because the single basic constructs change.
- Have *fillings*, which are other eye-tracking measures, such as fixation durations or dwell time, that fill the basic constructs and decide their height. More of the measure means a higher basic construct. The full attention map gets its shape from the additive effect when many basic constructs of varying heights pile up.
- Appear in *visualizations* as heat maps, luminance maps or contrast maps, and in *measures* as their basic mathematical forms, and in normalized versions called probability density functions (pdf:s).

In the remainder of the chapter, focus will be on the smooth representations of attention maps, since they dominate the literature.

7.3 Hands-on advice for using attention maps

If you plan to use attention maps to exemplify results, make exploratory investigations of your data, perform statistical tests between groups, or because heat maps are a deliverable to your customer, the following list shows issues that you should consider.

- Attention maps represent the *spatial distribution of data* and nothing else.
- Visualizations such as heat maps tend to inspire less experienced viewers to jump to conclusions about *why* participants look at the hot spots. A heat map can only show where participants look, not why they look there (p. 71).
- Attention maps ignore the underlying semantic areas of your stimulus. Use areas of interests (AOIs) if you want to relate eye-movement data to semantic areas.
- Attention maps collapse over time and often also over participants, which means that you lose much information. If you plan to use attention map-based statistics, see to it that your hypothesis compares the information retained, namely the overall spatial distribution.
- Visualizations such as heat maps can exemplify, support, and even nuance quantitative results, but should be published on their own only after careful consideration.
- There are virtually no guidelines or systematic investigations of the effects of settings for the colour mapping. A σ value of around $2°$ visual angle (diameter) will give an indication of what is looked at with the point of highest visual acuity—the fovea, but note that this can be misleading because items can still be attended in peripheral vision outside of this area. Blignaut (2010) has recently addressed this issue by incorporating perceptual span into attention map settings.
- Do not make a habit of changing values up and down between heat map visualizations of your different groups, participants, or conditions. If you do, your visualizations will not be comparable. In fact, you will be producing art rather than data visualizations. Select one setting and stick to it throughout all the heat maps you make, so you know that any difference that you see in the heat map is actually an effect in your data and not in your settings.
- When you publish your attention map visualization, always report type of eye-tracker and its sampling frequency, analysis software version, settings for the basic constructs, settings for the mapping of colour, luminance or contrast to the height of the map, the time segment that the visualization was created from, whether you use fixations rather than raw data samples, and the criteria for fixation detection.
- Make sure to have sufficient amounts of data for your visualizations.
- If you have data from a low-speed eye-tracker with not so good precision, use fixations for building your attention maps. If you have a high-end eye-tracker, you can also use raw data.
- If you are having participants look at a central fixation cross before stimuli onset, make sure to remove the first fixation in your recordings. Otherwise your attention map may have an artificially large hot-spot in the centre.
- Attention maps are much more versatile than generally believed, and can also be used scientifically. Figure 7.6 illustrates the range of possibilities.

Addressing applied users of eye tracking, Bojko (2009) lists similar but not identical advice.

7.4 Challenging issues: interpreting and building attention maps

Attention maps are challenging for somewhat different reasons compared with event detection algorithms and AOIs. Their major advantage is that they provide a more simple and intuitive overview of large data sets than any other form of visualization. This is also their major disadvantage: the heat maps in particular look so simple that it is tempting to immediately draw conclusions from them that often can not and should not be drawn. In this section, we will look at two challenges related to attention maps, and present them in the order people typically encounter them: interpretation and construction.

7.4.1 Interpreting attention map visualizations

"The hot-spots in the heat map show us what participants found most interesting" seems to be a straightforward, sound observation one could make from a heat map visualization. However, is this assumption always correct, or does the heat map really tell us something else? Let us start by looking at an example from reading.

Notwithstanding the complications with attention maps, their major advantage is that they very quickly give an easily digestible overview of the total data from a large number of participants. This they do much better than any other data visualizations. Take for example the ten non-native readers visualized as scanpaths in Figure 7.7(a). Such a scanpath visualization looks like a complete mess of fixations and connection lines, and it is not possible to see if some words attracted more attention than others. Figure 7.7(b) shows only the fixations and no connection lines. The circles representing fixations have also been made smaller and with thinner lines. It is difficult but not impossible to see that some words have indeed been looked at more than others. The words 'magician' and 'sorcerer' in the heading, for instance, and several of the first words in each line. We cannot see how these individual fixations add up to a total group gaze on the words, however, nor compare between the words. This is where the attention map shows its strength. The heat map in Figure 7.7(c) shows that the words 'Culliton's', 'sorcerers', and 'may' have attracted more total gaze than the words higher up, but also that 'extent' and 'this fits' appear under the highest peaks.

Now, reading researchers have altogether avoided using attention maps in their studies. This is not only because attention maps ignore the important temporal order which is the basis for detecting for instance regressions. Nor is the major problem that heat maps ignore the small effects that reading researchers typically look for. Rather, heat maps and the other visualizations of attention maps do not provide any method for systematic and statistical comparison between conditions. How should we reason over a heat-map visualization? Suppose that we are linguists pondering over the heat map in Figure 7.7(c). We can see that certain words are hot, and, since we are curious about the result, immediately try to look for explanations: 'Culliton's' could be an unknown proper name, and 'mythical', 'sorcerers', and 'diseases' are infrequent words that the readers had to take some time to look at before they could understand them. And the hot-spot on 'this fits' must have something to do with the reference being difficult to understand, must it not? 'Though mythical' is perhaps also a difficult sentence start for these non-native readers? Throughout the data collection phase, we have looked forward to finding effects in the data of difficulties in understanding the text, and now we see them in the red-hot areas of the heat map. The hot-spots become confirmatory examples for our first explanation of whatever word or construction happens to be underneath it, making this study at best *exploratory* or at worst a confusing *fishing trip* (p. 66). We fail to look at the cool blue areas where less reader attention has been spent, and where similar references exist and where infrequent words are hidden counterexamples. The heat map sim-

(a) SMI BeGaze 2.2 scanpath visualization of ten non-native readers. The velocity algorithm with threshold 40°/s threshold and size of fixations proportional against fixation duration.

(b) Fixation point visualization of ten non-native readers; with no lines between fixations.

The Marketer: Alchemist, Magician, Sorcerer and Medicine Man

Is marketing an art or a science? Perhaps marketing is more like sorcery. Think of a sorcerer collecting ingredients from different sources and mixing them into a potion, accompanied with the magical effect of a flash of light and the illusion to follow. To some extent this fits with Culliton's vision of a marketer as a 'mixer of ingredients'. Of course sorcerers are more mythical than real, but if we stay with this myth it may help to dispel some of the myths surrounding 'marketing'.

Though mythical, sorcerers were far from perfect. Not all their potions and spells succeeded. When they tried to cure diseases, the patient often died through severe poisoning -- and the fate of the sorcerer was anyone's guess. Perhaps the same could be said of alchemists. Alchemy was the medieval dream of using a 'philosopher's

(c) SMI BeGaze 2.2 heat map visualization of ten non-native readers. Kernel width 99 pixels, maximal saturation 300 ms, and minimum saturation 0 ms.

Fig. 7.7 Heat maps give a good overview over data. Data from 10 non-native students of economy reading a management text, while being recorded with a towermounted high-end system.

ply does not invite systematic comparisons between all confirmatory and counter-examples, and so does not fit into the scientific method. Instead the heat map tends to invite to post-hoc interpretations that favour the researchers own hopes or favourite theory.

Are heat maps more helpful if we use them only to characterize the general viewing behaviour, rather than to explain it? In the eye tracking for web usability field, heat map visualizations are very commonly used to describe the general outcome of an eye tracking study. For example, Nielsen refers to the well-quoted so-called F-pattern (Nielsen, 2006): "Eyetracking visualizations show that users often read web pages in an F-shaped pattern: two

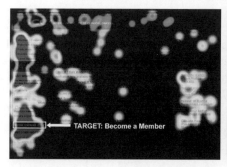 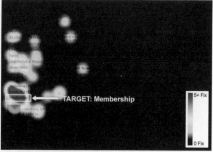

Fig. 7.8 Two designs of the same web page. Participant task was to find the membership link. ©UPA, *Journal of Usability Studies,* Volume 1, Issue 3, p. 117; Bojko, A.A. (2006), Using eye tracking to compare web page designs: A case study.

horizontal stripes followed by a vertical stripe". Wulff (2007) uses heat maps to investigate how viewers explore a web page and concludes:

> Only the very first links are looked at and our test confirms—as do some Google tests—that the user does not read much on the page. The first 1-2 hits are read to the end. However, lower down in the list, it is only the first part of the line that is looked at. At the bottom we find only scattered glances. It is important that the most relevant hits are placed at the top of the page as is also the case in Google.

Similarly, Bojko (2006) compares two web page designs (Figure 7.8), using the heat map only to show that in the one case the gazes of participants were focused only on the task-relevant target, while in the other web page design, gazes were spread out. As long as the conclusion refers to *the viewing behaviour itself*, rather than *explanations to it*, the heat map is not tricking us. Compare this with the use of a heat map over a web page to conclude that: "Bottom half of page—ineffective line-height spacing and lack of white-space reduce reading. Most of the content is being missed".[25] Yes, the content is being missed by many; this a heat map can show. But to prove that it is missed *because of* ineffective line-height spacing rather then due to position, reader interest in the content, or long-term evolved reader expectations of where to look at web pages; that requires a much larger undertaking in terms of experimental design (p. 71).

   In summary, the hot-spots in a heat map can point out the regions that attracted people's gazes, but it is highly speculative to draw any conclusions of what made people look there solely based on the heat map; it could be because these regions are interesting, but also because they are confusing, and people need to look twice to get the message.

Attention maps and effect sizes

Figure 7.9 shows a much quoted teaser from a commercial company promoting their eye-tracking services. The heat maps appear to show that when the woman looks at the product, the participants—real customers according to the company web page—look towards the product too. We can easily compare the two conditions, and immediately see the difference in heat maps, can we not?

   A particular uncertainty lingers on: how big is this difference, or *effect size*, really? The heat (i.e. the altitude in the attention maps) on the two product bottles may differ less than the heat map, with all its variable settings, suggests. The effect size in Figure 7.9 is much

---

[25]Citation from `http://blog.eyetools.com/2005/02/the-new-washington-post-homepage-design -an-eyetools-eyetracking-analysis.html`, retrieved Aug 31, 2010. The company owning the webpage is called eye-tools, and claim to be "The inventors of eyetracking heatmapping".

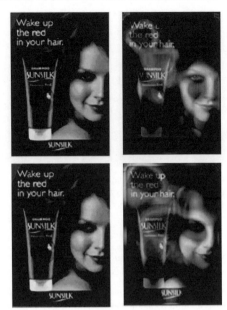

Fig. 7.9 Is this heat map convincing evidence that gaze direction in a face of the picture alters viewer gaze towards the product? From http://www.bunnyfoot.com/articles/not_focus_groups.htm, with kind permission from Bunnyfoot and Think Eyetracking.

easier to calculate using AOIs and the total dwell time measure (p. 389). The product bottle in Figure 7.9 would make an excellent AOI, and the statistical test should be easy. If this marketing analysis company had wanted to impress us, why not present dwell time data in AOIs instead, or at least as a complement to the heat map? The reason could be in their customers; applied eye-tracking practitioners that we have interviewed claim that most of their customers strongly prefer heat map visualizations to conclusions based on statistics.

In other cases, positioning AOIs onto the stimulus image is not always possible. In an elegant example, Pomplun et al. (1996) used attention maps to alter the luminance of an image to promote a certain perceptual interpretation (we call this luminance-based attention map a *luminance map*). Using pictures with two ambiguous interpretations, eye movements were measured and participants were asked to press one of two different buttons to indicate which interpretation they currently perceived. Attention maps built on the collected eye movements belonging to each interpretation were used to modify the luminance such that frequently viewed regions were retained in high luminance, whereas other regions were reduced in luminance. Hence, two new versions of each stimulus image were generated, one for each subjective interpretation. Figure 7.10 exemplifies data for one stimulus image. The difference between the two luminance maps can quickly be seen in the figures, and we tend to easily accept that these images show that the subjective experience of an ambiguous picture is closely related to gaze position. However, on closer inspection, it is also obvious that there is a considerable overlap between the two luminance maps. In fact, the only part of the king in 7.10(b) that is not visible in the animal version 7.10(c), is the small area around the mouth. If we want to calculate effect sizes (how big the difference really is) using a dwell time measure, how do we position the AOIs? On the mouth, or on the king as a whole, or somewhere in between? Every position is a poor compromise. What we would want is a comparison that takes the attention map as a whole and compares it to another attention map as a whole.

Lacking a statistical method for comparing attentions maps, Pomplun et al. (1996) had

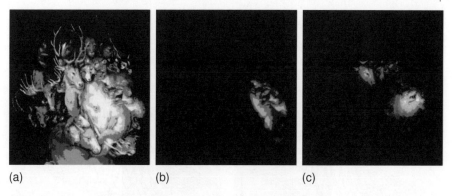

(a)   (b)   (c)

Fig. 7.10 The painting 'Earth' by Giuseppe Arcimboldo. a: Original: b: luminance maps of data samples from participants who (clicked to) report that they see the king. c: luminance map of data from participants who report that they see the animals. Reprinted from *Perception, 25*(8), Pomplun M, Ritter H, Velichkovsky B, Disambiguating complex visual information: Towards communication of personal views of a scene, ©1996, pp. 931–948 with permission from Pion Limited, London.

other participants look at the luminance maps in Figures 7.10(b) and 7.10(c), and judge which interpretation they experienced in each. This difference proved to be strong. Such indirect tests are rarely applicable, however.

Bojko (2006) compares two web designs using heat maps, as a complement to the other two measures: entry time in number of fixations (defined on page 437), and total duration on the page. Participants had various tasks, for instance to find the 'How to become a member' link on the page. The purpose of using heat maps was to visualize the spread of search across the page up until the correct link was found. Figure 7.8 on page 241 shows heat maps that indicate a fairly clear difference between the two designs, but how do we quantify the difference? As the heat maps are used to illustrate the spread of search, AOI analysis could not easily do the job, but the relatively new dispersion and similarity measures in Chapter 11 would be able to quantify the deviation we see in the heat maps of Figure 7.8, adding an effect size to what is otherwise only a difference in visualizations.

There is one virtually never used benefit of attention maps, in relation to effect size measures with AOIs and other quantitative statistical tools: suppose that we use AOI measures, and get a significant effect that participants indeed look more at one part of the image than another, or more at an object in one image than in the other (as in Figure 7.9). Normally, a significant effect makes us trust that the effect is robust and worthy of publication. But a significant effect only shows that the difference is systematic and stable, not its magnitude. An attention map visualization such as a heat map allows us to estimate the magnitude of the effect in the context of the entire data: are the peaks in the selected areas really that big in comparison to the rest of the data?

7.4.2 How many fixations/participants?

As mentioned earlier in the chapter, attention maps are helpful to visualize large amounts of eye-tracking data. But when is it useful to switch from e.g. a scanpath view to a heat map? How many fixations/participants do we need in order to produce a robust visualization, i.e. one that does not change significantly if more data is added to it, or if the same amount of data from another group of viewers is used to produce it? Unfortunately, there is no single answer to these questions. Pernice and Nielsen (2009, p. 19) propose that usability studies should contain at least 30 participants if heat maps are "the main deliverables", and/or used in drawing conclusions. To motivate this heuristic, Pernice and Nielsen (2009) correlate a heat

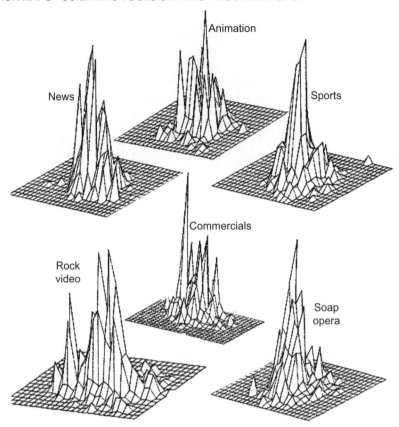

Fig. 7.11 Attention map visualization showing the cumulative gaze distribution from three participants watching five videos. Reprinted with permission from Elias, Sherwin, and Wise (1984), ©1984, SMPTE.

map built from 60 viewers with another heat map built from a subset of these 60 viewers, and conclude that a subset of 30 people suffices to obtain a robust correlation between the maps. However, in the general case, the number of participants required closely depends on:

- your experimental hypothesis and the exact implementation of the heat map
- whether you have recorded a heterogeneous participant group
- the width of your basic construct (e.g. σ in a Gaussian function)
- whether the task at hand leads to increased inter-participant gaze dispersion

7.4.3 How attention maps are built

Yet another challenge is to decide what raw material to build the attention map from, i.e. the 'basic construct'. As we saw earlier in the chapter, different constructs are used across analysis software. The good news is that if you have a large enough set of data, most attention map implementations will produce heat maps that look more or less the same.

Figure 7.11 shows what are perhaps the first visualizations of attention maps. The maps summarise the gaze distribution from three viewers watching video clips with different contents, and the authors conclude that the viewers seem to have a strong bias towards the centre of the display on which the videos were shown. However, the implementation is not described in the paper.

Another early usage of attention maps for scientific purposes, Pomplun et al. (1996), used Gaussian functions as basic constructs. Metaphorically, a Gaussian function is equivalent to a little hill of sand. Adding a new fixation to an attention map more or less equals pouring another bucket of sand over the stimulus picture. Gaussians are not said to be poured, however, but are dropped onto the stimulus image. As an alternative metaphor, the Gaussian can be seen as a rubber sheet, which with a given elasticity is being dropped on a pole located at the position of a fixation or raw sample point. The height of the pole would then correspond to the fixation duration.

The SMI BeGaze 2.1 implementation of attention maps first scales each image pixel in proportion to the durations of all fixations landing on it. Typically, this results in a very sparse 'fixation hit map', since only a small proportion of the pixels have been 'hit'. Then this 'hit map' is convolved with a Gaussian kernel with a certain width; a wider kernel gives a smoother, less pointy appearance to the attention map. The reason for dividing the attention map creation into two steps—one to produce the 'fixation hit map' and one to perform the convolution—is simply because the latter can be done directly on the computers graphics card, and therefore speeds up the software significantly and shows attention map visualization in real time, e.g. as video replay. The end result, however, is largely the same as using the Gaussian functions directly. The Tobii Studio software version of 2009 does not appear to have this setting, nor is it clear from the Tobii documentation of that time whether they use Gaussians or some other mathematical form. The heat map visualizations suggest that the Tobii Studio of 2009 uses cones with soft tips and constant widths.

In fact, using Gaussians is not the only way to mathematically represent the buckets of sand poured for each fixation. Wooding et al. (2002) proposes using *cylinders* to approximate the Gaussian. For small numbers of participants, cylinders give attention maps with very sharp edges, but when the number of participants is large, the many cylinders soften each other and the difference from a real Gaussian landscape will diminish. The Tobii cones of 2009 have softer edges, but do not gradually continue out into the periphery as does the Gaussian. Also, neither cylinders nor cones share the mathematical elegance of the Gaussian.

Formally, the Gaussian is defined as

$$G(x,y) = \exp\left(-\frac{(x-x_i)^2 + (y-y_i)^2}{2\sigma^2}\right) \tag{7.1}$$

where (x_i, y_i) is the centre point of the fixation or data sample at which we drop it. (x,y) typically span the dimensions of the stimulus image. The overall attention map is generated by dropping one Gaussian function at each such centre point, and then summing all such dropped Gaussian functions into a single function.

There is only one important choice to make in the definition of the Gaussian, namely its *variance*, σ^2. In our sand metaphor, σ^2 is a measure of the sand's resistance to sliding. A small value on the variance σ^2 gives thin pointy Gaussian peaks, as though the sand resisted sliding to the sides and only formed a higher and higher peak at the very position where it was poured (Figure 7.12(a)). A high value on σ^2 makes the sand slide very much to the side, so that the Gaussians of different fixations completely merge and a map with a much smoother surface will be generated (Figure 7.12(b)). If the σ^2 is high enough, there is no resistance to sliding, and the Gaussians will be so wide and low that the attention map will look as though we were pouring water rather than sand: completely flat. If we look at the heat map visualization, a very low σ^2 setting will give many but narrow intense hot-spots with large cool areas between them. Very high values will yield a uniformly coloured heat map with one or two vague and very distributed hot-spots. Sigma corresponds to kernel width in manufacturer software.

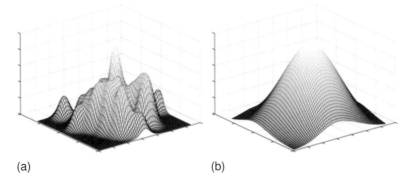

(a)   (b)

Fig. 7.12 Pointy and smooth Gaussian-based attention maps generated from the same eye-tracking data, but with different σ.

So what is so great about the Gaussian function? There are at least three reasons why we should use them:

- The Gaussian can be used to *approximate the acuity fall-off* away from the point of fixation. It can then be argued that the value of the attention map corresponds to what a viewer can visually resolve at that position. Taken one step further, the attention map can be thought to reflect the amount of attention a viewer spends at each image location. As we already know, fixation is not identical to attention, nor does the Gaussian perfectly match the fall-off in acuity,[26] but seen from a mathematical perspective it is one of the simplest, most well-known and well-behaved functions there is that approximates this fall-off.

- A smooth, Gaussian-based attention map can be used as a probability density function that gives a good estimate of where a new viewer, having the same image and task, is likely to look.

- Because of its desirable properties, a powerful suite of mathematical tools can be used to derive measures from the Gaussian-based attention map (p. 359–376).

The few researchers who have used Gaussian-based attention maps have suggested that the variance σ^2 should be set so that at the half-height of the Gaussian peak, the width of the hill at that altitude corresponds to the size of the foveal projection on the stimulus image (Rajashekar, Cormack, & Bovik, 2004; Nyström, Novak, & Holmqvist, 2004). The foveal size is approximately two degrees of visual angle (p. 21). If the geometrical set-up of the experiment is known (or can be estimated), the $2°$ variance setting can easily be calculated. As mentioned above, this setting of σ^2 does not make the attention map mimic the fall-off of acuity on the retina precisely, but it does approximate both the size of the foveal projection and the further decrease in acuity outside. There is in fact not much point in precise modelling of retinal acuity, since attention maps almost always incorporate several participants whose data are not perfectly aligned. The variance has also been adjusted to compensate for the lack in precision of the eye-tracker; the higher the precision the smaller the variance and vice versa. Following this rule, data from a remote eye-tracker would produce a smoother attention map than data collected from a tower-mounted high-end system.

Raw data samples or fixations?

Either raw data samples or fixations can be used to generate the attention map. The attention map, and the visualizations made from it, will differ depending on your choice. This is

---

[26]The true fall-off appears to follow an exponentially decreasing function (Geisler & Perry, 1998).

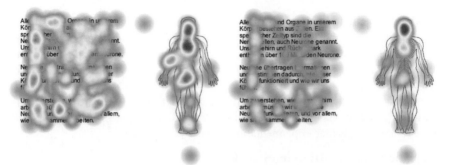

(a) Filled with number of fixations   (b) Filled with fixation duration

Fig. 7.13 The role of filling with fixation duration becomes clearer when fixation durations differ in different parts of the scene. Here fixations on the text are short, but longer on the image, in particular the face. Data recorded using a very common but slightly outdated 50 Hz remote and visualized using Tobii Studio.

particularly true for the Gaussian attention map, so we will focus on it here.

If you have reason not to trust the fixation algorithm, either because it is simply not a good algorithm, or because you are uncertain of its settings, or because you use animated stimuli that elicit smooth pursuit (Chapter 5), then using raw data to generate the attention map is the only proper alternative. If the attention map is built from raw data samples, then each sample contributes with the same small height, simply because a data sample is always of the same duration.

Commercial implementations of attention maps typically use fixations as input when building attention maps. This way, the input is preprocessed, avoiding adding saccades and various noise to the visualization. Using fixations as input is beneficial also in terms of computational processing, since fixations are substantially less voluminous than raw data; about 250 times smaller when recorded at 1000 Hz. Consequently, it becomes quicker to generate and update an attention map that is built with fixations instead of raw data.

With fixations, there is a choice: either each fixation yields the same height in the map, or we scale the fixation with its duration. Using the manufacturers' terminology, this is often referred to as 'unscaled' or 'scaled' heat maps. In an attention map filled by fixation duration, each peak will represent *fixation time* on an area and therefore look more like an attention map generated from data samples than will an attention map filled by numbers of fixations. The peaks in the attention map then rather represent the *number of fixations* in an area. As dwell time is more related to the level of cognitive processing and number of fixations rather than to repeated interest, the two attention maps also represent different types of analysis. For instance, Figure 7.10 from Pomplun et al. (1996) uses attention maps filled with fixation duration to visualize differences in processing. In practice, filling attention maps with fixation duration does not generally differ much from filling with number of fixations. Only if fixation durations differ, as in Figure 7.13 where fixations are short on the text and long on the image, does this choice makes a difference.

There are situations when the choice between using raw data and fixations becomes particularly relevant. If you are using an eye-tracker with low sampling frequency and poor precision, individual data samples can significantly impact the appearance of the heat map, making it look very different from one generated from fixations. This case is nicely illustrated by Bojko (2009), who recommends users to always generate heat maps from fixations. If you on the other hand use data recorded at higher speed and good precision, heat maps look more or less the same regardless of how they were generated.

One exception is if the width of the basic construct is small; Figure 7.14 shows heat map visualizations generated from the same raw data samples using the unprocessed data directly (column 1) and filled with fixation durations (column 2). As illustrated in the figure, the magnitude of difference between the rows depends on the width of the basic construct (σ in the Gaussian function), with a very narrow width more clearly emphasizing the difference between maps.

In summary, to fully understand an attention map visualization, a certain minimum amount of knowledge about the nature of the eye-tracking data (accuracy, precision, and sampling frequency) and the particular implementation you use is necessary.

Normalization: harmonizing map scale

Depending on the later usage of an attention map *normalization* is sometimes necessary. Normalization changes the scale of the attention map, but retains its form. Two kinds of normalization have been used by researchers, with slightly different properties.

1. The simpler type of normalization is done by scaling the altitude of the attention map, so that the maximum peak has the altitude value 1. This allows two attention maps to be compared even if one has a higher maximum peak than the other, which is the case if it is built on a much larger participant population or on longer recordings with more fixations than the other (Wooding, 2002a).

2. The other type of normalization scales the altitude so that the volume underneath the attention map (the total volume of sand poured) is 1 unit. This allow for the same kinds of comparisons across maps as the simpler normalization, but additionally opens up for use of the normalized attention map as a *probability density function* (pdf).

The pdf representation of attention maps has a range of properties that allow us to use well-established mathematical tools from information theory, such as the Kullback-Leibler distance (KLD) on page 376. Normalization is particularly important when two attention maps are to be compared with each other, removing differences due to unequal viewing times.

7.5 Usage of attention maps other than for visualization

More than for any other purpose, attention maps are used to visualize data. Visualization is what commercial eye-tracking software offers for us to do with attention maps. But there are other possibilities: you can use the attention map to manipulate the stimulus in a variety of ways, and look at effects of manipulation. Under certain conditions, attention maps may also be used to define AOIs. Moreover, viewing behaviour can be *quantified* using attention maps; new measures based on attention maps are continuously finding their way into the analysis of eye-tracking data.

7.5.1 Using attention maps to define AOIs

Attention maps give "an opportunity for defining objectively the principal regions of interest of observers when they view an image", according to Wooding (2002a). There are two ways to describe the operation that does this. Imagine that the sand metaphor of the attention map that we formed above has solidified, and that it is flooded to a level so that only some of the peaks are above the waterline, as mountainous islands in an archipelago. In this metaphor, the coastline of each island defines the form of an area of interest. An equivalent metaphor with no water is to slice the attention map at the same altitude as reached by the flood, and let the slice areas comprise the AOIs. We then project the slice areas (or the equivalent coastlines) down to the stimulus image at the bottom of the attention map. Given an attention map with eye-tracking data, two things decide the size and form of the generated AOIs:

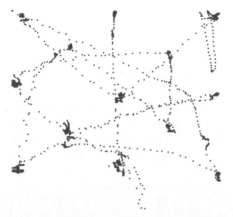

(a) Raw data samples (one participant looking at 13 dots)

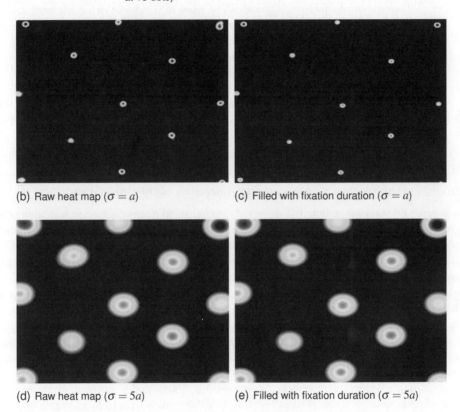

(b) Raw heat map ($\sigma = a$)

(c) Filled with fixation duration ($\sigma = a$)

(d) Raw heat map ($\sigma = 5a$)

(e) Filled with fixation duration ($\sigma = 5a$)

Fig. 7.14 Heat map visualization from raw data samples (column 1) and filled with fixation duration (column 2). Notice how raw data samples from very short periods of stillness outside of the central fixation point give rise to bleak spots (for instance inside the ring) in the raw heat map at setting $\sigma = a$, while at $\sigma = 5a$, these raw outlying data samples are hidden under the wide Gaussian distribution. Eye movements were tracked at 500 Hz with a tower-mounted eye-tracker.

- The level of the slice/flood. Wooding (2002a) does not suggest how this value should be selected, nor does anyone else. The AOIs become smaller (and typically fewer) as the level of water increases, i.e. as the height of the slice increases.

- What value of σ is selected in Equation (7.1); a large value of σ gives wider AOIs, and vice versa.

Notice also, that the attention map method to define AOIs suffers from a number of disadvantages.

1. The AOIs do not necessarily encapsulate objects in the stimulus image, and if they do, parts of the objects may be outside of the AOIs. Just like with the gridded AOIs on page 212, the AOIs generated from attention maps do not correspond to semantic entities in the stimulus image, and when they do, it is largely by coincidence. In contrast, most of the analyses that would make use of the AOIs assume that the AOIs are meaningful semantic units (p. 216).

2. Second, small local peaks in the attention map may be incorrectly disregarded (under the water/slice level), even though they could define regions that attract many viewers' gazes. One suggestion to overcome this problem is given by Nyström (2008), where 'slicing' is repeated after the highest peaks in the attention map are removed. Another approach to solving this problem is to multiply the attention map with a 'squashing' function which remaps the attention map, such that values above average grow, whereas other values are suppressed (Itti, 2004).

3. Third, using an attention map to define AOIs often means defining the AOIs in a post-hoc manner. Whether this is a problem or not depends on the precise research question, and what AOI measures are then employed using the generated AOIs (p. 216). Probably, measures utilizing transition and string representations of data make more sense to use with these AOIs than dwell time and the various fixation number measures.

7.5.2   Attention maps as image and data processing tools

Stimulus manipulation and the effects thereof

For a range of purposes and across different research fields, attention maps has been used to manipulate an image such that luminance, resolution, frequency, or contrast are modified according to the height dimension of the map (see e.g. Pomplun et al., 1996; Wooding, 2002b; Nyström, 2008). We have already seen some examples of this earlier in the chapter. For example, Figure 7.10 is one of the earliest uses of attention maps to manipulate images. After having produced the luminance maps in this figure, Pomplun et al. had another group of viewers looking at them, and found that the perceptual interpretation participants saw was very much influenced by image manipulation.

Attention map-based image manipulation has been widely used in both engineering and psychology; in engineering to speed up graphics rendering and improve image and video communications (see e.g. Parkhurst & Niebur, 2002; Kortum & Geisler, 1996; Z. Wang & Bovik, 2001; Z. Wang, Lu, & Bovik, 2003; Nyström, 2008), and in psychology to measure the perceptual span in scene perception (Loschky, McConkie, Yang, & Miller, 2001) and to investigate the possibility of manipulating viewers' gaze behaviour and perception (Dorr, Jarodzka, & Barth, 2010; Dorr, Vig, Gegenfurtner, Martinetz, & Barth, 2008), to name just a few examples.

Girod (1988) argued that if you know where a person looks, this information can be used to make image and video communications more efficient. Since people cannot see with high detail in their peripheral visual field, it would be enough to have high quality only where the person looks and reduce the quality elsewhere. Such quality reduction typically makes a video smaller in size after compression. More recently, this way of manipulating video quality has been dubbed 'foveation', and has been adapted by a number of people working with image and video compression (Juday & Fisher, 1989; Stelmach & Tam, 1994; Kortum &

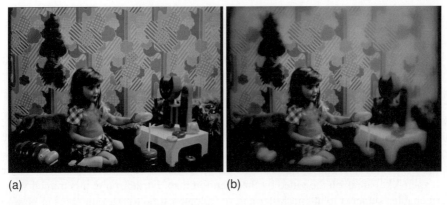

(a)   (b)

Fig. 7.15 An example of image foveation. Fixations have been collected from (a), and the attention map created from the fixations has been used to control the amount of foveation in (b). Notice the quality reduction in regions where no or few people fixated.

Geisler, 1996; Geisler & Perry, 1998; Duchowski, 2000; Z. Wang & Bovik, 2001; Z. Wang et al., 2003; Bergström, 2003; Nyström, 2008). Foveation-based techniques have been used both when a person's gaze position is measured online by an eye-tracker and offline when eye movements from one of several people are recorded beforehand. An example of the latter is given by Nyström (2008) where video regions are foveated in accordance with the attention map. Regions with small heights in the map were lowpass filtered more heavily than other regions, resulting in blurred quality with little contrast while regions corresponding to the peaks in the map were left in full quality. An example of such offline filtering is shown in Figure 7.15, where the left figure shows the original image and the right figure illustrates the image after foveation. In Nyström (2008), foveation showed a reduction in the number of bits needed to represent the video after compression, without a reduction in subjective quality. Watching the foveated videos, viewers tended to look at regions in high quality (where original viewers had looked) and avoided gazing at regions that has been heavily lowpass-filtered.

With the resolution (which typically reflects the quality) of an image being reduced in regions where people do not look, there is an obvious computational gain when generating foveated images instead of images with a high, uniform resolution (which is the typical case). Parkhurst and Niebur (2002) found this gain to reach 8.7 for a typical viewing set-up on a computer screen. This means that it requires 8.7 times more computational resources (or 8.7 times more time with the same resources at hand) to render an image with uniform resolution compared to a foveated image.

Besides the potential benefit of using attention maps to improve the efficiency in technical systems, there are several areas in psychology where such image manipulations have been shown to be useful. Loschky et al. (2001), for example, used gaze-contingent foveation to investigate how much you can reduce the peripheral quality of an image before it becomes visible to the observer, and also how such manipulations affect eye-movement parameters such as fixation duration. Moderate quality reductions did not affect either the impression of image quality or eye-movement behaviour. However, with an increasing degree of peripheral blur, quality judgements became lower, fixation duration increased, while saccade length decreased. For this set-up to work in real time, the image quality must be updated very quickly every time a viewer changes his position of gaze, otherwise quality impairments will be visible after a saccade. Loschky and Wolverton (2007) found that if the update is complete within 60 ms after the saccade has landed, viewers will not notice that change. These results tell us that caution should be taken if you plan to use foveated images in your experiment; depending on how the quality reductions are implemented and how quick your system is to update and display the foveated images, perception and eye movements can be affected in various ways.

Image manipulation based on attention maps has opened up some interesting possibilities to study the effects of gaze guidance, which refers to the hypothesis that manipulations can be used to control or guide a viewer's gaze towards certain parts of a display. There are several situations in which gaze guidance would be interesting to study. For example, eye movements from experts can be recorded on instruction videos in medicine, human factors, biological classification, and other fields where it is important to look at the correct position to make a correct diagnosis or classification based on visual observations. Novices studying foveated video examples based on an expert model's eye movements, are guided to the relevant (expert-like) areas on the video by the attention map. Furthermore, this trained viewing pattern enables students to attend faster and for a longer time to relevant areas in new—not foveated—videos and interpert these more correctly, compared to students learning from non-foveated videos (Dorr et al., 2010; Jarodzka, Balslev, et al., 2010; Jarodzka, Van Gog, Dorr, Scheiter, & Gerjets, forthcoming).

7.5.3 Using attention maps in measures

So far, attention maps predominantly become a tool for *visualizing* eye-tracking data. But attention maps are by no means limited to visualization, but can be used to *quantify* and *statistically test* the distribution of a group of fixations or data samples, or the position similarity between two different groups of fixations, even over time. A number of measures now exist that do this, either using just the set of points, Gaussians, or gridded AOIs, see Chapter 11.

7.6 Summary: attention map representations

Attention maps are used to describe the overall spatial distribution of eye-tracking data. They typically come in one of three representations:

- The **gridded AOI** with its grid size settings and its various fillings.
- The **Gaussian landscape** with its σ-setting.
- The normalized version of either of these, known as a **probability density function** or pdf.

Attention map visualizations, in particular heat maps, are today widely used to illustrate large amounts of eye-tracking data. With the current range of software tools, attention maps can be built in a variety of ways, each having its own concept of what an attention map is. They are so visually appealing that less careful viewers may easily misinterpret them, but these visualizations are nevertheless important complements to quantitative data. Settings for attention map visualizations always contain a width or σ but are otherwise diverse: before you make any decisions on the basis of a heat map, check carefully how it has been calculated and what settings were used. If you publish a heat map, always report the form and size of the basic contructs, whether height is scaled by fixation durations or any other measure, whether raw data or fixation position were used, and the precise mapping of colour to altitude. Otherwise your heat map may be a piece of art suited for gallery exhibitions but hardly a tool for the scientific study of human behaviour.

8   Scanpaths—Theoretical Principles and Practical Application

Previous chapters explained how to process raw data samples into fixations, saccades, and smooth pursuit (Chapter 5), how to divide stimulus space into areas of interests (AOIs) (Chapter 6) that give rise to events such as dwells and transitions, and also how to build representations of overall spatial distribution called attention maps and their visualizations such as heat maps (Chapter 7). In this chapter, we discuss the *scanpath*—a trace of a participant's eye-movements in space and time—and its events and representations.

Using and analysing scanpaths raises many questions, some very practical, and some deeply abstract. This chapter consists of the following sections, and we suggest selective reading:

- The first Section 8.1 (p. 253) presents a formal definition of scanpaths and relates it to visualizations and representations of scanpaths.
- Section 8.2 (p. 255) provides condensed hands-on advice for research with scanpaths.
- In Section 8.3 (p. 256), we present the most common usages of scanpaths.
- Common events that occur in scanpaths are defined in Section 8.4 (p. 262): The *backtrack*, the *regressions*, the *look-back*, the *look-ahead*, *local versus global* scans, and the *reading versus scanning* events.
- Section 8.5 (p. 268) describes by what means a scanpath may be represented: *strings*, Euclidean *vectors*, and sequences of *attention maps*.
- Scanpath representations are typically used for the purpose of comparing two or more scanpaths. The principles for scanpath comparison are outlined in Section 8.6 (p. 273).
- Section 8.7 (p. 278) discusses whether scanpaths can be related to specific cognitive processes. It addresses scanpath theory and the related role of memory and task to scanpath planning and inhibition of return. The section further discusses the average scanpath and the challenging issue of how to develop and evaluate better scanpath comparison methods. This section ends with open issues in scanpath comparison.
- Finally, Section 8.8 (p. 284) summarizes the chapter and the scanpath events and representations that we will use throughout the rest of the book.

8.1   What is a scanpath?

The term 'scanpath' originates from the work by Noton and Stark in the early 1970s (Noton & Stark, 1971a, 1971b). Other common terms for scanpaths are 'scan pattern', 'search pattern', 'scan sequence', 'gaze sequence', 'fixation track', 'inspection pattern', and 'eye-movement pattern'. About 70% of the journal papers and 84% of Google hits write scanpath as a single word ('scanpath'), and the rest use separate words ('scan path').

Noton and Stark's scanpath term refers to the fairly abstract concept of a fixed path that is characteristic to a specific participant and viewing pattern. In contrast, the term scanpath is today used to very concretely describe how the eye physically moves through space, typically but not exclusively for one participant. In agreement with the physical definition of other common terms in this book, we define a scanpath as the *route of oculomotor events through space within a certain timespan*. This assumes that the 'path' has a beginning and end, and therefore a length.

The most accurate estimate of a scanpath that an eye-tracker can provide is the spatial coordinates of a participant's gaze on a stimulus taken every $1/F_s$ second, where F_s is the sampling frequency of the eye-tracker. Space is usually confined to two dimensions x and y, and a scanpath of length L can then be described by a sequence of coordinates $S_i = (x_i, y_i), i = 1, 2, \ldots, L$. This is what we can see if we plot a raw data sample scanpath.

A *scanpath function* $f(\cdot)$ is given one or many scanpaths as input and computes a representation of those scanpaths. For example, one output from f would be a sequence of attention maps which can then be seen as a Gaussian-based scanpath function, which encodes the probability that a certain spatial position will be a part of the scanpath. Another output would be vectors representing the fixations and saccades of which a scanpath is comprised. Figure 8.1 shows four different scanpath representations of the same data.

The most common previous definitions of scanpaths have followed Noton and Stark (1971a) in saying that scanpaths consist of a sequence of *saccades*. *Fixation positions* are part of several scanpath definitions, but *fixation durations* are seldom utilized in any of the measures of scanpaths. *Smooth pursuit* is completely absent from most researchers' working definition of what a scanpath is, with rare exceptions, such as Boccignone, Caggiano, Marcelli, Napoletano, and Di Fiore (2005), who conduct an analysis of eye-tracking data on video stimuli.

The minimum requirement of a scanpath representation is that it is a sequence that *takes ordinal information into account*. This means that any representation of a specific scanpath must transform into a representation of *another* scanpath whenever the order between elements in the representational sequence is changed.

Static and dynamic visualizations

Recorded scanpaths are typically projected onto the stimulus or an empty space representing the stimulus. Visualizations of data that are not projected onto a 2- or 3D stimulus space, for instance a space–time diagram of (x, y)-coordinates, are not generally considered to be scanpath visualizations.

Most analysis softwares offer scanpath visualizations in a number of varieties, and the possibility to export or print them. Scanpath visualizations are either *static*, of which previous chapters have had many examples, or *dynamic*, which comes out well on computers but not on paper. Both these allow for direct inspection of the data from a single participant and a single trial. Most software packages support viewing four types of static visualizations: raw data sample scanpaths, which depict the entire set of raw (x, y) coordinates; fixation-based scanpaths, with fixations plotted either with or without circles of different size to indicate their duration, and with the option to print sequence numbers next to fixations.

In the static visualizations, the dynamic aspect of the scanpath is supported by connection lines and fixation numbering. Without these, the static scanpath visualization is reduced to a density plot: the same set of unconnected points that underly the attention maps of Chapter 7. The dynamic visualizations in the software additionally emphasize the sequential order of scanpaths in a variety of ways depending on the manufacturer. The basic dynamic scanpath is a single gaze cursor that is played back. This type of visualization is often used to replay participants' eye-movement data in order to elicit verbal data from them (pp. 99–108). Moreover, this type of visualization may also be depicted for many participants at a time. Scanpaths of multiple participants typically become very cluttered, except in dynamic gaze replay, whereby multiple gaze cursors are played back against a stimulus.

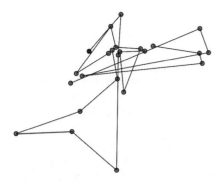

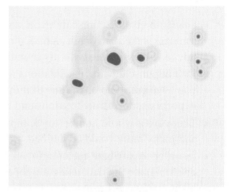

(a) Fixations as dots on positions and undirected connection lines for saccades.

(b) Attention map visualizations with just position information.

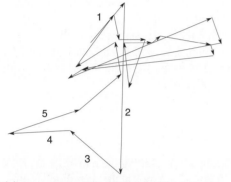

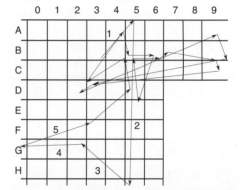

(c) A sequence of directed vectors for saccades, first five of which are numbered.

(d) Gridded AOIs over the vectors in (c), yielding the AOI dwell string representation B3 A5 I5 G2 G0 F3 D5 B4 D3 A4 . . . .

Fig. 8.1 Visualization of the four different scanpath representations of the same data.

Scanpath representations

The three scanpath representations that are more than sole visualizations are all designed to cope with what visualizations are poor at; namely providing a representation of data that can be used for computational analysis and statistics. The AOI strings—in particular the dwell string—are the most common non-visualizing scanpath representation, but sequences of Euclidean vectors and attention maps are also beginning to be used.

Besides visualization, the commercial analysis software packages of 2010 are only just beginning to add functionality for scanpath analysis. If you want to use the existing scanpath measures, you therefore need to export data such as raw data samples, fixations, saccades, and/or AOIs, and then implement the measures yourself. The alternative is to use non-commercial applications (e.g. West, Haake, Rozanski, & Karn, 2006; C. H. Tsai, 2010; Foulsham, 2010; Cristino, Mathôt, Theeuwes, & Gilchrist, 2010).

8.2   Hands-on advice for using scanpaths

Scanpaths are used so variably that only a few general pieces of advice can be offered. If you plan to use scanpaths as visualizations, or calculate statistics from scanpath representations you should consider the following issues:

- Scanpath visualizations are excellent for first inspections of data, answering questions such as: is the data quality good, did the fixation detection algorithm do a good job, is this recording in line with my hypothesis?
- Do not put scanpath visualizations in your papers just as decoration. Ask yourself why you have put it there, and see to it that the scanpath visualization aligns well with your hypothesis, operationalizations and results.
- There are a whole number of scanpath events ready to be used in statistical analyses, and many more could be defined.
- In order to attribute meaningful interpretations to individual scanpaths, you need to disambiguate the data using a tight experimental design, verbal data, or other complementary data recordings.
- All scanpath representations used in measures reduce the level of detail in the scanpaths, for example in terms of spatial and temporal accuracy. Other properties such as fixation duration are sometimes ignored completely. Be sure to use a scanpath representation that retains the properties that you want to measure.
- If you are using measures that utilize scanpath representations, be aware that raw data quality, event detection algorithms and their settings, as well as all issues around AOI identification may introduce noise in the values you get from the measure. Scanpath events and representations are at the top of the hierarchy.

8.3   Usages of scanpath visualization

There is little doubt that the most common use of scanpaths is plotting them in order to check the quality of data immediately after a recording. "Let's have a look at the recording" is often synonymous with "Let's look at the scanpath", even though other data quality visualizations exist. We can recapitulate several down-to-earth usages of scanpath *visualizations* as:

Data quality checks   In Chapters 4 and 5, we made ample use of scanpath visualizations for this purpose. It shows you if there are offsets or poor precision in the data, and whether fixation and saccade detection worked properly.

Preliminary impression of the data   Often a scanpath is visualized to receive a quick first impression of where the participants looked, and in which order. During piloting, such inspection can be used to check whether the task elicits the desired eye-movement behaviour, and to give a first impression of whether your hypothesis will be supported.

Offset compensation   If your data has an offset, some software allows you to perform manual offset compensation and drift correction watching scanpath visualizations, as described on page 224.

Manual data analysis   Scanpath analysis by visual inspection is hopefully decreasing as methods and software become more capable, but has been the main form of analysis in previous years (e.g. Josephson & Holmes, 2002; Holsanova, 2001; Buswell, 1935).

Illustrating scanpaths in publications   There are a variety of reasons why scanpaths are shown, from showing off some good data on the background of a stimulus, to using the scanpath visualization to clearly demonstrate the experiment and/or the analysis.

Cued retrospective thinking aloud   Participant's thoughts may be difficult to access through eye-movement data and tight experimental designs alone. It has become increasingly common to show the scanpath to a participant just after his data has been recorded, and ask him to retell what he was thinking of during the initial inspection of the stimulus. This method is described in-depth on pages 99–108.

In the next sections, we present and discuss three of the most common usages of scanpath visualizations: checking the data quality, analysing the data manually, and exhibiting scanpath visualizations in publications.

8.3.1 Data quality checks

Checking data quality is undoubtedly the most common, yet informal and quite undocumented use of scanpath visualizations. We have already looked extensively at data quality issues in Chapters 2 and 4, and only reiterate the major points here. Visual inspection of eye-movement data for quality checking should not be a problematic issue, unless your software does not allow you to visualize scanpaths with raw data samples. Data quality checks can tell us a lot about the data:

- Is the data accurate or is there an *offset* in any part of the stimulus image? Offsets can often be seen as mismatches between actual data and semantic entities in the stimulus picture that were likely fixation targets given the task. Accuracy tests are easier to do with text than with general images. The upper scanpath in Figure 8.2(a) provides an example.
- Are there many *optic artefacts* in the data, as in Figure 8.2(a)?
- Are many *data samples lost*? This could indicate that the eye image is poor and the pupil and corneal reflection therefore cannot be properly detected. It could also occur if the participant is closing his eyes or is turning his head away from the eye-tracker.
- Is the *precision* low (noise levels high) in the recording, as seen in the spread of raw samples contained within fixations? For example the fixations of six participants in Figure 8.2(b).
- Is the event calculation algorithm doing a proper job? Plot the raw sample scanpath next to the fixation-based scanpath, and compare. Figures 8.2(c) and 8.2(d) from Chapter 5 provide an example where fixations were lost during fixation and saccade calculation.

8.3.2 Data analysis by visual inspection

There are many reasons why researchers would want to use scanpath visualizations for their data analysis.

First of all, a manual, participant-by-participant analysis may be what is needed for *pedagogical reasons* in the publication, for instance in Buswell (1935), who starts his book with a long commentary to the scanpath visualization from the data of the participant called "Miss W.", focusing on the order and position of individual fixations, and on what has not been fixated. This manual analysis and the description of the scanpath serve a particular pedagogic purpose that quantitative analyses could not easily provide.

In other cases the *software is inadequate*. For instance, Buswell (1935) reports statistics using what we today call gridded AOIs, constructed by manual analysis from scanpath visualizations. It took many decades until software supported such AOI analyses.

Even fairly recently, researchers have had to retreat to manual analysis because *statistical tools are inadequate*. For instance, Josephson and Holmes (2002) give a thorough description of the string-edit method (p. 348), and additional methods that can be used to further a string-edit analysis. They conclude, however, that statistical results based on string-edit calculation are currently not possible, and end up eyeballing their data. Similarly, Tzanidou, Minocha, and Petre (2005) discuss the problem of identifying metrics that compare scanpaths across many participants and many stimuli, concluding that there is no such measure, and decid-

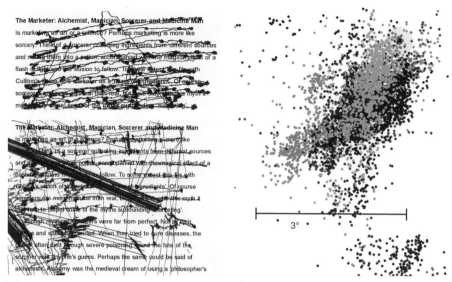

(a) Above a scanpath with corner offset due to problems during calibration; and below extreme optic artefacts due to mascara.

(b) Noisy recording showing raw samples (scanpath without connection lines) from six participants fixating a corner point on the stimulus monitor. Notice that the noise is large and oblique.

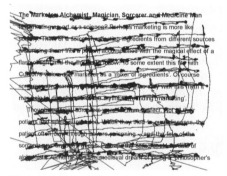

(c) Raw data samples. Fixations are seen as black blobs.

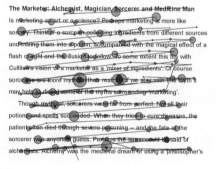

(d) After fixation and saccade analysis, some fixations have disappeared.

Fig. 8.2 Data quality checks using scanpaths.

ing to analyse their own scanpath data over web pages using visual inspection and manual categorization.

Arguing that *the types of analysis provided by the academic fields of eye tracking are not useful* for usability research, Ehmke and Wilson (2007) set out to find types of scanpaths that coincide with a specific cognitive process, but since so little is known about scanpaths and possibly meaningful subscans, manual analysis of scanpaths against retrospective interviews—that is verbal data—appears to be the only way forward.

As Holsanova (2001, 2006, 2008) studied the eye-movements of participants freely describing pictures, she examined patterns in scanpaths and speech that jointly indicated specific cognitive processes, using a manual transcription method to finds alignment between sub-scans and spoken items. More precisely, Holsanova (2001) built what are known as *multimodal score-sheets*, in which several tiers of temporal data share one common timeline. As shown in Figure 8.3, one tier was the sequence of dwells in AOIs, while another tier listed the

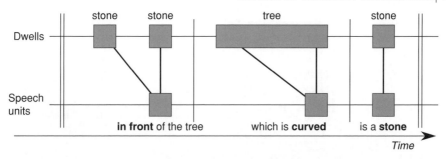

Fig. 8.3 Multimodal score-sheet resulting from manual co-analysis of synchronized speech and eye–movement data. The final dwell on the 'stone' AOI is a lookback, coinciding with the participant naming the stone, and thus most likely due to the planning and development of speech. Adapted from Holsanova (2001).

development of speech units over time. As this was a picture description task, gaze travelled across the same AOIs that speech referred to, and so the multimodal score-sheet indicated patterns of temporal alignment of speech to gaze.

Using an adapted variety of the method in Holsanova (2001), Johansson et al. (2006) compared scanpaths during scene perception with scanpaths during subsequent imagery, and needed to take into account shrinking and repositioning of scanpaths, as well as synchronization to speech. Again, this could only be done manually.

Land, Mennie, and Rusted (1999) recorded scene videos with overlaid gaze cursors of participants making tea. Their analysis of task behaviour led to a multimodal score-sheet similar to Figure 8.3, but instead with tiers representing actions rather that speech. This video-based analysis could only be made manually.

How should a manual analysis be carried out? In all the above cases, manual scanpath analysis aims at finding the sequence of fixations or dwells in AOIs, that is a list of the objects looked at, with information about when and for how long gaze stayed there. Today many softwares can output this list, but not when data consist of gaze-overlaid scene videos, and not always with dynamic stimuli or in mental imagery studies where AOIs are difficult to define. Since in these cases the scanpath needs to be played back, the coding methods for gaze-overlaid scene videos in Chapter 6 (p. 227) can be utilized, with small adaptions to take advantage of the more advanced playback control features in scanpath visualization software.

8.3.3   Exhibiting scanpaths in publications

All quantitative results in Buswell (1935) and Yarbus (1967) were based on manual analysis from scanpath visualizations. Both publications make extensive use of scanpath illustrations, both for illustration of data and presentation of actual results.

Many authors still publish selected scanpath visualizations in their papers and books, for a variety of reasons. First, some publications simply address an audience new to eye-movement data and the scanpath is needed to explain what eye-movement data are. Second, when the presented analysis includes an important *qualitative description* of the scanpath (Buswell, 1935; Holsanova, 2008), a scanpath visualization is obviously needed. *Difficulties in operationalizing the concept* under study in terms of computational measures could be another major reason why we find scanpath visualizations in research publications. Methodology papers and papers that discuss measures, such as Goldberg and Kotval (1999), Rötting (2001), and Underwood, Humphrey, and Foulsham (2008a) present many scanpath visualizations to illustrate concepts and operationalizations, and the same is true in this book.

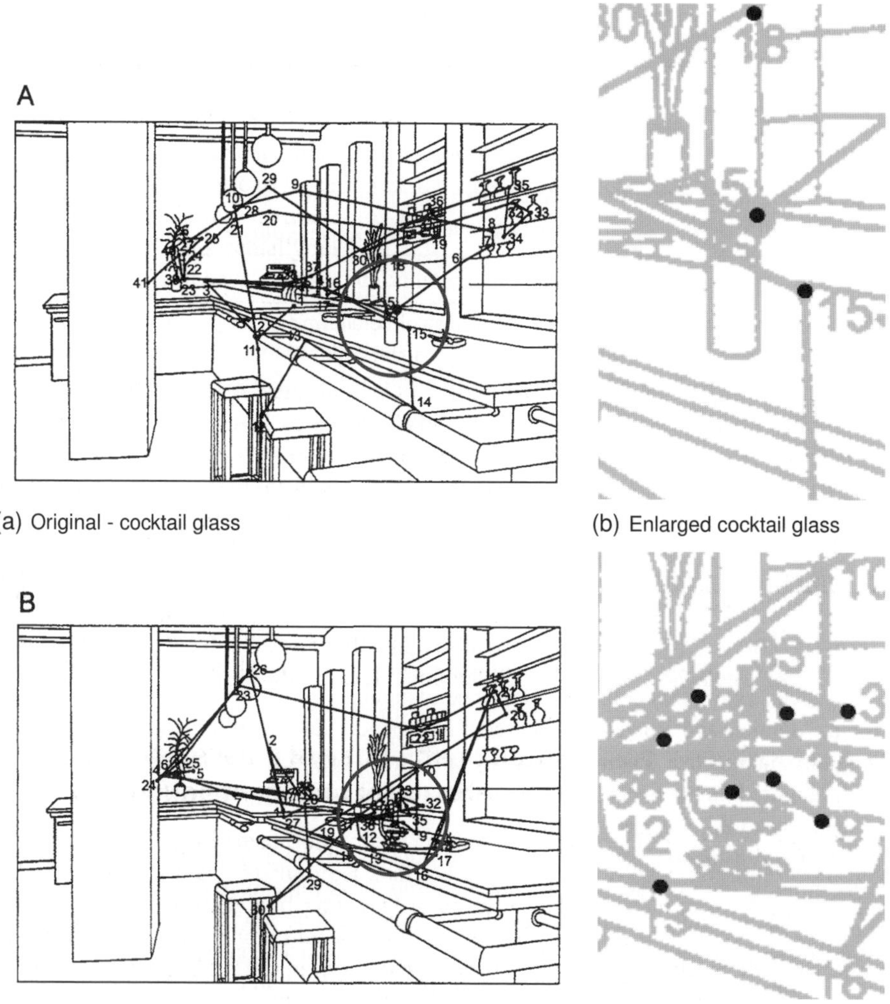

A

(a) Original - cocktail glass

(b) Enlarged cocktail glass

B

(c) Original - microscope

(d) Enlarged microscope

Fig. 8.4 This "typical viewing pattern" in fact proves to be an outlier. The circle in (a) and (c) denotes the cocktail glass and microscope respectively, which are then blown up with dimmed background in (b) and (d) to indicate fixation clustering (note, this is a visualization only, and fixation dots in (b) and (d) may not reflect the exact number of fixations in the recorded data). Reprinted from *Journal of Experimental Psychology: Human Perception and Performance, 25*(1), John M. Henderson, Phillip A. Weeks, and Andrew Hollingworth, The Effects of Semantic Consistency on Eye Movements During Complex Scene Viewing, pp. 210-228, Copyright (1999), with permission from Elsevier.

In other cases, when the audience of the paper knows about eye tracking, when the operationalizations are clear and quantitative results do not rely on visualizations, why then use scanpaths for illustrations?

Our first example is taken from J. M. Henderson, Weeks, and Hollingworth (1999). It has been selected because it is a well-known paper with many citations, but also because the scanpath visualization the authors choose to include in the paper is in line with their hypotheses, but deviates from the statistical results. More precisely, they present two "typical viewing patterns" (stated in the last paragraph of page 213 in their article) over almost identical bar room scenes, but where a cocktail in one is replaced by a microscope in the other.

Their Figure 2, here reproduced as Figure 8.4 depicts this. The concept under investigation is 'semantic consistency', and it is a natural hypothesis that participants will look earlier, more often and longer at the inconsistent microscope compared to the consistent cocktail. Indeed, this is also what the included scanpath visualization shows. When counting the fixations in the scanpaths of their Figure 2, we find 7 or 8 fixations near the microscope, but only one or two next to the cocktail glass. However, a scanpath visualization is not a result. For one thing, a scanpath is descriptive data from one single participant, usually in one single trial. Therefore, J. M. Henderson et al. (1999) make a statistical analysis of the data, over several participants, using a number of AOI measures, including number of fixations on the target, number of entries, first-pass and second-pass dwell time, and several others.

After we have seen the impressive example in the scanpath visualization of the authors' Figure 2, the reported overall difference in number of fixations is somewhat disappointing: 9.7 versus 10.7, which was found to be a non-significant difference. The large difference in the scanpath visualization from this particular participant is not even close to the reported nonsignificant 9.7 versus 10.7 averages. In fact, this "typical viewing pattern" is an outlier.

Maybe scanpath visualizations are often superfluous additions to the results presented in current-day journal papers. They may distract some readers to look for confirmation of the hypothesis, and even to start counting fixations in the single scanpaths visualization, rather than to look at the overall data analysis and the quantitative results. The authors appear to add these scanpaths with unclear but probably quite different intent, for instance proof that data were actually recorded and not just made up, or that data quality—as judged from the included scanpath—was good, or perhaps just as decoration or in tribute to Buswell (1935) and Yarbus (1967).

In our second example, however, we should trust the published scanpath illustration rather than the given quantitative data. In schizophrenia research, there has been much discussion about 'restricted' scanpaths to facial stimuli, which have consistently been reported in studies of schizophrenia patients (for instance, M. J. Green, Waldron, Simpson, & Coltheart, 2008; M. J. Green, 2006; Benson, Leonards, Lothian, St Clair, & Merlo, 2007; Loughland, Williams, & Gordon, 2002, just to mention a few). Similarly, participants with social phobia tend to exhibit 'hyperscanning' when watching faces, (Horley, Williams, Gonsalvez, & Gordon, 2004). 'Restricted' and 'hyperscanning' are definitely characteristics relating to scanpaths. Figure 8.5 shows examples with such (fabricated) data.

Operationalizing 'semantic (in)consistency' with reference to 'looking earlier, more, and longer', as did J. M. Henderson et al. (1999) in our first example, is relatively uncomplicated. There is a direct connection between the concepts used in their hypothesis, and conclusion, and the measures used. There is one AOI only, and the measures in use are simple and well-known, and nothing is really said about the general shape of the scanpaths that motives a scanpath visualization in the paper. In contrast, operationalizing 'restricted scanpaths' puts much larger demands on data representations and measures, and eye-tracking-based papers in schizophrenia and social phobia research are consequently richly decorated with scanpath visualizations illustrating restrictedness and hyperscanning.

M. J. Green et al. (2008) and other schizophrenia researchers attempt to construct quantitative tests that approximate a 'scanpath restrictedness' measure, using a combination of two measures:

1. *Scanpath length* (p. 319) should be shorter for more restricted scanpaths in almost all cases. There are unfortunate exceptions however. Many short fixations at the circumference around the nose could add up to quite a long scanpath, while a small number of long fixations at the eyes and mouth could give a shorter scanpath length.

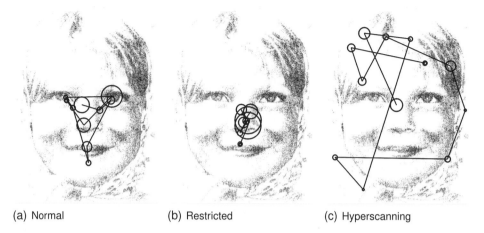

(a) Normal   (b) Restricted   (c) Hyperscanning

Fig. 8.5 Examples of normal, restricted and hyperscanning scanpaths on the well known face image used by Yarbus (1967), here faded to increase scanpath visibility. The scanpaths are fabricated for the purpose of illustration.

2. Therefore, the authors additionally compared *number of fixations* (p. 412). In particular, if the number of fixations were equal and the scanpath lengths still differ, the probability increases that the shorter scanpath would indeed be restricted (in the sense of the presented scanpath visualizations).

Operationalizing the 'restrictedness' concept using the combination of scanpath length and number of fixations is not intuitive, but requires careful mathematical thinking of why this operationalization could work. The scanpath visualizations are included to explain what 'restrictedness' really is, and in effect define the concept ostensively, rather than through the measures.

Generally, if it is difficult to make the operationalization of the study intuitive with the use of scanpaths and their visualization, then it is advisable to shop around for other measures in collections such as Part III of this book. For instance, the variability measure known as convex hull (p. 364), the Kullback–Leibler similarity measure (p. 376) and related measures on pages 359–376, could have provided the authors with a single measure that would be closely aligned with the restrictedness concept.

8.4   Scanpath events

Just as fixations and saccades are eye-movement events that can be detected from raw data samples, *scanpath events* are temporally restricted patterns that occur in eye-movement sequences. Typically, scanpath events comprise subscans of length two or more in a sequence of fixations, saccades, or other events (such as smooth pursuit). A scanpath event can be associated with any type of form or pattern, and therefore an almost unlimited number of scanpath events may exist. Reading researchers, and some usability researchers have defined the few scanpath events that have been used in published research, and these are the ones discussed here.

8.4.1   The backtrack

A *backtrack* is the specific relationship between two subsequent saccades where the second goes in the opposite direction of the first.

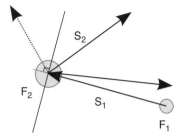

(a) The backtracking saccade, for instance S_2, must deviate by more than 90° from the previous saccade S_1.

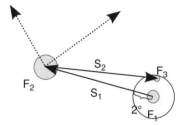

(b) The last fixation F_3 must be within 2° of the first fixation F_1.

Fig. 8.6 Two definitions of backtracking. Dashed lines indicate saccades that are *not* counted as backtracks. In (a) the definition by Goldberg and Kotval (1999), and in (b), the one by Renshaw et al. (2004).

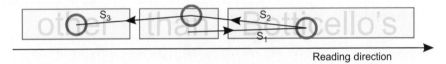

Reading direction

Fig. 8.7 Backtracking versus regressions: Saccade S_2 is a regression, because it moves in the opposite direction to the text, and also a backtrack because it moves in the opposite direction to the previous saccade. Saccade S_3 is only a regression, but not a backtrack in the sense of Figure 8.6. If a fourth saccade S_4 continued backwards, S_2–S_4 would count as backtracks according to Murray and Kennedy (1988).

There are two operationalizations of backtracking saccades outside of reading research. The original definition by Goldberg and Kotval (1999) counted all saccades deviating more than 90° from the previous, making many saccades backtracks. Renshaw, Finlay, Tyfa, and Ward (2004) gives a more restrictive definition of backtracking, which requires the fixation ending the backtracking saccade to be within a minimal distance (set to 2°) for the event to count as a backtrack. Figure 8.6 illustrates the two operationalizations. When comparing their own definition to that of Goldberg and Kotval, Renshaw et al. found, in data collected from a usability evaluation task, that their more restrictive measure was more sensitive, arguing that it is a better measure for finding differences in usability studies.

In reading research, backtracks have been defined as "sequences of three or more left-going saccades, each of which is no greater than 13 character spaces in extent. Typically, these comprise a series of short saccades directed to a sequence of words, which are, as a result, inspected in reverse order." (Murray & Kennedy, 1988). It is interesting to note that Tatler and Vincent (2008) found that reversal of direction in a scanpath is preceded by a longer than average fixation.

8.4.2 The regression family of events

The closely related term *regression* refers to events that are similar to backtracks but not the same. In order to be a regression, the saccade needs to move in the opposite direction to the text, but not necessarily the opposite direction to the previous saccade. Figure 8.7 illustrates the difference.

Regression events exist in different sizes: an *in-word regression* is a small movement

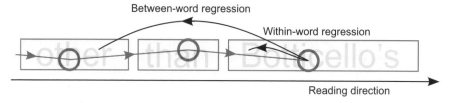

Between-word regression

Within-word regression

Reading direction

Fig. 8.8 A short in-word regression that does not leave the word just looked at, and a long between-word regression.

broom many times over and provides the replicants with arms and hands to carry the buckets Having given the command to the brooms to fill the well he promptly falls asleep only to be woken by the flow of

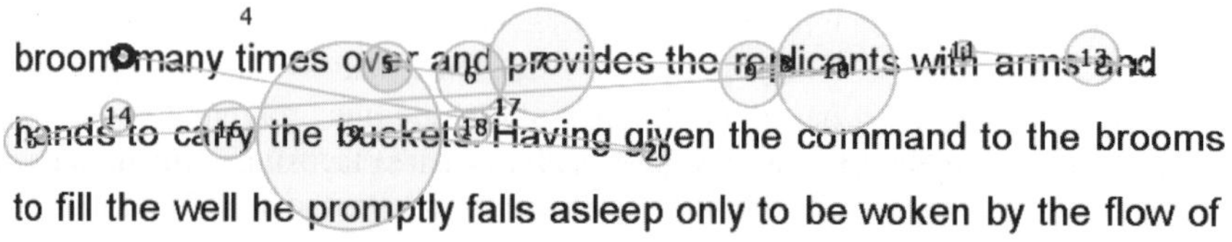

(a) Fixation number 20 at 'given' is the foremost fixation in the text. Then the regression starts with a saccade back to 'broom many' at the beginning of the previous line.

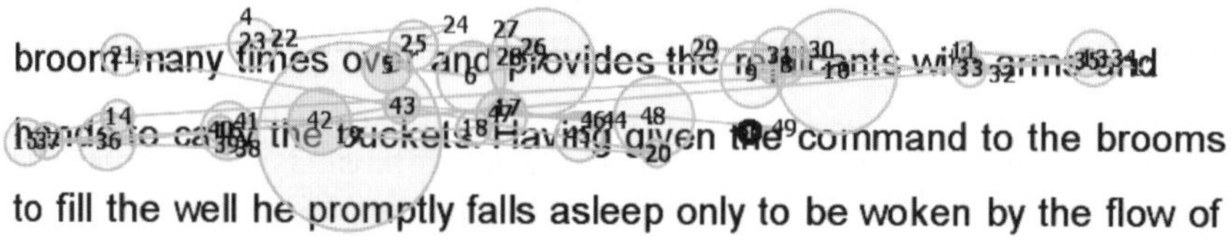

broom many times over and provides the replicants with arms and hands to carry the buckets Having given the command to the brooms to fill the well he promptly falls asleep only to be woken by the flow of

(b) The regression scanpath continues as the participant re-reads one and a half lines, until fixation number 49 at 'the', just before 'command', passes fixation number 20.

Fig. 8.9 A regression scanpath is a reading event, defined as going back in the text (a) and re-reading a passage. The regression scanpath ends when the point of departure from forward reading is passed and the participant resumes reading left-to-right (b).

backwards within a single word, a *between-word regression* moves further back in the sentence, to a previously fixated word (Figure 8.8).

The regression scanpath is a scanpath event in reading research. Figure 8.9 shows a regression scanpath starting after fixation number 20. Not until fixation number 48 is gaze back at the same word, so this regression scanpath has a length of 28 fixations.

Hyönä, Lorch Jr, and Kaakinen (2002); Hyönä et al. (2003) furthermore differentiate between *re-inspections* (when re-reading parts of the currently fixated sentence) and *look-backs* (when re-reading parts of another previously read sentence). Each of these are events from reading data.

8.4.3 The look-back and inhibition of return

Both backtracking and regressions differ from *look-backs*. Look-backs are operationalized as saccades to AOIs already looked at; they are also known as 'returns' and 'refixations'. The term look-back more pertains to spatially extended viewing behaviour, outside the field of reading research, for example searching for a target in a visual array or a link on a web page.

Look-backs are closely related to the concept of *inhibition of return* (Posner, Rafal, Choate, & Vaughan, 1985), which is the observation that attention is unlikely to be re-directed to previously inspected areas within a transient temporal window—in short, we do not look back to places we have just looked. Although considered a well-established phenomenon,

T. J. Smith and Henderson (2009) found only little support for a general inhibition of return mechanism in scanpaths during scene viewing. They provide empirical evidence that saccades frequently go back to previous fixation locations. It therefore seems that inhibition of return is not sustained enough to account for extended viewing scanpaths. This is not to undermine the importance and validity of inhibition of return however. There is a large corpus of literature examining the phenomenon. Its effects are more subtle and are likely masked when viewing visually complex stimuli like scenes.

"Returning to a previously fixated item constitutes a failure of memory", Gilchrist and Harvey (2000) write, but working memory has a limited temporal capacity, and it should matter how long ago the AOI was previously looked at for fixations there to count as look-backs. If the AOI content is no longer in working memory, is a look-back then different from looking at an object that has not yet been fixated? With this in mind, Mennie, Hayhoe, and Sullivan (2007) limited the operational definition of look-backs to within a 10 s window (after a reach and grasp sequence had been completed). Gilchrist and Harvey (2000) instead measured the number of "between-refixation intervals"—the periods between visits of the same AOI—at different durations in a visual search task, finding them to be below 8 seconds for one participant, and below 3 seconds for the two others.

8.4.4 The look-ahead

Look-aheads are saccades forward towards, and resulting fixations upon, objects that will soon be used, picked up, or in other ways be part of future planned actions.

Mennie et al. (2007) define look-ahead fixations according to the following spatial and temporal properties. When a fixation lands upon an AOI corresponding to a container within the "10 second period before the initiation of a reach from the workspace to that container" it counts as a look-ahead fixation. They emphasize that guiding fixations coinciding with the reach are excluded from the look-ahead category.

Although not providing a precise definition of look-aheads, Pelz, Canosa, Babcock, and Barber (2001) propose that "look-ahead fixations represent a strategic deployment of attentional and visual resources to optimize information gathering during natural tasks". In this sense, look-aheads are highly task dependent. Pelz et al. (2001) reported that, in a hand washing task, 3% of all the fixations were look-aheads compared to only 1% in a less complex control task.

8.4.5 The local and global subscans

The idea of local scanpaths is that spatially confined saccades with a small amplitude—Zangemeister, Sherman, and Stark (1995) suggest the thresholds $1.6°, 4.6°, 7.9°$, or $11°$—belong to a local scan of the particular details in a small patch of the stimulus. Larger saccades are assumed to belong to global overview scanning. Viewers tend to alternate between global and local scans when inspecting visual scenes, and tend to start with a global overview scan directly after onset of the scene.

Overview scans appear to be associated not only with longer saccadic amplitudes but also with shorter fixation durations (Unema, Pannasch, Joos, & Velichkovsky, 2005). These authors, amongst others, propose that global and local scanpaths are indications of two different types of cognitive processing: *ambient* and *focal*, respectively. The distinction is based on the well-known observation that fixation durations gradually increase from the time of stimulus onset, while saccadic amplitudes decrease. Participants initially exhibit scanning of the salient features of the image—long saccades, short fixations (ambient processing)—and later inspect the local areas in more detail—using short saccades and long fixations (focal

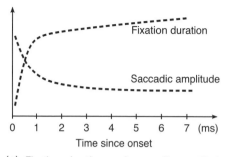 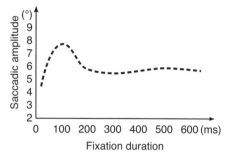

(a) Fixation duration and saccadic amplitude over bins of time

(b) Fixation duration against saccadic amplitude

Fig. 8.10 Short fixation durations combined with long saccades are characteristic of ambient processing, according to Unema et al. (2005), while longer fixation durations and shorter saccades are indicative of focal processing. These principal drawings are adapted from data presented by Unema et al. (2005), and Tatler and Vincent (2008).

processing).

The local versus global distinction indicates that clustering, for instance on saccadic amplitude, may separate data into events belonging to two qualitatively different categories. The need for a threshold is its major drawback.

On a more theoretical level, Groner, Walder, and Groner (1984) argue that local scans are not necessarily comprised of short saccades, and global scans long saccades. Rather, local scanpaths are seen to be driven by cognitive processing real-time, whereas global scanpaths are driven by an *overall* search strategy, or purpose. The former is bottom-up mediation of scanpaths, while the latter reflects top-down control.

8.4.6 Ambient versus focal fixations

Ambient and focal are two different cognitive states that a fixation with its preceding saccades is believed to correspond to. The distinction is operationalized as illustrated in Figure 8.10: a fixation with duration below a threshold d following a saccade with amplitude above threshold a is ambient (overview scanning), while the fixation is focal (focused inspection) when the fixation duration is above d and the preceding saccadic amplitude is below a. The thresholds do not have clearcut settings, but Velichkovsky, Rothert, Kopf, Dornhöfer, and Joos (2002) argue that d should be in the vicinity of 250 ms, and a around 4°. In principle, an event detection algorithm could categorize fixations into ambient and focal.

Alternative operationalizations exist. The *saccade/fixation ratio* from Goldberg and Kotval (1999) is argued to compare search time (saccades) to processing time (fixations). This variety uses saccade duration rather than amplitude, which is of little importance, as both correlate strongly. The global to local (g/l) ratio measure on page 338 quantifies the overall amount of global scanning versus detailed inspection, but does not classify the fixations.

The interpretation stems from Buswell (1935), who noted that the earliest fixations in a picture are shorter (around 210 ms) than later (around 360 ms). Also, saccadic amplitudes are longer in the initial scan and decrease over time (Figure 8.10). Several studies have repeated both these findings, and interpreted them as indicative of an early orienting period, followed by a more scrutinous inspection of informative details.

Unema et al. (2005) argue that a model for saccade generation with two visual processing systems, ambient and focal processing, can be supported with data on this relation. Ambient processing is characterized by long saccades and short fixation duration, corresponding to the peak in 8.10(b). Ambient processing is thought to be a process that is bottom-up driven and which creates an overview for later focal processing. Their speculation is that ambient processing is linked to what is known as the where/how system of the dorsal stream. Focal processing, which takes place at the flatland in Figure 8.10(b), conversely reflects top-down-driven scrutinous inspection of details which may be associated with the corresponding 'what' system.

When participants searched for possibly camouflaged military vehicles in photos, their mean saccade amplitude decreased and mean fixation duration increased gradually as a function of the ordinal saccade and fixation number (Over, Hooge, Vlaskamp, & Erkelens, 2007), independent of whether they knew that the target was the only unknown part of the scene or not. Over et al. interpret the result as showing that the coarse-to-fine search strategy is used even when it is not optimal.

8.4.7 The sweep

Aaltonen, Hyrskykari, and Räihä (1998) define a 'sweep' as *a sequence of saccades that move in the same direction*, and compare downward and upward scanpaths (sweeps) of varying sizes. Aaltonen et al. do not present a computational method for detecting sweeps, but various computational operationalizations are possible (e.g. detecting sweeps has similarities with detecting reading; see the next section).

8.4.8 The reading and scanning events

Reading and scanning events can be loosely defined as scanpath patterns that correlate with the cognitive processes of reading and scanning (see Rayner & Fischer, 1996 for a distinction between reading and scanning). In practice, such patterns are detected by algorithms that follow a set of predefined criteria, much like those detecting fixations and saccades. As with the detection of other scanpath events, reading detectors identify physical properties of scanpaths, and do not assess cognitive processing in the participant; it is indeed possible to move the eye in a reading-like pattern, even though the mind is occupied with something else.

The simplest reading detectors use criteria for saccadic amplitude, which is quite short during focused reading, whilst when scanning across pages saccades are longer. More advanced versions of reading filters add requirements on saccades such that they must be horizontal in direction (within certain bounds), or fixation durations such that different timings correspond to reading rather than scanning.

Figure 8.11 shows the principle for a simple reading detector. It assumes that the current fixation is located at position ($curr_h, curr_v$), and imposes an area in which the next fixation must land for it to be part of a reading event. The area, indicated by a rectangle, spans about two words ahead horizontally, and a word back (in case of in-word regressions); there is also some margin for upwards and downwards movements along the line. A second return sweep detector finds long backward movements corresponding to line length; this also detects slightly downward movements, again with a delimiting area around the expected landing position at the start of the next line. Reading is assumed to have been detected if at least three fixations (two intermediate saccades) fulfill the detection conditions. The reading detector developed by Holmqvist et al. (2003) compared the amount of reading in paper newspapers compared to internet newspapers. It was found, in contradiction to popular expectation, that traditional newspapers give rise to more reading and less scanning, with the opposite being true of online news.

Several other detection algorithms have been published:

1. Attempting detection of online reading, Campbell and Maglio (2001) use three criteria

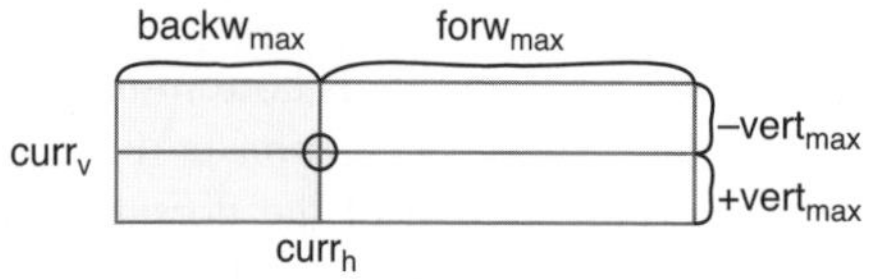

(a) Simple forward reading saccade detector with margin for in-word regression

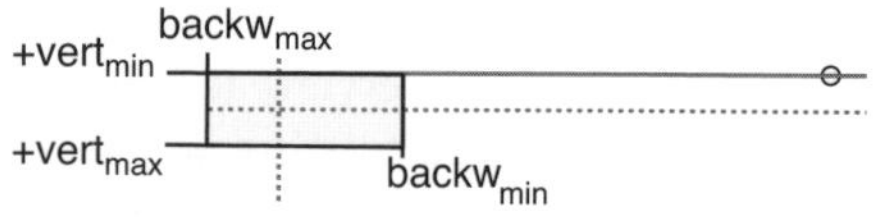

(b) Return sweep detection.

Fig. 8.11 Spatial requirements for the simple algorithmic reading detector used by Holmqvist et al. (2003). Successive saccades should move within or to restricted boxes to count as reading.

on saccades: amplitude (long versus short), direction (right, left, up, and down), and axis (x versus y). Using these criteria, each recorded saccade is given a total score that, when summed over all combinations of criteria, can then be compared to a threshold for reading. The authors report high classification accuracy and a detection latency of 1000 ms.

2. Simola, Salojärvi, and Kojo (2008) trained a 9-state discriminative hidden Markov model to differentiate between eye-movement data from three different reading tasks: (i) simple word search, (ii) finding a sentence that answers a question, and (iii) choosing the subjectively most interesting title from a list of ten titles. Their model has a 60% accuracy in determining the correct type of task.

3. Kollmorgen and Holmqvist (2009) used Markov models to train a version of the reading filter from Holmqvist et al. (2003) to detect reading in eye-movement data recorded from participants writing on computers (data shown on p. 291). This was also used to analyse the interplay between reading and writing activity in a number of other studies (see Johansson, Johansson, Wengelin, & Holmqvist, 2008; Wengelin et al., 2009; Johansson, Johansson, Wengelin, & Holmqvist, 2010). The 6-state hidden Markov model has a precision/recall of 0.88/0.87 on validation data.

4. Based on the work by Campbell and Maglio (2001), Buscher and Dengel (2009) implement a reading and skimming detector. Again, saccades are scored based on saccadic amplitudes such that a sequence of long saccades is likely to reflect skimming over the text.

8.5 Scanpath representations

Even a scanpath built from raw data samples contains so much information that calculations quickly become computationally complex. Therefore, several *representations* of scanpaths have been developed that take only selected aspects of the oculomotor behaviour included within scanpaths into account. In the following sections, we will describe how sequences of *symbols* (typically letters representing *AOIs*), *Euclidean vectors*, and *attention maps* are used to represent scanpaths.

Besides containing voluminous amounts of data, scanpaths generated from data samples may contain information that is largely irrelevant to the experimental questions at hand. The goal when building the scanpath representation is therefore to retain as much of the relevant information as possible while allowing the desired visualization or calculation. AOI strings, for example, have mainly been developed to render string-edit comparisons (p. 348) of scanpaths possible. However, this comes at the cost of decreasing the spatial and temporal resolution of the scanpath, since the positions of data samples are replaced with letter strings corresponding to larger areas.

Scanpath representations reside at the top of the hierarchy. A small error in the simpler components (such as fixation detection criteria) travels all the way up, thus affecting higher representations (such as scanpath length). For instance, M. J. Green (2006) calculated *scan-path length* on her data as the sum of all saccadic amplitudes. She used the I-DT algorithm with a minimal fixation duration setting of 200 ms however, which strongly reduces the number of detected fixations as well as the distribution of their durations (p. 159). Green includes a raw data sample scanpath (the sum of all distances between successive samples) "to ensure that potential group differences in fixation scanpath length did not simply reflect group differences in the number of fixations." (her page 87), or, we could add, the settings of the algorithm. Overall, the reported saccade-based scanpath length is about half the raw sample scanpath length. As another example, a scanpath represented by gridded AOIs is uniquely defined by the grid size. Consequently, scanpaths that are judged as similar using one grid size may become dissimilar when using a smaller or larger grid size. Choosing an appropriate scanpath representation with carefully defined fixations, saccades, AOIs, and/or other entities is of crucial importance for the outcome of a study.

Three formal scanpath representations have been devised for algorithmic comparison of pairs of scanpaths, and the calculation of a few other measures. These are: strings, vectors, and attention maps. They make use of the representations defined in Chapters 5–7.

8.5.1 Symbol sequences

Symbol sequences refer to a string of symbols, typically letters, that represent selected aspects of a scanpath with or without relation to AOIs. By far the most common type is the *AOI string*, where each symbol represents either fixations or dwells in an AOI. Other types of strings are based on properties such as *fixation duration*, *saccade amplitude*, or *saccade direction*. These representations are mainly developed for the purpose of calculating scanpath similarity using the string-edit (Levenshtein, 1966), or related methods.

AOI-based fixation and dwell strings

Several scanpath measures, the most known of which is the string-edit measure, represent scanpaths with a string of fixations or dwells in areas of interest (AOIs), as defined in Chapter 6. The important difference between *gridded AOIs* and *semantic AOIs* should be taken into account in this type of representation. Figure 8.12 shows both varieties. The gridded AOIs are constructed by putting a grid of equally sized areas across the stimulus, ignoring whatever semantic parts the stimulus consists of. When a scanpath runs over the gridded AOIs, each fixation or dwell is replaced by the name of the AOI it hits. The scanpath in Figure 8.12(a) will be represented by the string: A6 C5 F0 I1 J1 K2 I3.

Each letter is a representation of a single fixation position within a whole AOI area, which is known as *spatial downsampling*. As a consequence, a small difference in gaze pattern would be enough to alter the string, but interestingly, other small differences would result in the *same* string. That is, some small differences matter, whereas others are ignored. Fixation and dwell string representations thus introduce a form of noise in your scan path data that may occlude actual results.

A division of stimulus space into semantic AOIs adopts the natural semantic parts of the stimulus. In Figure 8.12(b), the semantic AOIs are taken from Josephson and Holmes (2006), who used them to analyse viewing behaviour on a television screen. Semantic AOIs have different sizes, so in Figure 8.12, the scanpath example would be represented by the string MMTCCHGM (where M = 'Main' etc., and each letter denotes a fixation). The three Ms in the string represent fixations with very different positions in the stimulus, which means we have a very coarse position representation. This can be motivated if the 'Main' AOI is a

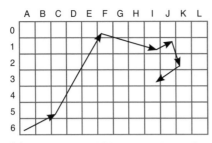

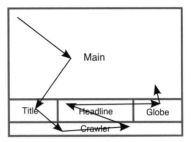

(a) Using gridded AOIs to approximate fixation position with AOI hits. The first fixation is approximated with the AOI A6, then C5, F0 etc.

(b) Semantic AOIs used by Josephson and Holmes (2006) to approximate fixation position with AOI hits. Both first and last fixation are approximated with AOI 'Main'.

Fig. 8.12 Gridded versus semantic AOIs for representing scanpaths.

semantically homogeneous area from the viewpoint of the hypothesis, analysis and theory. Otherwise, *very* different scanpaths will be represented as equal when using semantic AOIs.

As an alternative to gridded and semantic AOIs, data driven methods where recorded eye-movement data are used to define AOIs are only beginning to emerge for scanpath representations (see Santella & DeCarlo, 2004; Hooge & Camps, 2009). As pointed out earlier (pp. 219–220), data-driven AOI representations should be used with appropriate care.

Since our sample scanpath has two subsequent fixations in each of 'Main' and Crawler', we have a repetition for M and C in the string MMTCCHGM. Brandt and Stark (1997) use a variety of the AOI-string representation of scanpaths that ignores such repetitions, or in other words, they represent the scanpath with dwells rather than with fixations. The dwell-based AOI-string for the same scanpath would be MTCHGM. Removing consecutive repetitions is referred to as "compressing" the string; several fixations (CC) are replaced by one dwell (C).

The major advantages of the AOI string representation of scanpaths are that it retains an approximate *sequence* representation of the order of fixations, and that the string is a rough representation of the *shape* of the scanpath. The major drawback is the reliance on AOI segmentation, which necessarily introduces noise in the measures that rely on it.

Saccade amplitude and direction based strings

While being most frequently used, AOI strings represent scanpaths only in relation to spatial areas. If we are more interested in other aspects of a scanpath, strings can be constructed from other properties of eye-movement data such as the amplitude and direction of saccades, or the durations of fixations.

Gbadamosi (2000) and Zangemeister and Liman (2007) developed a string representation of scanpaths that combines one number for amplitude with another for direction. They use 16 (hexadecimal) numbers for each, as illustrated in Figure 8.13. Each saccade is therefore represented by a pair of (hexadecimal) numbers, and a scanpath with a sequence of pairs, such as D6 23 71 28 73 B3 54. This representation of scanpaths does not require a segmentation of space into AOIs; in fact, it completely abandons positional and semantic information, and instead focuses on representing our subjective perception of the overall shape of a scanpath. Still, it is based on segmentation (of direction and amplitude) and therefore again introduces noise when used in measures.

Letter strings with fixation durations have been proposed in the literature (Jarodzka, Nyström, & Holmqvist, 2010; Goldberg & Helfman, 2010), although they are only just beginning to appear (see Cristino et al., 2010 and p. 353).

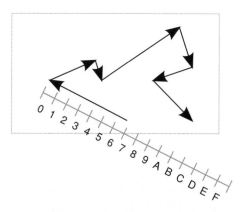

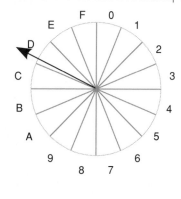

Fig. 8.13 To the left, the amplitude (length) of the first saccade is measured using a hexadecimal (16 unit) ruler. To the right, a discreet 16 region segmentation of saccadic direction, and the same first saccade has been placed so its direction is measured. With a 6 unit amplitude and a D for direction, the first saccade is represented by D6, where the first (hexadecimal) number in each pair represents direction and the second amplitude. The whole scanpath is represented by the string: D6 23 71 28 73 B3 54.

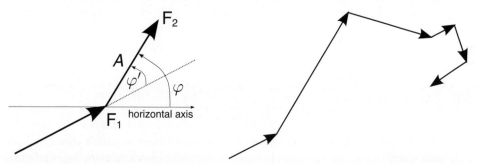

(a) A single saccade with amplitude A from fixation F_1 to fixation F_2 as a vector in a Euclidean space, with the absolute direction φ and relative direction φ'.

(b) A scanpath represented by a series of vectors.

Fig. 8.14 We can think of a scanpath as a sequence of vectors in space (b). Each vector is described by its origin F_1 and endpoint F_2. We can immediately derive its amplitude A, its angular deviation from the previous saccade φ', and its direction φ relative to the horizontal axis.

8.5.2 Vector sequences

Because of the reliance on the string-edit similarity calculation, few non-symbol representations have evolved. However, Jarodzka, Nyström, and Holmqvist (2010) argued that Euclidean vectors were suitable to represent ideal saccades, i.e. those that take the shortest distance between subsequent fixation positions.

A vector is a mathematical entity with length (A) and direction (φ), as shown in Figure 8.14(a). Apart from curvature, it thus approximates two major properties of a saccade. In addition, the vector representation does not require a segmentation of space, but retains the original detail of the ideal saccade and hence introduces no additional noise in future calculations. As shown by Jarodzka, Nyström, and Holmqvist (2010), a similarity calculation can nevertheless be made, using geometric calculations instead of letter identity checks.

Using vectors for single saccades, a scanpath can be represented as a *sequence of vectors*,

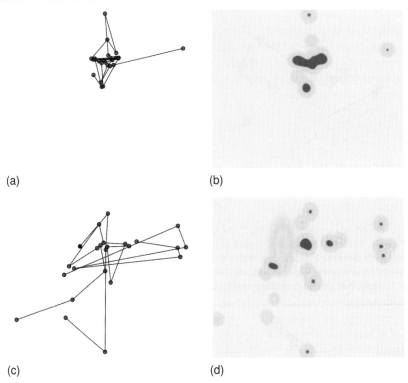

(a) (b)

(c) (d)

Fig. 8.15 Scanpaths (a) and (c) and their corresponding attention maps (b) and (d). The stimulus is the Mona Lisa painting (not shown).

as shown in Figure 8.14(b). Given the position of the initial fixation, such a vector sequence completely describes a fixation–saccade based scanpath. If saccadic start- and end-points explicitly encode fixation positions, we can attribute a duration to them, and utilize them in calculations as well. This way, a vector-based representation contains the same information as the recorded data after event detection. A vector-based representation can additionally be visualized in an intuitive manner very similar to the scanpath visualizations from most manufacturer software.

8.5.3 Attention map sequences

Attention maps, introduced in Chapter 7, are two-dimensional functions or 'maps' that represent the spatial distribution of a scanpath(s). Examples are shown in Figure 8.15 where the left pictures illustrate scanpaths connecting fixation sequences with lines, and the pictures on the right illustrate the corresponding attention maps. Attention maps are generated from either data samples or fixations, and ignore the order of these. According to the scanpath definition in this book, an attention map therefore does not qualify as a scanpath representation, because it does not signify the route, or order, of oculomotor events through space.

Nevertheless, the attention map measures of pages 359–376—including the Mannan distance measure developed by Mannan, Ruddock, and Wooding (1996)—are often referred to as 'scanpath metrics' in the literature (for example, by Cerf, Harel, Huth, Einhäuser, & Koch, 2009; Boccignone et al., 2005). Similarly, in their overview over what they refer to as scanpath analysis metrics, Underwood et al. (2008a) discuss both the Mannan distance measure and fixation maps, before settling for the string-edit analysis, which uses fixation and dwell string representations of scanpaths.

It is however straightforward to generate a *sequence of attention maps* from a scanpath, thus retaining order information. In the simplest case, each position $S_i = (x_i, y_i)$ in a scanpath can be replaced with an attention map $G = f(x, y)$, where $f(\cdot)$ denotes a function that generates an attention map G from the position (x_i, y_i). The most common function used for this purpose is the Gaussian

$$f(x,y) = \exp - \left(\frac{(x - x_i)^2}{2\sigma_x^2} + \frac{(y - y_i)^2}{2\sigma_y^2} \right) \tag{8.1}$$

where σ_x and σ_y denote the horizontal and vertical standard deviation, respectively. Given just one scanpath, its attention map equivalent carries the same spatio-temporal information, since peaks in the attention maps correspond directly to positions in the scanpath. An alternative is to think about the attention map sequence as a probabilistic scanpath that encodes the probability that a certain spatial position will be visited by a participant's gaze. However, as more scanpaths are used to build the attention map sequence, the 'path' in each individual scanpath is lost, but not the ordinal, collective eye-movement behaviour. In this sense, an attention map sequence does not violate our definition of what a scanpath is.

More generally, we can define a *scanpath function* $g(x, y)$ that represents any mapping from a set of scanpaths to an alternative representation, regardless of whether it is based on Gaussian functions or not. This concept is closely related to the average scanpath discussed on page 282.

8.6 Principles for scanpath comparison

We should stress here that this section deals with the *principles* of comparing scanpaths only, and by this we mean the different processing steps necessary before scanpath comparison can be carried out. The exact measures of quantitative scanpath comparison are covered in detail in Chapter 10, where we also discuss other measures of movement in eye-tracking data, besides the movement inherent in a scanpath representation.

According to J. M. Henderson and Ferreira (2004, p. 42), one of the reasons for reduced research interest into 'scan patterns', as they refer to them, is the lack of appropriate scanpath similarity measures for calculating commonalities in viewing behaviour both within- and between-participants: "it may be that with more careful examination, more consistency in scan patterns will be found, especially as analysis tools become more sophisticated". Indeed, scanpath comparison is needed in fields from neurological schizophrenia research (Benson et al., 2007), over to mental imagery (Johansson et al., 2006) and scene perception (Underwood, Humphrey, & Foulsham, 2008b), but also including applied areas such as evaluating web page design (Josephson & Holmes, 2002), and in expertise task analysis (Jarodzka, Scheiter, et al., 2010). See the unresolved issues section towards the end of this chapter (p. 278) for further discussion.

Methods to compare two or more sequences have long been used in bioinformatics to align DNA and protein sequences. In this field they have been used to test, for example, whether mutated sequences have evolved from the same original sequence, or to match a test sequence against a database.

In eye-movement research, the majority of sequence comparison methods have been used to compare pairs of scanpaths comprising AOI-strings. For example, Brandt and Stark (1997) compared scanpaths from participants viewing checkerboard patterns with scanpaths from subsequent visual imagery of the same stimuli. Similarly, Foulsham and Underwood (2008) compared scanpaths from participants viewing the same pictures twice; the initial viewing was followed by a later recognition test.

Scanpath similarity calculation is typically performed in four sequential steps:

1. *Representation*. A scanpath representation is chosen that best fits the experimental questions at hand.
2. *Simplification* is performed to remove parts of the scanpaths that are irrelevant to the hypothesis or that decrease subsequent computational power.
3. *Alignment* aims to optimally map entities between scanpaths.
4. *Calculation* of similarity between the aligned scanpaths then generates the final similarity score(s).

Only the last step is required to actually compute a similarity score, whereas the first three steps are performed to prepare the scanpaths to best address the experimental questions.

As noted, we discuss the principles of scanpath comparison here, and leave the implementation details of specific algorithms, as well as the calculation of similarity scores, for Part III.

8.6.1 Representation

The first step concerns choosing a suitable representation of the scanpath. The most common representations are data samples (x, y, t), AOI letter strings, vector sequences, and attention maps sequences. By definition, a representation does not retain all oculomotor information contained within the scanpath, but provides a more crude approximation of some of its features.

8.6.2 Simplification

Scanpaths are sometimes subjected to a process that typically is called *compression*, or *simplification*. Compression further simplifies the representation such that detail considered superfluous by the designer of the measure—such as several small fixations next to one another in Figure 8.16—is removed, and the output is a simplified version of the original scanpath. For AOIs strings, ABC would be a compressed version of the original string ABBBC, since the repetitive Bs have been removed. This type of simplification is suitable when order of AOI visits is of relevance, but not when dwell time or number of fixations within an AOI is of importance.

8.6.3 Sequence alignment

Sequence alignment originates from bioinformatics and aims to arrange two or more sequences in such a way that their elements (e.g. amino acids) optimally match. For very short sequences, the optimal match is usually easy to identify simply by looking at the sequences. However, as they get longer, alignment become an increasingly harder problem that needs to be addressed computationally. Then optimality is defined by a set of scoring parameters, and alignment is reduced to the problem of finding the optimal solution (e.g. the maximum or minimum score) based on the scoring scheme. Common scoring parameters consist of costs to insert, delete, and substitute sequence elements or blank spaces (gaps).

Alignment is typically *global* or *local* in nature. Global alignment intends to optimally match whole sequences with each other, whereas local alignment aims to identify shorter subsequences that are shared between the sequences being aligned. As an example, consider the following sequences:

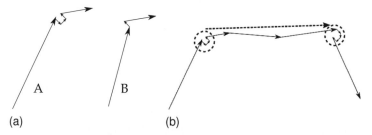

Fig. 8.16 Simplification of a vector-based scanpath representation as a prerequisite for successful alignment. In (a), four fixations in scanpath A with small saccades between them should be aligned to two fixations in scanpath B. Our intuition tells us that these small saccades are irrelevant for the comparison, and algorithmic simplification provides a firm tool to justify this judgement. Figure (b) shows two types of simplifications: small saccades are removed (dashed circles), and sequences of saccades in the same direction are removed (dashed arrow).

$$
\begin{array}{lll}
\text{Global} & \text{FTFTALILLAVAV} & S_1 \\
& \text{F--TAL-LLA-AV} & S_2 \\
\text{Local} & \text{FTFTALILL-AVAV} & S_1 \\
& \text{--FTAL-LLA\,AV--} & S_2
\end{array}
$$

Fig. 8.17 Sequence alignment between a short and a longer scanpath represented as strings. *Global* sequence alignment creates several gaps, indicated by –, in the shorter AOI fixation string, while *local* sequence alignment maximizes the length of substrings. Example from Wikimedia Commons.

$$S_1: \text{FTFTALILLAVAV}$$
$$S_2: \text{FTALLLAAV}$$

These are aligned according to Figure 8.17. Gaps or blank spaces, denoted by –, have been introduced at locations where matching between elements has not been possible. They correspond to one participant looking at some extra AOI, for instance, that the other participant skipped. A *gap penalty* is then paid for every such unmatched element. Notice that the number of possible alignments becomes huge as the sequence length increases, and that the optimal alignment is not necessarily unique.

A concise way to express the cost associated with matching one sequence element to another is the *substitution matrix*. Table 8.1 shows such a matrix for the sequences in Figure 8.17. Thus, the cost of matching I in one string with T in another is given by the value c_{35}. The diagonal is zero, and the reason for this is because there should be no cost associated with replacing an element with itself. Most substitution matrices are symmetric, that is $c_{ij} = c_{ji}$, but nothing prevents you from assigning higher costs for alignments in one direction and building an asymmetric similarity measure. The substitution matrix is particularly useful since it encodes the relationships between sequence elements. Translated to AOIs, this means that costs can be directly related to how similar two AOIs are with respect to each other in terms of spatial (e.g. Euclidean distance) or psychological (e.g. semantic similarity) aspects. Together with the gap penalty, the substitution matrix defines the optimal sequence match.

The matching process often utilizes a *comparison matrix*, in which the two strings being compared form the column and row divisions in the matrix, as shown in Table 8.2. Again, substitution costs can be added that allow the computation of an optimal path through the

	A	F	I	L	T	V
A	0	c_{12}	c_{13}	c_{14}	c_{15}	c_{16}
F	c_{21}	0	c_{23}	c_{24}	c_{25}	c_{26}
I	c_{31}	c_{32}	0	c_{34}	c_{35}	c_{36}
L	c_{41}	c_{42}	c_{43}	0	c_{45}	c_{46}
T	c_{51}	c_{52}	c_{53}	c_{54}	0	c_{56}
V	c_{61}	c_{62}	c_{63}	c_{64}	c_{65}	0

Table 8.1 A substitution matrix for the sequences in Figure 8.17. The cost of aligning I in one string with T in another is given by the value c_{35}. The Levenshtein measure has $c_{ij} = 1$ for all cells except the diagonal, where $c_{ij} = 0$.

	F	T	A	L	L	L	A	A	V
F	c_{22}	c_{25}	c_{12}	c_{24}	c_{24}	c_{24}	c_{12}	c_{12}	c_{26}
T	c_{25}	c_{55}	c_{15}	c_{45}	c_{45}	c_{45}	c_{15}	c_{15}	c_{56}
F	C_{22}	c_{25}	c_{12}	c_{24}	c_{24}	c_{24}	c_{12}	c_{12}	c_{26}
T	c_{25}	C_{55}	c_{15}	c_{45}	c_{45}	c_{45}	c_{15}	c_{15}	c_{56}
A	c_{12}	c_{15}	C_{11}	c_{14}	c_{14}	c_{14}	c_{11}	c_{11}	c_{16}
L	c_{24}	c_{45}	c_{14}	C_{44}	c_{44}	c_{44}	c_{14}	c_{14}	c_{46}
I	c_{23}	c_{35}	c_{13}	C_{34}	c_{34}	c_{34}	c_{13}	c_{13}	c_{36}
L	c_{24}	c_{45}	c_{14}	c_{44}	C_{44}	c_{44}	c_{14}	c_{14}	c_{46}
L	c_{24}	c_{45}	c_{14}	c_{44}	c_{44}	C_{44}	C_{14}	c_{14}	c_{46}
A	c_{12}	c_{15}	c_{11}	c_{14}	c_{14}	c_{14}	c_{11}	C_{11}	c_{16}
V	c_{26}	c_{56}	c_{16}	c_{46}	c_{46}	c_{46}	c_{16}	c_{16}	C_{66}
A	c_{12}	c_{15}	c_{11}	c_{14}	c_{14}	c_{14}	c_{11}	c_{11}	c_{16}
V	c_{26}	c_{56}	c_{16}	c_{46}	c_{46}	c_{46}	c_{16}	c_{16}	c_{66}

Table 8.2 A comparison matrix for the sequences in Figure 8.17. The path for local alignment is outlined with Cs.

comparison matrix, from the upper left corner to the lower right corner. With the optimal path for local alignment, denoted by C in the comparison matrix, vertical and horizontal movements are treated as gaps, whereas diagonal movements represent matches.

The popular string-edit algorithm uses three types of operations for sequence matching: insert, delete, and substitute (Levenshtein, 1966), usually with equal weights. Therefore, it can be seen as optimal sequence matching to use a very simple substitution matrix containing only ones in the cells c_{ij}.

Recently, more flexible algorithms have been adapted into eye-movement research and scanpath comparison, mainly the Needleman-Wunsch algorithm (Needleman & Wunsch, 1970) and Dijkstra's algorithm (Dijkstra, 1959). The Needleman-Wunsch algorithm is a method to align two sequences globally and allows a flexible scoring scheme. It performs best for sequences with already high similarity and similar lengths. Dijkstra's algorithm operates on representations known as *graphs* to find the shortest path from one node in the graph to another. The use of Dijkstra's algorithm presupposes that the comparison matrix is first transformed to a graph representation.

Note that a substitution matrix is only of practical use when the number of possible sequence elements is finite and small. In the case of sequences with infinite alphabets (i.e. an unlimited number of unique elements), costs have to be calculated directly in the comparison matrix. This is the case for example when scanpaths are represented by a sequence of vectors,

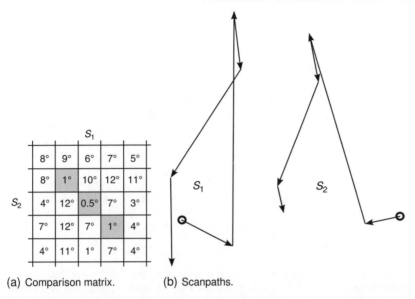

(a) Comparison matrix.   (b) Scanpaths.

Fig. 8.18 Pairwise vector comparison of all saccades in two vector representations $S_1 = \{u_1, u_2, u_3, u_4, u_5\}$ and $S_2 = \{v_1, v_2, v_3, v_4, v_5\}$ of scanpaths. Circles denote the onset of a scanpath. The comparison matrix (a) shows, for each pairwise vector comparison, the length of the differential vector $||u_i - v_j||$ in degrees of visual angle. If the two vectors are similar in amplitude and direction, this value is low. Figure (b) shows the scanpaths used in the comparison. Grey matrix cells indicate consecutive mappings that would produce a good alignment for a subset of the saccades.

which can have a large number of possible amplitudes and directions. Figure 8.18 illustrates a situation where saccade vectors u_i and v_i are compared to each other and the substitution cost equals the length of the differential vector $||u_i - v_j||$.

Closely related to the comparison matrix is the visualization known as a *dot-matrix plot* or simply *dotplot*. Instead of assigning each value in the matrix with a substitution cost, it adds a dot at positions where elements match, while keeping other matrix cells empty. This is visualized in Figure 8.19, which shows a dotplot for self-similarity where one string is matched with itself to point out commonly *recurring* subsequences. Two identical strings with a unique set of elements (i.e. without recurrences) would generate a diagonal in an otherwise empty dotplot. A collection of dots located off the main diagonal represent matching subseqences. However, more than being a method to align and quantitatively compare sequences, dotplots are typically used to subjectively inspect and interpret similarity.

8.6.4 Calculation

Finally, we *calculate the similarity* between the two scanpaths. Given the aligned scanpaths and the similarity metric, this is usually a simple and quick operation. For example, when the optimal alignment represented by a path in the comparison matrix is found, the similarity score is typically found by summing all cost and gap penalties along the path.

Scanpath similarity is a complex multidimensional concept, yet all similarity measures proposed so far have had at their heart the design criterion that they should output a single similarity value between 0 and 1. This could be a problem when scanpaths are very similar in some aspects, but dissimilar in others. For a multidimensional approach, which takes account of scaling, spatial and temporal offset, as well as fixation duration amongst other components which are important in the comparison of scanpaths. Details are given in Jarodzka, Nyström,

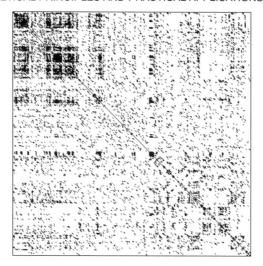

Fig. 8.19 Dot-matrix plot for visual evaluation of regional self-similarity between two identical strings. Similar repetitive patterns within the same string are seen as black regions. This is particularly common in the first 25% of string, in the upper left corner of the plot. From Wikimedia Commons (File:Zinc-finger-dot-plot.png).

and Holmqvist (2010) and on page 354.

8.6.5   Pairwise versus groupwise comparison

The comparison measures that exist for scanpaths, irrespective of their representations, are mainly pairwise and output a single value. Methods to compare groupwise similarity between scanpaths are only beginning to surface, in particular those that allow statistical testing of similarity. Feusner and Lukoff (2008) attribute the lack of statistical methods to the fact that a scanpath itself does not produce a numerical value, but only a pairwise comparison between two scanpaths. This disqualifies the use of traditional statistical methods such as the t-test, which require one value for each group entity (scanpath).

A way to approach groupwise scanpath comparison is first to calculate the *average scanpath* for each group (p. 265), and then compare this pair. However, if the comparison only results in a single value, statistical analysis is still not possible.

Feusner and Lukoff (2008) provide one solution to this problem by calculating the average pairwise similarity between ($d_{between}$) and within (d_{within}) two groups of scanpaths. Then they calculate the difference between these two values,

$$d^* = d_{between} - d_{within} \qquad (8.2)$$

for all possible group divisions where one group has n scanpaths and the other one has m scanpaths ($m + n$ is fixed), yielding a symmetric distribution of d^* with zeros mean. If the groups contain random scanpaths, we would expect a d^*-value around zero. Significance tests of group similarity are then possible using permutation tests.

8.7   Unresolved issues concerning scanpaths

There are several important but unresolved issues that it is useful to be aware of when working with scanpath representations of eye-movement data. One is the question of whether there is a direct relationship between scanpath patterns and specific cognitive processes. Another is the validity of scanpath theory, and its prediction that participants will re-produce a spatial model of the same scanpath when looking at an identical stimulus anew. Closely related is the issue of scanpath planning; that is the question of what drives the eyes to the successive locations along the route of a scanpath, and whether *inhibition of return* (Posner & Cohen, 1984) decreases the likelihood of the eyes going back to their previous location. Another unresolved issue is whether it is possible, or even meaningful, to build an 'average scanpath' from a group of scanpaths. The final unresolved issue revolves around open problems concerning how to compare the similarity of two scanpaths computationally and statistically, adopting the framework(s) outlined earlier in the chapter.

8.7.1 Relationships between scanpaths and cognitive processes

It is easy to agree with Yarbus (1967) who wrote:

> Eye-movements reflect the human thought processes; so the observer's thought may be followed to some extent from records of eye-movements (the thought accompanying the examination of the particular object). It is easy to determine from these records which elements attract the observer's eye (and, consequently, his thought), in what order, and how often.

Often, Yarbus' findings raise the question of whether "thought processes" can reflect more specific cognitive states such as interest, difficulty, or confusion? Is there a specific scanpath pattern that directly and uniquely corresponds to a cognitive process?

There is indeed a general consensus that scanpaths are determined to a large extent by idiosyncratic cognitive factors (as claimed by Choi et al. (1995) and others). Very few studies however have targeted what a specific cognitive process (like a "thought") looks like when appearing in a scanpath. The attempts by Goldberg and Schryver (1995b), Goldberg and Kotval (1999), and Salvucci (1999) to infer intent from eye movements, led to the definition of several new measures, but none of them could be directly and systematically linked to specific cognitive processes.

Usability analysts using eye tracking are in need of a method to investigate the relationship between scanpaths and cognitive processes; Ehmke and Wilson (2007) argue that the measures used by academic researchers are of little help to someone looking at scanpaths for signs of interest, confusion, hesitation, or poor computer interface design. They argue that the usability analyst needs to be able to draw concrete conclusions from scanpaths. For instance when seeing a scanpath comprised of "many short fixations across a page where information might be expected", can she conclude that "expected information is missing"? Is it scientifically justified to ask the participant if they expected content to be present at certain points along the route of this scanpath?

There are several dangers to such manual assignment of cognitive processes to scanpaths. For instance, it is not unlikely that a scanpath described as "many short fixations across a page" will co-occur with many different cognitive states, and will not be uniquely determined by any one of them. The usability analyst may easily fall prey to guesswork, and the participant to inadvertently confirming the guesses (compare p. 105). Moreover, many of the scanpath-based concepts (such as 'regularity'), referred to by Ehmke and Wilson (2007), are vague and difficult to accurately capture in a measure. Trying to relate vague scanpath-based concepts to guessed cognitive processes is not scientific, and is unlikely to be revealing for research purposes.

While it is very difficult, if possible at all, to define a general relationship between a cognitive process and a prototypical scanpath pattern, there are ways to associate a cognitive process with a scanpath that is specific to a situation. One way is to use an experimental

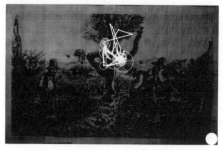
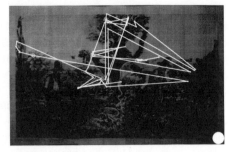

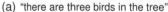

(a) "there are three birds in the tree"   (b) "it looks like ... early summer"

Fig. 8.20 Two scanpaths and concurrent speech. Reprinted from *Human Cognitive Processes, 23,* Holsanova, J., Discourse, vision, and cognition, Copyright (2008) by, and re-printed with kind permission from, John Benjamins Publishing Company, Amsterdam/Philadelphia, www.benjamins.com.

design that constrains the number of possible interpretations of the scanpath. This requires control over stimuli, task, and even background of participants, however. Another option is to include complementary data sources, such as speech, neurophysiological data, or body-movement data.

For example, Holsanova (2008, 2006, 2001) had participants describe complex scenes and then segmented the spoken discourse into a series of what Chafe (1994) calls "idea units"; sections of thought expressed as speech and delimited by prosodic features, speech timing, and a particular form of words called "discourse markers". The flow of idea units in speech is considered to correspond to the flow of thought in the speaker's mind. Holsanova then temporally matched the idea units to scanpath patterns, so that it became clear what participants looked at while speaking a particular idea.

Figure 8.20 shows two of the clearest simple patterns from Holsanova's research. In Figure 8.20(a), "three birds in the tree", a limited picture element, corresponded very well to the idea in speech. In Figure 8.20(b), the idea in speech, "it looks like early summer", was not located at any particular position, but spread out in the image, at places where there is evidence of summer. These examples suggest a tight coupling between sub-scanpaths and cognitive processes in free description, complementing the more well known visual world paradigm of Tanenhaus et al. (1995) and others. However, it still only means that scanpaths reflect ideas, not that ideas or cognitive states can be uniquely identified from scanpaths. It also shows that the particular stimulus partly determines the scanpath, so it might be difficult to find general stimulus-independent scanpath patterns for the same cognitive processes.

What does Holsanova's research tell us about interpreting all those scanpaths from non-experimental freeviewing tasks that have no concurrently recorded speech? Without the idea units from speech and their temporal on- and offsets, we have no method to find the on- and offset in the scanpath, i.e. event, that corresponds to the start and end of a thought, and we have no content of the thought either. Without speech or other complimentary data, we are simply left guessing.

8.7.2 Scanpath Theory

It is rare for discussions about scanpaths to circumvent scanpath theory as devised by Noton and Stark (Noton & Stark, 1971a, 1971b). From two reported studies, which use two participants in the first and four in the second experiment, the authors conclude that when a participant looks through an image already seen, the remembered spatial model (which the authors term "the feature network") from the first viewing directs him to look at the stimulus in the

the same way the second time around. In essence the scanpath theory predicts that:

> ...for each pattern with which he is familiar, each person has a fixed and characteristic path which he follows from feature to feature, both when viewing the pattern and when matching it with its internal representation during recognition. (Excerpt from Noton & Stark, 1971b.)

Note that the scanpath according to this theory is a fixed, theoretical path that has a representation in the brain. The main implication of scanpath theory is that scanpaths will be re-capitulated, not being driven by image content, but by a stored internal representation.

Scanpath theory has been re-considered, for instance by J. M. Henderson and Ferreira (2004), who review a number of studies in contradiction to the predictions of Noton and Stark. In particular, participants can recognize a scene without making eye-movements (Biederman, Rabinowitz, Glass, & Stacy, 1974), and there is usually very little sequence similarity between repeated viewings by the same participant; even if looking at the same positions a second time, the order is different, according to these authors. In fact, some authors completely refrain from the term 'scanpath' in order to dissociate themselves from scanpath theory, for instance Underwood, Foulsham, and Humphrey (2009) and J. M. Henderson (2003).

On the other hand, scanpath theory is to some extent supported by empirical evidence. When recording eye movements from participants viewing pictures during encoding and later recognition, Foulsham and Underwood (2008) found higher than chance similarity between scanpaths. Moreover, *mental imagery* studies from the late 1990s and onward repeatedly find that participants shown a blank screen and asked to retell a previously shown scene, largely reiterate the same eye-movement sequences on the blank screen as when viewing the scene itself (Zangemeister & Liman, 2007; Johansson et al., 2006; Brandt & Stark, 1997). In these studies scanpath theory has been replaced by newer theoretical explanations, however.

8.7.3 Scanpath planning

Research on *scanpath planning* investigates whether, when, and to what extent participants plan their scanpaths ahead, and which information is involved in this planning.

An appealing argument in favour of scanpath planning is the frequent occurrence of one or a series of short fixations (< 100 ms); considering that the time it takes to program a saccade by far exceeds these 100 ms, some of the saccades in the sequence must be pre-programmed (Becker & Jürgens, 1979).

Zingale and Kowler (1987) proposed that a scanpath results from an organized plan that is retrieved from memory before the scanpath is initiated. Using simple visual arrays, they asked participants to fixate a sequence of 1–5 static targets and found the latency of the first saccade to increase with the number of targets. Zingale and Kowler attributed the increase to the additional planning required to encode a longer scanpath.

Findlay and Brown (2006) identify three possible scanning strategies which they go on to test empirically: *systematically directional*, raster-like as in reading or back and forth scanning; *locally perceptual*, based on low-level information acquired at the current point of fixation; and *globally perceptual*, considering global stimulus features such as shape. Asking participants to sequentially fixate each item in a visual array, they found empirical evidence only for the strategies to scan items in a raster order (directional), and to use the global external contour to guide eye-movements, making saccades towards the centre, but still using the contour as a guide. Supposedly, a systematic strategy such as a raster scan can be pre-planned, but there is no need to encode the whole scanpath into memory (Gilchrist & Harvey, 2006). In contrast, a scanpath guided by global contour requires some initial global processing of the stimulus, where the scanpath is first encoded and stored in some way.

Both Zingale and Kowler (1987) and Findlay and Brown (2006) argue that it is likely that bottom-up information can modify the scanpath, and make it deviate somewhat from the pre-planned scanpath. In visual search, for example, backtracks were found to be more common to items that resembled the visual search target (Peterson, Kramer, Wang, Irwin, & McCarley, 2001). Interestingly, using very reduced stimuli with a small set of equal-sized objects, some researchers have suggested that when there is no bottom-up information to distinguish between objects, attentional deployment is random (Horowitz & Wolfe, 2001) and no memory is retained of what objects have (and have not) been visited.

An important part of scanpath planning is to keep track of previously visited locations, and prevent revisits to these. This mechanism is known as *inhibition of return*, and is argued to serve as a 'foraging facilitator' in visual search (Klein & MacInnes, 1999), preventing inefficient returns to areas already inspected. It has been suggested that at least five spatial objects can be kept in memory (Synder & Kingstone, 2000), and that this information is used when planning future scanning (Findlay & Brown, 2006).

Other research has concluded that memory not only guides the selection of targets along a scanpath (Gilchrist & Harvey, 2000), but that this memory can also prevent *revisits* of earlier targets for fairly large sets of objects (Dickinson & Zelinsky, 2007). This research has developed into the question of whether visual search is like foraging, carried out over chunks of space that can then be successively dismissed.

Using real-world stimuli and tasks, such as letting participants make sandwiches, avoid non-animate targets, or meet other people approaching in a narrow hallway, Land and Hayhoe (2001); Hayhoe and Ballard (2005); Rothkopf, Ballard, and Hayhoe (2007), and others show that scanpath planning is tightly connected with the ongoing task and the immediate visual surroundings. In particular, *look-ahead* fixations during real-life tasks, for instance looking at the jam jar four or five seconds before it is actually time to grab it, show how the eye-movement system is used in the planning of future sub-activities in the overall task (Mennie et al., 2007). In this view, task-driven plans lie behind virtually all eye movements, and random scanpaths would only occur when participants feel they have no task, and bottom-up features are free to pull the eyes—even then, however, we quickly apply meaning to what we look at.

8.7.4 The average scanpath

Although some researchers find the 'the average scanpath' difficult to calculate due to the unique unfolding of each scanpath (for instance, Hornof, 2007, p. 317), others make an attempt to take a number of scanpaths and build an average from them (Josephson & Holmes, 2002; Hembrooke, Feusner, & Gay, 2006; Torstling, 2007).

Josephson and Holmes (2002) first calculate the pairwise string-edit distance between all AOI-based scanpaths, and then define 'the most central scanpath' as the sequence with the smallest average distance to all other sequences. Using multiple sequence alignment, Hembrooke et al. (2006) construct the average scanpath from global similarities among the scanpaths.

A slightly different definition of the average scanpath was suggested by Holsanova et al. (2008). It is illustrated in Table 8.3 with a hypothetical example including five AOIs and five participants. The AOIs in this table have been ranked in the order that they were visited by each of the five participants. Participant 1, for instance, looked at AOI 1 first, then at AOI 3, etc. Revisited AOIs are not counted, only first visits. AOIs that are not visited by a participant receive the highest remaining rank or the average of the highest remaining ranks.

Finally, a sequence of attention maps can be considered to represent an average scanpath in the sense that each attention map in the sequence describes spatial distribution for all participants.

The term 'averaging' implies calculating one single entity out of several, so that the single

Table 8.3 Average scanpath as the average order of entry for five AOIs seen by five participants (fictitious data).

Participant	AOI 1	AOI 2	AOI 3	AOI 4	AOI 5
1	1	3	2	4	5
2	2	1	3	5	4
3	1	2	3	4	5
4	3	1	2	5	4
5	1	3	2	4	5
Average	1.60	2.00	2.40	4.40	4.60

average is somewhere near the middle, and accepting that the variance information from the averaged group of scanpaths is lost. This makes the average scanpath alone unsuited for statistical calculations. Moreover, if two participants consistently look at different sides of a monitor, their average scanpath will be in the centre of it, where none of the participants have ever looked. These are severe limitations when using averaging scanpath representations and measures.

8.7.5 Comparing scanpaths

The general principles for scanpath comparison were outlined earlier in the chapter. However, many challenges still need to be addressed. At a conceptual level, there are a large number of desirable pairwise scanpath comparisons. For instance, we would like to detect the degree to which:

- the *overall shape* is the same between two scanpaths, and whether both scanpath shapes exhibit the same temporal sequence. The string-edit measure has approximated a shape comparison for some cases, while many measures completely ignore temporal order.
- two scanpaths are *similar in shape but different in scale*. A half-sized but otherwise identical scanpath should be considered similar by a measure to be useful in for instance mental imagery studies, but no current measure can do this.
- two scanpaths have a difference in *spatial extent*. This can be studied with measures utilizing attention map representations of scanpaths.
- there is a *similarity in position but reversal of order*. This could in principle be detected using the sequence alignment method described above.
- one participant executes his scanpath faster than another participant, although to the exact same positions, by investigating how the *temporal alignment* differs.
- the *fixation duration profiles* between two scanpaths differ, even if position and sequence order is identical.
- *similar sub-scans* exist in either of the two scanpaths (even though the sub-scans may appear in a different order).

Any proposed scanpath comparison measure must eventually be validated. There are two main methods for validating scanpath similarity: *absolute* and *relative*. Absolute validation can only be made by comparing the output from the proposed measure to a baseline that expresses the true similarity between scanpaths. One such baseline can be established by showing people a large number of scanpath pairs and asking them to judge the similarity for each pair on some scale. However, setting up this baseline both requires and allows us to answer many open questions: Should we show static or dynamic scanpath pairs (i.e. is dynamics a part of scanpath similarity)? Should our judges rate the similarity using a single or multiple scales? Is human judgement of the similarity between pairs of scanpaths really systematic across individuals? Is it possible for a human to judge the degree of similarity between any two scanpaths at all?

Validating relative similarity is much easier. Take for example any scanpath and create distorted versions of it by adding an increasing amount of noise. Since we know that scanpath similarity between the original scanpath and its distorted version should increase with the level of noise, this is something that should be reflected in a valid scanpath similarity measure. Still, we cannot tell whether the absolute differences in similarity between noise levels are sensible.

Given a substitution matrix, another open issue is how to choose appropriate costs. Although the matrix offers a flexible scoring scheme, it is up to the researcher herself to choose costs that are suitable to the experiment in hand.

Finally, it is important to distinguish between scanpath comparison in picture- and video viewing; objects, and therefore fixations, in video stimuli are largely associated with a particular temporal span. Therefore, scanpaths recorded from videos do not critically require sequence alignment prior to comparison. Moreover, since the duration of a video is always fixed, different sequence lengths are not a large problem in the comparison.

8.8 Summary: scanpath events and representations

Scanpath events are specific subscans that occur within a limited chunk of a scanpath. Six such events have been defined in this chapter:

- **backtracks**, saccades going in the opposite direction to the previous one.
- **regressions**, which exist as *in-word* and *between-word* regressions, *regression scanpaths*, and *re-inspections*.
- **look-backs**, which are also known as *returns*.
- **look-aheads**, saccades towards items that are important in the immediate action plan.
- **local versus global**, a categorization of the scanpath into two types of subscans; this is very similar to *ambient versus focal*.
- **sweeps**, a sequence of saccades in the same direction.
- **reading versus scanning**, events in reading of larger texts such as newspapers.

Furthermore, a scanpath can be represented in a number of ways:

- **Sequences of symbols** aim to represent selected features of a scanpath by means of symbols. The most different types of symbol sequences are
  * **Fixation strings** where fixations are represented by letters denoting names of the AOIs where they reside. An example of a fixation string is MMTCCHGM.
  * **Dwell strings**, which are fixation strings where consecutive, repetitive fixations are merged. The dwell string of the example string above would thus become MTCHGM.
  * **Direction/amplitude strings** of saccades such as
    D6 23 71 28 73 B3 54,
    where the first hexadecimal digit in each pair is segmented saccadic direction and the other digit segmented saccadic amplitude.
  * **Duration strings** where symbols represent quantized fixation duration. However, these have been used very sparingly in the literature.

- **The vector sequence** represents a scanpath by a sequence of Euclidean vectors. Typically, the vectors represent saccades, and the start and end position of saccade vectors represent fixations.
- **Attention map sequences** represent one of many scanpaths as a sequence of attention maps. Sequence information but no participant identity are retained in this representation.

Scanpaths and their representations are also commonly used in visualizations. They are for example useful for exemplifying data in journals, for checking data quality, and to see what the fixation algorithm did, and have often been used for manual analysis. Scanpath visualizations can be used as elicitation in retrospective speech.

This chapter also outlined the principles for scanpath comparison, which include choosing a suitable scanpath representation, simplifying the scanpath, and aligning scanpaths with each other before calculating a similarity score. When selecting between 'scanpath comparison measures', of which there are many, be certain that you use a representation that retains the information you want in the comparison.

Finally, a number of open issues that researchers dealing with scanpaths should be aware of concerning scanpaths were discussed.

9 Auxiliary Data: Events and Representations

This data analysis chapter differs from the earlier ones by adding to the eye-tracking data other data recorded from the participant. Recording auxiliary data along with eye tracking is a technical pursuit currently in its infancy, therefore there is only limited advice available on the complex details surrounding the combination of equipment and complementary data representations. Becasuse of the structure of this book, you will find information on how to deal with auxiliary data in two other parts of this book: if you *plan* to use auxiliary data, see pages 95–108. If you want to *record* auxiliary data, please read the section on pages 134–139. This chapter deals only with *analysing* auxiliary data *in addition to* eye-tracking data. Please note that the analysis of auxiliary data in isolation from eye-movement data is out of the scope of this book. If you are interested in analysing auxiliary data in itself, please adhere to a large body of already existing literature, such as Ericsson and Simon (1993) and Chafe (1994) for verbal data, and Luck (2005) for EEG data.

Co-aligning the data streams over time should be the first step. The continued analysis depends on whether the other data source has events, or whether their analysis requires processing data over a period of time. The chapter is structured as follows:

- In Section 9.1 (p. 286), we exemplify two common methods for co-analysis of data: first, using the eye-movement data as an onset marker, and analysing the data in the other channel from that onset. Second, when there are events in the auxiliary data that can be associated with events in the eye-movement data, latencies can be calculated. We exemplify this analysis using studies combining eye-movement data with EEG, fMRI, motion tracking, verbal data, and keystroke data.
- Section 9.2 (p. 290) introduces a content-oriented co-analysis of eye-movement and verbal data. In this type of analysis, the eye-movement data have only been used to stimulate the elicitation of verbal data and are not intended for further analysis. Recording verbal data along with eye-movement data, however, also allows the researcher to co-analyse the two types of data as a form of methodological triangulation.

9.1 Event-based coalignment

Whether the auxiliary data consist of motion tracking, EEG, speech, or GSR recordings, the analysis with eye-tracking data starts by placing the two synchronized data streams side by side, and then executing some form of latency analysis. Typically, the onset of an event in one of the two data streams is taken as time 0.

For auxiliary data where events cannot be detected, the analysis takes its starting point as the onset of an event in the eye-tracking data, most commonly a fixation or a saccade. Figure 9.1(a) illustrates this case. Around the selected event, periods of analysis are defined, often called 'epochs' in EEG and fMRI terminology. Specific types of analysis are then done for the auxiliary data within those periods.

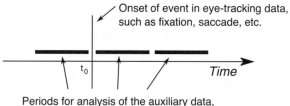

(a) When the auxiliary data have no events, alignment is made at the point in time of the onset of an eye-tracking event (t_0), such as fixation, saccade, micro-saccade, smooth pursuit.

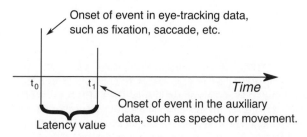

(b) When there are events in the auxiliary data, the two time lines can be aligned. The duration $t_1 - t_0$ is calculated and defines the latency between the two events.

Fig. 9.1 Principles for the two types of co-alignment of eye-tracking and auxiliary data.

However, the selected 0-time event can just as well reside in the other data channel. For instance, Diderichsen (2008) investigated dwell times to AOIs in collaborative puzzle building just before and after the onset of the indefinite pronoun 'one'. Often, a latency analysis is made between the onset of eye-tracking events and the corresponding events in the auxiliary data. Latency analysis was first performed by Buswell (1920), and in this book Chapter 13 is entirely dedicated to latency measures. A crucial question when there are many events in both eye-tracking and auxiliary data is which event in one stream should correspond to which in the other stream. Solving this often requires using objects in the stimulus as *alignment mediators*.

Note that co-alignment and latency analyses require that both recording systems, the stimulus presentation tools, and the stimulus monitor are synchronized, and that there are no internal system latencies in either type of recording system.

9.1.1 Alignment of eye-tracking events with auxiliary data

The simplest type of co-analysis is to take the onset of an event in one of the data streams as the onset for analysis of the other data stream. EEG co-analysis with eye-tracking data is shown in Figure 9.2. A fixation event starts at time 0, and during the period of its duration and for some time after it has ended—a total of 300 ms in this case—ERP components are analysed. This simple synchronization ties the ERP components to the object looked at during the fixation (Baccino & Manunta, 2005), allowing identification of what is known as EFRPs (eye fixation related potentials). Alternatively when analysing ERP components in a window just after a saccade onset, the measurement is called SEMRPs or saccadic eye-movement

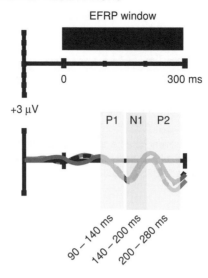

Fig. 9.2 The principle for EFRPs (eye-fixation-related potentials), a form of co-analysis of EEG data with fixation data. The 0 in the top half of the figure represents the onset of a fixation. EEG data are investigated in a window starting at 0 ms up to 300 ms ahead in time. The EFRP consists of the positive (down) and negative (up) voltage deflections (or 'components') in the EEG data called P1 (first Positive, at 100 ms), N1 (first Negative, at 150 ms) and P2 (second Positive, at 200 ms). The EFRP analysis takes the onset of the fixation as the beginning of the processing of the item looked at. Adapted from Simola, Holmqvist, and Lindgren (2008).

related potentials (Jagla et al., 2007).

EEG data need to be averaged over several trials, in order to improve the signal to noise ratio. Each fixation in the eye-movement data is related to a subsequent EEG period, and these periods must be aligned on the basis of the onset of the fixations that they belong to. It is important to note that these fixation events that are used to obtain such an average are caused by comparable stimuli in the experimental design.

The window size of 300 ms in Figure 9.2 was selected to analyse ERPs during a fixation period. Co-registration for longer time windows can be used to study higher-order cognitive processes, but you need to be careful with ocular artefact correction if you analyse over time windows including saccades. Also note that the EFRPs of successive short fixations may be overlaid if fixations land on areas which each evoke a reaction and the ERP reaction of the previous fixation has not yet terminated. The same is true of SEMRPs, of course.

The same method for finding co-aligned periods is used in combination with fMRI data. For instance, Ford et al. (2005) compared what is known as BOLD activity in fMRI data between correct and incorrect antisaccades and prosaccades. They divided the preparatory period into an early period, which lasted from task-cue onset to 4 s into the preparatory period and a late period lasting from 5 s into the preparatory period until the end of the preparatory period (Figure 9.3). After the launch of the saccade, a period of 4 s covers the neurological aftermath. Analysis of the fMRI data is then done within each period, using an analysis that suits fMRI data over epochs. Because fMRI data are of a very low frequency, typically one sample per second, many brain-situated processes governing the planning and execution of saccades take place during each of these samples. Also, for tasks with a higher saccade rate than this anti-saccade task, with up to several saccades per second, the temporal resolution in fMRI data of one Hz is much too low. The reason that it works in the saccade task is that saccades can be launched with very long fixation intervals between them.

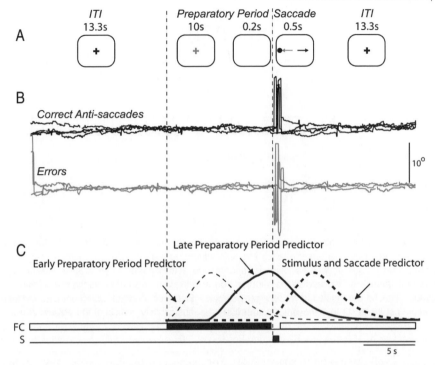

Fig. 9.3 Principle for alignment and co-analysis of fMRI data (C) with antisaccades (B). Three fMRI epochs were analysed: early preparatory, late preparatory, and stimulus and saccade epoch, shown in C. Epochs were aligned with the start of the saccades. ITI means 'inter-trial interval'. Figure 1 from Kirsten A. Ford, Herbert C. Goltz, Matthew R.G. Brown, and Stefan Everling. Neural Processes Associated With Antisaccade Task Performance Investigated With Event-Related fMRI. *Journal of Neurophysiology*, 2005, *94*, 429–440.

9.1.2 Latencies between events in eye-tracking and auxiliary data

In the EEG and fMRI examples, eye-movement data could be immediately aligned with the auxiliary data using the time stamps in each data type, under the assumption that synchronization during recording was technically successful. In other cases a mediator is necessary for alignment. For instance, Figure 9.4 shows how motion tracking data from a violin player are aligned with gazes on the score of notes. The notes are the proper mediators in this analysis because notes are linked both to the motion tracking data (the bow playing the note) and to the eye-movement data (the eye is looking at the note).

The need for a mediator is even more clear when combining eye-movement data with verbal data. We will illustrate it using the Speech-AOI method of synchronized verbal and eye-movement data (Holsanova, 2008; Griffin & Spieler, 2006). In an AOI-analysis, we segment the audio signal into 'Speech AOIs' much like the spatial AOIs of Chapter 6, only in one dimension rather than two. That is, a speech AOI has an onset and an offset time, and covers the entire period in-between.

If the participant has been speaking, each participant has his own audio file, and speech AOIs need to be individually assigned to each participant. If the participants have instead been listening to the same sound, the same synchronized AOIs can be used across all participants.

In some analysis software, a 'Speech AOI editor' can be used to set these on- and off-sets and to give names to the speech AOIs. In practice, speech AOIs are likely to be words, phrases, and sentences or fragments thereof. As a participant is speaking about a stimulus, the

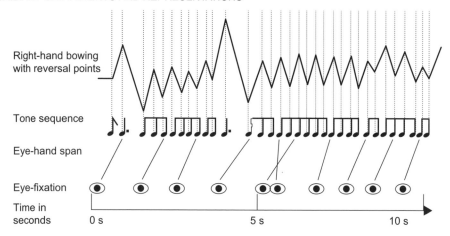

Fig. 9.4 Motion tracking data aligned with eye-movement data on a score of notes. The top line shows violin bow strokes (top). The onset of each stroke is aligned to the tone played (middle) as indicated by the dashed lines. Tones as well as fixations (bottom) are both aligned to synchronized recording time. The eye-hand latency is analysed as the duration from eye-fixation on a note until the note is beginning to be played. With kind permission from Springer Science + Business Media: Experimental Brain Research Sight-reading of Violinists: eye movements anticipate the musical flow, *194*(3), 2009, Pascal Wurtz.

speech AOIs will often refer to spatial AOIs. For instance, if the participant says "the stone", there is likely to be a stone AOI in the stimulus that the participant is referring to. However, speech and spatial AOIs do not always have a one-to-one relationship. There may be *many* stones in the scene that the speech AOI can refer to.

In this case, the mediator between the speech AOIs and the objects in the scene are of course the meanings of words. For this reason, the speech AOI editor must be at least partly manual, both because computational segmentation of speech will always be imperfect and in need of human control and postprocessing, but also because algorithms have no understanding of reference in speech to visual objects.

In data recordings from complex real-life scenarios, the number of possible latency calculations may become very large. Figure 9.6 shows a recording of eye-movement data from a participant writing on a computer. The different tiers show when the participant looks at the keyboard and the monitor, but also synchronized data about keystrokes on the monitor. Two tiers show periods of reading, and at the bottom, for validation of the reading detection filter, the (x,y) coordinates over time.

A myriad of possible latencies appear in such rich data. For instance, the duration from the last keystroke in a sequence to the start of reading, or the duration from looking up at the monitor until first reading, or from the onset of looking at the keyboard until the first keystroke.

9.2 Triangulating eye-movement data with verbal data

Eye movements are often co-recorded with verbal data not to investigate the eye–voice relationship, but for use as a form of methodological triangulation. Another common possibility is to use the eye-movement data as an intermediate form of data that is dropped once the verbal data has been recorded and becomes the data of preference (pp. 99–108 and 134–139, and also Van Gog, Paas, Van Merriënboer, & Witte, 2005). This use of verbal data in conjunction with eye-movement data is known as 'cued retrospective reporting'.

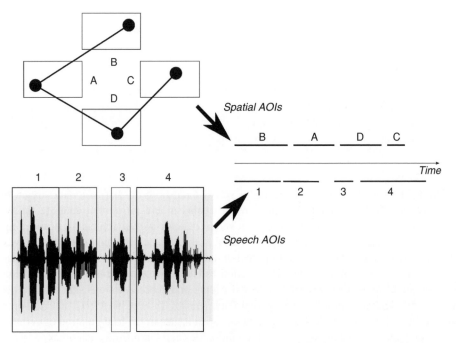

Fig. 9.5 The principle for co-analysing 'speech AOIs' with spatial AOIs over time. Each type of AOI is overlaid separately onto the data, with numbers indicating speech AOIs and letters spatial AOIs. The two are then combined using their common, synchronized time stamps, so that we can put them on the same time line (right). A similar co-analysis is shown on page 259.

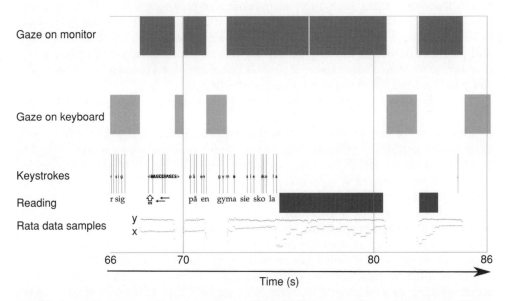

Fig. 9.6 A complex latency situation: data from a participant writing a text, the recording situation shown on page 54. The tiers show gazes on the monitor and keyboard, keystrokes writing the end of a sentence, periods of reading as detected by a reading detector (p. 267), and at the bottom, the (x,y)-stream of raw data samples.

Table 9.1 Example of transcribed and segmented speech from a description of poor building quality in bathrooms.

(38)	but it's a piece/ a part of the basin ...
(39)	and it is placed *on* the bench ...
(40)	which means that if water runs over here
(41)	then you have to force it over the edge ... back again ...
(42)	which is very natural ... for us ...
(43)	so the sink actually rests on ...
(44)	so if you have a cross section here ...

Eye-movement data are very similar to verbal data: both consist of a data stream over time, and both are composed of events. While events in eye-movement data are the well-known fixations, saccades etc., the events in verbal data are words, sentences, or meaningful parts. In this section we will see how these verbal events can be detected in verbal data, which is called 'transcribing and dividing into idea units', and how representations can be built out of these events, known as 'coding'. This section ends by reviewing measures that can be used based on such transcribed and coded verbal events and representations. For further detail on the event-detection procedure in verbal data, see M. T. H. Chi (1997) or Ericsson and Simon (1993). Finally, this section will address open issues in the triangulation of verbal and eye-tracking data and what both research communities can learn from each other.

9.2.1 Detecting events in verbal data: transcribing verbalizations and segmenting them into idea units

When analysing the audio recordings, there are two possibilities. The first is to code the audio files by listening to them. Such direct analysis of audio files is only possible for very simple coding schemata, such as if you want to check whether certain terms were mentioned, by listening through the audio files and tick the mentioned terms on a checklist or in a software program designed for this purpose. Several software packages support this function (e.g. Crutcher, 2007). With a large number of possible verbal events and complex verbal processes, you quickly run the risk of losing the overview of your data.

The other option is to transcribe the verbal data into written text. This has many benefits: it is easier to grasp the context of single statements, easier to segment the data, and easier to compare ratings of multiple coders (see next section). In particular, if you are interested in more detailed analyses of your data, you cannot forgo a time-consuming transcription. The transcriptions can be done in two ways: by typewriting or by the use of speech recognition software. If you are good at typewriting, this is the preferred choice. Using a pedal that controls the sound player you are using (pausing and playing) frees your hands for writing. Current speech recognition software may be helpful but needs to be trained on the voice to be transcribed, and also has problems with surrounding sounds or different dialects.

Just as fixations are aggregated into dwell or scanpath events such as regressions and sweeps, the single words of verbal data are also aggregated into larger units. These segments may be of different granularity: an entire paragraph, a sentence, a turn between different people speaking, or a meaningful idea unit. For instance, Table 9.1 shows a piece of verbal data which has been transcribed and segmented into idea units. Segmenting verbal data into idea units is only one of several possibilities, but it gives units that are not only easy to read but are argued to correspond both to the flow of conscious ideas and to eye-movement data (Holsanova, 2001; Chafe, 1994).

Table 9.2 Some sub-types of speech, adapted from Chafe (1994). Substantive speech relates solely to factual information; Contextual regulation indicates the speaker is remaining 'on topic'; Interactional utterances signify engagement with another; Cognitive verbalizations reflect thinking directly, possibly arrival at a solution; Validational utterances reflect judgement of the likelihood that the information being conveyed is accurate.

Type of speech	Example
Substantive	"the voltage is very low"
Contextual regulation	"and then...", "well..."
Interactional	"mhm", "you know"
Cognitive	"let me see", "oh"
Validational	"maybe", "I think"

9.2.2 Coding of verbal data units

In eye-tracking data analysis, eye movement events, like fixations, are usually aggregated into representations, like different AOIs. A comparable procedure is usually chosen when dealing with verbal data. The transcribed and possibly segmented verbal data must be coded and may be scored in a next step. *Coding* refers to assigning each verbal data event into a category within a coding schema. This coding schema provides an overview over categories that are important for investigating a certain research question. You can either re-use an existing coding schema from other researchers who have investigated a similar research question or you can develop your own by means of task analysis.

After the verbal data have been coded, these coded events may be *scored*, i.e. positive or negative values may be assigned within a code. An utterance that is relevant for the task is a correct statement versus an incorrect statement would be an example. In that, "utterances relevant for the task" would be a category within a coding schema, while "correct versus incorrect" would be the score.

How the transcribed data are coded and scored depends on the purpose of the study in which the data are recorded, and the decision is part of your overall experimental design: what is the question your study wants to answer, and what verbal events would confirm or refute your hypothesis? Hence, verbal data can be coded and scored according to very different systems, depending on the research perspective, as stressed in the following.

Examplary coding schemas

The verbal data can either be recorded as performance or as process data. If they are recorded as performance data, the data should be scored according to whether the utterances are correct or wrong, complete or incomplete, and whether the relevant technical terms are mentioned. This is often the case, for instance, for free recall or self-explanation data.

If verbal data were recorded as process data, they can be coded in several ways. They may be coded according to their verbalization level, to the level of processing, to learning and other cognitive processes involved, or based on a cognitive task analysis. The following bullet points expand on these terms along with the tables that accompany them.

- A very common way to code the verbal data is to code them according to a prior *cognitive task analysis*. In his study of software users, J. P. Hansen (1991) categorized (substantive) speech events into three different categories ('cognitive', 'visual', 'manipulative'), and the same were used by Hyrskykari et al. (2008) and Holmqvist and Hanson (1999). Van Gog, Paas, Van Merriënboer, and Witte (2005) used 24 different categories for an electrical circuit problem-solving task. In a study where participants

Table 9.3 Major types of idea units appearing in speech when describing a scene; adapted from Holsanova (2008).

Function	Types of foci
Presentational	*substantive foci*: speakers describe the referents, states, and events in the scene. *summarizing foci*: speakers connect scene elements with similar characteristics at a higher level of abstraction and introduce them as a global gestalt. *localizing foci*: speakers state the spatial relations in the scene.
Orientational	*evaluative foci*: speaker judgement of the scene as a whole, the properties of the scene elements or relations between picture elements. *expert foci*: speaker judgements of scene genre or scene composition.
Organizational	*interactive foci*: speakers signal the start and the end of the description. *introspective foci* and *metatextual comments*: thinking aloud; memory processes; procedural comments, monitoring; expressing the scene content on a textual met-alevel; speech planning; speech recapitulation.

evaluated machine translation outputs, Doherty and O'Brien (2009) used five categories ('positive', 'negative', 'mixed', 'silent', and 'N/A'). Based on a task analysis where steps need to be performed to execute the task of classifying fish locomotion, Jarodzka, Scheiter, et al. (2010) coded verbal data according to categories of knowledge and understanding. In sum, if verbal data are scored according to a cognitive task analysis, the categories will vary across tasks and research questions.

- A coding schema based on *cognitive processes* in speech, as in Table 9.2, was devised by Chafe (1994), which subdivides utterances into different categories, e.g. substantive, contextual regulation, interactional, cognitive, and validative. Holsanova (2001), based on Chafe's system, used seven different types of 'ideas units' (substantive, summarizing, localizing, evaluative, expert, interactive, and introspective), in her study of picture viewing (Table 9.3).

- Another possibility is to score the data according to the three *verbalization* levels in Table 9.4 (Ericsson & Simon, 1993). Note that the higher the verbalization level, the more it interferes with the primary task and slows it down.

- Verbal reports may also be scored according to the different *levels of processing* (Craik & Lockhart, 1972). The exemplified levels of verbalizations in Table 9.5 can be used to indicate whether a content was processed on a surface or on a deep level.

- Furthermore, verbal reports may be scored according to *learning strategies* used: rehearsal, elaboration, overall control strategies, confirming comprehension, comprehension failure, and planning for further learning (Lewalter, 2003).

Irrespective of which coding system you use, you have to keep in mind that at least part of it needs to be coded by two independent raters. Only if the inter-rater reliability is high,

Table 9.4 Verbalization levels. Adapted from Ericsson and Simon (1993).

Level-1-verbalizations	The thoughts of the participant were verbalized directly. The content of the working memory existed already in a verbal code. Thus, the verbalizations represent the direct content of the working memory, without interposed processes in between attending to the working memory content and its verbalization.
Level-2-verbalizations	The content of the working memory existed initially in a non-verbal code. Thus, it needed to be converted into a verbal code before being verbalized. One example is verbalizations of mentally animating a picture of a dynamic system, like pulley systems. This level of verbalization is important to all research dealing with pictures, like scene perception, learning with multimedia, or inspecting advertisements.
Level-3-verbalizations	The participant's thoughts were filtered before verbalizing (most likely by instruction). In that, search and selection processes were interposed before the actual verbalization in order to compare the content of the working memory to the to-be-reported information. This level of verbalizations also occurs in verbalizing motor activities, like car driving, because those activities are normally not accessible to verbalizations.

Table 9.5 Surface and deep levels of processing. Adapted from Craik and Lockhart (1972).

Surface level of processing	For instance, pure verbalizations where no higher level of understanding is inferred, e.g. reading a text word-for-word.
Deep level of processing	Verbalizations which indicate recognizing the concepts referred to in an abstract sense. Comprehension, and the ability to extract meaning and relatedness between concepts referred to are necessary requisites of deep levels of processing.

may the remaining files be coded by one rater. Otherwise you have to re-think your coding schema.

9.2.3 Representations, measures, and statistical considerations for verbal data

Besides simple counting of the verbal unit, data representations similar to those in eye-movement data can be built. As a coded verbal event is a state similar to an AOI dwell, transitions between verbal codes can also be counted, for instance the number of instances in which a contextual verbal event is followed by a validational verbal event. A transition matrix which holds the number of each such transitions can easily be calculated, and measures we know from eye tracking applied to it. Also, both eye-movement data and verbal data count and numerosity data such as frequency, rates, etc. can be reported and different experimental groups can be compared statistically. To do so, you have to keep the following in mind.

The coded verbal data can have different levels of measurement, depending on the coding. If you have a coding without a certain order, the level of measurement is nominal, for instance if you code whether the participant mentioned one of n possible objects. If you have a coding that can be arranged into a meaningful order, the level of measurement is ordinal. This is the case if you assigned school marks (i.e. A, B, C...) to the verbal codes, since you used them as a performance measure. If you have a coding that has not only an order, but also the difference between two codes is always equal, then the level of measurement is interval. This might be the case, for instance, if participants have to recall a certain number of items. If your coding has an absolute zero point, then you have a ratio level of measurement. This is the case, for instance, in counting word numbers. Note that only in the case of interval and ratio data can you use parametric statistical tests. In other cases you have to use non-parametric tests (p. 90).

It is currently not systematically investigated exactly how extensive the similarity in analysis methods really is between eye-movement and verbal data.

9.2.4   Open issues: how to co-analyse eye-movement and verbal data

As we have seen, both data types pass through a similar procedure, from raw data over event detection and representations to measures. On each of these levels both data types can be compared. The first section in this chapter referred to a comparison on an event level, namely eye–voice latencies. Other research often triangulates both data types on a representation level. For instance, it may be compared whether participants verbally mention an area as often or in the same order as they look at it (e.g. Jarodzka, Scheiter, et al., 2010).

This said, it has to be kept in mind that both data types are very rich and require a vast amount of skills, effort, and time from the analyst. Hence, a researcher usually places an emphasis on one of these data sources, and very seldom are data sources investigated to their full potential. The big open issue in co-analysing verbal and eye-tracking data is to successfully triangulate both in an equally elaborate manner. Therefore, the eye-movement and the verbal data communities must start to recognize each other's presence far more and to learn from each other.

9.3   Summary: events and representations with auxiliary data

We have learned from this chapter that eye-tracking and auxiliary data sources can be analysed in conjunction. In that, the following steps are taken:

- Both data sources are aligned, either according to their onset or offset, or via a mediator.
- The **latency** events are established, with their onset time, duration, and references to the two events between which the latency is calculated.

Moreover, we learned that eye-tracking and verbal data can be triangulated. The triangulation can in principle take place on each level of the alike data preparation:

- As raw data, verbal data are audio files, while eye-tracking data are timestamps and (x, y)-coordinates. While in eye-tracking data events like fixations are detected with algorithms, in verbal data the event detection is usually done manually by identifying so-called idea units.

- Next, the verbal data are coded according to a schema selected (or developed) by the researcher.
- Finally, representations can be built of verbal data, and measures calculated on these representations.

Part III

Measures

In Part II we gave detailed descriptions of how to go about calculating oculomotor events from raw data samples, and also how to build meaningful representations from these eye-movements events. Part III of this book provides a comprehensive taxonomy of eye-movement measures. 'Measures' can be thought of as precisely quantifiable data which can be calculated taking events and/or representations as input. Measures are the *dependent variables* we explained in Chapter 3. From here statistical analysis can be performed, allowing you to understand what your data means in relation to your experimental design. Measures are thus more quantitative counterparts complimenting events and representations that are more qualitative in nature. Some 120 measures are discussed and evaluated in Part III from a vast literature search. The measures covered are grouped thematically according to commonalities in metrics. There are many overlapping and interchangeable terms concerning eye-movement measures, and our aim is to envelope the vast majority of terms and come up with the most appropriate "fit" in our taxonomy. It is therefore likely that if the reader does not find a measure addressed in a particular chapter of Part III, then it will be addressed in another chapter, and the reasoning for this placement has been thoroughly considered (see p. 463).

10   Movement Measures

The chapters in the first two parts of this book provide detailed information about the technology and skills necessary to conduct eye-tracking research (Part I), and how to process eye-tracking data after recording (Part II). In Part III, we cover the vast range of measures which can be calculated on the basis of the events and representations described in Part I. Measures of eye *movement* are many and diverse, and this is where we begin.

Eye-*movement* measures, as defined in this chapter, refer to different properties of movement events during a finite period of time. The properties of movement are *direction, amplitude, duration, velocity,* and *acceleration*.

Movement measure group	Uses	Page
Movement direction measures	*In what direction did the eye move?*	301
Movement amplitude measures	*How far did the eye move?*	311
Movement duration measures	*For how long did the eye move?*	321
Movement velocity measures	*How fast did the eye move?*	326
Movement acceleration measures	*How fast did the eye accelerate?*	332
Movement shape measures	*What is the shape of the eye movement?*	336
AOI order and transition measures	*How similar are movements in AOIs?*	339
Scanpath comparison measures	*How similar are two or more scanpaths?*	346

Also, all movements have the more ill-defined property *shape*. These six general properties of movements have generated the measures that are listed in Sections 10.1–10.6.

In Sections 10.7 and 10.8, we classify measures that quantify the order of movement through space: AOI visits and transition sequences between AOIs, and methods to calculate the similarity between pairs of eye-movement sequences (i.e. scanpaths).

Many of the movement measures have a ratio value type, which makes their usage statistically straightforward. However, some measures in the later sections require the use of more advanced statistics.

10.1   Movement direction measures

Movement direction measures pertain to single instances of movement events such as saccades, glissades, drifts, microsaccades, smooth pursuits, and scanpaths. Some but definitely not all of these events move along a straight line, but by no means always and definitely not all. The movement of saccades, glissades, and smooth pursuits can be curved, i.e. altering direction along the event. When we refer to a scanpath's direction we refer to its *overall* direction, if it has any directionality at all.

The resulting values are *direction of movement* (φ) in stimulus space or towards specified AOIs. Direction should not be confused with the angular distance (measured in degrees of visual angle (°)) the eye moves during the saccade, which is referred to as the *amplitude of movement*. The difference between these two parameters is illustrated in Figure 10.1.

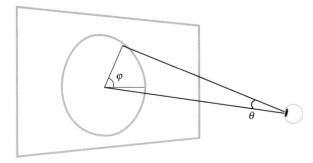

Fig. 10.1 For a saccade, the saccadic direction φ is the angle between the saccade and the horizontal axis in the coordinate system of the stimulus. The saccadic amplitude θ is the angular distance the eyes move during the saccade.

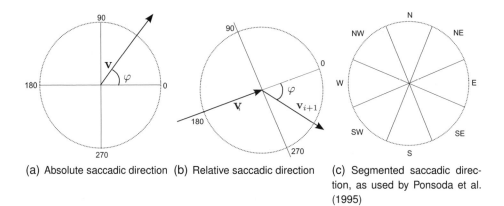

(a) Absolute saccadic direction   (b) Relative saccadic direction   (c) Segmented saccadic direction, as used by Ponsoda et al. (1995)

Fig. 10.2 Saccadic direction, sometimes also referred to as orientation.

Note that direction is a *circular*—angular—dimension (see Figure 10.2), and that this requires the use of circular statistics (see Batschelet, 1981 and Drew & Doucet, 1991 for the calculation of many sorts of descriptive and inferential statistics). While circular statistics have been widely used on eye-tracking data in neurological and biological studies (for instance, Snyder, Batista, & Andersen, 2000), they appear not to be an established analysis tool in the psychological and applied fields of eye-movement research.

10.1.1 Saccadic direction

Target question	*In what direction does the saccade take the eye?*
Input representation	*A saccade*
Output	*The direction φ (degrees)*

The saccadic direction, sometimes known as 'saccadic orientation', is the direction of any saccadic movement. Figure 10.3 describes how this calculation is done when zero is to the right and orientation order is counter-clockwise (the trigonometric version). Some studies instead use $0°$ for upward and a clockwise ordering of directions (the clock and compass version), which alters the calculations slightly.

There are several operational definitions of saccadic direction:

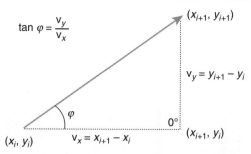

$$\tan \varphi = \frac{v_y}{v_x}$$

(x_{i+1}, y_{i+1})

$v_y = y_{i+1} - y_i$

φ

$0°$

(x_i, y_i) $v_x = x_{i+1} - x_i$ (x_{i+1}, y_i)

Fig. 10.3 Absolute saccadic direction φ for a saccade between fixations (x_i, y_i) and (x_{i+1}, y_{i+1}) can be calculated using basic trigonometry. Note that many saccades are curved and hence have varying directions along the trajectory. The saccadic direction only represents an ideal straight line from start to end point.

1. *Absolute saccadic direction* can be calculated based on the coordinates of the immediately preceding and consecutive fixations using simple trigonometry, if it is not already available from the event detection software (see Figure 10.2(a)).
2. *Relative saccadic direction* is calculated as the difference between the absolute saccadic directions of the current and the previous saccade (see Figure 10.2(b)).
3. *Segmented saccadic direction* means dividing—quantizing—the absolute saccadic direction into discrete bins. Ponsoda et al. (1995) and S. P. Lee, Badler, and Badler (2002) use eight segments as in Figure 10.2(c), while Gbadamosi (2000) uses 16 segments.
4. *Adduction, abduction, centrifugal,* and *centripetal* movement are common direction distinctions in binocular research (Collewijn et al., 1988). Adduction refers to saccades towards the nose; abduction refers to saccades away from the nose; centrifugal movement refers to saccades away from the central line of fixation; and lastly, centripetal movement refers to saccades towards the central line of fixation.

Other varieties of saccadic direction measures exist, for instance segmented relative direction, but they appear not to have been used.

Histograms of saccadic direction have previously been presented linearly. In the twenty-first century, they have gradually been replaced by circular histograms known as 'rose plots' (sometimes 'polar' or 'angular' plots). Figure 10.4 shows a linear histogram, as well as a rose plot from reading data.

Many studies that have used saccadic direction measures have been vision experiments with a central fixation cross surrounded by peripheral targets at fixed saccade angles. A linear histogram can show how many saccades are launched in each direction, and classical non-circular statistics can be used, since in such a study there is no need to calculate the average saccade direction or to compare distributions of saccade directions between tasks or conditions.

Another large user group of saccade direction measures are neurologists. The preparation and execution of saccades in different directions can then be compared to neuronal discharge or brain activation. These researchers use both rose plots and circular statistics.

Over the past ten years, a few studies of saccade direction have emerged in general picture or scene viewing. Rose plots are then an informative way of illustrating the results. The following are general observations about saccadic direction:

Reading conventions decide the predominant saccadic direction when viewing written text.

Scene viewing Most saccades are aligned with the picture horizon (Foulsham, Kingstone, & Underwood, 2008). Pictures of natural scenes are more affected by picture rotation

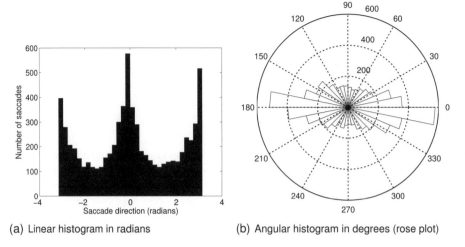

(a) Linear histogram in radians (b) Angular histogram in degrees (rose plot)

Fig. 10.4 Saccadic direction histograms for reading data. First a classical linear histogram, then an angular histogram (rose plot) for the same data. Bin size is π/16 radians (11.25 degrees).

than pictures of fractals (Foulsham & Kingstone, 2010). There is a clear tendency in scene viewing to make either horizontal or vertical, but more seldom oblique saccades (Tatler & Vincent, 2008; S. P. Lee et al., 2002; Mackworth & Bruner, 1970); horizontal saccades are more frequent, however.

Oblique saccades The few oblique saccades are pulled by dual muscle pairs, which are not always in perfect sync, and therefore tend to have a larger curvature than horizontal and vertical saccades (Viviani, Berthoz, & Tracey, 1977).

HV-ratio

Target question	Are saccades predominantly horizontal or vertical?
Input representation	A set of saccades
Output	The ratio of horizontal to vertical saccades

The horizontal to vertical (HV-) ratio is defined as the sum of all horizontal saccade amplitude components v_{hi} in a trial, divided by the sum of all vertical saccadic components v_{vi} in the trial. It is calculated as

$$\text{HV-ratio} = \frac{H}{W} \cdot \frac{\sum_i v_{hi}}{\sum_i v_{vi}} \tag{10.1}$$

where the H and W are the height and width of the stimulus, and the ratio $\frac{H}{W}$ normalizes for stimulus proportions.

Lau, Goonetilleke, and Shih (2001) used the HV-measure to study the difference in search direction between mainland and Hong Kong Chinese participants, finding that the search pattern differed significantly. They interpreted this result as reflecting the differences in reading direction between the two areas. This has implications for design where populations have differing reading directions.

Overall fixation vector

Target question	*Where are the fixations relative to the central gaze line?*
Input representation	*A set of fixations and a central gaze point*
Output	*Direction (degrees) and length (mm or pixels) of the overall fixation vector*

The overall fixation vector is an average direction of fixation positions from a central gaze point, which for monitors is simply the centre of the monitor. The fixation vector takes the number, position, and duration of fixations into account and indicates, on average, which part of a stimulus has received most attention. Given N fixations, the measure is calculated as

$$\text{Overall fixation vector} = \sum_{i=1}^{N} t_i v_i \qquad (10.2)$$

where $v_i = (x_i - x_c, y_i - y_c)$ represents a vector from the centre point (x_c, y_c) to the fixation position (x_i, y_i), and t_i is the duration of fixation i.

The measure was introduced by C. F. Chi and Lin (1997), who recorded data from participants viewing pre-recorded videos of car-driving situations. They argue that the overall fixation vector indicates visual workload. On urban roads, for instance, the overall fixation vector had an average length of 499 inches and a direction of 163° during daylight, while at night, the length was 751 inches and the direction 190°. The latter case would indirectly imply a greater workload.

The antisaccadic metrics

Target question	*To what degree can the participant inhibit reflexive saccades to suddenly appearing targets?*
Input representation	*Raw data samples recorded during antisaccade trials*
Output	*Proportion of errors in saccade direction and saccade latency (ms)*

Antisaccade metrics are a whole family of measures related to a specific task, and the core measure is saccade direction. The task is simple: have your participants looked at a central fixation cross, flash a peripheral target on one side, at which the participant must immediately look in the *opposite* direction. Antisaccade tasks can cause fatigue, so it is especially important that trial orders are randomized when the experiment is long.

The antisaccade metric is comprised of a collection of six measures illustrated in Figure 10.5(b). They all relate temporally to the onset of the target in the periphery which corresponds to time 0, marked in the figure with a dashed line. The *error latency* (A) is the time in ms it takes to launch a saccade towards the target. The *error amplitude* (B) is the saccadic amplitude towards the target. The *time to correct* (C) is the fixation duration (or dwell time if there are more fixations) at or near the target before the participant corrects himself by a saccade in the opposite direction. The *final eye position* (D) is the closest the eye reaches to the direct opposite mirror position of the target during the trial. *Correct antisaccade latency* (E) and *amplitude* (F) are the time from onset of the target until the correct saccade is launched, and the amplitude of that saccade, respectively. An additional metric is the *number of correct trials*.

The gap condition variety of the antisaccade task is when the the the central fixation cross offsets some time before the appearance of the peripheral target (so as to release attention from the centre, p. 430). As Hutton and Ettinger (2006) point out, in the gap condition, antisaccade errors are more common and correct antisaccade latencies are shorter.

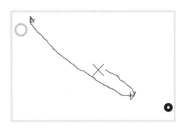

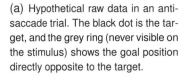

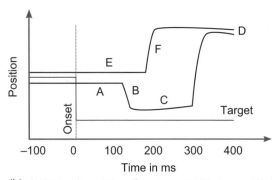

(a) Hypothetical raw data in an anti-saccade trial. The black dot is the target, and the grey ring (never visible on the stimulus) shows the goal position directly opposite to the target.

(b) Antisaccade metrics. One correct trial (upper black line) and one incorrect trial (lower black line). A: Error latency. B: Error amplitude. C: Time to correct. D: Final eye position. E: Correct antisaccade latency. F: Correct antisaccade amplitude. Modified from Hutton and Ettinger (2006).

Fig. 10.5 Antisaccade trial and measures.

Ettinger et al. (2003) found a between- but not within-session practice effect on the antisaccade task, and point out that this has to be considered with repeated testing of the same participants on different occasions. There are trial-by-trial effects also, as found by Tatler and Hutton (2007). For instance, after a successful trial, if the target appeared in the same hemifield on the next trial, the error rate is low and the primary saccade latency (E) is slightly reduced. Trial-by-trial effects call for a careful design of the experiment, or the introduction of more advanced statistical methods such as multilevel modelling.

Data validity in the antisaccade task also depends on how well participants' states are known. For instance, a large number of drugs and medications affect antisaccade behaviour. A precise and accurate diagnosis of participants is also crucial to the validity of antisaccade studies.

Poor participant performance may indicate that (prefrontal) voluntary control, and hence inhibition of reflexive saccades to the periphery, is poor, possibly due to a neurological impairment. The antisaccade paradigm is widely used in the field of neuropsychiatry (next to smooth pursuit tests), but is also used in several other areas of psychological research concerning eye-movement control.

Psychiatric disorders There is considerable evidence that genetic predisposition to schizophrenia can be diagnosed using antisaccadic metrics. Similarly, affective disorders, polar disorders, psychosis, obsessive compulsive disorder, Tourette's syndrom, attention deficit hyperactivity disorder, Alzheimer's desease, Huntington's disease, Lewy body dementia, palsy and Parkinson's disease show atypical effects in antisaccadic metrics (list from Hutton & Ettinger, 2006, p. 309). Prosaccades seem to be more impaired in neurological disorders than in the psychiatric ones. The precise neural and cognitive mechanisms underlying antisaccadic metrics are under debate, and the interpretation of data—as always—relates to how they were recorded.

Drugs and medication Many drugs have an effect on antisaccade performance, but not always in the way one would naturally assume. For instance, low levels of ethanol increase the proportion of correct antisaccades (Khan, Ford, Timney, & Everling, 2003), and nicotine reduces antisaccadic errors in participants who suffer from schizophrenia (Kumari & Postma, 2005).

Minor neurological damage The observation that greater distraction resulting from whiplash—experienced during a car crash most commonly, where the head is violently flung
backwards then forwards—may benefit from specific rehabilitation using the antisaccade task was tested by Mosimann, Muri, Felblinger, and Radanov (2000). Moreover,
very prematurely born children, although having largely normal control over saccades
and smooth pursuit as adults, make significantly more antisaccadic direction errors
(Newsham, Knox, & Cooke, 2007).

Age Children perform more poorly than adults on the antisaccade task, but error rates and
latencies will decrease as their prefrontal control develops. Older adults appear to make
more direction errors, and/or exhibit longer saccadic latencies for correct antisaccades
(Eenshuistra, Ridderinkhof, & Molen, 2004).

Working memory Several studies have shown that antisaccade measures are sensitive to
variations in working memory capacity (e.g. Kane, Bleckley, Conway, & Engle, 2001).

Direction of regressions, backtracks, look-aheads, and leading saccades

Target question	*Did the saccade bring the eye to a task relevant AOI?*
Input representation	*A saccade and an upcoming action*
Output	*Binary*

Regressions by definition are directed *in the opposite direction of the text*, and backtracks
in the opposite direction *of the previous saccade* (pp. 262–265). Their directions are not used
as measures but only as part of the event definition. Look-aheads are instead movements
towards upcoming activities, such as looking at the soap some time before reaching towards
it in order to make sure that it is there for later hand-washing use. The direction of a look-
ahead saccade is given by the task and not by established (reading) conventions or absolute
angular directions. Although researchers talk about 'look-ahead fixations', it is the saccade
that moves the eye to the look-ahead position.

The look-ahead concept assumes that look-ahead fixations are limited in time and number,
and that tasks preceding the use of the object which receives a look-ahead fixation require
visual attention. If using a greasy tool like a spanner, for instance, this task requires attention
up until completed, even though the next planned action is to wash your hands, indicated by a
look-ahead fixation to some soap near the the the sink. The following factors have been observed
regarding the direction of look-aheads:

Speech planning Participants describing a picture often look ahead to objects soon to be
described (Holsanova, 2008).

Physical task requirements Within a hand-washing task, participants looked ahead at a
soap dispenser, towel dispenser, and waste bin significantly more often than with a
cup-filling task (Pelz & Canosa, 2001). Similar task-dependency has been observed
with tea- and sandwich-making actions (Land et al., 1999; Hayhoe, 2000).

Accuracy in guidance Mennie et al. (2007) found that look-ahead saccades may facilitate
the accuracy of the future eye movement that guides the upcoming action.

Leading saccades are another type of eye movement linked to an upcoming action. These
are saccades with an amplitude over $1°$ that occur during smooth pursuit. A leading saccade
is directed *in the direction that the participant expects of the target motion*, but the leading
saccade skips over the target, and is followed by a period of slow pursuit so that the target
can catch up with the eye. In other words, the eye's movement is slower than the target's so

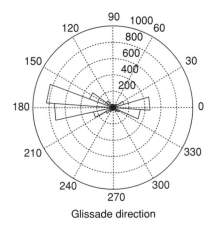

Glissade direction

Fig. 10.6 Direction of glissades, in circular degrees, during reading. Glissades were calculated using the algorithm described in Nyström & Holmqvist, 2010.

that the two can become aligned. Like many smooth pursuit measures, 'leading saccades' are used in research on schizophrenia (e.g. R. G. Ross et al., 1999).

10.1.2 Glissadic direction

Target question	*In what direction does the glissade take the eye?*
Input representation	*A glissade*
Output	*Direction φ (degrees)*

Glissadic direction is a measure of the orientation of the small movement appended to many saccades that we call glissades (p. 182). Just like saccadic direction, it can be calculated from the start and end points, although in reality glissades are very curved, even more so than saccades. Figure 10.6 shows a rose plot of glissadic direction during reading of English (study 1 on page 5). It can been seen that the majority of glissades go in the opposite direction of forward reading saccades; this is what should be expected since a glissade is an event that often swings the eye backwards compared to saccade direction.

10.1.3 Microsaccadic direction

Target question	*In what direction does the microsaccade take the eye?*
Input representation	*A microsaccade*
Output	*Direction φ (degrees)*

Microsaccade direction is a measure of the orientation of transient, fixational micro-movements of the eye. Once the start and end point of the movement have been found, the direction can be calculated the same way as for saccades and glissades.

The distribution of microsaccade orientation is very similar to ordinary saccades, with a strong dominance for horizontal and vertical directions, as data in Figure 10.7 from Engbert (2006) illustrate. Interestingly, vertical microsaccades seem to be largely monocular.

Studies making use of the microsaccade direction measure are common in neurology, and scarce elsewhere. Rolfs, Engbert, and Kliegl (2005) found that when playing sounds on one side of the participant, microsaccades moved in the opposite direction of the sound within 100–200 ms. But when additionally showing visual stimuli on the same side, a second

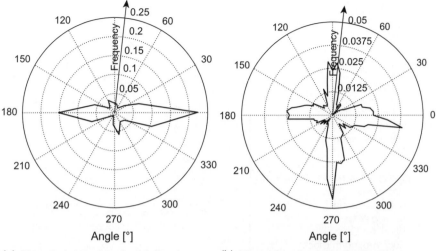

(a) Binocular microsaccade direction. (b) Monocular microsaccade direction.

Fig. 10.7 Distributions of microsaccade directions for binocular (a) and monocular (b) microsaccades. Reprinted from *Progress in Brain Research, 154*(1), Ralf Engbert, pp. 177–192, Copyright (2006), with permission from Elsevier.

microsaccade moves the eye back towards the visual stimulus. Rolfs et al. conclude that auditory and visual information are integrated even at the microsaccadic level. Engbert and Kliegl (2003) found that microsaccade direction reflects the locus of visual attention, a view that is not shared by Horowitz, Fine, Fencsik, Yurgenson, and Wolfe (2007). In fact, there is an ongoing debate concerning how biases in microsaccade direction are related to covert attention shifts and motor programming (Martinez-Conde et al., 2009).

10.1.4 Smooth pursuit direction

Target question	In what direction does smooth pursuit take the eye?
Input representation	A period of smooth pursuit
Output	Average or individual smooth pursuit direction (degrees)

Smooth pursuit direction is a measure that may appear to attribute a single direction to a characteristic of eye movements which is considerably varied—smooth pursuits can track a stimulus as it moves between a multitude of locations, thus giving a range of directions within one smooth pursuit. It is only possible, therefore, to attribute an objective measure of smooth pursuit direction if we allow the direction value to change along the smooth pursuit path. From the point of view of smooth pursuit detection, this is often achieved by dividing long periods of pursuit into smaller pursuits, interleaved with catch-up saccades. As an alternative, a momentous direction value between any two points ((x_i, y_i) and (x_{i+1}, y_{i+1})) along the path, can be calculated as in Figure 10.3 by replacing fixations with raw data samples. High precision data is required or the measure will have very noisy values.

Smooth pursuit has directional preference: most humans and primates tend to be better at horizontal than vertical smooth pursuit. This is defined by the ability to initiate smooth pursuit quickly and to pursue smoothly without making catch-up saccades, which is worse when the required pursuit target moves along the vertical axis. For these vertical pursuits, moreover, most humans are better at downward than upward pursuit (Rottach et al., 1996). Horizontal

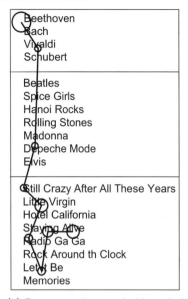

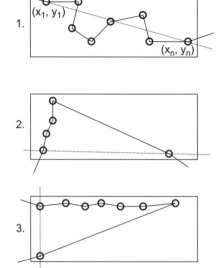

(a) Free scanpath 'sweep' with vertical direction, adapted from Aaltonen et al. (1998).

(b) Scanpath direction in AOIs. Dashed lines indicate the operational definition by Renshaw et al. (2003).

Fig. 10.8 Scanpath directions. An example of a free vertical downward scanpath (a). Illustration of the operational definition of scanpath direction as the dotted line through the first and the last fixation in the AOI (b; 1). Examples of when the definition is not intuitive (b; 2 and 3).

superiority of smooth pursuit in the visual system is often related to the extensive experience of following objects in motion along the horizontal meridian (Collewijn & Tamminga, 1984).

The ability to elicit smooth pursuit in many directions is commonly studied in the assessment of neurological disorders. The neurological sites that subserve smooth pursuit mechanisms, or the effect of medication on smooth pursuit in neurological conditions, can therefore be examined. However, very few studies have made use of smooth pursuit direction as a measure in its own right.

With the purpose of developing a detection algorithm, Agustin (2010) used relative sample-to-sample directions within a moving window to, after saccade detection, separate pursuit samples from fixation samples. When the variance of relative sample-to-sample directions was low, pursuit was more likely than fixation and vice versa.

10.1.5 Scanpath direction

Target question	*In what direction did the scanpath take the eye?*
Input representation	*A scanpath (and sometimes an AOI)*
Output	*The direction of the scanpath (degrees)*

Scanpath direction is a measure of the *general* direction of a sequence of fixations and saccades while scanning a stimulus. Like smooth pursuit, the whole scanpath can change its direction many times over time. Therefore, it is more common to measure direction on smaller, local parts of the scanpath. If these smaller parts consist of individual saccades, the scanpath direction measure simplifies to a standard saccade direction measure.

There exist at least two different ways of quantifying scanpath direction. First, detecting sweeps (p. 267) and calculating an average direction for it. In lack of sweep events, a second way of quantifying scanpath direction is to operationalize it in terms of direction through AOIs. Renshaw et al. (2003) define a measure of scanpath direction through AOIs, and refer to this with the term 'gaze orientation', defined according to the following equation:

$$\text{Scanpath direction} = \frac{y_n - y_1}{x_n - x_1} \tag{10.3}$$

where (x_1, y_1) and (x_n, y_n) are the coordinates of the first and last fixations in the AOI respectively. Figure 10.8(b) shows the principle. Scans with a ratio of up to 1 were designated as horizontal whereas those with ratios greater than 1 were designated vertical. Using the trigonometric calculation in Figure 10.3 would instead give the direction in degrees. In either case, this operational definition is very sensitive to the positions of the first and last fixations, which may be misleading, as Figure 10.8(b) exemplifies.

Scanpath direction is indicative of search strategy according to Aaltonen et al. (1998), an interpretation which is shared by Renshaw et al. (2003), Poole and Ball (2005) and other usability researchers. The scanpath direction measure appears to be used sparingly, however.

10.2 Movement amplitude measures

Movement amplitudes concern events such as *saccades, scanpaths, smooth pursuit, glissades,* and *microsaccades. Amplitude* has two common operational definitions (Figure 10.9). The first refers to the shortest distance between the start and end point of a movement, i.e. the displacement, and the second is the total distance along the trajectory of the movement between the start and end points. The latter can be approximated by multiplying the average velocity of the movement by its duration. Since many types of eye movements do not follow a straight path, these operational definitions are often different.

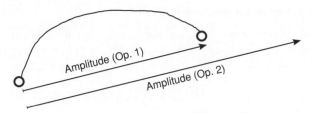

Fig. 10.9 The two definitions of saccade amplitude. Amplitude according to the first operational definition (Op. 1) is the shortest path between the end points, known as the Euclidian distance, whereas the second (Op. 2) refers to the total distance covered by the saccade along its trajectory. Amplitude according to Op. 2 can be seen as taking the end points of a curved saccade, and stretching the saccade until it forms a straight line.

Both operational definitions are used in journal articles and research reports, but only occasionally is it explicitly stated which is meant. For example, Smeets and Hooge (2003) use the Euclidian definition 1 in Figure 10.9, as do the earlier SR Research manuals from around year 2000, while later EyeLink manuals (SR Research, 2007) and SMI Technical Notes (SMI, 2007) propose a calculation according to definition 2, namely:

$$\theta = \frac{1}{1000} (t_{\text{offset}} - t_{\text{onset}}) \dot{\theta} \tag{10.4}$$

where $\dot{\theta}$ [°/s] is the average velocity of the saccade, and $(t_{\text{offset}} - t_{\text{onset}})$ the saccade duration in ms. If you have not written your own software for calculation of amplitude, beware of whether the program you use calculates amplitude according to the first or the second operational definition.

10.2.1 Saccadic amplitude

Target question	*Across what distance did the saccade take the eye?*
Input representation	*A saccade*
Output	*The amplitude of the saccade (pixels or degrees)*

The saccadic amplitude (earlier 'magnitude', and in reading research, 'size') is the distance travelled by a saccade from its onset to the offset. The unit is typically given in visual degrees (°) or pixels, but has also been segmented into 16 discrete categories by Gbadamosi (2000). Saccadic amplitude is much used in itself, as well as in combinations to form complex measures.

If glissades are appended to preceding saccades in your event detection algorithms, the saccadic amplitude will be somewhat shorter, while adding it to the following fixation will make the amplitudes longer. Event-detection algorithms with too high a threshold also leave out raw data samples that could be argued to belong to the saccade and hence underestimate saccadic amplitude.

'Interfixation distances' are a coarse approximation of saccadic amplitudes. Interfixation distances are calculated as the Euclidean distance between fixation points (Megaw & Richardson, 1979), and are typically used on low-speed, low-precision eye-trackers, or when for other reasons, saccade measurements cannot be made. There is always a danger that some event other than saccades, such as a blink or lost data samples, is hidden between what the detection algorithm considers to be fixations, and then interfixation distances do not equate to saccadic amplitudes.

Important properties of saccadic amplitude

Saccadic amplitude is *idiosyncratic* for most participants, like fixation durations and several of the other basic oculomotor measures. This means that one person's parameters are different from another person's, irrespective of task. For instance, although data from the reading to music study (study 2 on p. 5) have highly significant ($0.90 < r < 0.98$) correlations *within the individual* across all four reading tasks, there is much less consistency *between individuals*. Participants have their idiosyncratic defaults.

Saccades larger than about 15° are often inaccurate, failing to reach the intended target; in such cases they are commonly followed by another, corrective saccade (Becker & Fuchs, 1969). This difficulty in making longer saccades is a motor property of the saccadic system, which has been studied using the amplitude-based measures saccadic gain (p. 452), and the main sequence (p. 316).

Large saccades are often followed by small corrective saccades, but otherwise there appears to be no systematic relationship between the amplitudes of successive saccades (Motter & Belky, 1998). It is worth noting, however, that this conclusion is based on primate eye-movement research, and may not generalize. Tatler and Vincent (2008) found some evidence for sequences of short amplitude saccades in scene viewing (see p. 266), indicative of focused inspection of details. This was not the case for long saccades, which showed no consistent patterns in terms of sequences.

Saccadic amplitudes can be made shorter by flashing a light at the time of the onset of the saccade. This is known as 'saccadic compression' (J. Ross et al., 1997), and reveals the mechanisms by which we update our perceptual experience of what we are viewing so that it

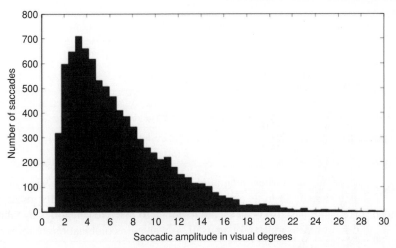

Fig. 10.10 Histogram over saccadic amplitudes (bin size 0.6°) during scene viewing (natural photographs shown on a computer screen). Recorded with a tower-mounted system at 1250 Hz, and saccades derived using the velocity-based algorithm in BeGaze 2.1 with a peak velocity setting of 40°/s.

remains consistent across eye movements.

The size of the stimulus image influences the mean and median saccadic amplitudes (Von Wartburg et al., 2007). When there is no stimulus, as in mental imagery studies, Zangemeister and Liman (2007) found that saccadic amplitudes are shorter than during real picture viewing. Humphrey and Underwood (2008), however, found the opposite trend when comparing amplitudes from imagery to picture encoding.

When recording binocular eye movements, the saccades recorded from each eye often have slightly different amplitudes (Kenyon, Ciuffreda, & Stark, 1980).

Amplitude values and usage of the measure

Saccadic amplitudes from scene viewing are distributed with a very clear rightward skew, as illustrated in Figure 10.10. This means that participants are more likely to saccade towards a location within the proximal vicinity of the last fixation, with large exploratory saccades to new locations being increasingly rare. For reading data, the skew is even larger (Figure 10.11).

Saccadic amplitude is one of the most used eye-movement measures. During reading, for instance, saccadic amplitude is known to adapt to combined physical, physiological, and cognitive factors. Reading saccades are limited in length by the visual spanwidth, which is around 7–8 letters (2°) in the average reading situation (Rayner, 1998). It would be detrimental to understanding to make such long saccades that you fail to see some parts of the words, and therefore reading saccades must be on average 7–8 letters long.

When using other stimuli than text, saccadic amplitudes also adapt to task demands, workload, the stimulus, and the needs of the current cognitive process. *Decreased saccadic amplitudes* have been found in relation to:

Search task difficulty Saccadic amplitudes are shorter in more difficult search tasks (e.g. Zelinsky & Sheinberg, 1997). Using a search task and studying performance improvements, Phillips and Edelman (2008) found that saccade metrics (primarily saccade amplitude) accounted for much more of the variability and improvement in performance than did fixation duration.

Increased cognitive load With increasingly demanding counting complexity, May, Kennedy,

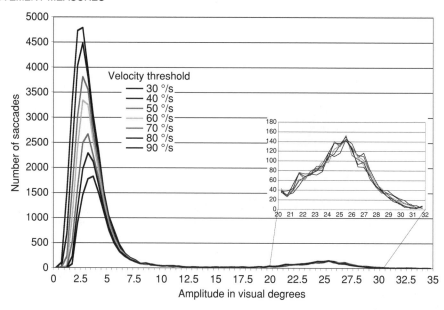

Fig. 10.11 The distribution of saccadic amplitudes with 10 participants while reading (study 1 on page 5). Bin size 0.5°. For larger velocity threshold settings, the velocity-based event detection algorithm outputs much fewer saccades in the lower amplitudes, in particular the many short reading saccades below 5°. Longer saccades, here exemplified by the return sweeps at around 25°, are not affected at all, since their velocity peaks are far above any of the thresholds.

Williams, Dunlap, and Brannan (1990) found a reduction in saccadic amplitude. Ceder (1977) and Troy, Chen, and Stern (1972) also found that when task time increases, the number of saccades with amplitudes above 9.5° decreases. Car drivers who perform cognitive operations unrelated to driving have a smaller 'saccadic extent' (Recarte & Nunes, 2003). Reduced saccadic extent has implications for mobile phone use when driving because this may encourage engagement in mental activity about things which are not physically present, or task relevant. These findings have been interpreted as an effect of cognitive load, resulting in 'tunnel vision' (L. J. Williams, 1988), which restricts the amplitude of saccades.

Careful inspection versus meaningfulness When a participant inspects an object carefully, saccades are shorter than during overview scans (Buswell, 1935). This observation has developed into the scanpath event ambient/focal (p. 266), but it is also part in the focal/global measure (p. 338). Interestingly, in usability research, larger saccadic amplitudes have been interpreted as a sign of *more* meaningful visual clues than shorter ones (Goldberg et al., 2002).

Adaptation to memory load When stipulated to do so, large saccadic amplitudes can be avoided by participants. Moreover, visual memory usage increases to compensate for the less often updated access to visual information (Phillips & Edelman, 2008; Inamdar & Pomplun, 2003). The avoidance of making long saccades is the effect of a cost, which the authors do not specify clearly, but which could relate to the main sequence measure described on page 316.

The onset of brain injury If saccadic amplitudes become inaccurate, due to neurological injury or growth, the brain adapts and corrects the saccades back to correct amplitude sizes (McLaughlin, 1967). This has given rise to neurobiological research on 'saccadic adaptation' that is focused on understanding the neural site for saccadic plasticity.

High-frequency visual information When free-viewing natural scenes, shorter saccades ($<$ 8°) appear to be driven by high-frequency information at the landing position, while longer saccades are scale independent (Tatler, Baddeley, & Vincent, 2006). Basically, our eyes are drawn towards areas containing detail near to where we are already looking. Longer saccades are more exploratory, because peripheral vision cannot disambiguate coarse and fine visual detail further away from the fovea.

A lower error tolerance in pursuit Catch-up saccades in smooth pursuit are made to compensate for participant tracking error, and many short saccades have been taken as an index of low tolerance for position error, while long saccades are made after a large tracking error has occurred, according to the overview in O'Driscoll and Callahan (2008).

Beginning, poor, and dyslexic readers When children first learn to read, saccades have an amplitude corresponding to the distance between letters. Poor readers and readers with dyslexia also exhibit shorter than average amplitudes (Rayner & Pollatsek, 1989).

Oral reading In oral reading, average saccadic amplitude falls to around 6 letters (1.5°), while during music reading and typing, saccades are a mere 1° on average (Rayner & Pollatsek, 1989).

Decreased musical tempo For participants reading musical scores, Kinsler and Carpenter (1995) found that the mean saccadic amplitude increased as the tempo of the music increased.

Lower participant age Young children exhibited shorter amplitudes than adults when examining pictures of familiar scenes (Mackworth & Bruner, 1970).

When the distances are very small, it may be detrimental to make saccades (Kowler & Steinman, 1977). In this study participants were asked to count thin bars 7–14 arcmin apart. The results showed that participants performed better if they made fewer saccades (Kowler & Steinman, 1977). The authors hypothesize that at this scale, attention can move without accompanying saccades. In other words, in some circumstances it may be favourable to preserve the image on the retina and tune attentional resolution than to make saccades.

The skewness of saccadic amplitude distribution

Target question	*Do shorter or longer saccadic amplitudes dominate?*
Input representation	*A set of saccades from a trial or whole recording*
Output	*A skewness value for the frequency distribution*

Skewness refers to the degree of asymmetry in the distribution of saccadic amplitudes. It should not be confused with the skew of the saccadic velocity profile, the 'saccadic skewness' (p. 333). As Figures 10.10 and 10.11 show, saccadic amplitude distributions are heavily skewed, and the degree of skewness is task dependent. Characteristic for a skewed distribution is that the mode, the median, and the mean do not coincide. For saccadic amplitudes, fixation durations, and many other eye-movement measures, the distribution tends to be skewed to the right (positive skew), indicating that the portion under the curve is larger on the right side of the mode than on the left side. There are several ways of calculating skewness, and, unfortunately, it is not always clear from journal papers which mathematical definition was used. One definition is based on the distance between the sample mean and the sample median. Another definition is based on the difference between the sample mean and the sample mode. In both cases, the larger this distance, the more skewed is the distribution. A third common definition is (Crawley, 2005)

$$\text{skewness} = \frac{\sum(X - \overline{X})^3/N}{s^3} \tag{10.5}$$

where $X, \overline{X}$ and N represent an amplitude value, the average amplitude, and the number of amplitude values, respectively. Often this value is divided by the approximate standard error $\sqrt{\frac{6}{N}}$, yielding a standard score. A non-significant value (roughly between -2 and $+2$) indicates that the distribution is normal. A value that falls outside that range is an indication that the distribution is skewed. The standard error may also be used to estimate the confidence interval of a distribution's skewness, and, consequently, also be used as an indication of whether one distribution is significantly more skewed than another.

As a hypothetical example, consider distribution A with a skewness of 0, with a standard error equal to 1. Distribution B has a skewness of 1.5 and a standard error of 2. Since there is considerable overlap in the two confidence intervals[27] $[-1.96, 1.96]$ for A and $[-2.42, 5.42]$ for B, we can not conclude that the distribution in B is significantly more skewed than that in A.

Reported values for the skewness of the saccadic amplitude distribution range from 0.5 to 1.2. Many of the effects on saccadic amplitude are likely to also affect this skewness measure, but few of them have been examined. Two exceptions are:

The task may change the skewness (Welchman & Harris, 2003).

The monitor size does effect the skewness value (Von Wartburg et al., 2007).

Inflection point of main sequence

Target question	At which amplitude are motor neurons bursting at full throttle?
Input representation	A set of saccades
Output	An inflection point

The *main sequence* is a systematic relationship between specific pairs of saccadic parameters, in particular the saccadic amplitude and the peak velocity (Bahill et al., 1975b). The shorter saccades form a dense set with an almost linear relation to peak velocity. Above a certain velocity—called the *inflection point*—longer saccades have another slope, and in naturalistic data also often a more variable velocity. Such data are illustrated in Figure 10.12(a).

Some authors argue that if another event (such as a microsaccade) adheres to the same main sequence as the saccade, then that other event is also of a saccadic nature. Figure 10.12(b) shows that microsaccades obey the main sequence, and Figure 10.13 that glissades do also.

The *inflection point* is the point on the main sequence curve where this systematic relationship ends. It is typically reached for saccades with amplitudes between 15° and 20°. This inflection point has been interpreted as the point at which motor neurons are bursting at full throttle, after which further increase will require greater effort, and saccadic gain will be lower (Bahill et al., 1975b).

Van Opstal and Van Gisbergen (1987) and Smit, Van Gisbergen, and Cools (1987) argue that the data used to study the main sequence need to take into account both the saccadic skew and the slow-moving saccades, which had previously been ignored and removed from analysis. Note that when recording with search coils, the saccadic velocity is reduced for longer amplitudes. In the worst case scenario, this could undermine a correct main sequence calculation (p. 326 and Träisk et al., 2005).

The main sequence has been used to build and test neurological models of saccade generation, and appears virtually unused in other research using eye movements. The measure

---

[27] As the z value for a 95% confidence value equals 1.96·standard error.

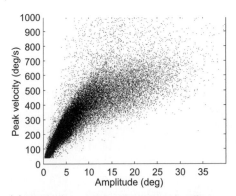

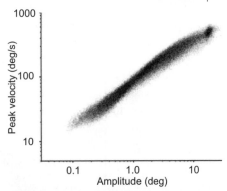

(a) Illustration of the main sequence effect using 57668 saccades. An inflection point can be seen at around 10°. The saccades are generated with the velocity algorithm and a threshold of 40°/s. Data from the mathematical problem solving project, number 4 on page 5.

(b) Microsaccadic main sequence to left (below circa 0.8°) softly overlap with the lower end of the saccadic main sequence. Reprinted from *Trends in Neurosciences, 32*(9), Susana Martinez-Conde, Stephen L. Macnick, Xoana G. Troncoso, and David H. Hubel, Microsaccades: a neurophysiological analysis, pp. 463–475, Copyright (2009), with permission from Elsevier.

Fig. 10.12 The main sequence.

is often used in combination with the saccadic gain/accuracy measure (Ciuffreda & Tannen, 1995).

Epelboim et al. (1997) showed that participants who tapped sequences on 3D targets located on a table in front of them exhibited a different main sequence than when they were just looking at the objects.

Main sequences for humans and monkeys are significantly different during free viewing of dynamic stimuli (D. J. Berg et al., 2009). For all amplitudes in this study, monkeys had faster velocities than humans.

10.2.2 Glissadic amplitude

Target question	*How far did the glissade bring the eye?*
Input representation	*A glissade*
Output	*An amplitude (degrees)*

The glissade amplitude is the length of the small movement that is often appended to saccades. Amplitude calculation is identical to that of saccades (p. 312). As Figure 10.13 shows, glissades have similar dynamics to saccades, and extend the saccadic main sequence. Glissadic amplitudes are typically less than 1°, and glissades "appear to serve no useful purpose" (Kapoula et al., 1986, p. 386). Neither does there seem to be a correlation between the amplitude of a saccade and its subsequent glissade (Nyström & Holmqvist, 2010).

10.2.3 Microsaccadic amplitude

Target question	*How far did the microsaccade bring the eye?*
Input representation	*A drift or microsaccade*
Output	*An amplitude (degrees)*

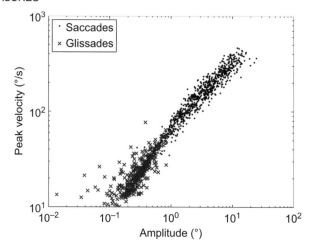

Fig. 10.13 Glissades extend the main sequence of saccades. Reading data at 1250 Hz. Saccades and glissades detected with the algorithm developed by Nyström and Holmqvist (2010).

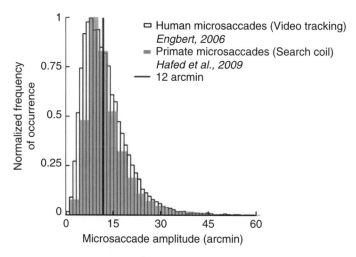

Fig. 10.14 Microsaccade amplitudes have a similar skewed distribution to ordinary saccades. 60 arcmin = 1°. Reprinted from *Trends in Neurosciences, 32*(9), Susana Martinez-Conde, Stephen L. Macnick, Xoana G. Troncoso, and David H. Hubel, Microsaccades: a neurophysiological analysis, pp. 463–475, Copyright (2009), with permission from Elsevier.

Microsaccadic amplitude calculation is identical to that of saccades (p. 312). The distribution of microsaccadic amplitude very much resembles that of saccades, only smaller in scale, as illustrated by Figure 10.14.

In the dark, both drift and microsaccades are 2–3 times larger than in light, while torsional drift remains the same as in light. Morisita and Yagi (2001) interpret this difference as showing that foveal displacement is necessary to detect and correct drift. Torsional drift alone implies peripheral displacement but not foveal displacement, which would not be enough.

Rolfs, Kliegl, and Engbert (2008) found a significant decrease in microsaccadic amplitude owing to the inhibition induced shortly after the onset of a visual stimulus, and argue that this could reflect activity in the central motor map.

10.2.4 Smooth pursuit length

Target question	*How long is the smooth pursuit event?*
Input representation	*A smooth pursuit event*
Output	*Length (degrees or pixels)*

The length of a smooth pursuit period is the distance travelled from pursuit onset to off-set. With natural stimuli, the measure is operationalized either as the sum of all distances between raw data samples along the path or as the product of the pursuit duration with its average velocity. As with saccades, the amplitude of smooth pursuit can also be calculated as the shortest distance between the points of on- and offset. However, this assumes that the smooth pursuit direction remains relatively constant. Square-wave jerks, catch-up, back-up, and leading saccades may all occur during smooth pursuit, and may cause the detection algorithm to miscalculate the length.

'Smooth pursuit amplitude' sometimes refers to the distance between the extreme points of the pursuit path with sinusoidal stimuli.

When the recording is made with a controlled stimulus target, the length of perfect pursuit should equal the distance that the target travels. However, poor tracking is usually measured with the smooth pursuit gain measure (p. 450). In studies with natural stimuli, smooth pursuit can go on and off many times, resulting in a multitude of events of varying lengths.

Since general smooth pursuit detection algorithms have been difficult to develop, the smooth pursuit length measure is very little used.

10.2.5 Scanpath length

Target question	*How long is the scanpath?*
Input representation	*A scanpath*
Output	*Length (degrees or pixels)*

Scanpath length is often defined as the sum of all saccadic amplitudes in a scanpath. As many studies using this measure record data that do not allow for saccade curvature measurements, the Euclidean distance (Op. 1 in Figure 10.9) of saccadic amplitude is used in scanpath length calculations. In order to account for saccadic curvature, and to circumvent peculiarities in event detection algorithms, scanpath length can also be calculated for raw sample scanpaths as the sum of distances between samples. Note however, that when using raw data samples for scanpath length calculation, the result is dependent on the sampling frequency of the eye-tracker, much in the same way that the length of a coastline depends on the length of the yardstick used to measure it. Moreover, a poorer precision in the data increases the scanpath length. For these reasons, reported absolute length values cannot always be trusted.

As an example of this, in studies of the face viewing behaviour of schizophrenic, autistic, and socially phobic patients, some researchers present both versions of scanpath length, one based on raw samples, and the other based on fixation/saccade data (Loughland, Williams, & Harris, 2004; M. J. Green, 2006; M. J. Green et al., 2008). These authors all report large differences between the scanpath length calculated from raw data samples compared to when calculated from fixations. Horley et al. (2004) write that "raw scanpath length [was] included to ensure that group differences in fixation scanpath length were not simply due to group differences in the number of fixations." The authors detected fixations using the I-DT algorithm using a minimum duration criterion of 200 ms with a dispersion criterion of 1°, and report that fixation based scanpaths are between 25–40% of the raw scanpath length. Much of this difference can probably be explained by the very high duration threshold, which undermines the detection of many fixations and hence makes the scanpath shorter (p. 148).

If trials—or separate tasks—have different durations, it may be necessary to divide the scanpath length by the duration of the trial. In principle, this results in an eye-movement speed measure (in the unit °/s), closely related to average saccadic velocity (p. 330). If scanpath length is not calculated over trials in full, a major challenge to an accurate calculation of scanpath lengths is in choosing the starting and ending points of the scanpath portion measured. In longer or self-paced tasks, the choice of scanpath start and end fixation is not obvious, and care must be taken so you can properly justify your cut off points.

Scanpath length as a measure has been used to:

Evaluate interfaces The optimal scanpath for a given task should be a straight line to a desired target. An unduly long scanpath could indicate non-meaningful representations or poor layout. With these assumptions, Goldberg and Kotval (1999) did observe a significant difference between scanpath lengths in good and poor user interfaces for a writing and drawing task. Renshaw et al. (2003) likewise also observed a strong significant difference in scanpath lengths between a poor and a good visual design of a graph. In both cases, the better design gave a smaller total scanpath length. Simonin, Kieffer, and Carbonell (2005) tested four different designs of digital photo albums, presenting photos either radially (star-formed), elliptically, as a square matrix, or just randomly positioned. The shortest scanpath length was found for elliptical layouts, which (together with a shortest search time) made the authors interpret it as being the most visually comfortable.

Approximate more complex concepts The term 'restricted scanpath' has been operationalized using scanpath length (p. 259). Generally, results show that participants with schizophrenia have a shorter—hence restricted—scanpath, and those with social phobia a significantly longer raw scanpath when looking at faces compared to controls.

10.2.6 Blink amplitude

Target question	*What distance does the eyelid travel during the blink?*
Input representation	*A blink*
Output	*An amplitude (mm)*

Blink amplitude is defined as the distance travelled by the eyelid, as illustrated in Figure 10.17 on page 325. This distance is not accurately measured with pupil and corneal reflection eye-trackers, but needs to be measured electro-oculographically or using dedicated eyelid trackers. Note that if the eye is slightly closed when the blink starts, the blink will have a smaller amplitude than if the blink starts from a fully open position. This fact is the foundation for using blink amplitude as a measure of workload, fatigue, and drowsiness.

According to Carney and Hill (1982) and Wolkoff, Nøjgaard, Troiano, and Piccoli (2005), for 80% of blinks, the descending upper eyelid covers more than two thirds of the cornea. For about 18%, the descending eyelid covers less than that; and around 2% of blinks are twitch blinking (flutter).

When blink amplitude decreases, performance errors in flight simulators increase for sleep deprived pilots (Morris & Miller, 1996). Blink amplitude was found to be a better predictor of performance than either blink rate or blink closure.

10.3 Movement duration measures

Movement duration measures all pertain to the time the movement took. Given the onset and offset, duration is trivial to calculate. The major challenge instead lays in detecting proper start and end points of the movement event.

10.3.1 Saccadic duration

Target question	*How long does the saccade take?*
Input representation	*A saccade*
Output	*Duration (ms)*

Saccadic duration ('transition time'; not the same as transitions between AOIs) is defined as the time the saccade takes to move between two fixations or instances of smooth pursuit. Onset of saccades is easy to calculate, but offset is ambiguous due to glissades, which can increase or decrease the duration of single saccades by up to 50% (Nyström & Holmqvist, 2010). Blinks also interfere with saccadic durations: when 20° saccades co-occur with a blink, their durations increase on average by 36% (Rottach, Das, Wohlgemuth, Zivotofsky, & Leigh, 1998) (horizontal only) and (Rambold, Sprenger, & Helmchen, 2002) (both horizontal and vertical).

Saccadic duration (in milliseconds, ms) is closely related to saccadic amplitude (in degrees visual angle, °). This relation has been found by Carpenter (1988) to be

$$duration = 2.2 \cdot amplitude + 21 \qquad (10.6)$$

The measure is sensitive to the same weaknesses as saccadic amplitude of event detection algorithms. Collewijn et al. (1988) report that centrifugal saccades larger than 15° have significantly longer durations than corresponding centripetal saccades, and provide an adjustment to Carpenter's relationship:

$$centripetal\ duration = 2.5 \cdot amplitude + 27 \qquad (10.7)$$
$$centrifugal\ duration = 3.9 \cdot amplitude + 13 \qquad (10.8)$$

Saccadic duration is bimodally distributed during reading. Figure 10.15 shows a sharp peak for the short saccades between words and a softer hill for the return sweeps. There are no saccades with durations below 21 ms, corresponding to the constant in Equation (10.6). Also note how sensitive the measure is to the threshold setting of the velocity algorithm, not only for small saccades but across all durations. At a 30°/s setting there are twice as many saccades in the 50–100 ms interval as there are for the 90°/s setting. High peak velocity settings lead the algorithm to omit a considerable number of saccades.

The duration of a saccade has largely been thought of as a period with no visual intake (p. 379 and Dodge, 1900; Volkmann, 1986). During a saccade, stimuli can be manipulated without the participant noticing. Somewhat in opposition to the complete blindness view on saccades, a number of studies have been conducted to find out whether some cognitive processes can nevertheless take place during the progress of saccades. D. E. Irwin and Brockmole (2004) review these studies, the main findings of which we summarize below:

- Stimulus encoding is blocked during saccades
- Mental rotation appears to be suppressed
- It is unclear whether memory comparisons are suppressed
- Response selection is not suppressed

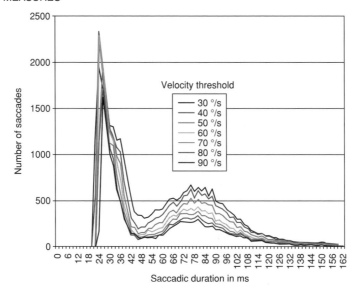

Fig. 10.15 Distribution of saccadic duration in reading at different peak velocity settings for the velocity algorithm. Bin size 1 ms. Study 1 on page 5. Recorded with a tower-mounted system at 1250 Hz with a high data quality. Saccade durations were calculated with BeGaze 2.1.

- Letter priming is not suppressed
- Lexical processing is not suppressed

In practice, saccadic duration is a measure frequently used in neurology and pharmacological papers, and only occasionally in human factors. The following factors have been found to increase saccade duration:

More difficult tasks For instance, saccades to remembered targets as well as antisaccades have strongly reduced peak velocities coupled with markedly increased durations compared to stimulus elicited saccades (Smit et al., 1987). Saccade duration increases with increasing blur in an image, and can be used for evaluation of image quality, according to Vuori, Olkkonen, Pölönen, Siren, and Häkkinen (2004).

A decreased processing capacity Independent of stimuli, participants with schizophrenia and bi-polar disorder have longer saccade durations (Bestelmeyer et al., 2006). 60 hours of sleep deprivation resulted in a 24% prolongation of saccade durations in a study conducted by S. Green and Farnborough (1986). McGregor and Stern (1996) report time on task effects on saccade duration. Saccadic duration is also increased by alcohol (Lehtinen, Lang, Jäntti, & Keskinen, 1979), but the changes in velocities and durations correlated more closely with feelings of intoxication than with blood alcohol concentrations. A large group of pharmacological and neurological journals use the saccadic duration measure to investigate the effect of drugs, psychological illness, and neurological injuries.

Cumulative transition time between fixations

Target question	*What is the cumulative duration of all saccades, as a percentage of the trial?*
Input representation	*A collection of saccades*
Output	*Percentage of time occupied by saccades*

In absolute terms, the cumulative transition time is defined as the sum of all saccade durations in a trial. The pragmatic idea behind the measure is that since vision is effectively shut down during saccades, a user interface or a pilot cockpit should be designed so that the cumulative transition time is minimized. Since saccade duration and amplitude correlate closely, this equates to having a user-interface design which results in producing few long saccades. For the same reason, cumulative transition time and scanpath length measures can be used interchangeably.

Cumulative transition time is a rare measure, used in human factors and ergonomics research. Abbott, Nataupsky, and Steinmetz (1987), who introduce the measure, found significant differences in the measure between two different designs (averages 18.6 versus 12.6% of trial time).

10.3.2 Scanpath duration

Target question	How long did the scanpath take, from onset to offset?
Input representation	A scanpath
Output	Scanpath duration (s)

Scanpath duration is defined as the time from onset of the scanpath until offset. The major challenge is to decide the exact points at which the scanpath starts and ends.

In usability research, scanpath duration measurements, including on- and offsets, are defined as "the sum of all the fixation duration times whilst completing a task" (Cowen, Ball, & Delin, 2002). The originators of the measure, Goldberg and Kotval (1999), do not specify the on- and offset conditions in sufficient detail. In practice, therefore, this means that scanpath duration more or less equals task completion time—but then the question becomes, how can we be sure when engagement in the task has commenced and ceased?

In reading research, several varieties of the scanpath duration measure have been developed for the study of sentence and global text processing. The following two examples are taken from Hyönä et al. (2003) and Liversedge, Paterson, and Pickering (1998), which both provide a methodological discussion on scanpath duration measures in reading. Note how elaborate the conditions for scanpath on- and offset are.

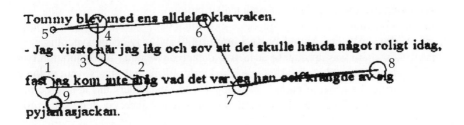

Fig. 10.16 Piece of data from a participant reading a longer text. Fixation number 2 on the word (ihåg) is followed by a regression scanpath two lines up. The regression scanpath ends at the 7th fixation, when the eye reaches a word beyond the last new one looked at. In this case go-past duration is the duration of the regression scanpath from after the second until the seventh fixation. Recorded 2000 with an SMI RED II, 50 Hz. Fixations detected with the I-DT algorithm using a 60 ms duration threshold.

Go-past duration is defined as the duration from first entering an AOI—in this case a word—until moving *forward* beyond the AOI, in the direction of the language read. Figure 10.16 shows a go-past scanpath with four fixations, where the difficulty was in resolving the

Swedish pronoun 'jag' ('I' in English), the second word on the third line, and overcoming it required looking back at the proper name 'Tommy' (this interpretation of the scanpath was verified by a retrospective interview with the participant immediately after recording). The closely related measure 'regression path duration' is part of the go-past duration; this is because go-past duration also includes eye movements which return to parts of the sentence already read. The go-past duration is considered to reflect difficulties in integrating a word within a context. This may be an early effect of inadequate initial processing, but it may also reflect overcoming comprehension difficulty despite sufficient processing initially, in which case it should be seen as a late effect (Clifton, Staub, & Rayner, 2007).

The *Extended first-pass fixation time* is the dwell time on a sentence or word AOI including the duration of regression scanpaths. The idea is that inconsistencies in the AOI can be better verified in eye-tracking data if the regression time—time to resolve the inconsistency—spills over to that AOI. In our example, the dwell time of the word 'ihåg' ('remember'), underneath the second fixation, would be increased by the duration of the entire regression scanpath (up until fixation 7). Be careful that the measure may be misinterpreted as 'the participant needed to read all this to understand the text they left', while in fact he has only lost a term from working memory.

10.3.3 Blink duration

Target question	*For how long is the eye closed during the blink?*
Input representation	*A blink*
Output	*Blink duration (ms)*

Blink duration is the complete time from when the eyelid starts moving down until it is fully up again. Real eyelid trackers record data as shown in Figure 10.17. Blink duration is only one of a number of duration measures that can be defined with data from an eyelid tracker. Data and software from pupil and corneal reflection eye-trackers operationalize blinks differently (p. 176), and typically underestimate blink duration. In addition, the commercial algorithms calculating blink duration tend to interpret noise in the data as blinks. High-speed optic artefacts in particular may cause an abundance of very short blink durations, as can be seen in Figure 10.18. Summary statistics such as average calculations should not be made before removing the artefactual part of such a distribution.

Blink duration values exhibit considerable individual variation across all drowsiness levels (Ingre, Åkerstedt, Peters, Anund, & Kecklund, 2006) and may be idiosyncratic.

In the 1940s, there was an intense academic debate on whether blink duration could be associated with anything like visual fatigue. Luckiesh (1947) and others were at the centre of this, supporting the association, while Tinker (1945) and others did not agree that this association was valid. Today, blink duration is considered to increase due to the following factors:

Drowsiness Blink duration and its close relative 'eye cleft' are among the most reliable camera readable signs of drowsiness. Re-opening time, in particular, changes reliably with increasing drowsiness. As an example, bus drivers with the obstructive sleep apnea syndrome have significantly longer blink durations compared to controls (Häkkänen, Summala, Partinen, Tiihonen, & Silvo, 1999).

Loss of vigilance There is an increase in blink duration during sustained attention tasks that correlates with decreased performance (Morris & Miller, 1996).

Mental workload Blink duration is highly correlated with object tracking errors of participants (Van Orden et al., 2000), in agreement with research conducted by Stern, Boyer,

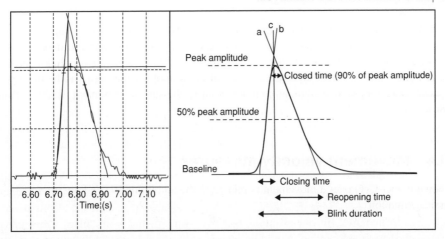

Fig. 10.17 To the left a plot of a blink recording, with the lid closure as the vertical amplitude dimension. To the right, blink duration and other blink measures defined on the background of a blink amplitude curve. With kind permission from Springer Science+Business Media: *European Journal of Applied Physiology*, Experimental evaluation of eye-blink parameters as a drowsiness measure, *89*(3), 2003, Phillipp P. Caffier.

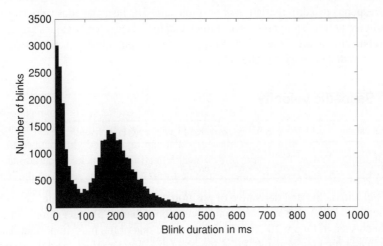

Fig. 10.18 The histogram of blink durations during mathematical problem solving, as measured with a tower-mounted 1250 Hz system, and analysed in BeGaze 2.3. Bin size 10 ms. Total number of blinks in this histogram is 32700, of which 203 are above 1000 ms in duration. The peak below 80 ms shows that this particular blink detection algorithm accepts various measurement noise as blinks.

and Schroeder (1994). Morris and Miller (1996) found that blink duration increases as a function of time on task. However, Veltman and Gaillard (1996), in a study of pilots, conclude that blink duration is affected by the visual demands of the task rather than by the cognitive workload in general.

Alcohol and anaesthetic sedation Blink duration appears to be sensitive also to low levels of sedation (Jandziol, Prabhu, Carpenter, & Jones, 2006) and alcohol (Biederman et al., 1974).

Like saccadic suppression, where visual intake is reduced before the physiological movement of the eye begins, there is a similar phenomena for blinks known as *blink suppression*. Ridder III and Tomlinson (1995) propose that these mechanisms are produced by similar underlying systems. According to Volkmann, Riggs, and Moore (1980), blink suppression starts around 50–100 ms before the blink onset, and lasts until 100–150 ms after offset. However, others have found that full acuity is not recovered until 200–500 ms after a blink (Ehrmann, Ho, & Papas, 2005). In addition, the amount of blink suppression seems to be directly influenced by factors such as blink amplitude and task (Stevenson, Volkmann, Kelly, & Riggs, 1986).

10.4 Movement velocity measures

Average velocity ($\bar{v}$) over a movement is related to the amplitude (θ) and duration (t) by the classical equation

$$\bar{v} = \frac{\theta}{t} \qquad (10.9)$$

Velocity levels can change along a movement, and that is why average velocity for one eye movement event (e.g. a saccade) is only of marginal use. Instead the instantaneous, *tangential velocity* ($\dot{\theta}$) is approximated by the distance between consecutive raw data samples (θ) multiplied by the sampling frequency of the eye-tracker $f_s = \frac{1}{\Delta t}$. Mathematically, this calculation of ($\dot{\theta}$) corresponds to a differentiation of position data. The instantaneous velocity is typically lowpass filtered before being processed further, and the exact velocity values are therefore intimately related to the properties of the lowpass filter (Inchingolo & Spanio, 1985). Note that filters *may* introduce latencies in the velocity data.

10.4.1 Saccadic velocity

Target question	*What was the peak/average velocity of the saccade?*
Input representation	*A saccade*
Output	*Saccade velocity (degrees/s)*

Saccadic velocity is the first derivative of position data with respect to time. Saccadic velocity is typically calculated as part of event calculation (Chapter 5). An example of a velocity plot can been seen in Figure 10.20. Velocity plots are one of the most important data inspection tools in eye-tracking research. Precision problems, optic artefacts, and the successes and failures of event detection algorithms can be readily inspected in them.

   Träisk et al. (2005) showed that search coils reduce the velocity of saccades, in particular for longer amplitudes. Saccades are therefore probably most accurately recorded with video-based pupil and corneal reflection eye-trackers. Furthermore, McGregor and Stern (1996) found that saccades occurring during a blink were significantly slower than those occurring independently of a blink. An example of a blink-accompanying saccade is given in Figure 10.19.

   In Figure 10.20, we can see the velocity curves for three saccades that develop very differently in time. The first saccade is a fairly common type. The velocity peak appears slightly before the middle of the saccade, so that the acceleration phase is faster than the deceleration phase. Two small glissadic movements are appended to this saccade. The middle saccade in Figure 10.20 is what has often been considered the ideal velocity curve. It has a clear velocity peak with only a slightly faster acceleration than deceleration. The glissade is minimal. The third saccade has multiple velocity peaks, of which the first two are saccadic and the last one possibly a glissade. The eye moves in spurts, but is never completely still between each burst. Zivotofsky, Siman-Tov, Gadoth, and Gordon (2006) report very similar data from

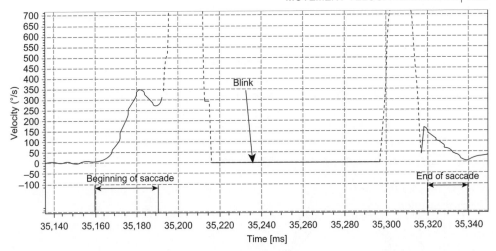

Fig. 10.19 180 ms saccade (black velocity) coinciding with a blink (dashed velocity). The saccadic velocity peaks at 35,180 ms, and the blink takes over at 35,190 ms (dashed artefactual velocity line). At 35,340 ms, note how the now prolonged saccade ends, around 180 ms after starting. Recorded during the mathematical problem solving task, number 4 on page 5, using a tower-mounted system at 1250 Hz. The data quality was high.

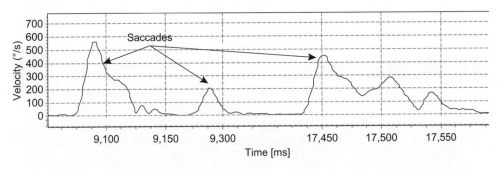

Fig. 10.20 Three saccades by one participant shown in a velocity over time diagram. Data taken from the mathematical problem solving task, number 4 on page 5, recorded with a tower-mounted 1250 Hz eye-tracker. The data quality was high.

a participant with Stiff-Person Syndrome, where the multiple peaks are most likely a result of incomplete muscle control. Rucker et al. (2004) link these multi-step saccades to Tay-Sachs disease. The data in Figure 10.20 are from a presumably healthy participant—a young student—but he was the only person from over 300 participants in this reading study who exhibited this pattern. The saccade is curved, and different velocities occur along the curved trajectory, possibly as the three pairs of eye muscles alternate controlling the eye.

Three common values are derived from velocity data such as in Figure 10.20:

1. Average saccadic velocity is an average of velocities over the entire duration of a saccade. Averages are however poor representations of the Gaussian-shaped saccadic forms.

2. Peak saccadic velocity is the highest velocity reached during the saccade. Average peak saccadic velocity reported by your software may be heavily affected by the peak velocity threshold in the event detection algorithm, as Figure 10.21 illustrates. Not only are saccades with a peak velocity lower than the threshold excluded—a large

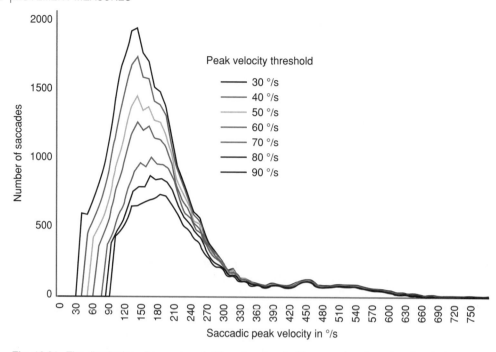

Fig. 10.21 The distribution of saccades at different peak velocities, as a function of peak velocity threshold. Note that a higher threshold reduces the number of saccades also at peak velocities *above* the threshold, due to the additional conditions on saccades in this implementation (p. 173). Bin size 10°/s. 10 participants reading for 10–15 minutes each, recorded with a tower-mounted system at 1250 Hz with high data quality. Saccades detected with the velocity algorithm.

number of the saccades with velocities from the threshold up until around 300°/s are also eliminated by the higher settings. Similar results were found by Bahill et al. (1981), but this also depends on the exact implementation of the detection algorithm.

3. Time to peak is the duration from the onset of a saccade until the peak velocity is reached.

The highest recorded peak saccadic velocity tends to be around 1000°/s, as Figure 10.12 on page 317 shows for a large saccade population during mathematical problem solving. Such fast saccades are very rare, however. In the peak velocity histogram in Figure 10.21, even the fastest reading return sweeps across the entire monitor have velocities no larger than approximately 700°/s.

The lower end of peak saccadic velocities is less investigated, although of great importance in event detection algorithms. On page 171–172, we concluded that a proper setting is about 30–40 °/s for a high-speed system with good precision. If there are long fixations in the data, there is a certain risk that occasional microsaccades will be detected, as a few microsaccades have peak velocities above 50°/s (Engbert, 2006).

Saccadic velocity has been used as a measure of cognitive activation level, or what is often called arousal level. Circumstances and factors that influence saccadic velocity include:

Arousal levels and sleepiness Low vigilance decreases saccadic velocity (Galley, 1989), and so does tiredness (McGregor & Stern, 1996; Becker & Fuchs, 1969) and sleep deprivation (Russo et al., 2003; Bocca & Denise, 2006). However, McGregor and Stern (1996) present results that suggest caution in interpreting saccadic velocity change as an index of 'fatigue', since the reduction in average saccadic velocity may be secondary to increases in blink rate.

Anticipation Anticipatory saccades, made to targets that are so predictable that the saccade can be launched before target onset, have lower velocities than reactive saccades (Smit & Van Gisbergen, 1989; Bronstein & Kennard, 1987).

Task Saccadic velocity increases as the difficulty of the task increases (Galley, 1993) and decreases with an increasing time on task (McGregor & Stern, 1996). When the task requires a higher saccadic rate (greater frequency of saccades), the saccadic peak velocity increases (C. J. Lueck, Crawford, Hansen, & Kennard, 1991).

Age Saccadic velocities are of the same size in children as with adults (Salman, Sharpe, Eizenman, et al., 2006), and Abrams, Pratt, and Chasteen (1998) found velocities not to differ between younger and older adults. However, Moschner and Baloh (1994) found velocities to be 20% slower for participants older than 75 years compared to participants younger than 43.

REM sleep During sleep, REM saccades—i.e. rapid eye movements—are about half the velocity of equal amplitude saccades made when awake (Aserinsky, Joan, Mack, Tzankoff, & Hurn, 1985). However, a more recent study could not confirm this finding (Sprenger et al., 2010).

Melancholia This is a disorder of low mood and lack of enthusiasm, and is associated with a difficulty in increasing peak velocities as target amplitudes increase (Winograd-Gurvich, Georgiou-Karistianis, Fitzgerald, Millist, & White, 2006).

Neurological disorders Slow saccades can be an indication of lesions in the pons, the midbrain, or the basal ganglia. Low saccade velocities also occur with Alzheimer's disease, AIDS, certain drugs, and a few other specific diseases. See the excellent summary in Wong (2008) for details.

Drugs and alcohol Peak saccadic velocity has for a long time been one of the prime oculomotor measures when studying the neurological and behavioural effects of drugs and alcohol (Abel & Hertle, 1988; Griffiths, Marshall, & Richens, 1984; Jürgens, Becker, & Kornhuber, 1981; Lehtinen et al., 1979; Franck & Kuhlo, 1970).

10.4.2 Smooth pursuit velocity

Target question	*What was the peak or average velocity of the smooth pursuit event?*
Input representation	*A smooth pursuit event*
Output	*Velocity (degrees/s)*

Smooth pursuit velocity is calculated just like saccadic velocity. Velocity plots on pages 169 and 179 show smooth pursuit velocity from a participant watching a pendular movement. We differentiate between average and peak smooth pursuit velocity.

It is generally thought that smooth pursuit velocity, peaking at 25–40°/s, is much slower than saccadic velocity (Boff & Lincoln, 1988; L. R. Young, 1971). However, C. H. Meyer et al. (1985) recorded 100°/s smooth pursuit on ordinary participants. Measuring professional baseball players who simulated hits on a baseball, Bahill and LaRitz (1984) recorded smooth pursuit velocities of up to 130°/s. According to Bahill and LaRitz, p. 235, "The success of good players is due to faster smooth pursuit eye movements, a good ability to suppress the vestibulo-ocular reflex, and the occasional use of an anticipatory saccade". Due to their large overlap in velocity range, smooth pursuit and saccades may be hard to separate by considering velocity alone. When the smooth pursuit follows targets moving with velocities of greater than about 30°/s, there tend to appear catch-up saccades in the data.

Smooth pursuit velocity has been argued to reflect the following:

Path curvature When the target moves in curved paths, smooth pursuit velocity decreases with decreasing radii of the curves (De'Sperati & Viviani, 1997).

Age Smooth pursuit velocity is slower for older participants (mean 67 years) than for younger (mean 42) (J. A. Sharpe & Sylvester, 1978). Newborn children have an undeveloped smooth pursuit, and have difficulty tracking targets even at low speeds such as 25°/s (Kremenitzer, Vaughan Jr, Kurtzberg, & Dowling, 1979).

Drugs Few studies have been conducted on the effects of drugs, and often with negative results. For instance, Tedeschi, Bittencourt, Smith, and Richens (1983), contrary to expectations, found no effect of amphetamine on smooth pursuit velocity.

Disorders Children with autism (Takarae, Minshew, Luna, Krisky, & Sweeney, 2004), adults with a childhood history of physical and emotional abuse (H. J. Irwin, Green, & Marsh, 1999), as well as patients with schizophrenia and post traumatic stress disorder (Cerbone et al., 2003) all show a decreased ability to smoothly track targets at higher velocities.

10.4.3 Scanpath velocity and reading speed

Target question	*What was the velocity of the scanpath?*
Input representation	*A scanpath, consisting of a sequence of saccades*
Output	*Velocity (degrees/s)*

Scanpath velocity (which you may also see referred to as 'average saccadic velocity', 'eye movement speed', or 'eye velocity') is defined as the product of average saccadic amplitude (in °) of saccades of which the scanpath is comprised, and saccadic rate (in 1/s). Apart from being a measure of scanpath velocity, this measure allows for a crude approximation of average saccadic velocity for data collected with such low sampling frequency and poor precision that actual saccadic velocities cannot be calculated.

The measure was defined by Saito (1992), who compared monitor work (23°/s) with similar work without a monitor (9°/s).

In reading studies, an alternative calculation of the same scanpath velocity has been made as the product of reading speed (in characters per second) and letter size (in visual degrees per character). The originators of this calculation, Krischer and Zangemeister (2007), investigated optimal conditions for reading, and conclude that the best skill- and acuity-matched letter size gives an eye movement speed of 8°/s during reading. Small letters, in particular, slow down the eye movement speed.

Beymer, Russell, and Orton (2005) instead divided text distances read by the time it took to cover them. This velocity measure was used to compare paragraph widths, and the authors found that a 4.5 inch monitor text is read only slightly faster than a 9.0 inch text.

An ambitious operational definition of reading speed (RS) was provided by Bullimore and Bailey (1995), who defined it as

$$RS = FR \frac{\#forward\ saccades}{\#total\ saccades} (average\ saccadic\ amplitude\ in\ letters) \qquad (10.10)$$

where FR is fixation rate (p. 416). The measure was used to study participants with macular degeneration and the effect of luminance, which both have effect on reading speed.

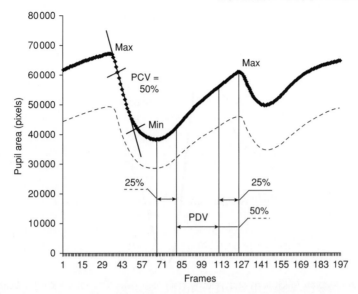

Fig. 10.22 Broken line, left eye; unbroken line, right eye. Max, maximum pupil area; Min, minimum pupil area. PCV, pupil constriction velocity, is calculated from the middle portion of the curve between Max and Min; PDV, pupil dilation velocity, is calculated from the middle portion of the curve between Min and Max. Data from a healthy participant about 60 years of age watching a variable light source. Recorded using a custom-built 60 Hz pupillometer. With kind permission from John Wiley and Sons: *Acta Ophthalmologica*, Relative afferent pupillary defect in glaucoma: a pupillometric study, *85*(5), 2007, Lada Kalaboukhova, Vanja Fridhammar, and Bertil Lindblom pp. 519–525.

10.4.4 Pupil constriction and dilation velocity

Target question	What was the velocity of the pupil closure or opening movement?
Input representation	Raw sample data
Output	Velocity (mm/s or mm²/s)

In pupillometry, pupil velocity is an established dependent variable. Pupil constriction velocity is approximately three times faster than dilation velocity (C. J. Ellis, 1981), so these should be measured separately. Figure 10.22 shows a pupillometric recording, and demonstrates what portions of data should be selected for pupil velocity calculations.

Average pupil velocity is calculated by selecting a constriction or dilation period with constant velocity and dividing the change in pupil diameter or area by the duration of the period (Figure 10.22). *Tangential pupil velocity* is calculated either by differentiating the horizontal diameter by time (Bitsios, Prettyman, & Szabadi, 1996), or by differentiating the pupil area by time (Figure 10.22). After tangential velocity has been calculated, *maximum pupil velocity* can easily be calculated.

Pupil velocity measurements have mainly been used clinically, for instance to assess pupil parasympathetic function, effects of medication, or the effect of glaucomas on pupil dilation. Age differences are known. For instance, Bitsios et al. (1996) found a smaller maximum dilatation velocity in an elderly compared to a younger group.

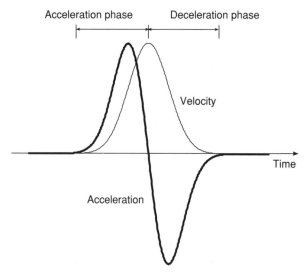

Fig. 10.23 Acceleration (thick line) and velocity (thin line) over time for an ideal saccade. Note that acceleration rises before velocity; and that acceleration is 0 when velocity peaks. Also note that during the deceleration phase, acceleration is negative.

10.5 Movement acceleration measures

The instantaneous, tangential acceleration $\ddot{\theta}$ is calculated by differentiating velocity $\dot{\theta}$ with respect to time:

$$\ddot{\theta} = \frac{d}{dt}\dot{\theta}$$ (10.11)

Mathematically, acceleration is therefore the second derivative of position data. Peak and average acceleration can be retrieved from the continuous acceleration data. Deceleration—slowing down—can be seen as negative acceleration (Figure 10.23). Jerk ($\dddot{\theta}$) is the third derivative, measuring the change in acceleration over time.

Movement acceleration is necessary to start a movement and to increase the velocity of it. Acceleration and jerk drive velocity, and therefore a change in acceleration are accompanied by a change in velocity. Unfortunately, numerical differentiation magnifies noise in the signal, and may require additional filtering.

10.5.1 Saccadic acceleration/deceleration

Target question	What was the peak/average acceleration of the saccade?
Input representation	A saccade
Output	Acceleration (degrees/s²)

Saccadic acceleration is the derivative of saccadic velocity with respect to time. Acceleration thresholds are used in some of the saccade detection algorithms (most prominently in the EyeLink parser from SR Research), and are valuable to separate smooth pursuit movements (low acceleration due to small variation in velocity) from saccades (high acceleration/deceleration at onset/offset).

Saccadic acceleration rises very fast, and reaches a maximum peak of up to $100000°/s^2$, with typical peak values ranging between $6000–12000°/s^2$. Extremely high acceleration values may be an indication of optic artefacts in the data. As Figure 10.24 shows, the distribution has a rightward skew.

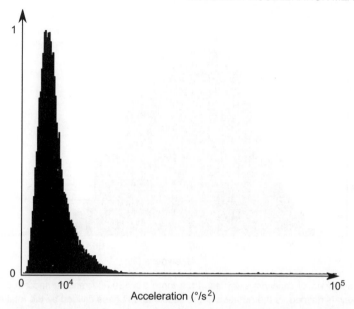

Fig. 10.24 A normalized distribution of saccades at different peak accelerations. Acceleration is calculated using the algorithm by Nyström and Holmqvist (2010). Ten participants reading for 10–15 minutes
each, recorded with a tower-mounted 1250 Hz system. Data quality is high.

Acceleration and deceleration were found by Collewijn et al. (1988) to increase as a function of saccade amplitude; however, data were recorded with coils, not the type of commercial
video-based eye-trackers in common use in research today.

Saccadic acceleration is a very uncommon measure that appears to have attracted mainly
neurologists with an interest in the cerebellum and superior colliculus (important saccade
programming areas of the brain). All participants in Straube and Deubel (1995) showed an
idiosyncratic pattern of saccadic acceleration and deceleration.

The existence of glissades and saccades with multiple velocity peaks means that some
saccades have more than one acceleration phase. Whether this also means that the eye muscles are actually pulling the eye during all acceleration phases, or whether some acceleration
phases are the consequence of eye lens inertia during deceleration still remains an open question.

10.5.2 Skewness of the saccadic velocity profile

Target question	*How much of the saccadic duration is taken up by acceleration and deceleration phases, respectively?*
Input representation	*A saccade*
Output	*Skewness*

The skewness of the saccadic velocity ('saccadic skewness') is defined as the degree
of skewness of the velocity plots of saccades. It attempts to measure the duration of the
acceleration versus deceleration phases in saccades, as shown in Figure 10.23.

The measure has been operationalized in at least three different ways: First, Collewijn et
al. (1988) define the skewness value as the acceleration phase (time to peak velocity) divided
by the total saccade duration. A symmetrical saccade therefore has a skewness of 50%. Figure

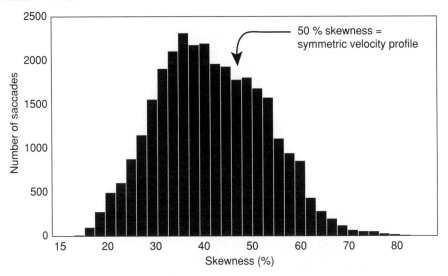

Fig. 10.25 Histogram of saccadic skewness from more than 30,000 reading saccades from project 1 on page 5. Skew is defined as the duration of the acceleration phase divided by the total duration of the saccade. Bin size 2%. Recorded with a tower-mounted eye-tracker at 1250 Hz. Saccades detected using the velocity algorithm at a threshold setting of 30°/s. Glissades are largely included in saccades.

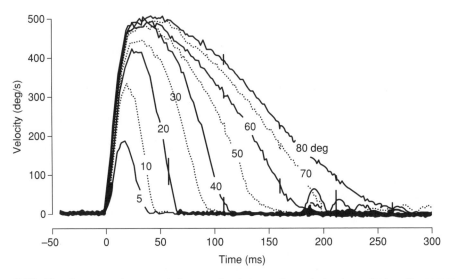

Fig. 10.26 The skewness of a saccade has previously been shown to be dependent on the saccadic amplitude. Data recorded with a coil system. Reprinted with kind permission from John Wiley and Sons: *Journal of Physiology*, Binocular co-ordination of human horizontal saccadic eye movements, *404*(1), 1998, Collewijn, H., Erkelens, C.J., & Steinman, R.M., pp. 157–182.

10.25 shows a histogram of saccadic skewness using this calculation. A similar operational definition used by Straube and Deubel (1995) and others is to calculate the acceleration phase divided by the deceleration phase. Symmetrical saccades in this case have the value 1; right-skewed are lower, and left-skewed (the few that exist) have a value above 1. Using this, the distribution of skewness values in Figure 10.25 will be even more skewed than as depicted. A third operational definition was provided by Van Opstal and Van Gisbergen (1987) who approximated a gamma function to the velocity profile of the saccades. By finding values for α, β, and γ that optimize the fit of

$$v(t) = \alpha \cdot \left(\frac{t}{\beta}\right)^{\gamma-1} e^{-\left(\frac{t}{\beta}\right)} \tag{10.12}$$

to the velocity curve $v(t)$, the skewness can be calculated as

$$\text{Skew} = \frac{2}{\sqrt{\gamma}} \tag{10.13}$$

Skewness is a little used measure. Anticipatory (or predictive) saccades were found to be slightly more skewed than visually guided saccades (Smit & Van Gisbergen, 1989). Liao et al. (2006) found that head saccades (turning the head) have a constant skew of 0.5, while the skew of eye saccades varies. Soetedjo, Kaneko, and Fuchs (2002) found that injection of the substance muscimol in the superior colliculus of monkeys increased the skewness since the duration of the deceleration phase increased more than the duration of the acceleration phase.

In previous research based on scleral coil recordings, the acceleration phase has been shown to be of approximately the same duration across all amplitudes, while the deceleration phase increases rapidly with increasing amplitudes up to 90° (Figure 10.26). However, using the data described on page 5, from video-based eye-trackers, we have not been able to find any correlation between amplitude and the skewness of the saccadic velocity profile for saccades up to 40°.

The many glissades that exist in video-based eye-trackers (but are suppressed with coil systems) are categorized with the saccades by some of the detection algorithms. In effect, this means that glissadic saccades of whatever amplitude will be heavily skewed. In fact, the skewness measure will itself have a skewed distribution, as shown in Figure 10.25. The skew of the skewness distribution *may* indirectly reflect the amount of glissadic saccades, depending on your particular event detection algorithm.

10.5.3 Smooth pursuit acceleration

Target question	*What was the peak/average acceleration of the smooth pursuit event?*
Input representation	*A smooth pursuit event*
Output	*Acceleration (degrees/s^2)*

Using targets moving at 40°/s, Kao and Morrow (1994) found smooth pursuit acceleration values of up to 350°/s^2. Acceleration values were significantly higher when the target motion was predictable, yet more evidence of the anticipatory nature of smooth pursuit. Moschner et al. (1999) reported smooth pursuit accelerations between 43–128°/s^2 across individuals over the first 60 ms of "visually guided smooth pursuit". During smooth pursuit with constant velocity, the acceleration is zero.

10.5.4 Saccadic jerk

Target question	*What was the peak/average jerk of the saccade?*
Input representation	*A saccade*
Output	*Jerk (degrees/s^3)*

The saccadic jerk ($\dddot{\theta}$) is the derivative of saccadic acceleration, and thus the third derivative of gaze position. For this reason, expect jerk data to be noisy. Alternative terms are 'jolt', 'surge', and 'lurch'. Wyatt (1998) proposes a saccade detection algorithm based on jerk instead of velocity or acceleration. Since saccades mostly start off very sharply, jerk is particularly useful for determination of precise saccadic onset; Wyatt suggests the simple jerk threshold of $200,000°/s^3$. Jerk is not very helpful in determining saccadic ending, because of the slow glissades that are often appended to saccades.

10.6 Movement shape measures

Shape refers to the form and figure of movements, such as the *curvature* of saccades and glissades, the *smoothness* of pursuit, the *selfcrossing* of scanpaths, and shapes associated with specific cognitive processes such as *reading*, or *local versus global* scanning. Although shapes are easily discernible for human viewers, 'shape' is a vague concept, and can therefore be hard to define precisely. No attempts have been made to categorize or quantify all possible movement shapes. There are undoubtedly countless possible shapes of movements, but so far only occasional shape measures have been developed.

10.6.1 Saccadic curvature

Target question	What is the curvature of the saccade?
Input representation	A saccade
Output	Curvature (degrees or more complex units)

Saccadic curvature is a measure of the overall spatial shape of the saccade. Few saccades are perfectly linear, and some really large saccadic curves can be elicited by having a participant circle their gaze quickly between four dots in a square, which is how the saccades in Figure 10.27 were generated.

There are several different operational definitions of saccadic curvature. Port and Wurtz (2003) use standard circular statistics, and define the saccadic curvature as the angular standard deviation of the tangential direction of the saccade. The curvature unit will then be in orientation degrees (like φ, p. 302). Attempts have also been made to use polynomial curve fitting, and Ludwig and Gilchrist (2002) found a quadratic curvature metric to provide a robust fit, where the polynomial coefficients describe the curvature. Harwood, Mezey, and Harris (1999, p. 9098) define a measure called the *spectral main sequence*, which is claimed to be "exquisitely sensitive to the saccade trajectory and should be used to test objectively all present and future models of saccades."

It is clear however, that curved saccades often have multiple velocity peaks, since changes in saccadic direction co-occur with local velocity minima.

The properties and influences on saccadic curvature as known from research can be summarized as follows:

Oblique saccades These are more curved than horizontal and vertical saccades. The curvature of oblique saccades compensates for the divergence of the initial direction from the direction called for by the target (Becker & Jürgens, 1990). Note that in oblique saccades two pairs of muscles are involved, and may change their relative influence on the movement over time.

Curve direction This is dependent on the *location of the target* and the *type of saccade* (Smit & Van Gisbergen, 1990; Viviani et al., 1977).

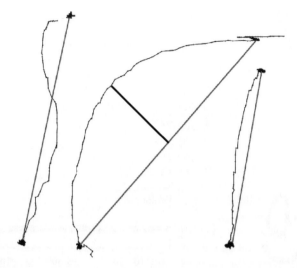

Fig. 10.27 Three saccades with varying degrees of curvature. Grey lines show the shortest distances from saccadic origin to endpoint. The thick black line shows the operational definition of saccadic curvature by Nummenmaa, Hyönä, and Calvo (2008). Recorded with a tower-mounted eye-tracker at 500 Hz; data quality is high.

Irrelevant distractors When near the saccade target, visual distractors also cause curved saccades. Curvature is always directed *away from* the distractor, and this finding also holds for verbal distraction (Doyle & Walker, 2001). Even emotional content may curve a saccade (Nummenmaa et al., 2008).

Instructions When told to look at something other than the saccade target, instructions also affect saccadic curvature (Sheliga, Riggio, Craighero, & Rizzolatti, 1995).

Pharmacological effects For example, injection of muscimol into the superior colliculus was found by Aizawa and Wurtz (1998) to increase the curvature of saccades in monkeys. The authors argue that this can been taken as evidence that the superior colliculus is critically involved in regulating the trajectory of saccades during their execution.

10.6.2 Glissadic curvature

Target question	What is the curvature of the glissade?
Input representation	A glissade
Output	Curvature in ° or more complex units

Glissadic curvature refers to the path of a glissadic eye movement, as exemplified in Figure 10.28. Glissades are typically more curved than saccades, perhaps since they may lack controlled and prototypical programming, and hence can take on a variety of shapes.

Calculation of glissadic curvature is in principle the same as for saccadic curvature. However, the greater degree to which glissades curve must be taken into account. Average circular variance certainly works, using polynomial curves is a possible option, but one cannot use the maximum distance from the saccade to the line spanning the Euclidean distance between glissadic onset to offset, as with saccades (see Figure 10.27, middle curve).

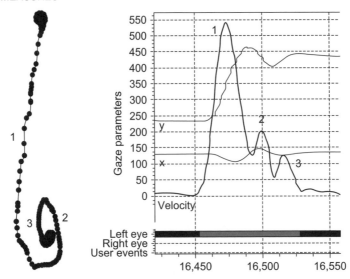

Fig. 10.28 Glissadic curvature: A saccade (1) followed by a double glissade (2 and 3), shown as raw data sample plot over stimulus (left), and velocity plot (right), recorded with a tower-mounted system at 1250 Hz; data quality is high.

10.6.3 Smooth pursuit: degree of smoothness

Target question	*How 'smooth' is the pursuit event?*
Input representation	*A smooth pursuit event*
Output	*Smoothness value*

The degree of smoothness of a smooth pursuit refers to whether the pursuit movement is smooth, or jagged (e.g. as in square-wave jerks). Smoothness ratings are typically performed by experts, and inter-rater reliability is then reported. They normally do not take into account catch-up saccades, but if catch-up saccades are included, the frequency of these can also be used as a measure of smoothness. This strategy was used by Mather and Putchat (1983) to evaluate pursuit in patients with schizophrenia.

Diefendorf and Dodge (1908), and Holzman, Proctor, and Hughes (1973) provide evidence that schizophrenic patients and their relatives demonstrate disordered smooth pursuit eye movements. Later studies have shown that schizophrenia-related smooth pursuit deficits are more likely due to an inability to correctly *execute* eye movements which track a stimulus, rather than an inability to correctly *encode* velocity information (Avila, Hong, Moates, Turano, & Thaker, 2006). Studies using the smoothness of pursuit have developed into a paradigm of eye-movement research.

10.6.4 Global to local scanpath ratio

Target question	*How much overview scanning and detailed inspection?*
Input representation	*All saccades in a scanpath*
Output	*Ratio*

First introduced by Groner et al. (1984), the ratio of global to local saccades (g/l) of which a scanpath is comprised is calculated as the number of saccades *longer* than a threshold amplitude, divided by the number of saccades *shorter* than a threshold amplitude. The former threshold is set to determine 'global' scanning saccades, while the latter is set to identify 'local' saccades indicative of more detailed inspection. Zangemeister, Sherman, and Stark (1995) suggest $1.6°, 4.6°, 7.9°$, or $11°$ as possible thresholds, while Zangemeister and Liman (2007) use $1.1°$ to separate the two types of saccade. Since saccadic amplitude correlates strongly with saccadic velocity, this type of threshold operates much like the velocity-based saccade detection algorithms in Chapter 5.

A larger g/l ratio indicates a longer scanpath, fewer local fixations, and faster average eye movement speed.

The downsides of this measure are the arbitrary settings, and the fact that saccades scale with the size of objects in the stimulus scene; making a local scanpath on a large object not comparable to a global scanpath covering lots of small objects.

Small saccades, nevertheless, are generally assumed to be the result of detailed inspection of the stimulus, while longer saccades are eye movements *between* areas inspected—this is usually referred to as scanning. Thus the g/l ratio is synonymous with a comparison between scanning and detailed inspection, and has been used for:

Finding expert versus novice differences In a study of art perception, Zangemeister, Sherman, and Stark (1995) found that professional art viewers had a g/l ratio of 2.8, while non-professionals had a ratio of 1.3. Hence the authors conclude that the measure is capable of distinguishing between levels of cognitive skill.

Comparing imagery versus real stimulus perception The g/l ratio was found to be higher during stimulus viewing by Zangemeister and Liman (2007), who also found effects of *task* and *stimulus type*.

A similar definition was given by Krischer and Zangemeister (2007), who defined a 'global scanpath length' (sum of all long saccades) versus a 'local scanpath length' (sum of all small saccades), and found that the global scanpath length in picture viewing makes up around 95% of the total length.

10.7   AOI order and transition measures

AOI order and transition measures take the sequential order of movement into account. A 2D transition matrix is used exclusively for single transitions between two AOIs, and does not in any way represent what happened before or after those transitions. Each limited sequence in a transition matrix therefore, only has a 'history' of two dwells in two AOIs—this is its trace. Similarly, a first-order Markov model predicts the occurrence of a state (fixation, saccade, or AOI hit) on the basis of the preceding state, and does not include earlier states in the prediction. There are few measures that take longer intervals of a sequence into account, but the practical length of intervals seems to be around 2–10 dwells.

10.7.1   Order of first AOI entries

Target question	*Do participants look earlier at some AOIs than at others?*
Input representation	*AOI strings with first entries*
Output	*p-value for order effects*

The order of first AOI entries allows us to have significance tests for the difference in entry order between AOIs visited early and AOIs visited late. We form the same sort of table (such as Table 10.1) as in the calculation of average scanpaths (p. 282).

Table 10.1 Order of first entries for five AOIs seen by five participants (fictitious data). In this example, participant 2 first enters AOI 2, then AOI 1, then AOI 3 and so on.

Participant	AOI 1	AOI 2	AOI 3	AOI 4	AOI 5
1	1	3	2	4	5
2	2	1	3	5	4
3	1	2	3	4	5
4	3	1	2	5	4
5	1	3	2	4	5
Average	1.60	2.00	2.40	4.40	4.60

The average rankings, given in the bottom row of the table, indicate the average order in which the participants visited the five AOIs. On average, they visited AOI 1 first, AOI 2 second, and so on. Note that the amount of variation between the average rankings reflects whether the participants tended to visit the AOIs in the same order or not. If there had been no systematic ordering of the rankings across the five AOIs, the average rankings would be approximately the same. Since this is not the case in Table 10.1, the variation between the average rankings is relatively large.

The amount of variation between the average rankings is used to calculate W, Kendall's coefficient of concordance (Siegel & Castellan, 1988). If the AOI $i = 1, 2, \ldots, n$ is first visited at order $r_{i,j}$ by participant $j = 1, 2, \ldots, m$, then

$$W = \frac{12S}{m^2(n^3 - n)} \qquad (10.14)$$

where

$$S = \sum_{i=1}^{n} (K_i - \bar{K})^2 \qquad (10.15)$$

$$\bar{K} = \frac{1}{2} m(n+1) \qquad (10.16)$$

$$K_i = \sum_{j=1}^{m} r_{i,j} \qquad (10.17)$$

The coefficient W was originally used as a measure to determine whether a number of objects (here: AOIs) receive similar ratings (here: are visited in the same order) by a number of judges (here: participants). The value of W may vary between 0, indicating absence of agreement, and 1, indicating perfect agreement. In the example, W is equal to 0.784, suggesting that the AOIs were visited in more or less the same order by the participants.

If there is a high degree of agreement between the participants, then it is the case that one or more AOIs were visited before the other AOIs. The researcher may ask, then, whether the difference in average ranking between two AOIs is significant or not. A test that can be used for answering that question is Friedman's chi-square for related samples, which is the non-parametric alternative to a one-way within-subjects ANOVA. The resulting chi-square calculated on the data in Table 10.1 is 15.680, which, with four degrees of freedom, is significant. A procedure, Nemenyi's procedure, for doing pairwise comparisons is available (Heiman, 2006).

Since there is a direct relation between the amount of agreement and the differences between the average ratings, it is not surprising that the values of Kendall's W are also related to these. Friedman's chi-square may be used to determine whether W is significant or not. Computationally, the relation between W and Friedman's chi-square is:

$$\chi^2 = n(m-1)W \tag{10.18}$$

in which n is equal to the number of AOIs, and m is equal to the number of participants.

In spite of its simplicity, this method has been surprisingly little used. One exception is Le, Raufaste, and Demonet (2003), who found that a participant with prosopagnosia (a neuropsychological disorder in which patients are unable to recognize faces) still looked at the parts (AOIs) of normal and scrambled faces in an order that could not be differentiated from the control group.

10.7.2 Transition matrix density

Target question	Is the scanpath across AOIs directed or randomly distributed?
Input representation	A transition matrix
Output	A sparseness value

Transition matrix density was defined by Goldberg and Kotval (1999) as the number of non-zero entries in the transition matrix divided by the total number of cells. It is better to divide the number of non-zero entries by the number of real cells in the matrix (see p. 195), in particular for dimensions (string lengths) higher than two.

A low transition density is an indication of efficient and directed search, while a dense matrix would imply random search, Goldberg and Kotval say. They apply gridded AOIs to two very different computer interface designs, and study the extent of search behaviour. The significant difference in the measure is argued to show that the two interfaces are differently searched. Note that this is true for two-dimensional transition matrices. For longer strings, a low transition density means that the participants have preferred paths through the AOIs of the stimulus and that many other possible paths are avoided.

10.7.3 Transition matrix entropy

Target question	Is the scanpath across AOIs directed or randomly distributed?
Input representation	A transition matrix
Output	Entropy (bits)

Entropy, originally defined by Shannon (1948), is a measure that calculates the uncertainty in a random variable, in our case a transition matrix. To explain entropy, we are going to run through an example illustrated in Figure 10.29 and Table 10.2.

Assume that we have a normalized transition matrix according to the figure. This is a fairly non-random transition matrix, since half of the transitions are of the type $B \rightarrow C$. The entropy H is then calculated as the negation of the sum of the last column, or in our example, 2 bits. More generally, entropy is defined as

$$H(R) = -\sum_{r_i \in R} p(r_i) \log_2 p(r_i), r_i > 0$$

where R is a normalized transition matrix and r_i are the cell values of that matrix with probabilities $p(r_i)$.

Entropy can be calculated for any dwell map or transition matrix. The lowest possible value is zero (0), which is only reached if there is just one cell in the matrix, i.e. when there

	A	B	C
A		0.0625	0.0625
B	0.0625		0.5
C	0.25	0.0625	

Fig. 10.29 Fictitious transition matrix with normalized values.

Table 10.2 Step-by-step entropy calculations for the transition matrix in Figure 10.29.

Transition	$p(r_i)$	$\log_2 p(r_i)$	$p(r_i)\log_2 p(r_i)$
$A \to B$	0.0625	-4.0	-0.25
$A \to C$	0.0625	-4.0	-0.25
$B \to A$	0.0625	-4.0	-0.25
$B \to C$	0.5000	-1.0	-0.50
$C \to A$	0.2500	-2.0	-0.50
$C \to B$	0.0625	-4.0	-0.25

is no uncertainty about what type of transition will occur. The maximum value for entropy is when all cells have the same value. In our example with six cells, the maximum value would be $-6\frac{1}{6}\log_2(\frac{1}{6})$, which equals 2.59 bits. 'Bits' is not a very intuitive unit, however, but by dividing the $H(R)$ value with the theoretically maximal value for the system (in our example 2.59), we arrive at a *normalized entropy* that allows for comparisons of results across groups and stimuli.

Calculating the entropy of a transition matrix, Shic, Chawarska, and Scassellati (2008) argued that a high resulting value is aligned with a preference for exploration, while low values indicate data with transitions mainly between a few of the AOIs. Jordan and Slater (2009) interpreted a drop in scanpath entropy over time as an indication that the virtual environment they tested "had cohered into a meaningful perception" (p. 185). They calculated entropy from transition matrices created from 1-second intervals, and collapsed data from all participants to estimate the total change in entropy over time.

10.7.4 Number and proportion of specific subscans

Target question	How common is a specific subscan?
Input representation	AOI-processed data
Output	The number or proportion of each subscan, commonly determined in a histogram

This measure counts the number of unique subscans in string representations of scanpaths. Groner et al. (1984) decided "in a compromise between theoretical considerations and statistical arguments" (p. 529) to analyse subscans with a length of three AOIs. As their face stimuli had seven AOIs (Figure 10.30(b)), they found the total number of possible subscans of length three to be 210 (see Equation 6.1 on page 195). Interestingly, the 20 most common subscans subsumed 57% of the total number of subscans. The two most common subscans moved between the eyes, but there was considerable individual variation (Figure 10.30(a)). Each subscan corresponds to a cell in a 3D transition matrix as the one on page 194.

TRIPLETS   S U B J E C T S

	1. RU	2. ME	3. BR	4. BK	5. WI	6. TR	Total
2-3-2	7	9	13	36	0	<u>68</u>	133
3-2-3	20	9	10	25	1	<u>46</u>	111
7-2-3	13	2	5	4	0	<u>31</u>	55
2-3-4	8	6	3	<u>19</u>	0	<u>17</u>	53
4-2-3	10	9	3	<u>10</u>	3	17	52
5-2-3	14	<u>13</u>	3	6	3	6	45
2-3-5	21	<u>1</u>	2	8	2	9	43
3-2-4	5	7	0	12	3	13	40
5-4-3	3	2	0	0	15	8	28
3-2-5	5	4	3	7	<u>3</u>	6	28
4-3-2	6	1	0	5	7	8	27
7-5-4	9	2	0	0	<u>8</u>	8	27
4-5-4	1	3	0	4	<u>11</u>	2	21
2-4-3	4	3	1	4	<u>3</u>	4	19

Table 1: The 14 most frequent triplets. Numbers indicate frequencies of observation. Under linings symbolize significant higher frequency than expected by independence (Chi-square test, p< .01)

(a) Subscan 'triplet' frequency table for six participants looking at faces.

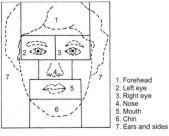

(b) Stimulus and the seven AOIs.

1. Forehead
2. Left eye
3. Right eye
4. Nose
5. Mouth
6. Chin
7. Ears and sides

Fig. 10.30 Subscan frequency analysis. Reprinted from *Advances in Psychology*, Volume 22, Rudolf Groner, Franziska Walder, and Marina Groner, Looking at Faces: Local and Global Aspects of Scanpaths, pp. 523–533., Copyright (1984), with permission from Elsevier.

Again using subscans of length three, Koga and Groner (1989) compared non-native learners of Japanese Kanji sign sequences before and after training using two different presentation modes. Based on the 20 most common subscans, they conclude that subscan frequency is not influenced by the presentation mode.

When analysing eye-movement data from participants picking up and dropping block objects, Ballard et al. (1992) found that the most common subscan sequence consisted of four AOIs. Tasks and participant strategies definitely influence the prevalence of longer subscans.

10.7.5 Unique AOIs

Target question	*Does the scanpath over AOIs represent a focused or an overview scan?*
Input representation	*AOI strings*
Output	*Proportion of scanpaths in each category*

The unique AOI measure counts how many unique AOIs there are in a substring, but is not concerned with the exact order of the AOI visits. For example, the strings ABB and BBA of length three both have two unique AOIs (A and B) but different AOI order. Since the unique AOI measure does not have to consider all possible subscans in a transition matrix, substantially fewer data need to be processed, and longer subscans become easier to investigate. However, the price is that sequential information within the subscan is completely disregarded. The measure resembles the local versus global and ambient versus focal of pages 265–267, but differs by using AOIs rather than amplitudes.

The unique AOI measure is calculated by letting a window of length ℓ slide over the recorded AOI sequence, and counting the number of unique AOIs in the window. Suppose for instance that for a hypothetical participant and trial, we record an AOI sequence IAIBACIAIABCDIAIAI. Repetitions are not allowed, and are collapsed to include only a single letter (as in compressed string edit representation). Unique-AOI sequences are then defined by letting a window of size 5 travel along the AOI sequence. First the window will

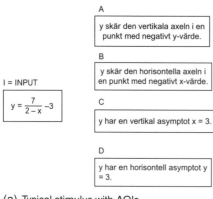

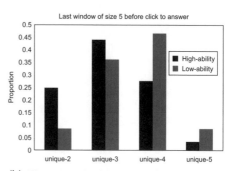

(a) Typical stimulus with AOIs.

(b) Histogram of uniqueness values, all participants and the last five AOIs before clicking to answer.

Fig. 10.31 Unique-AOI data. Sequence length $\ell = 5$, number of AOIs $n = 5$. High-ability participants clearly made more pairwise AOI inspections compared to low-ability participants.

encounter IAIBA, and see that there are *three unique AOIs* (i.e. I, A, B). Next, we move the window one step, and find AIBAC, which has four unique AOIs. We continue like this, until we have reached IAIAI at the end, which has only two unique AOIs. In total we will have 14 AOI-uniqueness numbers from the recorded sequence of 18 AOIs, namely 3–4–4–4–3–3–3– 4–5–5–5–4–3–2. We now count how many unique-2, unique-3, unique-4 and unique-5 there are in this sequence and we find: 1 unique-2, 5 unique-3, 5 unique-4 and 3 unique-5.

Figure 10.31 shows a mathematical problem and the unique-AOIs values resulting from the last five AOIs looked at before participants clicked on the alternative they thought was correct (experiment described on p. 5). During this decision phase, high-ability students (defined as those solving a larger proportion of problems compared to the whole student group) made 25% pairwise comparisons—that is cases with five consecutive dwells, in which only two unique AOIs were visited—and another 43% unique-3 sequences. Low-ability students have a higher tendency to make overview scans.

When the uniqueness values calculated from each window are not collapsed over time, they can be used to study the relation between focus and overview looking over time. Calculations of the chance levels for each uniqueness group give chance probabilities of 0.0156 for unique-2, 0.328 for unique-3, 0.562 for unique-4, and 0.0938 that participants will sequence all five AOIs consecutively. Holmqvist, Andrà, et al. (2011) present calculations of chance probabilities for a whole variety of numbers of AOIs and window sizes, and describe how significance calculations should be carried out.

10.7.6 Statistical analysis of a transition matrix

Target question	*Are some transitions significantly more common than others?*
Input representation	*A transition matrix*
Output	*Significant transitions and p-values*

In this section, we illustrate the use of log-linear statistical analysis for the analysis of the transition matrix given in Table 6.1 on page 194. The principles behind log-linear analysis are briefly explained on page 90.

Table 10.3 Adjusted residuals for the data in Table 6.1 on page 194.

	LS	LF	RF	RS	I	E	O
Left Side (LS)	.	**8.58**	-1.93	**−2.04**	-1.41	-1.90	**−4.45**
Left Front (LF)	**5.50**	.	0.42	-1.93	**3.35**	-1.57	**−4.39**
Right Front (RF)	-1.34	1.67	.	**5.92**	-1.58	-1.44	-1.88
Right Side (RS)	-1.84	**−5.21**	**9.58**	.	**−2.07**	**5.90**	1.65
Instruments (I)	-0.60	0.58	**−2.53**	-1.63	.	-0.28	1.74
Engine (E)	-1.84	**−4.89**	**−2.82**	-0.29	0.85	.	**8.21**
Other (O)	-1.06	1.57	**−2.49**	0.31	-0.22	-0.25	.

In a two-dimensional table, as in Table 6.1, the first step in the analysis is to exclude the two-way interaction from the model, and to calculate the expected number of transitions based on only the two main effects. Note that the calculation of expected number of transitions in tables that contain structural zeros is realized by means of an iterative procedure, and should be left to a computer. The resulting value of chi-square indicates whether or not the expected numbers of the more parsimonious model are still reasonably close to the observed frequencies. In the case of Table 6.1, they are clearly not, since the chi-square value of 473.411 with 29 degrees of freedom[28] is highly significant.

The fact that chi-square is significant indicates that the two factors are dependent on one another. Translated to transition matrices, this means that transitions between certain AOIs were either significantly more or less likely than expected.

The natural question that follows is, of course, which transition numbers in the matrix deviate significantly from expected. Cells for which the expected number deviates significantly from the observed number may be identified through examination of the adjusted residuals, given in Table 10.3. Adjusted residuals are indications of the distance between an observed and an expected value, similar to standard scores. Positive values indicate that the observed number of transitions is higher than the expected number, whereas negative values indicate that the observed number is lower than the expected number. Absolute values that are larger than 1.96 are significant with $p < 0.05$. These are marked in bold in Table 10.3. The table shows, for instance, that the number of transitions from left side to left front was significantly higher than expected, whereas the transitions from left side to other were significantly fewer than expected.

If you have an a-priori interest in one or more transitions, the analysis of adjusted residuals may be pursued further (Bakeman & Gottman, 1997). Suppose that the transitions from left side to left front in cell (1,2) were of particular interest for the study. The effect of these transitions on the overall chi-square can be evaluated by declaring cell (1,2) structurally zero, and then recalculating the expected numbers. In the above example, the exclusion of this cell results in a new value of chi-square of 395.666 with 28 degrees of freedom. This is a reduction compared to the earlier value, but obviously, the new value is still highly significant.

In the case where transitions are being examined within the context of an experimental design, the situation becomes more complicated. A direct comparison of transition numbers across groups is not allowed. Instead, however, the researcher may choose to use a measure of the strength of association within the table as the dependent variable within the design. One such measure that is suitable for the analysis is the log odds ratio (Bakeman & Gottman, 1997). A restriction to this measure is that it is based on a two-by-two table. Therefore, the researcher either needs to incorporate this in the design of the experiment, or collapse across

---

[28](Number of columns–1) * (Number of rows–1)–Number of structural zeros = Degrees of freedom for a two-dimensional transition matrix.

multiple rows and columns in a larger table. If the cells of a 2×2 table are designated as F_{11}, F_{12}, F_{21}, and F_{22} respectively, the log odds ratio can be calculated as,

$$\ln \left(\frac{F_{11}/F_{12}}{F_{21}/F_{22}} \right) \tag{10.19}$$

Log odds ratios may be calculated for the individual items and participants in the experiment, and the resulting values are used as the input to a statistical test.

Two other methods have been used for the analysis of transition matrices: Markov modelling and correspondence analysis. Markov models were introduced on page 196. This method has been used within eye-tracking research by Liu (1998) and others. Correspondence analysis has not been applied often for the analysis of eye-tracking data. An exception is found in Loslever, Popieul, and Simon (2007). Correspondence analysis is an exploratory technique that may be used to see which rows or columns in the table are similar. Usually, the degree of similarity is visualized in a so-called biplot that shows which rows or columns are at close distance within a two-dimensional space. For an introduction to correspondence analysis, we refer the reader to Greenacre (2007).

10.8 Scanpath comparison measures

Scanpath comparison measures are used to estimate the similarity between two or more scanpaths. They draw on the methods for scanpath representation, simplification, and sequence alignment that we introduced in Chapter 8. In this section only measures that take into account the *ordinal* aspect of scanpaths are listed, and therefore position-based measures like attention map difference, Kullback-Leibler distance, and Mannan distance can be found in Chapter 11, devoted explicitly to gaze position.

Many of the measures described here perform mainly pairwise comparisons, but there are measures that allow for groupwise comparisons as well. For example Feusner and Lukoff (2008) describe a method for calculating statistical significance between groups of scanpath comparisons, even if the basic comparison measure is only pairwise. Moreover, several groupwise similarity measures have been devised using attention map sequences.

10.8.1 Correlation between sequences

Target question	Do participants visit the AOIs of your stimulus in the same way, or in the particular order that you predict?
Input representation	AOI strings
Output	Correlation value [-1,1]

The correlation between sequences takes two numerical representations of AOI strings and correlates them. The simplest is to correlate the strings of two participants or conditions. An alternative is to have a predicted order and correlate each participant's string to the string representing the predicted order.

Table 10.4 shows fictitious data from a participant looking at two different designs, one after the other, each having nine AOIs (named 1 to 9). Data in the table only include the *first* entries into an AOI. Calculating the correlation between the observed and predicted order of the AOI entries then gives us an estimate of the accuracy of the prediction. In the example, Design 1 has a correlation value of 0.95 and Design 2 the value -0.017. This indicates that Design 1 better triggered the predicted eye-movement behaviour from this participant.

Table 10.4 Order of predicted AOIs above, and below the fictitious AOI sequences of one participant looking at two different designs.

Predicted	1	2	3	4	5	6	7	8	9
Design 1	2	1	3	4	6	5	8	7	9
Design 2	8	7	2	3	6	1	5	4	9

Suppes (1990) used this measure to compare a normative model of arithmetic problem solving against eye-tracking data, finding average correlation values ranging from 0.583 to 0.874 for the different participant groups. Holsanova et al. (2008) used the measure to compare a serial versus a radial design of information graphics, finding an average correlation of 0.95 between predicted and actual reading behaviour for the serial information graphics, and no correlation for the radial design.

10.8.2 Attention map sequence similarity

Target question	Do individual participants, or groups of participants, sequence the AOIs of your stimulus in a particular order?
Input representation	Raw data samples
Output	Similarity value

Attention maps are typically static entities. However, attention maps can evolve over time and become *map sequences* (Wooding, 2002a). Such sequences can be seen as a collection of scanpaths from one or many participants that preserve ordinal information. As such, an attention map sequence is a three-dimensional scanpath function $f(S)$, as defined on page 253.

If we have a still image as a stimulus, we can generate different attention maps, each for a separate time interval along the trial duration. The resulting map sequence gives insight into how the attention map evolves over time, information which cannot be extracted from the final attention map collapsed over the entire trial. In fact, initial attention and overall attention can differ significantly in distribution, as Figure 10.32 shows (from Nyström, 2008).

Since map sequences can be generated from single and multiple scanpaths, both pairwise and groupwise scanpath comparisons are possible. Nyström et al. (2004) used the harmonic Kullback-Leibler distance (p. 376) to compare map sequences generated from two videos: an original video and a foveated, compressed version of it. Comparing the eye movements predicted by their well-known computational model of saliency to the real eye movements of human observers, Itti (2004) devised a metric that evaluated each recorded data sample on the saliency map, and then calculated the resulting average value over all data samples and frames. Itti found the saliency model to predict gaze locations better than chance. Grindinger, Duchowski, and Sawyer (2010) proposed a similar groupwise measure where fixation samples from all viewers in one group were compared to an attention map built from all viewers in another group. To validate their approach, a classifier was used to test whether experts' scanpaths were more similar to other experts' scanpaths than they were to novices', and vice versa. Grindinger et al. (2010) used still images as stimuli, and reported that their method achieved higher classification-accuracy than did the string edit distance (adapted for groupwise comparison).

Given two map sequences, any of the attention map based measures in Chapter 11 can be used to compare the maps at a certain time instant (or ordinal position). Then all similarity values can be added to find the overall scanpath similarity. This approach can be generalized to all point-based measures that compare two or more sets of data samples over time.

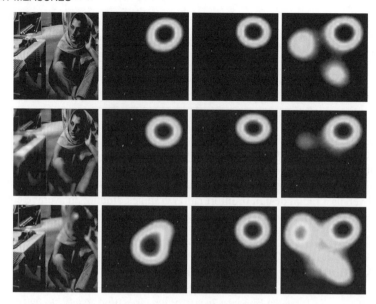

Fig. 10.32 The heat maps visualize how recorded data sample positions from seven viewers are distributed over different time intervals when viewing three different versions of an image. The second column shows where attention is located between 300–350 ms, the third column where attention is located between 600–650 ms, and the fourth column shows the overall attention. The photo is reproduced here with permission from the Signal Compression Lab, University of California Santa Barbara.

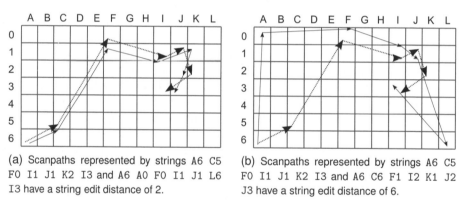

(a) Scanpaths represented by strings A6 C5 F0 I1 J1 K2 I3 and A6 A0 F0 I1 J1 L6 I3 have a string edit distance of 2.

(b) Scanpaths represented by strings A6 C5 F0 I1 J1 K2 I3 and A6 C6 F1 I2 K1 J2 J3 have a string edit distance of 6.

Fig. 10.33 Examples showing a major weakness of the string edit measure: the sensitivity to AOI borders.

10.8.3 The string edit distance

Target question	What is the AOI sequence similarity between two scanpaths?
Input representation	AOI strings of dwells
Output	String edit distance (string symbols)

Comparing two scanpaths and giving a distance value for them, the string edit measure (known as the 'Levenshtein distance' in computer science after originator Levenshtein, 1966) assumes that both scanpaths are represented with an AOI string of dwells. Both gridded and semantic AOIs are being used with the string edit distance measure (see p. 206 for the distinction between these AOI types).

Distance is calculated as the minimum number of *insert*, *delete*, and *substitute* operations needed to transform one string into the other. A smaller distance means that fewer transformations have to be made, and therefore the scanpaths should be more similar. For instance, if we have two scanpaths

$$S_1 : \text{A6 C5 F0 I1 J1 K2 I3}$$

$$S_2 : \text{A6 A0 F0 I1 J1 L6 I3}$$

we need to substitute A0 with C5 and L6 with K2. This gives us a total editing distance of two (2) for the comparison of S_1 against S_2. If instead we compare S_1 to a very different string S_3,

$$S_1 : \text{A6 C5 F0 I1 J1 K2 I3}$$

$$S_3 : \text{A6 C6 F1 I2 K1 J2 J3}$$

we need to substitute the last six AOIs in one string, giving an edit distance of six (6). This pair of scanpaths is thus three times more dissimilar than the first pair.

In order to compare two scanpaths of lengths m and n, the string edit distance d is often normalized against the maximum string length, which equals the largest possible edit distance.

$$\hat{d} = 1 - \frac{d}{\max(m,n)} \qquad (10.20)$$

Thus, $\hat{d}$ varies from 0 to 1, where 1 signifies two identical strings. In our example, we would have a $\hat{d}$ of 0.71 for the more similar pair, and 0.14 for the less similar pair.

The string edit measure is undoubtedly the most employed measure for pairwise scanpath similarity. In the literature, it has been used to study:

Scene perception versus subsequent imagery For instance, Brandt and Stark (1997) and Gbadamosi and Zangemeister (2001) both compare imagery theories.

First viewing versus a second viewing L. Holm (2007) studied the role of expectations on the perception of an upcoming stimulus.

Website scanning Josephson and Holmes (2002) tested the scanpath theory with repeated viewings of the same web content. Also see Pan et al. (2004) who investigated behaviour when viewing webpages using the string edit method.

The validity of different theories about scanpaths Privitera and Stark (2000) and Foulsham and Underwood (2008) compared the fixation sequences of human viewers of a scene versus the scanpaths predicted by saliency-based models of eye movements. Hacisalihzade, Stark, and Allen (2002) investigated the relative role of deterministic and probabilistic influences on scanpaths, and the originators of this research, Choi et al. (1995), directly questioned the "usefulness of using string editing algorithms as a tool to quantify the similarity of fixation sequences for human participants searching a quasi-natural stereoscopic three-dimensional environment".

Moreover, the string edit algorithm is implemented in the publicly available software programmes of West et al. (2006) and Myers and Schoelles (2005).

Privitera and Stark (2000) denoted the edit distance 'sequential similarity' and complemented it with a 'locus similarity' measuring the proportion of letters in one string that were present in the other string, regardless of order. To represent the large number of similarity scores within and between participants and stimuli, they proposed what they call parsing diagrams, where only the average score for each combination was given. Comparing computer generated and human fixations, Privitera and Stark (2000) conclude that the algorithms they test do a poor job at predicting human fixation sequences.

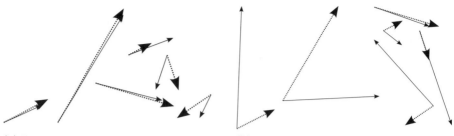

(a) Pairs of vectors from scanpath (a) in Figure 10.33.

(b) Pairs of vectors from scanpath (b) in Figure 10.33.

Fig. 10.34 The length of the differential vector in each pair equals the distance between the two arrow tips.

String editing is not limited to data representations based on two-dimensional AOIs, but can be extended to handle vectors. The *vector string* is calculated based on the amplitude and direction of the scanpath saccades, as described on page 269. In short, each vector is represented by two values: one for amplitude and one for direction. Using the same example as in Figure 10.33, the three vector strings will be:

- Left side thin scanpath: 23 1B 46 34 83 92
- Dashed thick scanpath: 24 1B 47 22 83 A3
- Right side thin scanpath: 0D 3A 46 52 7A E9

Since the example uses hexadecimal values, only 16 possible amplitudes/directions can be represented.

As in standard AOI-string editing, two strings are compared using editing operations, and the result is an editing distance. Since the strings represent real vectors, Gbadamosi (2000) added geometrical costs to the comparisons:

- *Insertion* or *deletion* equalled the amplitude of the inserted or deleted vector.
- *Substitution of vector u by vector v* added a cost equal to the length of the differential vector $\|u - v\|$.

In our example, there are no insertions or deletions but only substitution in the minimal edit distance, so the cost consists of a sum of the differential vectors. Figure 10.34 shows the pairs of vectors. For each pair, the differential vector equals the Euclidean distance between the tips of the arrows. For the pairs in (a), the tip distances are 7.95, 5.83, 12.14, 20.37, 20.6, 21.09, which gives a total editing cost (i.e. similarity) of 87.98. In the (b) pairs, the tip distances are 116.05, 106.16, 11.09, 26.08, 74.10, 97.33, with a total editing cost of 430.81.

Gbadamosi (2000) suggests normalizing all distances (d) against the maximum d_{max} (in our case 430.81) to yield a value span of between -1 and 1, giving the normalized edit cost

$$\hat{d} = 1 - 2\frac{d}{d_{max}} \qquad (10.21)$$

Vector string editing handles scanpath *shape* much better than the classical AOI string editing. The major weakness of the vector string editing method is that it completely ignores spatial position. For example, two scanpaths which produce the same vectors—or angles—when connecting fixations, will give identical similarity scores when using vector string editing, even if the overall scanpath is focused in a different area, if it is spatially scaled, or if the amplitudes between saccades in the sequence are completely different (see Figure 10.35). Vector string editing per se therefore needs to be complemented with a position comparison method.

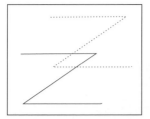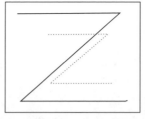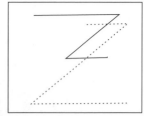

Fig. 10.35 Pairs of scanpaths where the first fixation in each begins in the top left. Vector-based string editing omits any comparison of position: each scanpath (thick line) and its pair (dashed line) are identical in terms of vectors, but completely different in terms of overall spatial position (left panel), scaling (middle panel), and amplitude between fixations (right panel).

Design issues with the string edit measure

Originally, the string edit distance algorithm by Levenshtein (1966) was developed to be a string comparison method that is extensively used on one-dimensional strings in computer communication theory and genetic research. The method was imported into the eye-tracking world around 1990 by Lawrence Stark and collegues (compare Choi et al., 1995). Was the import successful? Does the string edit measure correspond to our subjective feeling of similarity? Figure 10.33 shows the scanpaths represented by the strings we used earlier. As we can see, the pair of scanpaths found to have distance 2 appear much less similar than the pair with distance 6.

It is easy to create other examples showing non-intuitive results of this measure. One fundamental weakness of the measure is that it was originally designed for single-dimensional strings and not for a two-dimensional space with its built-in Euclidean distance. Therefore two AOIs at a far distance are considered equally similar to two AOIs in immediate proximity. That is the reason why we constructed the example in Figure 10.33(a) with the A0 and L6 fixations in it. In Figure 10.33(b), we placed fixations close to each other, but on either side of a border, to make two very similar scanpaths appear very dissimilar in the string edit measure. In Figure 10.33(a), we placed fixations as far away as possible from each other, yet within the same AOI, to make two dissimilar scanpaths appear similar to the measure.

The weaknesses illustrated in Figure 10.33 are not uncommon, as the probability for two fixations to be located on either side of a border is not very low. Noise and poor precision increase the danger that two fixations that should be at the same position are in different AOIs. However, over many scanpath comparisons, the effect can be expected to be somewhat milder. Also, some users of the string edit measure, for instance Foulsham (2008), ran the same similarity calculations over several different grid sizes (Figure 10.36), to reduce the arbitrariness of the division of space into gridded AOIs.

If semantic AOIs with very varying sizes are used, the intuitiveness of the string edit measure is even lower. Figure 10.37(a) shows two widely different scanpaths that would be classified as identical, even though this is clearly not the case.

Apart from the size of AOIs, the semantic content of the AOI matters. If each AOI is semantically homogeneous, as in Figure 10.37(b)—where every AOI has only one semantic object and it does not matter where we look—then semantic AOIs give more intuitive results with the string edit measure, than if AOIs contain many different semantic elements. Also, the distance between the AOIs should not be of the same kind as the distance within the AOIs. In Figure 10.37(b), there is no meaningful semantic or spatial distance in the stimulus between the bottle and the glasses that can be expressed in terms of the height of the bottle or the diameter of the glasses. The lack of such between-AOI distances eliminates the possibility that AOIs which seem distant to us are treated by the string edit measure as equally close

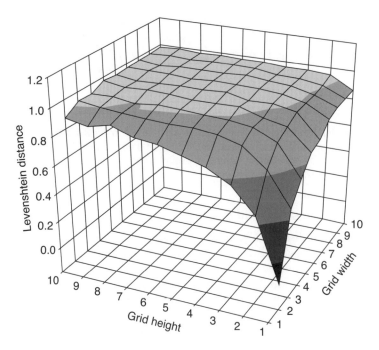

Fig. 10.36 The normalized Levenshtein string-edit distance for two random scanpaths as a function of size of the gridded AOIs. Grid dimensions vary from 1 x 1 (the stimulus is a single region where all fixations are evaluated as equal) to 10 x 10 (100 regions). The distance expected by chance increases as a finer grid is used. With kind permission from Springer Science+Business Media: HCI and usability for education and work, Knowledge-Based Patterns of Remembering: Eye Movement Scanpaths Reflect Domain Experience, *Lecture Notes in Computer Science* 5298, 2008, Andreas Holzinger, Figure 3.

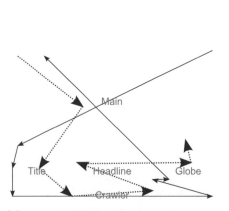

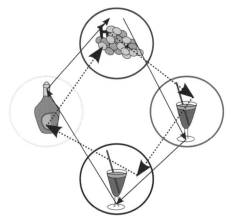

(a) Semantic AOIs and two scanpaths (big ar-rowheads and broken line, versus small arrow-heads and full line) that are considered identical by the string edit measure.

(b) The string edit measure best suits clearly delimited AOIs with a good distance between them, a generous margin and a single semantic unit inside each AOI.

Fig. 10.37 Poorer and better AOIs when using the string edit measure for scanpath similarity.

together as two AOIs which are in fact separated by only a small distance.

The third important AOI design issue is the proximity of the AOIs. Ideally, when the string edit measure is employed, AOIs should be clearly spatially separated, and have large enough safety margins, as in Figure 10.37(b), to reduce the danger that small variations in gaze position cause large differences in string edit distance.

10.8.4 Refined AOI sequence alignment measures

Target question	*How similarly have two scanpaths sequenced the AOIs?*
Input representation	*AOI strings*
Output	*Similarity score*

The limitations of the string edit algorithm call for more flexibility in adapting semantic and spatial relationships between AOIs, as well as cost parameters to match the specific question under investigation. To some extent the string edit algorithm can be extended by assigning different costs to operations. For example, Hacisalihzade et al. (2002) empirically found that 1 for substitution, 2 for insertion, and 3 for deletion were relevant costs with regard to their experimental questions.

In recent years, more advanced implementations of sequence alignment algorithms have been used for scanpath analysis; in particular the Needleman-Wunsch algorithm (Needleman & Wunsch, 1970) and the Clustal family of algorithms (Chenna et al., 2003). These algorithms use a comparison matrix combined with gap penalties to dynamically find the optimal alignment between two sequences (p. 274).

The Needleman-Wunsch algorithm is at the heart of the publicly available software packages ScanMatch (Cristino et al., 2010) and eyePatterns (West et al., 2006), and has been used to compare scanpaths when studying decision strategies (Day, 2010). Two implementations of the Clustal software, ClustalG (Wilson, Harvey, & Thompson, 1999) and ClustalW (Thompson, Higgins, & Gibson, 1994), have been used by Fabrikant, Rebich-Hespanha, Andrienko, Andrienko, and Montello (2008) "to systematically compare and summarise individual inference making histories collected through eye-movement analysis", and by Turano, Geruschat, and Baker (2002) and Turano, Geruschat, and Baker (2003) to quantify scanpath similarity during walking.

'ScanMatch' by Cristino et al. (2010) compares AOI strings in which duration has been taken into account by repeating letters in proportion to their fixation durations. It also allows AOIs to be labelled with two letters, allowing more AOIs than the 26 of the English alphabet. AOI strings are aligned with the Needleman-Wunsch algorithm, which appears earlier to have been used for scanpath alignment by West et al. (2006) in their 'eyePattern' software. Given a comparison matrix M and a gap penalty, the ScanMatch algorithm computes a similarity score (d) by summing values along the optimal path through the matrix. Each element in the comparison matrix represents a relationship between two AOIs, for example how far apart they are in space, or their semantic relationship.

To normalize for sequence length (ℓ_S), the final similarity score is computed as

$$\hat{d} = \frac{d}{\max(M)\max(\ell_{S_1}, \ell_{S_2})} \tag{10.22}$$

giving the best possible match the value 1.

Evaluating the algorithm in three experiments, Cristino et al. (2010) found ScanMatch to be more robust than the string edit distance in correctly classifying similar scanpaths, as well as identifying scanpaths recorded during a specific task.

Also using the Needleman-Wunsch algorithm, Day (2010) offers a slightly different way to compute similarity by dividing the number of identical letters N_I in the aligned sequences by the sequence length ℓ_S

$$d' = \frac{N_I}{\ell_S} \tag{10.23}$$

10.8.5 Vector sequence alignment

Target question	How similarly have two scanpaths sequenced through space?
Input representation	Saccade vectors, fixations, and input parameters
Output	A suite of similarity scores $[0, 1]$

Regardless of the method used to calculate similarity between AOI strings, string edit principles are inevitably limited by the fact that stimulus space is carved up, which only crudely represents the fullness of scanpaths. An alternative to AOI strings is to represent scanpaths with Euclidean vectors.

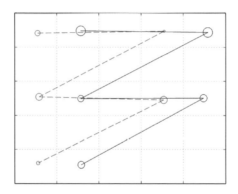

Fig. 10.38 Two example scanpaths where one is spatially shifted in relation to the other. Circle diameter represents fixation duration.

A scanpath can be seen as a collection of vectors, and hence comprise a vector space. This way of representing scanpaths was adopted by Jarodzka, Nyström, and Holmqvist (2010). Prior to comparison, the authors simplify scanpaths using thresholds for saccade direction and amplitude such that subsequent saccade vectors that go in a similar direction or have very short amplitudes are merged into larger vectors.

On the simplified representations, they propose the following sequential steps to compare two scanpaths:

1. Create a comparison matrix where each value corresponds to the similarity between two vectors in the scanpaths.
2. Create a graph (as in graph theory) from a set of rules defining how the matrix elements are connected. Assign each node in the graph with a weight proportional to the similarity value in the comparison matrix.
3. Calculate the shortest path from the top left element in the matrix to the bottom right element using Dijkstra's algorithm.
4. Align scanpaths along the shortest path such that each vector in one scanpath is matched with a vector in the other scanpath.

Then similarity is calculated on the aligned scanpaths with respect to five different aspects of the scanpaths: shape (length of vector difference), difference in amplitude between vectors, distance between fixation positions associated with saccades (equals the starting position for the saccade vector), difference in direction between vectors, difference in duration between fixations. Each measure is normalized with its largest possible value, to obtain values on the interval $[0, 1]$; 0 represents the best possible match and 1 the opposite.

Calculating similarity in several ways, the vector based algorithm has the potential to capture aspects of similarity that would otherwise be disregarded or hidden in the overall score. Figure 10.38 shows an example of two otherwise identical scanpaths, where one has been shifted in relation to the other. Given a 5×5 gridded AOI division of space as indicated in the figure, the string edit distance is 1 since no fixations do share the same AOI. However, calculating similarity according to the vector-based algorithm gives no difference in amplitude, direction, and shape, but clearly points out the difference in fixation position (0.15) and duration (0.32) (Jarodzka, Nyström, & Holmqvist, 2010).

11 Position Measures

The previous chapter presented measures of the movements of the eye. In this chapter, focus is on measures of stillness of gaze in one or many positions. The position measures pertain to where participants look, if they look at the same place, and to the properties, such as duration of fixations and dwells at that position. We differentiate between five groups of position measures.

Position measure group	Uses	Page
Basic position measures	*Where did the participant look?*	357
Position dispersion measures	*How focused versus distributed is the gaze data?*	359
Position similarity measures	*How similar are the positions of two groups of gaze data?*	370
Position duration measures	*For how long did gaze stay in the position?*	376
Position dilation measures	*What is the pupil dilation at the position?*	391

We begin this chapter by spelling out the basic properties of position, that is, simply where a participant looks in terms of raw data samples, fixations, and dwells. These *basic position measures* report the very (x, y)- and area of interest (AOI)-values of data, and where in a specific AOI the eye lands.

Next we go on to define measures which describe variability in basic position, that is, measures of *position dispersion*. Position dispersion measures calculate how focused versus distributed a collection of position data (which we will call $\mathscr{A}$) are. Note that the many dispersion measures are in fact not measures, but different mathematical definitions of the vague concept of dispersion. The reason that we list these definitions as measures is that the research community writes about them as measures, not as definitions. As a consequence, the target question and use of the measures are close to identical, and the measure descriptions are more mathematical, while less emphasis is placed on functional interpretations. Although they all define dispersion, each such 'measure' behaves differently, as the comparison on page 359 demonstrates.

From dispersion, questions arise as to how comparable different position data are, and therefore measures of *position similarity* come next. Position similarity measures compare one collection $\mathscr{A}$ of positions—say the fixations of one group of people—and give a value describing how similar the positions in $\mathscr{A}$ are to the positions in the collection $\mathscr{B}$. Again, these measures are rather definitions which attempt to capture the vague concept of position similarity. Also note that these measures only compare the similarity in position, not taking sequence information into account. A particular statistical quirk with the similarity measures is that they output one single value for the comparison.

In the next two sections of this chapter we consider the *properties* of position data. Measures of *position duration* focus on the temporal characteristics of eye movement events at specific positions in space. Fixation duration and dwell time are the foundation for all the other position duration measures (with the exception of the inter-microsaccadic interval, which we will come to).

Pupil dilation is another property of position data, giving the pupil size for the current position of the eye. These properties of position data are very important because they can reflect information processing with respect to the location a participant is looking.

As a whole, the position measures have very different units, from (x,y)-coordinates and percentages of AOI widths, to whole attention maps, and in the case of the Kullback-Leibler measure, a value without a unit. Consequently, statistical methods vary between the position measures. Note that many of the ratio measures in this chapter have values that are restricted by 0, 1, or by trial durations, and that this may give invalid outcomes from some statistical tests, for instance if used as outcome variables in a regression analysis, or in some cases, when performing ANOVAs on dwell times recorded with fixed trial durations.

There is much research on factors that makes us look at positions, which—if not taken into account when designing an experiment—may turn up as confounds, but which can also be actively manipulated in your experimental design. Therefore the final section of this chapter summarizes *potentially confounding factors* which may influence position data in unwanted or unanticipated ways (p. 394).

11.1 Basic position measures

The basic position measures address questions such as where a participant looks, and what areas of interest (AOIs) are not looked at.

11.1.1 Position

Target question	*Where did the participant look?*
Input representation	*Raw data, fixation data, or AOI-based data*
Output	*The position (pixels) or an AOI name (symbol)*

In eye-tracking data, *position* is given as Cartesian (x,y)-coordinates in a two (or three)-dimensional space; this is either the stimulus for remote and tower-mounted eye-trackers, or the scene video recording for head-mounted recordings. Typically, origo is located at the top-left corner (p. 61–64).

After we have run the raw position data through fixation analysis and related this to our AOIs, we are left with three types of data, each containing different position information:

Raw data samples These (x,y)-positions are the most reliable and detailed position data, their quality endangered only by low precision, inaccuracy, latencies, and real-time recording filters.

Fixations When transformed into events, the (x,y)-positions of the raw data samples are replaced by an average (x,y)-position for samples belonging to the fixation. Fixation position data are more commonly used than the raw data samples from which they are deduced. Fixation positions are additionally subject to the peculiarities of filters, the selected fixation detection algorithm and its settings.

Dwells The dwell event does not have (x,y)-positions. The value of a dwell position is its AOI, so dwells have a whole area as their position value. When AOIs are large, recording imprecision typically does not matter much, while inaccuracy can be problematic. As a consequence, the variable type is categorical.

When recording binocular data, position can be reported as (x, y, z) with z as a third dimension inferred from the relative distance between the eyes. Typically, z contains considerable noise since it is derived from a subtraction of two already noisy measurements. Therefore, it is used only rarely.

When recording data on gaze-overlaid scene videos, position is immediately visualized by the gaze cursor.

Quantifying basic eye movement position can be interesting to researchers for many specific reasons. For instance, Land et al. (1999) classified fixation position into different functions when participants completed the everyday task of making tea. Four categories could be identified: *locating*—where in space are the objects needed to complete the task, the kettle for instance; *directing*—just before contact the target direction must be relayed to the hand before the object is grasped; *guiding*—when several objects need to be manipulated in an action sequence, supervisory fixations facilitate this process; and *checking*—verifying whether the outcome is achieved or not, whether the kettle is full for instance. The researcher should keep in mind, however, that looking at a position does not necessarily mean full understanding of the information available there, as anyone who has tried to read a foreign language will know. In a study of squash players, Abernethy (1990, p. 63) conclude the same: "Not finding any differences between experts and novices provided further support for the conclusion that the limiting factor in the perceptual performance of the novices is not an inappropriate search strategy but rather an inability to make full use of the information available from fixated display features".

11.1.2 Landing position in AOI

Target question	*How far into an AOI A does the fixation land?*
Input representation	*A fixation in the AOI A*
Output	*Percentage of horizontal extension of A, or the letter position (pixels) in the word in A*

Landing position in AOI is mostly used in reading research. There, it not only assumes a conventionalized AOI order (word order), but also that the reading direction is manifest inside the AOIs. Landing position is typically reported as number of characters and sometimes also as a percentage of the AOI size. Early studies in the 1970s and 80s showed that reader gaze does not land randomly on words, at least not in single sentence reading. There are two 'positions' in the words that have attracted the interest of reading researchers:

1. The *optimal viewing position*, located slightly to the left of the centre of the word. This is the position that gives the shortest fixation durations and naming times, and therefore presumably the most effortless lexical activation. Naming time increases on average with 20 ms per character offset from the optimal viewing position. Also, the larger the distance is between a reader's landing position and the optimal viewing position, the more likely he is to make a refixation on the word (McConkie, Kerr, Reddix, Zola, & Jacobs, 1989).

2. The *preferred viewing location* is the position in a word where most readers land. Its average is located a bit further to the left from the optimal viewing position. McConkie, Kerr, Reddix, and Zola (1988) showed that the preferred viewing location in a word depends on the launching position in the previous word.

Vishwanath and Kowler (2004) used the measure outside of reading to investigate where saccades land inside AOIs outlining objects. They showed that saccades land either near the centre of gravity in a three-dimensional (3D) object, or near the centre of gravity in its 2D projection on the retina.

11.2 Position dispersion measures

Dispersion ('variability') refers to the extent to which data are spread out or scattered. Dispersion measures appear in the literature in different contexts and under several different names. For example, 'saccadic extent' is a measure of the extension of scanpaths in the vertical and horizontal dimensions during a task. 'Fixation density' is probably the most common term when fixations are the events under investigation, although that term more often refers to the counting measure number of fixations in an AOI (e.g. J. M. Henderson & Hollingworth, 1999). When measuring the extent of raw data samples contributing to fixations, the term 'fixation dispersion' is often used. 'Distribution of gaze intensity', 'spread of search' and 'scanpath area' are other common terms for the same variability.

Position dispersion could be seen as a single, somewhat vague measure with many operational definitions. However, the very mathematics of these definitions were developed; they were termed 'measures', and we adhere to this terminology.

The common denominator for all the dispersion measures presented in this section is that they operate on *one* group of samples, either raw data samples or fixations, that do not take time or order into account, i.e. all samples are either recorded at the same time, or collapsed over time. These samples can originate from different sources such as:

1. Raw data samples or fixations from one or many participants looking at a stimulus. In this case, the dispersion in where people look derives from factors discussed previously in the book such as task, viewer idiosyncrasies, and type of stimulus. Typical research questions include how large the inter-participant fixation variability is, i.e. whether viewers look at similar positions, and thus whether their fixations are constrained to a limited part of the stimulus.

2. Raw data samples within a fixation from one or many participants looking at a stimulus. The variation within a fixation depends on factors such as the precision of the eye-tracker, the fixation stability of the viewer and, of course, which algorithm was used to define the fixation. Intra-fixational dispersion is used, for example, for clinical purposes to detect differences in fixation stability across different patient groups. Unlike data from the first type of source, data samples within a fixation are less prone to outliers, which have been removed during fixation detection.

11.2.1 Comparison of dispersion measures

Examples of three hypothetical spatial distributions of eye-tracking data are shown in Figure 11.1. In Figure 11.1(a), all the data samples are located very close to each other, and the dispersion is hence low. The opposite situation, giving a high dispersion, is illustrated in Figure 11.1(c) where data samples are spread out evenly over the display. However, in Figure 11.1(b) it is no longer transparent whether the dispersion is low or high. On the one hand, the data samples tend to cluster in two distinct groups, each with a low dispersion. If all samples are treated as a whole, on the other hand, the sum of distances between them is quite large. While most measures of dispersion give largely similar results along the extreme cases (very low or high variabilities), the results produced from the intermediate range depend heavily on which measure is used, as illustrated in Figure 11.1(d).

As shown in Figure 11.1, most of the measures yield similar and consistent results when the dispersion is very high or very low. When the scattering of data is somewhere in between

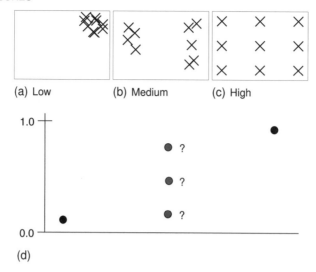

(a) Low   (b) Medium   (c) High

(d)

Fig. 11.1 For the position data in (a), dispersion is low, and for (c) it is high. But what dispersion value should the data in (b) give us?

low and high, however, less is known about how different measures behave. Here we provide a comparison of the different dispersion measures to give the reader an overview of how the definitions work (in particular with intermediate dispersion sources as input), before going on to describe the specifics of each measure of dispersion in full.

The properties of the dispersion measures which we will cover were investigated by im-plementing[29] each operationalization and comparing them using the data in Figure 11.2(b). The result can be seen in Figure 11.2(a), where values have been normalized to the interval $[0, 1]$ to better highlight differences across measures. Results show that some of the measures take more into account the fact that data with 'medium' dispersion forms two clusters, and therefore give lower dispersion values. Such examples are the nearest neighbour index (NNI), coverage, and average landing altitude. Conversely, standard deviation, range, and Kullback-Leibler distance (KLD) treat the medium- and high dispersion groups as being quite similar.

11.2.2 Standard deviation, variance, and RMS

Target question	*How much do the raw sample data or fixations in a set $\mathscr{A}$ vary from the position mean or from sample-to-sample?*
Input representation	*A set $\mathscr{A}$ of raw data samples, fixations, or angular distances θ between data samples*
Output	*Variance*

Standard deviation, variance, and root mean square are three statistical and mathematical ways of expressing variability in data. Standard deviation (SD) σ is defined as

$$\sigma = \sqrt{\frac{1}{N} \sum_{i=1}^{N} (x_i - \bar{x})^2} \tag{11.1}$$

---

[29] Our implementations, for practical reasons, differ slightly from how they are described in the text. All attention maps are generated with superimposed Gaussian functions using $\sigma = 0.10\times$ stimulus width. For coverage, the attention map was cut to half the maximum height, and the BCEA was calculated for $k = 0.5$. A symmetric version of the KLD was used (Rajashekar et al., 2004).

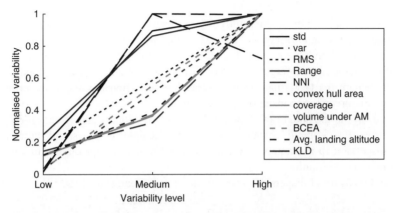

(a) Dispersion as calculated using the different operational definitions outlined in this chapter: Standard Deviation, Variance, Root Mean Square, Range, Nearest Neighbour Index, Convex Hull Area, Coverage, Volume under an Attention Map, Bivariate Contour Ellipse Area, Average Landing Altitude, Kullback-Leibler Distance. 'Low', 'medium' and 'high' corresponds to the synthetic data in (b), and a normalized variability closer to 0 indicates that the measure finds the positions to be less dispersed in space.

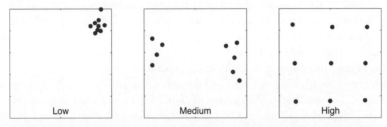

(b) Simple synthetic data sets representing fixation dispersions at two extremes (low and high), and the intermediate case where 'dispersion' is more subjective (medium). These data sets were input to the different dispersion measures, and position variability was calculated for purposes of comparison.

Fig. 11.2 The dispersion you come to report is very much influenced by the measure you chose. Simulated dispersion measures providing a heuristic for how your choice of dispersion measure will affect the dispersion output calculated. Values are normalized to the interval [0,1] to make relative comparisons easier. Note that the measures are in less agreement concerning low variability in position data, than high variability. This is a good index for the sensitivity of the chosen measure when, for instance, fixations are grouped in a spatially extended, yet local AOI on your stimulus display. It is logical that measures of dispersion in eye tracking are more sensitive to local differences in position since viewing is often restricted to monitors, and saccades are programmed to facilitate the acquisition of nearby visual information. Also note that KDL, one of the most widely used measures, finds dispersion to be lower in the 'High' case.

where $\mathscr{A}$ contains N data samples $x_i, i \in [1, 2, \ldots, N]$ and $\bar{x}$ denotes the average of all x-values.

Di Russo, Pitzalis, and Spinelli (2003) examined fixation stability in a group of professional shooters and a control group. They calculated average standard deviations of eye movements during a fixation task, and found that the shooters were more stable in their fixations (i.e. had lower standard deviations) than the control group. Furthermore, the participants in the control group were less able to keep their eyes fixated over time, since their standard deviations tended to increase after 30 seconds of fixating the target. Similarly, Edelman and Goldberg (2001) used standard deviation as a measure of the spread of saccadic endpoints (i.e. fixations) around the mean, in a study where the discharge in primate superior colliculus was compared to saccadic direction. This particular study revealed greater neuron activity to saccadic targets which were present at saccade execution (as opposed to when a saccade was made to a remembered target location). Firing rate remained constant regardless of the duration for which the target had been present, demonstrating the neural underpinnings of greater saccadic precision to visually present stimuli.

Variance, σ^2, is the square of standard deviation. Snodderly and Kurtz (1985) used the variance measure to compare fixation stability in macaque monkeys and humans, finding a greater dispersion in macaques, but also a larger between-trial variation in variance that reflected the type of stimulus.

A related measure of dispersion is the so called root mean square (RMS)

$$\theta_{RMS} = \sqrt{\frac{\theta_1^2 + \theta_2^2 + \cdots + \theta_n^2}{n}} \tag{11.2}$$

where θ denotes the distance in degrees of visual angle. It is commonly used when calculating the precision of an eye-tracker (p. 34–41).

Due to their sensitivity to outliers, and their inability to recognize cluster formations in a data set, these three measures are typically used to estimate the dispersion in samples from a fixation. Consider, for example, the case where data clusters in two well-defined groups containing the same number of points on opposite sides of a stimulus (as in Figure 11.1(b)). Arguably, the dispersion is low, but the variance becomes large since the mean lies in between the two clusters. This problem can be partly overcome by first identifying the two clusters, and then calculating the variance in each cluster separately.

Just like skewness (p. 384), the standard deviation, the variance, and RMS are summary statistics, that is, they summarize the amount of dispersion of an underlying variable. As such, these measures themselves should not be used as variables in a statistical test. Nevertheless, there are specific tests that may be used to compare the variance in two or more groups. One such test is the Levene's test, which is often used to establish whether the assumption of homogeneity of variance, that is equal variance across groups, in an ANOVA is violated or not.

11.2.3 Range

Target question	How large is the smallest box that covers the raw data samples, fixations or saccades in $\mathscr{A}$?
Input representation	A set of raw data samples, fixations or saccades $\mathscr{A}$
Output	Horizontal and vertical range /extension (pixels)

Range (R), also known as 'extent' is calculated as the distance between points in the horizontal and vertical meridians (left-to-right, and up and down directions).

$$R_h = \max(x) - \min(x)$$
$$R_v = \max(y) - \min(y) \tag{11.3}$$

Sometimes, but not always, the horizontal and vertical values are added to form an overall range $R = R_h + R_v$. Figure 11.3 illustrates the calculation. It can be seen that only four points (those that fall on the lines) are used in the calculation of range. This means that the distribution of other points within the boxed area does not affect the range, and it is therefore very

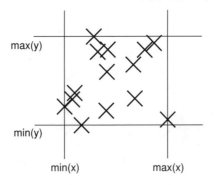

Fig. 11.3 Minimal box encapsulating all the fixations in $\mathscr{A}$.

sensitive to single outliers in the data. The maximum distance can be significantly larger if the maximal point becomes larger or the minimum point becomes smaller.

Range is a measure mostly used in human factors research, most specifically in the form of saccadic extent during car driving. Crundall and Underwood (1998) found that drivers have a saccadic extent varying from 38.7° to 82.4° in the vertical and 12.1° and 24.1° in the horizontal dimension. Saccadic extent is likely to be influenced by the *tunnel vision* that results from a heavier mental workload (see Godnig, 2003; Rantanen & Goldberg, 1999; L. J. Williams, 1988). For instance, when participants perform mental calculations and spatial imagery tasks while driving on highways, Recarte and Nunes (2000) observed significant decreases in saccadic extent.

Range has also been used to operationalize the variation in raw data samples during a fixation (this has also been termed 'fixation dispersion'), for instance in the I-DT fixation detection algorithm, to help define when a fixation begins and ends (see p. 154).

11.2.4 Nearest neighbour index

Target question	*To what degree are the points in $\mathscr{A}$ randomly distributed?*
Input representation	*A set of fixations $\mathscr{A}$*
Output	*Distance (pixels)*

The *nearest neighbour index* measure is an operational definition of dispersion originating from Di Nocera, Terenzi, and Camilli (2006), who attempt to distinguish between 'randomness' and 'order' in a distribution of fixations. Its value is calculated in three steps. First, for each point $(x_i, y_i), i \in [1, 2, \ldots, N]$ in $\mathscr{A}$, compute the Euclidean distance $d_{i,j}$ to the nearest neighbour among all the other points in $\mathscr{A}$. Then compute the average of all such distances $\frac{1}{N} \sum_{i=1}^{N} \min_j d_{i,j}$ and then divide that average by the expected value for random distributions $0.5\sqrt{\frac{A}{N}}$, where A is the area of the convex hull of the points. This gives a distance value D which can be calculated as

$$D = \frac{2}{\sqrt{AN}} \sum_{i=1}^{N} \min_j d_{i,j} \tag{11.4}$$

D approaches 1 when the distribution is more dispersed, whereas values smaller than 1 suggest more clustered distribution.

The originators of the measure calculate the NNI ratio for windows of duration 1 minute. The measure is used in human factors studies of mental workload. For instance, Camilli et al. (2008) showed that temporal attentional demand (items that need to be attended changing

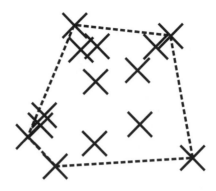

Fig. 11.4 The convex hull area is marked by a dotted line.

quickly in time) led to a more dispersed pattern, whereas visuospatial demand (the amount of information in space requiring attentional resources, irrespective of time) led to clustered pattern of fixations.

11.2.5   The convex hull area

Target question	What is the minimal convex area that spans all points in $\mathscr{A}$?
Input representation	A set of data samples $\mathscr{A}$
Output	An area (pixels^2)

The convex hull area is an operational definition of dispersion as the smallest convex polygon containing $\mathscr{A}$, illustrated in Figure 11.4. There are several algorithms for calculating convex hull for any set of points, the best known of which may be the 'divide and conquer' algorithm by Preparata and Hong (1977).

The convex hull area was adapted to eye-tracking analysis by Goldberg and Kotval (1999) to allow for crude comparisons of the overall form of a scanpath. Goldberg and Kotval give examples showing that a convex hull is a better representation of scanpath shape than just circumscribing the collection of fixations with a circle. Nevertheless, like the related range measure, the convex hull may ignore large empty areas inside the hull, and is very sensitive to single outliers; both of these are aspects of distributions that attention maps and their Gaussian landscapes readily account for (see Figure 11.5).

Some researchers still use convex hulls to analyse the spatial distribution of their eye-movement data. For instance, Sullivan, Jovancevic, Hayhoe, and Sterns (2005) had a Stargardt's disease patient, with bilateral central scotomata, perform three everyday activities: making a sandwich, catching a ball, and walking. Convex hulls were calculated from fixation data to visualize the extension of the preferred portion of visual field in each task. Ahlstrom and Friedman-Berg (2006) compare an air traffic controller weather interface with either a dynamic or a static representation of upcoming storms. Their data show that dynamic representations result in much smaller convex hull areas, and follow Goldberg and Kotval in interpreting this to mean that the static interface is poorly designed.

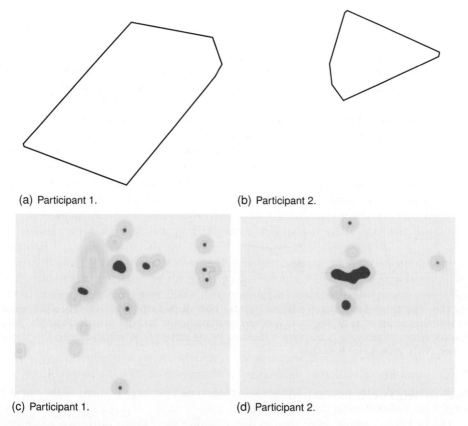

(a) Participant 1.   (b) Participant 2.

(c) Participant 1.   (d) Participant 2.

Fig. 11.5 Two participants viewing the Mona Lisa painting. Above, convex hulls around the scan path; below, heat maps for the same data.

11.2.6   Bivariate contour ellipse area (BCEA)

Target question	What is the dispersion measured as the area of an ellipse en-compassing the majority of data samples in $\mathscr{A}$?
Input representation	A set of raw data samples or fixations $\mathscr{A}$
Output	An area $(pixels^2)$

The bivariate contour ellipse area (BCEA) is calculated as the area of an ellipse that encompasses a given proportion $P = 1 - e^{-k}$ of points in a data set. It is calculated as

$$\mathrm{BCEA} = 2k\pi\sigma_h\sigma_v(1-\rho^2)^{1/2} \qquad (11.5)$$

where σ_h and σ_v denote the horizontal and vertical standard deviation of the data samples, and ρ is the Pearson's correlation coefficient between the x and y samples. As shown above, k then decides the proportion of samples (in %) to include in the ellipse area.

Crossland, Sims, Galbraith, and Rubin (2004) criticize the BCEA on grounds of not being able to differentiate between one dispersed fixation and two fixations very close to one another. Instead they opt for using a mixture of Gaussian functions to represent raw data samples in a fixation, in essence producing miniature attention maps for the raw data sample distribution within the fixation. This allows the authors to find (sub-) fixations as maxima in

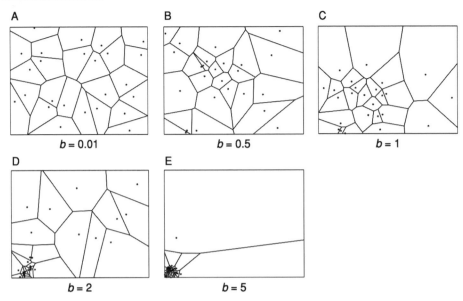

Fig. 11.6 Five stimulus spaces with fixations that have been divided into Voronoi cells. *b*-values indicate the skewness values of each. Reprinted with kind permission from Springer Science+Business Media: *Behavior Research Methods*, A quantitative measure for the uniformity of fixation density: The Voronoi method, *38*(2), 2006, Eelco A. B. Over.

the probability density function, and get information on how large portions of the raw data samples are included under each maximum.

The BCEA has mainly been used to operationalize the fixation dispersion ('stability') concept for clinical applications (Crossland & Rubin, 2002; Tarita-Nistor, Gonzalez, Mandelcorn, Lillakas, & Steinbach, 2009), but also in more applied fields to quantify the inter-participant dispersion across viewers watching video (Brasel & Gips, 2008).

11.2.7 Skewness of the Voronoi cell distribution

Target question	*What is the dispersion in a very large number of fixations, $\mathscr{A}$?*
Input representation	*A large set of fixations, $\mathscr{A}$*
Output	*A skewness value*

The skewness of the distribution of Voronoi cell sizes was introduced by Over, Hooge, and Erkelens (2006) who consider it an operational definition of 'fixation density'. In this measure each fixation is given one cell, as Figure 11.6 exemplifies. When fixations are sparse, cells will be large, while crowded fixations give small cell sizes. When fixations are equally distributed, cell sizes will be the same, and have an unskewed distribution. Voronoi tessalation is a simple calculation that exists in several softwares.

Skewness is calculated with Equation (10.5) on page 316 with cell sizes as input. Over et al. fitted mathematical probability density functions to the observed cell-size distributions in order to estimate confidence intervals. Although the skewness value can be calculated also when $\mathscr{A}$ contains few fixations, acquiring a confidence interval would require large numbers (at least 10,000) of fixations for high accuracy, Over et al. estimate.

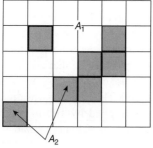
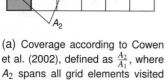

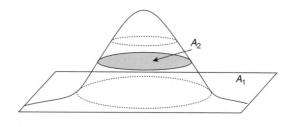

(a) Coverage according to Cowen et al. (2002), defined as $\frac{A_2}{A_1}$, where A_2 spans all grid elements visited at least once, and A_2 all non-visited areas.

(b) Coverage in attention maps: A_2 is the area of the cutoff region at a selected height, while A_1 is the area of the entire stimulus image. Coverage is defined as $\frac{A_2}{A_1}$, but is sensitive to the slice level. The volume under the map summarizes all slice levels in one value.

Fig. 11.7 Coverage versus volume under the map.

11.2.8 Coverage, and volume under an attention map

Target question	*How large is the area or volume covered by the attention map from $\mathscr{A}$?*
Input representation	*An attention map made from $\mathscr{A}$*
Output	*An area (pixels^2), a volume (pixels^3), or a proportion*

The coverage as well as the volume under an attention map are two closely related operational definitions of dispersion that deal with some of the drawbacks of extent and convex hull measures, but which have been too little used.

Coverage was proposed by Wooding (2002b) as a dispersion measure operating on attention maps to "measure the amount of the original stimulus covered by the fixations". Given a height at which the attention map is 'cut off', Wooding defines the coverage as the area of the cutoff region (A_2) divided by the area of the whole image (A_1)

$$\text{Coverage} = \frac{A_2}{A_1} \tag{11.6}$$

In Figure 11.7(b), the cutoff height is set to half the maximum height and the cutoff area is represented by the shaded, grey region. However, a major problem is that the coverage value depends heavily on an appropriate selection of slicing/cutoff level.

The volume under the map measure overcomes the settings problem by extending the calculation to three dimensions: normalize the height of the attention map to unity (p. 248), and then calculate the *volume* under the attention map using summation or integration. In addition to making the slice level setting unnecessary, the volume approach gives a more sensitive measure, since areas at all different slicing levels are integrated into one single value.

An appropriate smoothing factor for the attention map (e.g. σ if using Gaussian based attention maps) still remains to be selected, and this choice will affect the coverage and volume under the map measures. See page 245 for suggestions of how to select σ. Parallel analyses with several σs can be used to test whether the dispersion value is solely an effect of choosing the right σ, or if it reflects a systematic effect in your data.

Using a slightly different method to calculate coverage, shown in Figure 11.7(a), Cowen et al. (2002) first divided the stimulus into a grid, and then defined coverage as the number of visited grid elements divided by the total number of elements. One dwell into a grid element was sufficient to count it as a 'visit'. They interpret the measure to be indicative of 'focused efficient searching' versus 'widespread inefficient search'. Cowen et al. describe their method as follows: "A screenshot was taken and loaded into a graphics package so that a grid, with squares measuring 30×30 pixels, could be overlaid on the screenshot of the page. The number of squares containing one or more fixations was manually counted. This number was divided by the total number of squares covering the page and then multiplied by 100 to produce a percentage" (p. 329). Similar methods to calculate the dispersion of fixations had been proposed already in the 1960s by Mackworth and Morandi (1967).

A related coverage measure is the *weighted search area* (WSA) proposed by C. F. Chi and Lin (1997), who argue that the WSA "can describe concentrations of visual search patterns and potentially quantify the amount of visual load (p. 255)" [of participants engaged in a simulated driving task]. The implementation is described in 10 detailed steps in the paper, and is based on the ideas to 1) divide the stimulus space into quadrants and 2) represent fixations in each quadrant with a vector taking both the position and duration of fixations into account.

Taking stimulus features into account, coverage has also been defined as the percentage of objects in a scene looked at for more than a minimum duration (Yoon & Narayanan, 2004a).

11.2.9 Relative entropy and the Kullback-Leibler Distance (KLD)

Target question	How large is the dispersion in $\mathcal{A}$, when counted as the average distance between the attention map of each fixation in $\mathcal{A}$ and the attention map of all the other fixations?
Input representation	A set of raw data samples or fixations $\mathcal{A}$ per participant
Output	Dispersion value (bits)

Entropy was explained on page 341. The Kullback-Leibler distance (KLD), sometimes also called the Kullback-Leibler divergence or relative entropy, is an operational definition of distance—not dispersion, but we will come to that—between two groups of data according to the known information theoretic measure with the same name (Cover & Thomas, 1991). Input data have the form of probability density functions (pdf:s), a form of normalized attention maps. If $p(x)$ and $q(x)$ denote the input pdfs for sets of eye-tracking data $\mathcal{A}$ and $\mathcal{B}$, the KLD is defined as

$$\mathfrak{D}(p||q) = \sum_x p(x) \log_2 \frac{p(x)}{q(x)} \tag{11.7}$$

over the alphabet $\mathcal{X}$ and is measured in bits. Zero-values in $p(x)$ results in a mathematical error (the logarithm of zero), and therefore Onat, Libertus, and König (2007) replaced all zero-values with a very small constant ($c = 10^{-9}$).

The KLD can be interpreted as the penalty in bits when assuming that the distribution of a random variable is $p(x)$ when it is in fact $q(x)$. It is used in information theory to measure the 'distance' between two probability density functions, although it is not a mathematically true distance, since it does not fulfil what is known as the triangle inequality, and is asymmetric. Symmetrization of the KLD can be achieved by calculating, for example, the harmonic mean $1/[1/\mathfrak{D}(p||q)+1/\mathfrak{D}(q||p)]$. Another alternative symmetrization (and smoothing) of the KLD is called the Jensen-Shannon divergence ($\mathfrak{D}_{JS}$). It is defined as

$$\mathfrak{D}_{JS}(p||q) = \frac{\mathfrak{D}(p(x)||\frac{p(x)+q(x)}{2}) + \mathfrak{D}(q(x)||\frac{p(x)+q(x)}{2})}{2} \tag{11.8}$$

While the KLD is mathematically tractable it lacks intuitiveness; what does, for example, a dispersion of 14 bits mean? Moreover, a pdf cannot robustly be estimated from an attention map built from a few data samples, as pointed out by 't Hart et al. (2009).

The Kullback-Leibler distance can be transformed into a measure of dispersion, by calculating the KLD between the pdf of a single data point in $\mathscr{A}$, and the pdf generated from all other points in $\mathscr{A}$. This calculation is made repeatedly, by singling out each point in $\mathscr{A}$ and comparing the KLD to the others. The final dispersion value is the average of all these similarity measurements. This is a very general method, that can be applied to any similarity measures to make a dispersion measure out of it, and has also been done with the average landing altitude measure.

The KLD measure was first used as a dispersion measure for eye-tracking data by Tatler, Baddeley, and Gilchrist (2005), and was later adopted by 't Hart et al. (2009), for example. Tatler, Baddeley, and Gilchrist generated a gridded AOI with squares of $2° \times 2°$; fixations were binned accordingly into these squares, and then normalized into a probability density function before computing the KLD. Their study compares the consistency in fixation locations between observers over time (measured as number of fixations), finding that it is high in the early phase, but decreases already after 3–4 fixations. Using the standard definition of entropy, Sawahata et al. (2008) found in a study of children watching TV programmes that dispersion varied with programme comprehension.

11.2.10 Average landing altitude

Target question	What is the dispersion, measured as the average landing altitude, when dropping each data sample of each participant in $\mathscr{A}$ onto the attention map of all the other participants?
Input representation	A set of raw data samples or fixations $\mathscr{A}$ per participant
Output	A dispersion value

The average landing altitude (ALA) dispersion measure is closely related to the similarity measure with the same name on page 373. The average landing altitude is calculated as the height at which the eye-tracking data of each viewer landed on the attention map created from all other viewers' eye-tracking data. Formally, dispersion is defined as

$$D_{ALA} = \frac{1}{N} \sum_{i=1,2,...,N} \frac{AM_{max}^{i'} - AM^{i'}(x_i, y_i)}{AM_{max}^{i'} - AM_{avg}^{i'}} \qquad (11.9)$$

where $AM^{i'}$ denotes an attention map that has been generated by $N-1$ data samples; all excluding the ith sample. $AM_{max}^{i'}$ and $AM_{avg}^{i'}$ denote the maximum and average value of $AM^{i'}$, respectively. $AM^{i'}(x_i, y_i)$ represents the height at which data sample (x_i, y_i) 'lands'. Consequently, a random distribution gives a values close to 1, whereas a dense distribution has a dispersion close to zero.

The measure was developed by Nyström (2008) to overcome the lack in the KLD measure of an intuitive result unit. Inspired from the work by Itti (2005), Nyström used the measure to compare the dispersion across viewers' gazes before and after foveation of videos (where visual resolution is compressed at points at which the observer *did not* fixate), and found the dispersion to decrease when participants watched the foveated videos.

11.3 Position similarity measures

The similarity measures for position quantify similarity as the level of proximity between two sets of position data (raw data samples or fixations) with no particular order between them. They all take as input two sets of position data $\mathscr{A}$ and $\mathscr{B}$, and they output a single value for that comparison. A single value output for a comparison may make it difficult to perform statistical tests determining whether $\mathscr{A}$ and $\mathscr{B}$ are significantly different from one another.

Like dispersion, similarity is also a vague concept for which there are several operational definitions. These definitions, rather than the concept, are termed 'measures'.

11.3.1 Euclidean distance

Target question	*What is the distance between two positions?*
Input representation	*Two position points (x_1, y_1) and (x_2, y_2), either as raw data samples, fixations or dwells*
Output	*Euclidean distance (pixels or degrees)*

The Euclidean distance, a much-used general measure in eye-tracking research, has also been used to operationalize similarity in position between two sets of data samples (raw or fixations). Euclidean distance between two points is defined as

$$d = \sqrt{(x_1 - x_2)^2 + (y_1 - y_2)^2} \qquad (11.10)$$

where (x_1, y_1) and (x_2, y_2) are the coordinates of the two points in two-dimensional space. Rao, Zelinsky, Hayhoe, and Ballard (2002) use the Euclidean distance as an operational definition of position similarity. 't Hart et al. (2009) use Euclidean distance to quantify consistency between observers at each time instant. However, they argue that the KLD is better seen over a whole trial, since the Euclidean distances summed over time would give a low similarity value when all observers visit the same positions, but in different order.

11.3.2 Mannan similarity index

Target question	*How similar in position are the raw data samples or fixations in $\mathscr{A}$ to those in $\mathscr{B}$?*
Input representation	*Two sets of data samples $\mathscr{A}$ and $\mathscr{B}$*
Output	*A distance (pixels)*

An early attempt to operationalize the similarity between two populations of eye-tracking data was presented in Mannan et al., 1995, 1996 and Mannan, Ruddock, & Wooding, 1997. It is closely related to the nearest neighbour index. Given two sets of positions, $\mathscr{A}$ and $\mathscr{B}$ from raw data or fixations with M and N points, Mannan *et al.* used a measure where the squared Euclidean distance d^2 from each position i (of M) in $\mathscr{A}$ to the closest position j (of N) in $\mathscr{B}$ was calculated and vice versa. The similarity index was then calculated as the average of all squared distances

$$D_{\text{Mannan}} = \frac{1}{M+N} \left(\sum_{i=1}^{M} \min d_{i,j}^2 + \sum_{j=1}^{N} \min d_{i,j}^2 \right) \qquad (11.11)$$

As pointed out by Tatler, Baddeley, and Gilchrist (2005) as well as Underwood et al. (2008b), among others, this type of distance-based measure has a number of severe limitations. Individual fixations may have disproportional impact on the overall similarity index,

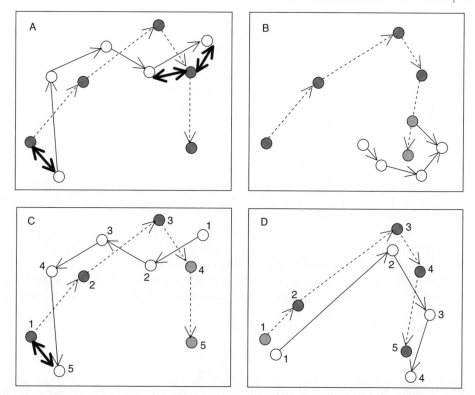

Fig. 11.8 Examples from Underwood *et al.* (2008b) pointing out limitations with the Mannan similarity index. A shows the basic case where fixations in $\mathscr{A}$ (grey) can be mapped to the closest fixation in $\mathscr{B}$ (white). Figure B exemplifies the problem that a single fixation in $\mathscr{A}$ will be mapped on all fixations in $\mathscr{B}$ and make the similarity value artifically low. Case C shows spatial mappings between the closest fixations in either distribution will ignore scanpath order, making the Mannan measure a pure position measure. Case D further exemplifies the need for scanpath simplification before alignment (pp. 268–273). With kind permission from Springer Science+Business Media: Knowledge-Based Patterns of Remembering: Eye Movement Scanpaths Reflect Domain Experience, 2008, Geoffrey Underwood.

and yield an index that is clearly not commensurate with the intuitive similarity. In extreme cases, the Mannan distance can be very unintuitive, as in Figure 11.8(B), where the positions in $\mathscr{B}$ are packed in a small region somewhere in the stimulus, whereas $\mathscr{A}$ covers the whole stimulus area. Since all distances to the closest point in $\mathscr{A}$ are low, the similarity index would indicate a good match between $\mathscr{A}$ and $\mathscr{B}$, although intuitively this is not the case. After the advent of improved similarity measures, the Mannan measure can be considered obsolete.

11.3.3 The earth mover distance

Target question	*What is the cost of transporting the total fixation durations from $\mathscr{A}$ to $\mathscr{B}$?*
Input representation	*Two sets $\mathscr{A}$ and $\mathscr{B}$ of fixations with position and duration*
Output	*A distance/cost (pixels)*

The earth mover distance (EMD) is a solution to the so-called transportation problem, which concerns minimizing the cost for moving any amount of matter from one set of source locations to another set of destinations. It can be solved by the Hungarian algorithm originally

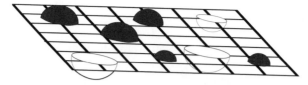

Fig. 11.9 Illustration of the earth mover distance: the five fixations in $\mathscr{A}$ are piles of earth, while the three fixations in $\mathscr{B}$ are holes. Both piles and holes have a volume corresponding to the fixation durations. The earth mover distance is the minimal cost (distance) for moving all the earth into the holes.

developed by H. W. Kuhn (1955).

In terms of eye movements, one set $\mathscr{A}$ of fixations are the origins, and the other set $\mathscr{B}$ the receivers. The durations of the fixations in $\mathscr{A}$ are taken to be 'piles of matter' (i.e. earth), and the durations in $\mathscr{B}$ are holes to be filled, as in Figure 11.9.

If $\mathscr{A}$ and $\mathscr{B}$ have different total duration, either earth or holes would remain after the transportation process ends. For this reason, Dempere-Marco et al. (2006) normalize each fixation by dividing it by the total duration of the set it belongs to.

The EMD solves the fundamental problem of the Mannan distance by making fixation durations a limited resource. This means that one single fixation in $\mathscr{A}$ cannot be the closest to all fixations in $\mathscr{B}$, because it will long be consumed.

Mathematically, the EMD similarity is calculated as

$$\text{D}_{\text{EMD}}(\mathscr{A},\mathscr{B}) = \frac{\sum_{i=1}^{m}\sum_{i=1}^{n} d(a_i, b_j) f_{ij}}{\sum_{i=1}^{m}\sum_{i=1}^{n} f_{ij}} \tag{11.12}$$

where $d(a_i, b_j)$ is the distance in stimulus space, and f_{ij} the minimal transportation distance found by the algorithm.

Dempere-Marco et al. (2006) applied this measure to compare visual search patterns of radiologists interpreting CT images where lung disease was suspected, but argue that their EMD measure has a broader applicability as a general similarity measure.

11.3.4 The attention map difference

Target question	*Where in a stimulus is the difference in attention map altitude between $\mathscr{A}$ and $\mathscr{B}$ large, and where is it smaller?*
Input representation	*Two attention maps $\mathscr{A}$ and $\mathscr{B}$*
Output	*An attention map or a similarity value*

The attention map difference is simple: just subtract the attention map for $\mathscr{A}$ from the attention map for $\mathscr{B}$, or vice versa. The originator, Wooding (2002a), proposed that this measure was appropriate to quantify the similarity after both maps were normalized to unit height. Figure 11.10(c) shows the difference map between the attention maps in Figures (a) and (b). To obtain a single value representing the similarity, the average value of the difference map can be calculated.

There are at least three varieties of operational definitions for this measure:

1. Simple subtraction of one map from the other.

$$AM_{\text{diff}} = AM_{\mathscr{A}} - AM_{\mathscr{B}} \tag{11.13}$$

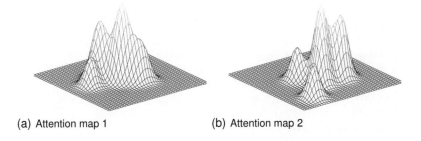

(a) Attention map 1   (b) Attention map 2

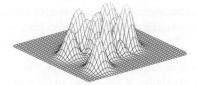

(c) Absolute difference between attention
maps 1 and 2.

Fig. 11.10 Calculating similarity by subtracting two attention maps.

This gives a difference map that can have both positive peaks and negative valleys. It shows the direction of the difference in addition to the magnitude.

2. The absolute difference between the two maps, which is always positive.

$$AM_{\text{AbsDiff}} = |AM_{\mathscr{A}} - AM_{\mathscr{B}}| \qquad (11.14)$$

Figure 11.10 exemplifies this case.

3. The *squared error* (SE), which squares the differences between the maps of dimensions $m \times n$.

$$AM_{\text{SE}} = (AM_{\mathscr{A}} - AM_{\mathscr{B}})^2 \qquad (11.15)$$

Very often the mean squared error (MSE) is used instead of the squared error

$$AM_{\text{MSE}} = \sum_{i=1}^{m} \sum_{j=1}^{n} (AM_{\mathscr{A}}(i,j) - AM_{\mathscr{B}}(i,j))^2 \qquad (11.16)$$

In spite of its simplicity, this measure appears not to have been used in actual research.

11.3.5 Average landing altitude

Target question	*What is the similarity in position between the two groups $\mathscr{A}$ and $\mathscr{B}$ of fixations or raw data samples?*
Input representation	*Two sets of position data $\mathscr{A}$ and $\mathscr{B}$ containing raw data or fixations*
Output	*A similarity value*

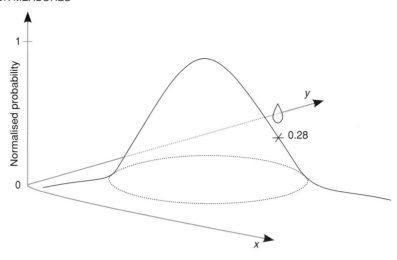

Fig. 11.11 Similarity as average landing altitude: for each fixation in $\mathcal{A}$, measure the landing height (for instance, 0.28) when dropping it on an attention map formed from $\mathcal{B}$, and then form an average over all such heights.

The average landing altitude has been used as both a dispersion (p. 369) and a similarity measure. When measuring similarity, it calculates the height at which the fixations (or raw data samples) from $\mathcal{A}$ land on the attention map created from the data in $\mathcal{B}$. This principle is illustrated in Figure 11.11, where the raindrop represents one fixation. Consequently, the similarity can be defined as

$$S_{\text{ALA}} = 1 - D_{\text{ALA}} \tag{11.17}$$

where D_{ALA} is the dispersion value given in Equation (11.9). *AM* in Equation (11.9) should now be interpreted as an attention map generated from set $\mathcal{A}$, whereas (x_i, y_i) represent data samples from set $\mathcal{B}$.

11.3.6 The angle between dwell map vectors

Target question	*How similar is the proportion of dwell time to AOIs between $\mathcal{A}$ and $\mathcal{B}$?*
Input representation	*Two matrices $\mathcal{A}$ and $\mathcal{B}$ of gridded AOIs with dwell time in each AOI cell*
Output	*A similarity value*

The angle between dwell map vectors is a mathematically elegant similarity measure first used by Pomplun et al. (1996). It uses the gridded AOI representation from page 212, in which a grid is put onto the stimulus image and dwell time is calculated for each cell. To understand the principle, we need a simplistic example. Figure 11.12 illustrates how vectors are formed from the gridded AOIs in a stimulus with only two AOIs, and how angles are formed between the vectors.

Since dwell times are always positive, the angle between the vectors can vary from 0° to 90°. Similarity is then expressed as the cosine of this angle, with a value of one indicating that the vectors are identical (0°), and a value of 0 indicating that the vectors are maximally different (90°).

Note that this measure only compares how similar proportions of dwell time are in each matrix. In particular, $\mathcal{A}$ and $\mathcal{B}$ would be considered equal by this measure if each cell value

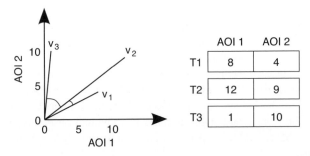

	AOI 1	AOI 2
T1	8	4
T2	12	9
T3	1	10

Fig. 11.12 Assume that there are three recordings, trial 1, 2, and 3 of data, now represented as T1–T3 in the figure. For each trial there are the same two AOIs in this simple example. There is a synthetic dwell time in each AOI for each trial. The *map vectors*, v_1–v_3 are based on using the dwell times in the grid AOIs as vector coordinates. An angle is formed between each pair of vectors. The similarity value between two recordings—trials in this case—is the cosine of that angle.

in $\mathscr{A}$ is twice the corresponding value in $\mathscr{B}$, since the two vectors would then be pointing in exactly the same direction. To test whether the dwell times in cells also equal in size, we need to calculate whether the two vectors are also of equal length.

DeAngelus and Pelz (2009) use dwell maps with normalized dwell time values (in %, with a sum of 1), which put the vectors on the unit circle. Their variety of the measure calculates the distance between (the tips of) the vectors, which roughly corresponds to the angle between vectors when the dwell map consists of normalized values.

Figure 11.12 shows gridded AOIs with only two cells. With matrices containing more cells, we have $n_x \cdot n_y$ number of cells, each with a dwell time value s_n within it. A vector $\mathbf{v} = s_1, s_2, \ldots, s_{n_x \cdot n_y}$ is then formed for each image and group of viewers. The similarity between groups 1 and 2 is defined as the cosine of the angle θ between the $n_x \cdot n_y$-dimensional vectors $\mathbf{v}_1$ and $\mathbf{v}_2$, and can be calculated as

$$\cos \theta = \frac{\mathbf{v}_1 \cdot \mathbf{v}_2}{||\mathbf{v}_1|| ||\mathbf{v}_2||} \tag{11.18}$$

Observe that when using a measures based on gridded AOIs, the output depends on the precise division of stimulus space into grids. Therefore Pomplun et al. (1996) calculated a final similarity by averaging over a number of different grid sizes.

11.3.7 The correlation coefficient between two attention maps

Target question	How similar are two sets of data samples $\mathscr{A}$ and $\mathscr{B}$?
Input representation	Two sets of data samples $\mathscr{A}$ and $\mathscr{B}$
Output	A similarity value

The correlation coefficient between attention maps uses attention maps in the form of gridded AOIs. Given two attention maps $AM_1(x,y)$ and $AM_2(x,y)$, the correlation can be computed as

$$r_{pq} = \frac{\sum_{x,y}(AM_1(x,y) - \bar{AM}_1(x,y))(AM_2(x,y) - \bar{AM}_2(x,y))}{\left[\sum_{x,y}(AM_1(x,y) - \bar{AM}_1(x,y))^2 \sum_{x,y}(AM_2(x,y) - \bar{AM}_2(x,y))^2\right]^{1/2}}$$

where $\overline{AM}(x,y)$ denotes the average value of $AM(x,y)$. This measure is closely related to the cosine from Equation (11.18). The only difference is that in Equation (11.18), the vectors have been shifted to have zero mean.

The advantage of using the correlation coefficient is that the results are intuitive and hence easy to interpret. Beside directly comparing two populations of eye-tracking data, the correlation coefficient and the KLD have been used to estimate the similarity between computationally generated *saliency maps* and attention maps from human observers (see Ouerhani, Von Wartburg, Hügli, & Müri, 2003; Rajashekar et al., 2004; Rajashekar, Van Der Linde, Bovik, & Cormack, 2008).

11.3.8 The Kullback-Leibler distance

Target question	*How large is the position similarity between the two groups of position data $\mathscr{A}$ and $\mathscr{B}$?*
Input representation	*Attention maps $\mathscr{A}$ and $\mathscr{B}$*
Output	*A similarity value (bits)*

The KLD similarity measure, mathematically defined on pages 368–369, appears to have been first used with eye-tracking data by Rajashekar et al. (2004), Nyström et al. (2004) and Tatler, Baddeley, and Gilchrist (2005). Rajashekar et al. (2004) used the symmetric KLD to quantify the distance between fixation predictions and recorded fixations from humans. Dempere-Marco et al. (2006) used the KLD measure in the feature domain in a study on mammography radiologists, to examine how similar features looked at were to visual features characteristic of malign changes. Bestelmeyer et al. (2006) compared the restrictedness of scanpaths in schizophrenia and bipolar patients using the KLD measure, as a diagnostic tool. Comparing fixation distributions on videos between humans and monkeys, D. J. Berg et al. (2009) found large differences using the KLD between distributions in a permutation test (Monte-Carlo simulation), which reveals how our visual systems differ from our closest evolutionary ancestors.

Levy, Bicknell, Slattery, and Rayner (2009) compared fixation distributions on a sentence before and after reading an ambiguous word. Fang, Chai, and Ferreira (2009) used the Jensen-Shannon divergence to investigate the change in dispersion in fixations on a scene before and after two adjacent utterances.

11.4 Position duration measures

The position duration measures all concern how long participant gaze stays within a position. The position stayed within is always either that of a fixation or an AOI. We call the fixation-based position duration *fixation duration* and the dwell-based position duration *dwell time*. With the exception of IMSI, the other measures are all varieties of fixation durations and dwell times.

11.4.1 The inter-microsaccadic interval (IMSI)

Target question	*How long is the inter-microsaccadic interval (IMSI)?*
Input representation	*An inter-microsaccadic interval*
Output	*A duration value (ms)*

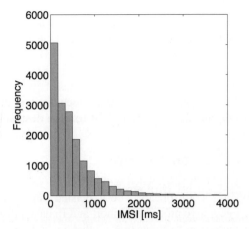

Fig. 11.13 Histogram over the distribution of inter-microsaccadic interval (IMSI), reproduced from Engbert (2006) with kind permission from Elsevier B.V.

The inter-microsaccadic interval (IMSI) is a very uncommon position measure, reported only by a few microsaccade researchers. The IMSI is to microsaccades what fixations are to saccades—periods of fixation-like ocular stability within the very small movements of microsaccades. Correctly detecting and calculating them puts high demands on both the eye-tracker hardware and filters and algorithms for event detection.

IMSI values have a distribution very similar to that of fixation durations, as Figure 11.13 shows.

11.4.2 Fixation duration

Target question	For how long was the eye still in a position?
Input representation	A fixation
Output	The fixation duration (ms)

Fixation duration is likely to be the most used measure in eye-tracking research. It is sometimes called 'fixation time', but also 'dwell time', or 'dwell time of the fixation', which may be confused with the most common use of the term dwell time as defined on page 386, which is the time from entering to exiting an AOI. Oster and Stern (1980) use the terms *saccadic reaction time* and *intersaccadic interval*.

There are a host of methodological issues surrounding the fixation duration measure, and we will go through them one by one.

The many different definitions

Informally, a fixation is defined as a period of time when the eye is relatively still (the oculo-motor definition), but some definitions add visual intake as an additional criterion on fixations (the processing definition).

In reality, fixation durations are calculated by the fixation detection algorithms described in Chapter 5, which do not care about visual intake, and have different definitions of stillness. As a result, we have a situation in which fixation durations are solely defined by the event detection algorithms and their settings. For example, there are the 'I-DT fixation durations', the 'velocity algorithm fixation durations', and the 'EyeLink fixation durations', and many more varieties due to settings, and these are related but different fixations. Researchers in general, however, have tended not to differentiate between the different algorithmic operational definitions, but surprisingly often treat the output of their own particular event detection algorithms as revealing generic true fixations that perfectly overlap with visual intake.

Data quality

As pointed out on page 161, the quality of the data affects fixation durations severely. Furthermore, if there is smooth pursuit in the data, most fixation detection algorithms will give faulty fixation durations.

Different fixations—different processing?

Different fixations are undoubtedly associated with different types of processing. In reading research, the first fixation on a word appears to be associated with lexical activation, and later fixations with discourse integrative processes. Inhoff and Radach (1998) note that it may be confounding to form averages over fixations that are that qualitatively different. This may be an issue for others than reading researchers, as the distinction between first and later fixations during scene viewing has been made by several researchers, for instance J. M. Henderson et al., 1999. Reading researchers and others furthermore differentiate between look-ahead (progressive) fixations and look-back (regressive) fixations, which may or may not be qualitatively different. Also, Land et al. (1999) classify fixations into four distinct functional types during everyday activities (see p. 358).

The different types of processing of fixations *may* be reflected in their durations. For instance, McConkie, Reddix, and Zola (1992) show that fixations *below but not above* 140 ms are affected by lexical properties of the text read. Buswell (1935):142 noted that the earliest fixations in a picture are shorter (around 210 ms) than later (around 360 ms) fixations. This has later been interpreted as an early orienting period, followed by a more scrutinous inspection of informative details, which could motivate a division of fixations according to *ambient* and *focal* processing modes (Unema et al., 2005).

Furthermore, J. M. Henderson and Pierce (2008) give evidence that one population of fixation durations is constant, while another is under the direct moment-to-moment control of the participants' ongoing scene analysis.

The participant idiosyncrasy

When a participant repeats a task, average fixation durations remain similar across trials; however different people have different average fixation durations (Andrews & Coppola, 1999, Rayner, Li, Williams, Cave, & Well, 2007, Johansson et al., 2011). These authors conclude that there is an endogenous component that correlates ($r = 0.5$–0.8) with fixation duration, requiring an adequate experimental design as well as statistical handling of data (pp. 83–85).

Dependency between successive fixations

Fixation durations are not entirely independent of one another: in scene viewing, long fixations are more often followed by other long fixations, and short fixations by short fixations (Tatler & Vincent, 2008). In visual search, Hooge, Vlaskamp, and Over (2007) found fixations on difficult search elements to be followed by long fixations on the next element, irrespective of its difficulty. Importantly, independence is required by many statistical tests.

Attention

Just and Carpenter (1980) formulated the influential strong eye–mind hypothesis, according to which there is no appreciable lag between what is fixated and what is processed. If this hypothesis is correct, then when a participant looks at a word or object, he also simultaneously processes it, for exactly as long as the recorded fixation. As can be seen below, to a large extent research supports at least a general eye–mind hypothesis.

However, visual attention—the spatial locus of intake and processing—moves slightly before the eye does. Deubel (2008) and others have shown that attention may be as much as 250 ms ahead of the eye, in particular in specially designed tasks called anti-saccade tasks (p. 305). It is not known whether this large temporal lag persists in more natural tasks, but most eye-tracking research is conducted and interpreted as though attention and fixation were synchronous events, and they probably are not.

It should be noted that there are several models of eye-movement programming in reading and scene perception (e.g. J. M. Henderson, 1992; Reichle, Rayner, & Pollatsek, 2004; Engbert, Nuthmann, Richter, & Kliegl, 2005) which attempt to capture and predict the proportion of fixation durations which can rightly be allocated to information processing, attention shifts, and saccade programming. The first two mentioned, by J. M. Henderson (1992) and Reichle et al. (2004) respectively, are strictly serial, arguing that attention does not shift until information processing is complete. However, Van Diepen and D'Ydewalle (2003) found that this does not hold across the board, since in scene viewing, masking the information visible in the visual periphery early during fixations using a gaze contingent window leads to increased fixation durations. This should not happen if a serial mechanism controls fixation duration, since information at fixation should always be processed first. The latter model cited, SWIFT, developed by Engbert et al. (2005), operates on the assumption that the attentional spotlight is more distributed, and a default timer regulates eye-movement triggering. Hence, SWIFT is a parallel model not a serial one, as attention (and thus fixations) can shift before information processing is complete.

There are many subtleties to the modelling of fixations and attention, and saccade programming. The main point is that there is a whole research literature on fixation duration and attentional shifts, regarding the two as distinguishable entities, therefore, if individual fixation durations are important for your results, it is worth bearing this in mind, and it should not just be assumed that the entirety of a fixation duration represents cognitive processing or 'visual intake'.

On the positive side, we can be fairly sure that attention and saccades are tightly coupled (Deubel & Schneider, 1996)—you can think of this like a rubber band, where stretching the rubber band to one point (the point where attention is allocated) means the other end of the rubber band (or the fixation point) will naturally follow. Therefore, when a participant executes a saccade to a target, you can be certain that attention has just moved to the same place. The fixation is only a short time behind attention, which indicates the metrics of the next eye movement.

Note that in real-world tasks, outside the laboratory from which the data and theorizing in this section derives, fixating something does not entail close attentive processing of it, and does not guarantee a trace in working memory of all the features of the object looked at (Triesch et al., 2003).

Finally, we must not forget that some processing trace of a fixated item may continue for a very long time after the eye has left the fixated position. This is evidenced by the fact that we learn from reading.

The duration of the intake period and saccadic suppression

Fixations produced by the event detection algorithms of Chapter 5 only concern the physical motion of the eye. The reason most researchers have for using fixation durations is that they are assumed to reflect perceptual intake and processing.[30] Generally speaking, this is a fair

---

[30] Although many researchers have devoted their careers to understanding the *functional mechanisms* of fixation durations on eye-movement programming it its own right; how and when a saccade is triggered, therefore not using

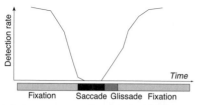

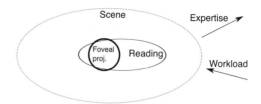

(a) Principle of saccadic suppression. Short flashes that are produced during a saccade are not reported by participants, and some of this effect spills over to neighbouring fixations.

(b) Principle for functional visual field. Visual intake takes place from an area larger than the foveal projection, expertise increases the area, and a higher workload decreases it. The functional field is asymmetrical for reading Westernised texts, and information may be gathered from a larger area during scene viewing.

Fig. 11.14 Visual intake does not coincide perfectly with fixations.

assumption *if* the intake period equals the period of stillness detected by the algorithms.

Most eye-tracking researchers know that their participants are effectively blind during saccades, but it is less known that this 'blindness' spills over to part of the fixation, and hence affects our use of the fixation duration measure, as illustrated in Figure 11.14(a). Typically *pre-saccadic suppression* shuts down visual intake for 30–40 ms preceding the start of a saccade, while *post-saccadic suppression* follows thereafter for a duration lasting around 100–120 ms (Volkmann, 1986). For a typical saccade of around 30 ms duration, some of the saccadic suppression spills over to the following fixation, so that in theory, intake and processing of the fixated position can start only after some 70–80 ms after the start of the fixation. The longer the saccade, however, the more of the suppression is consumed by the saccade, and the earlier the processing can start in the next fixation, which can thus be shorter. If fixation duration is used as a *precise* measure of processing, it is therefore advisable to measure also the duration of the preceding saccade, or at least refer to models of fixation control and saccade generation (e.g. Findlay & Walker, 1999, or some of the others mentioned in the previous section).

For a discussion as to *what* cognitive processes are suspended during saccadic suppression, see p. 321 and D. E. Irwin and Brockmole (2004). This is a large research area and full discussion is outside the scope of this chapter.

Glissades

Some authors argue that visual intake and processing starts not only directly when the fixation starts (the one detected by the algorithms), but already during the glissadic aftermaths of the saccade. For instance, Inhoff and Radach (1998) argue that there are good reasons for assigning the glissades to the fixation, since studies they quote have shown that brief flashes can be detected during the glissadic period. A counter argument is that the glissadic motion would smear the retinal image, making processing of fine texture difficult. As we saw on page 165, the glissadic velocity can be up to 130°/s, well above that of many saccades, so the smear is considerable, if intake is at all open. Event algorithms vary in what they assign the glissade to—saccade or fixation—and also in how systematically they assign them to one or the other. All in all, this contributes to making fixation duration values less comparable, at least between studies.

fixation duration simply as a measure which reflects processing of something else.

The functional visual field

How large is the area in which participants can take in meaningful information during a single fixation? In scene perception, this area has been given several names: 'functional field of view' (Mackworth, 1965), 'useful visual field' (Saida & Ikeda, 1979), 'functional visual field' (Nelson & Loftus, 1980), or 'visual span' (Reingold et al., 2001), while in reading research, the functional visual field goes under the name 'perceptual span', (Rayner & Pollatsek, 1989). Engel (1971) used the term 'conspicuity area' in visual search to describe "the retinal locus within which the object to be searched for was noticed in a single 75 msec exposure". The principle and several important factors are illustrated in Figure 11.14(b).

It is clear that the foveal projection of 1.5° of visual angle is not the only area in which intake is made. When reading, for instance, the perceptual span is asymmetric, stretching 3 degrees from the point of fixation into the direction of reading, and hardly 1 degree backwards. When radiologists scan for lung nodules, their functional visual field stretches over 5 degrees of visual angle (Kundel, Nodine, & Toto, 1991), but in general in picture viewing, it appears to be at least 10 degrees across (Shioiri & Ikeda, 1989). As with reading, a kind of expertise, the differences in span depend on what you are looking for and what you are practiced in. The larger functional visual field in scene viewing compared to reading perhaps means participants need to process more information in one fixation, which could be one explanation for why fixation durations on average are longer in scene viewing. Note, however, there are many other possible considerations: reading is highly automated with familiar words, while scenes in scene viewing experiments are likely to be comparatively novel, thus lacking in the same degree of automation as reading; moreover, participants are likely to have clusters of long fixations on objects in scene viewing, in between periods of scanning where no distinct object is fixated and fixation durations are short.

Note that the visual field is larger horizontally than vertically. Thus, human contrast sensitivity is better in the horizontal periphery than in the vertical (Banks, Sekuler, & Anderson, 1991), and detection is better in the horizontal compared to vertical dimension (Engel, 1977).

During many practical tasks, such as car driving, where peripheral vision is very important, the effective size of the functional visual field can be reduced by tasks or traffic situations that increase the *cognitive load* (Recarte & Nunes, 2000; Crundall, Underwood, & Chapman, 1999; Miura, 1992, 1990; L. J. Williams, 1988; Mourant, Rockwell, & Rackoff, 1969). For instance, car drivers' peripheral target detection decreases between 5 and 7 degrees of visual angle with increasing workload level, for all eccentricities (Crundall, Underwood, & Chapman, 2002). Furthermore, increased *driver age* further decreases the driver's peripheral detection between 8 and 24 degrees of visual angle (Gilland, 2004), while *expertise* in all tasks investigated have proven to increase the functional visual field.

Typical fixation duration values and how to interpret them

When you find the right algorithm and proper settings for your data, you will find that calculated fixations are frequently around 200–300 ms, but may be as long as several seconds (Karsh & Breitenbach, 1983; L. R. Young & Sheena, 1975), and as short as 30–40 ms, as exemplified in Figure 5.6 (p. 156). The distribution of fixation durations is not completely Gaussian; there is almost always a positive skew. Figure 11.15 shows the distribution of fixation durations in scene viewing (a) and during reading (b).

Average fixation durations definitely vary across different tasks and stimuli. Findings show one general pattern with several specific exceptions.

General finding—longer fixations equal deeper processing A longer fixation duration is often associated with a deeper and more effortful cognitive processing. This has been the conclusion in:

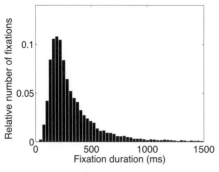 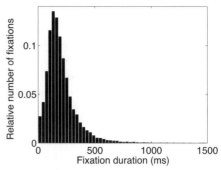

(a) Scene viewing—real still photographs from Nyström (2008).

(b) Reading for 10–15 minutes. From case study 1 (p. 5).

Fig. 11.15 Distribution of fixation durations. Data recorded with a tower-mounted high-end eye-tracker at 1250 Hz; fixations calculated with BeGaze 2.1 velocity algorithm at 40°/s.

> **Reading** Words that are less frequent, and would therefore require a longer lexical activation process, generally receive longer fixation durations (Rayner, 1998). More complicated texts give rise to longer average fixation durations, ranging from around 200 ms in light fiction to around 260 ms for physics and biology texts (Rayner & Pollatsek, 1989). More complicated grammatical structures give rise to longer fixation durations (Rayner, 1978). Also, longer fixation durations correlate with larger N400 amplitudes when taking ERP measurements (Dambacher & Kliegl, 2007), which is indicative of processing meaning and semantic content, particularly when the word is less frequently encountered.

> **Scene perception** Out-of-context objects generate longer fixations than objects which fit the context (J. M. Henderson et al., 1999; De Graef, Christiaens, & D'Ydewalle, 1990; Loftus & Mackworth, 1978). Finding the relevant information in blurred images increases fixation durations (Mackworth & Bruner, 1970).

> **Usability** R. L. Harris and Christhilf (1980) found that pilots fixate longer on critical instruments from which information had to be extracted, rather than those requiring a mere check. Unema and Rötting (1990) found longer fixations when participants made more difficult mental calculations than when they made simpler ones. Stager and Angus (1978) could show shorter fixation durations with increased experience of a task. After comparing several experimental tasks, Oster and Stern (1980) conclude that fixation duration is a consequence of task requirements rather than a property of the saccadic system. Car-driver fixations when negotiating high-incident curves on the road were longer than for non-incident curves (Shinar, McDowell, & Rockwell, 1977), and more than twice as long in curves at night compared to daytime (Mortimer & Jorgeson, 1974). Experienced drivers have shorter fixations (262 ms) compared to novices (296 ms) (Laya, 1992). Also Goldberg and Kotval (1999) and many other applied researchers interpret longer fixations as an indication of the difficulty a participant has in extracting information from a display.

All this indicates functional links between what is fixated and cognitive processing of that item—the longer the fixation the 'deeper' the processing. However, the following are exceptions to this rule:

> **Longer fixations mean shallow processing** In vigilance research, a long fixation is sometimes taken to indicate such a low arousal that participants are close to

daydreaming. This could be the reason why some have found that fixation durations of car drivers are longer on information-poor rural roads in comparison to information-dense urban roads (P. Chapman & Underwood, 1998). In this study however the I-DT algorithm was used with data containing smooth pursuit, and hence the concept of 'fixation' is different. Nevertheless, low arousal may in turn be the product of a non-demanding road requiring little search. In order to be able to use fixation duration as a measure of processing, it is therefore important to be able to argue that participants have not had tendencies to forget the task and start 'daydreaming'.

Higher stress results in shorter fixation durations In human factors, shorter fixations are indicative of a high mental workload (Unema & Rötting, 1990; Miura, 1990; Robinson, Erickson, Thurston, & Clark, 1972). Van Orden, Limbert, Makeig, and Jung (2001) developed a model using regression analyses from eye-movement data on a tracking task, showing that fixation duration was a robust and reliable predictor of tracking performance, again with short fixations correlating with high workload. The reader should be aware, however, that there is a distinction to be made between high workload which you complete successfully (giving longer fixations), and high workload which you struggle to engage with because you are too stressed (giving shorter fixations). Many short fixations across a web page are, according to Ehmke and Wilson (2007), indicative of the frequent usability problem, where a user goes to a page on the site, expecting to find specific details, but not finding them.

Expertise leads to longer fixation durations Expertise in a field such as chess, art, and goalkeeping result in longer (and fewer) fixations than for novices (Nodine, Locher, & Krupinski, 1993; Reingold et al., 2001; Savelsbergh, Williams, Van Der Kamp, & Ward, 2002; Reingold & Charness, 2005). In this case the longer fixation does not mean more processing, but rather a different kind, which involves a larger visual span. With expertise it can be a matter of processing efficiency; fixations may be longer for the expert, but there are less of them compared to the novice because, with increasing skill, more information is extracted around the point of fixation making eye movements overall more efficient.

Neurological impairment means longer fixations Schizophrenia patients have longer fixations the more disturbed their thoughts (Ishizuka, Kashiwakura, & Oiji, 2007). Alzheimer patients make longer fixations when reading (K. L. Lueck, Mendez, & Perryman, 2000). Alcohol intoxication results in longer fixation durations (Moskowitz, Ziedman, & Sharma, 1976; Moser, Heide, & Kömpf, 1998). This should not be interpreted as more or deeper processing, but rather as indicative of a hampered processor. Longer fixation durations in infants have been associated with a poorer cognitive performance, both concurrently, and later in life (Colombo & Frick, 1999), in a line of research that uses not eye tracking but videotaping and direct observation.

Inspected stimulus moves quickly A few studies of inspection workers and internet users have noted very long fixations on a stimulus that just passes in front of the participant (Moraal, 1975). This is interpreted as a deliberate strategy of experienced viewers/inspectors facing a fast-moving stimulus, where time constraints make it more efficient than fixation-saccade sequences.

11.4.3 The skewness of the frequency distribution of fixation durations

Target question	Do shorter or longer fixation durations dominate?
Input representation	A set of fixations from a trial or whole recording
Output	A skewness value for the frequency distribution

Skewness refers to the degree of asymmetry in the distribution of fixation durations. The skewness calculation was introduced on page 315.

In human factors, this measure is taken to indicate differences in information acquisition, that may either be due to design or to task. S. R. Ellis and Smith (1985) found values between 1.84 and 2.64 during different phases of air traffic control work. Abernethy and Russell (1987) finds the value 1.83 for expert badminton players, compared to 1.77 for novices.

R. L. Harris, Tole, Ephrath, and Stephens (1982) evaluate two different designs of vertical speed indicators in aircraft, and conclude that the higher skew in one of them, because of more short fixations, indicating a lower mental workload. Some of the studies referred to by Rötting (2001, pp. 114–119) found differences in the measure as an effect of different phases of work, for instance as a pilot goes through the different checking phases before take-off. Megaw and Richardson (1979) show histograms with large differences in skew between inspectors of different materials. If it can be assumed that different fixation duration values indicate different cognitive processes, then the skew value reflects the relative prevalence of those processes.

11.4.4 First fixation duration after onset of stimulus

Target question	How long was the first fixation on the stimulus?
Input representation	The first fixation on the stimulus after its onset
Output	The duration of the fixation (ms)

The first fixation after onset has a particular status, as it coincides with the *very first* intake and processing of the attended part of the stimulus, and its duration reflects the immediate information processing. The initial fixation duration typically reflects a latency in the sense that it measures the time between the onset of a stimulus and the initiation of a saccade (see figures 11.16(a) and 13.1). There are important issues to consider when using first fixation durations:

First, how to measure fixation onset? It is a mistake to think that fixation onset is aligned with the stimulus onset, since the oculomotor fixation very often starts before the stimulus onset, and later only continues. When the stimulus software switches trial during a fixation, many recording softwares will split the fixation into two parts, as illustrated in Figure 11.16(a). If you have many short trials, this may affect the average first fixation duration significantly. In addition, it is likely that processing associated with the last fixation in one trial will spill over to the first fixation in the next trial. One way to alleviate this effect is to show a blank (noise) display between trials.

Should you use the first or the second fixations? Since the fixation position at stimulus onset has not yet been influenced by the stimulus content, the initial fixation is often excluded, and the *first fixation after the initial saccade* is counted as the first fixation 11.16(b). This way, the duration reflects the processing at the first actively chosen fixation position.

As pointed out on page 378, some care should be taken before forming averages between first and other fixations, as they may represent different cognitive processes.

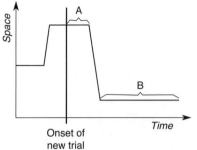

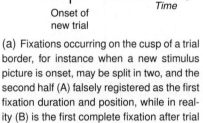

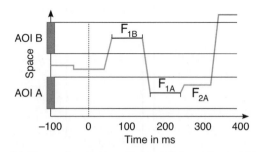

(a) Fixations occurring on the cusp of a trial border, for instance when a new stimulus picture is onset, may be split in two, and the second half (A) falsely registered as the first fixation duration and position, while in reality (B) is the first complete fixation after trial onset.

(b) The two first fixations, F_{1B} in AOI B and F_{1A} in AOI A, with their durations indicated in black. Note that F_{2A} in AOI A is not a first fixation.

Fig. 11.16 Examples of position duration measures, and a problem with trial borders for first fixation durations.

11.4.5   First fixation duration in an AOI, and also the second

Target question	*How long was the first (or second) fixation in an AOI?*
Input representation	*The first or second fixation on an AOI*
Output	*The duration of the fixation (ms)*

The duration of the first fixation in an AOI, the *first fixation duration*, or just *FFD*, is interpreted as reflecting the time taken for fast processes such as recognition and identification. Note that despite the similarity in name, this is a very different measure compared to the previous one, first fixation duration after onset of stimulus. The current measure is specifically reserved for the first fixation *on a part of* the stimulus image, whereas the former referred to the very first fixation per se.

Thus, with this measure the AOI resides in the same stimulus that the participant has already been looking at for a period of time (see Figure 11.17). It is likely that the participant has seen the AOI in question using peripheral vision, and to a small extent processed it and items in its immediate proximity, in particular if the AOI is a word. For the previous measure, the first fixation is only preceded by enough processing to launch a saccade.

In reading, where this measure was first developed, it is considered to reflect the *lexical activation process*. The word properties that affect first fixation duration include word frequency, morphological complexity, metaphorical status, orthographic properties, the degree of polysemy, and other linguistic factors (Inhoff & Radach, 1998; Clifton et al., 2007). The first fixation duration measure is now extensively used in reading research, second only to dwell time (also known as 'gaze duration').

There is also the *second fixation duration*, for instance F_{2A} in Figure 11.16(b). When a long word is hit by two subsequent fixations in the direction of reading, there is a systematic relationship between their landing positions and their durations. If the initial fixation hits the word on its initial few letters, it is short, and the subsequent fixation longer. If the initial fixation hits the centre of the word, it is longer, and the subsequent fixation shorter. According to Inhoff and Radach (1998), it is not clear whether this is an effect of different linguistic processes being computed. The second fixation duration is sometimes taken as a measure of

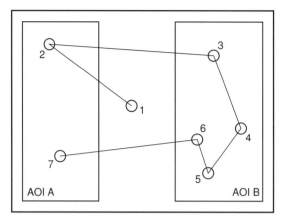

Fig. 11.17 Examplification of five related position duration measures. *First fixation* after trial onset: 1. *First fixations* in AOI: 2 and 3. *Fixation durations* of 1–7 are calculated on a fixation-by-fixation basis. *Dwell time* is the time from entry to exit, namely the durations of: 2, and 3+4+5+6, and 7, respectively. For *Total dwell time* in AOI A, add the durations of fixations 2 and 7.

serial processing of long compound words (Pollatsek & Hyönä, 2005).

In scene perception, Van Diepen, De Graef, and D'Ydewalle (1995), Van Diepen, Wampers, and D'Ydewalle (1998) and Van Diepen (2002) show line drawings of scenes, finding that first fixation durations are longer when the fixated area is masked or degraded using gaze-contingent technology, which indicates that first fixation duration would work as a measure on visual information acquisition from the fixated area. J. M. Henderson et al. (1999); De Graef et al. (1990) showed that first fixation durations on semantically inconsistent and low-probability (hence more informative) areas in a picture are longer than for fixations on more plausible objects. In this case, first fixation duration is used as a measure not just of object activation, but of overall scene integration.

11.4.6 Dwell time

Target question	*For how long, measuring from entry to exit, did gaze remain inside the AOI?*
Input representation	*A dwell in an AOI*
Output	*The duration of the dwell (ms)*

A dwell is defined as *one visit in an AOI, from entry to exit* (p. 190). Terminology for the dwell time measure varies. In some parts of human factors research, the measure is called 'glance duration', and Loftus and Mackworth (1978) used the term 'duration of the first fixation' for the first dwell in an AOI. Terms like 'observation' and 'visit' can also be found. In reading and some parts of scene perception research, dwell time is often called 'gaze duration', 'regional gaze duration', or even 'first-pass fixation time', and in psycholinguistics, Griffin and Spieler (2006) use the term 'gaze time'. Krupinski and Jiang (2008) use the term 'cumulative decision dwell time' for dwell time on lesions in medical images. Dwell time is used in most other eye-tracker-based research fields, and dwell is a more precise term than the ambiguous gaze.

The term 'attentional dwell time' is used for a completely different, non-eye-tracking measure, of the time it takes to release attention from a target that is being identified.

There are important distinctions between other measures, illustrated in Figure 11.17. First of all, returns to the AOI are counted as new dwells. Also, as dwell time measures from entry to exit, not over repeated visits, it is conceptually related to fixation duration, and sometimes the two are confused. However, dwells tend to be more dispersed than fixations, and are typically considerably longer in duration, as it usually comprises several fixations. Furthermore, fixations are completely independent of AOIs and are calculated exclusively on the raw data samples themselves, while dwells can only be calculated if the stimulus has been divided by AOIs.

Dwell time is often defined as the sum of all fixation durations during a dwell in an AOI, but the measure can just as well be based on raw data samples. The raw data dwell time measure will include the durations of non-fixations such as blinks, saccades, and glissades, as well as fixations shorter than your minimal fixation duration criterion. One may argue that a lot of non-fixations means a lot of non-processing time, and that the raw dwell time measure is unsuited as a measure of cognitive processing. That is true in special cases, for instance if you were to have an AOI that is never looked at but is passed over by saccades a great many times. In general, however, this non-processing time is small (up to 20% on top of fixation durations), and should equal out across AOIs and across conditions. Also, considering the current state of the various fixation analysis algorithms (see Chapter 5), a measure based on fixations may contain an equal amount of imperfections.

Furthermore, a distinction is sometimes made between the first and the second dwell in an AOI, in analogy to first/second fixation duration in the AOI. The difference, of course, is that the second dwell is preceded by an exit from the AOI, while the second fixation is not.

Hyönä et al. (2003) present the reading measure 'extended first dwell time' (or, 'extended first-pass fixation time'), which is the first dwell time in an AOI, but including regression to other AOIs (previous text), assuming that the AOI is again returned to. This also works if the other region is a pictorial element. The idea is that regressive excursions are part of forming the understanding of the word regressed from, and should therefore be included in the processing time of an AOI, and that the dwell time should not be terminated at the regressive exit from it.

In many tasks, dwell time distribution is heavily right-skewed, as in Figure 11.18, which shows a histogram over dwell times on photographs in paper newspapers. Such data are commonly log-transformed before applying statistical tests (pp. 87–90).

Dwell time distributions can be constrained by constant trial durations. For instance, a trial duration of 3000 ms could give a distribution peak at 2700 ms for an AOI. As part of the variance can be considered to disappear outside of the 3000 ms, variance analyses (such as ANOVA) on the data may be inappropriate (p. 83).

The recorded dwell time for an object depends on the semantics of the object, and the task of the participant. The following research findings illustrate this:

Interest and informativeness Dwell time indicates interest in an object, or higher informativeness of an object. A. Friedman and Liebelt (1981) found that objects with lower probability of occurrence (defined as higher informativeness), were looked at longer than objects with high-rated likelihood of being present. Pieters, Rosbergen, and Hartog (1996) also observed that on second viewings of print advertisements, the dwell time to advertisement elements decreases. When the contents of an AOI changes considerably in the midst of a trial, the first return dwell time to the AOI (after the change) is larger (J. D. Ryan & Cohen, 2004). All this indicates a strong relationship between consecutive fixations on an item and how much you need to mine information from it.

Uncertainty and poorer situation awareness A higher dwell time may be indicative of uncertainty and poorer situation awareness. Ottati, Hickox, and Richter (1999) found that in a navigational task, novice pilots had a higher dwell time on the outside (through the

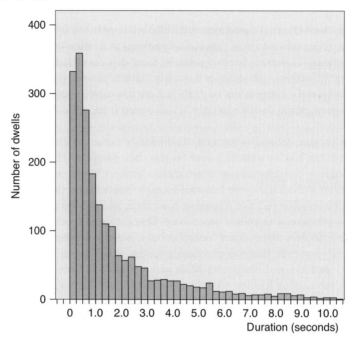

Fig. 11.18 Histogram with 2224 dwell times (unit: seconds) on newspaper photos during natural newspaper reading by 110 participants, using a headmounted eye-tracker at 50 Hz with Polhemus head-tracking. Bin size 250 ms.

window) than experienced pilots, which the authors attribute to uncertainty in locating navigational landmarks amongst pilots with less experience. Hauland (2002) in a large study of air traffic controllers, found that a higher dwell time on AOIs correlates with a poorer situation awareness.

Difficulty in extracting general information Longer dwell time may indicate difficulty in extracting information from a display, as put forward by Fitts et al. (1950), and Goldberg and Kotval (1999). Jacob and Karn (2003) note that dwell time is one of the most used measures in usability studies. In research on car driving for instance, a long-standing discussion is how long dwells to in-car instruments (radios, air control, and GPS etc.) can be without risk of accidents (Zwahlen, Adams, & De Bald, 1988; Rockwell, 1988)

Difficulty in extracting word information Rayner (1998), reviewing reading research using the fixation-based dwell time measure, concludes that dwell time ('gaze duration') is a good index both of word frequency—longer dwells relating to less frequent words—and of comprehension processes integrating several words. Dwell time on a word thus contrasts to first fixation duration, the other major reading measure. More generally, Rayner and Pollatsek (1989) argue that very fast cognitive operations, such as lexical activation and recognition, can be measured with first fixation duration, while slower cognitive processes affect dwell time. In spoken interaction, the dwell time on the interlocutor's (the speaker) mouth increases with the ambient noise levels, an indication that mouth movements play a role in hearing and understanding speech (Vatikiotis-Bateson, Eigsti, Yano, & Munhall, 1998).

An upcoming conscious choice When participants compared abstract, unfamiliar shapes for attractiveness, and were asked to select one, they gradually increased dwell time on the item that was eventually chosen, up until it was finally selected. This has been termed 'the gaze cascade effect' (Shimojo, Simion, Shimojo, & Scheier, 2003).

In gaze-based interaction with computers, dwell time is the predominant criterion for deciding whether gaze on a button AOI should cause activation of the button function. In the basic version, a dwell time threshold of some 400 or 500 ms is required before activation. When the dwell time threshold is too low, buttons activate prematurely, and users experience what is known as 'the Midas touch': everything they look at activates (Jacob, 1991). Research in this area is intense at present, and several new designs exist that combine other selection criteria with dwell time (see for instance, Tall, 2008).

11.4.7 Total dwell time

Target question	Over the whole the trial, how much time was spent in the AOI?
Input representation	A set of dwells on the same AOI
Output	The sum of dwell durations on the AOI (ms)

Total dwell time is the sum of all dwell times in the one and same AOI over a trial (or other specified period). This may sound simple, but so far terminology for and usage of this measure is confusing. Rötting (2001, p. 120) uses the term 'gaze duration', which is also used in the reading research community for the common single dwell time. Journal papers and manuals also exhibit the terms 'cumulative dwell time', 'glance duration', 'gaze', 'total viewing time', 'total fixation time', 'fixation cycle', and 'time in zone'. Clifton et al. (2007) use the term 'total reading time' for "the sum of all fixations in a region, both forward and regressive movements" (i.e. total dwell time). Inhoff and Radach (1998) point out that although total dwell time (which they call 'total viewing durations') seems to be sensitive to linguistic processes that operate after the word has been identified, the measure should be refined by separating dwell time during first reading from dwells on the same word in subsequent readings.

Total dwell time subsumes the whole duration of a trial, and should therefore be sensitive to slow and long-term cognitive processes, but the lack of terminological precision in much of the literature before 2010, in particular the lack of distinction between single and total dwell time, makes it almost impossible to review what the measure has been used for. However, J. M. Henderson and Hollingworth (1999) conclude in their review that studies on scene perception "show a clear effect of the meaning of a scene region on gaze duration [which here means total dwell time] in that region, but a less clear effect on first fixation duration".

Reading-specific varieties of total dwell time include 'look-back fixation time' ('second-pass fixation time'), which is the sum of all dwells to a text AOI except the first one, and 'regression time', the sum of all dwells upon an AOI that follow a regression (Hyönä et al., 2003).

When there are few AOIs, total dwell time suffers from the fixed trial duration restriction on variance analysis (p. 83) even more so than ordinary single entry dwell time.

11.4.8 First and second pass (dwell) times in an AOI

Target question	How long was the first dwell in the AOI, and how long the second?
Input representation	The first (or second) dwell $\mathcal{D}$ on an AOI
Output	The duration of $\mathcal{D}$ (ms)

First pass dwell time (also referred to as 'first pass gaze duration', 'first-pass fixation time', and 'duration of the first fixation') is the reading research communities' term for the duration of the *first* dwell in an AOI, which may be a word, a region, or a sentence. In Figure 6.3 on page 191, the first pass dwell time in AOI 1 consists of two fixations, while the first pass dwell time in AOI 2 has a single fixation. When there is only one fixation, first pass dwell time equals first fixation duration (plus saccades, in the raw data option). Both AOIs have second pass dwell times, also, made up of 3 and 5 fixations each.

First pass dwell time has been proposed as a candidate measure for *early processing and object recognition*. For instance, Liversedge et al. (1998) argue that for long words, which are hit by many fixations, not only the first fixation involves early processing (lexical activation), but also several fixations thereafter combine to do this, and then the first pass dwell time is a better measure than the first fixation duration. Loftus and Mackworth (1978) find that the measure increases for semantically informative objects and A. Friedman (1979) that it increases for unlikely objects in its context. J. M. Henderson et al. (1999) found both first pass dwell time and second pass dwell time to be longer for semantically informative objects. However, J. M. Henderson and Hollingworth (1999) estimate total dwell time to be a better measure than first pass dwell time for studying object recognition.

Second-pass dwell time is defined by Hyönä et al. (2003) (under the names 'look-back fixation time' and 'second-pass fixation time') as the summed durations of all returning dwells to an AOI.

11.4.9 Reading depth

Target question	*How 'deeply' is the text read?*
Input representation	*Text in an AOI and eye movement data*
Output	*A depth (in pixels) or proportion of the text looked at*

Reading depth, also known as 'reading ratio', is a vague measure with several possible operational definitions. When using newspapers or other everyday written material, readers read only portions of the text, and may skip parts to continue with later text, as in Figure 6.5 on page 192. The purpose of the reading depth measure is to quantify how much of the text has been read. The following definitions have been used:

Centimetres Manually measuring how many centimetres have been read from scanpath visualizations and scene-overlaid videos is one option. This operational definition was used by J. P. Hansen (1994), who found the following relationship between text length and reading depth in newspapers: Triple the length of the text—e.g. from 20 to 60 cm—and you will have half as deep a reading—10% rather than 20% of the whole text. Although this entails an increase of 2 cm reading in 60 cm compared to the 20 cm text, this 2 cm gain costs 38 cm of additional unread text space. The variable type is ratio.

Dwell time divided by AOI area Holmqvist and Wartenberg (2005) and Holsanova, Rahm, and Holmqvist (2006) showed that broadsheet newspapers are read less densely (34 ms/cm^2 over all pages) compared to tabloid newspapers (50 ms/cm^2 over all pages), and that the most read article had an average value of 207 ms/cm^2, with the ads hovering around 5 ms/cm^2. The major advantage with this kind of measure is that it works for all sorts of combined stimuli, not just for text, as you can have pictures and words presented together. The variable type is again ratio.

The number of fixations per word in a text AOI If the entire newspaper article is read, we expect a value of about 0.8 (since not all words are fixated), but if a participant reads less of the text, we get a lower number. Poole, Ball, and Phillips (2004), and Poole

(2003) found the values 1.08–2.41 fixations per word in bookmark phrases that participants searched for on web pages. The variable type is nominal, as the data can only
be counted; however, recalculation into a proportion is possible. Although not formally correct, ANOVA could be used if the data are normally distributed. A logit-
transformation may be appropriate.

Dwell time per word in a text AOI Processing time is included in this operational definition of the measure. We can expect a value of around 200 ms/word when the text in the
AOI is fully read, and lower values for a more shallow reading depth. This definition
exists also in the reading research community in the form of two rare measures 'first
pass reading times per character in a region' and 'total pass reading times per character
in a region'. The variable type is ratio.

Ratio to baseline Record a full reading of the stimulus, and use as a baseline. If a supermarket customer reads on a food package for 2.5 seconds, and we have previously
recorded a full reading at 20 seconds for the complete content on the package, then
the 2.5 seconds corresponds to a reading depth of 12.5%. This operational definition
is particularly useful for stimuli with very mixed content, such as food packages and
information graphics. The variable type is ratio.

Note that re-reading adds to the reading depth measure, even if the same text is read over
and over again, except in the centimetre length operational definition by J. P. Hansen (1994).
On the other hand, all varieties except Hansen's have no demands on consecutive reading, not
even that the participant sticks to conventional reading order.

Figure 11.19 shows one application of the reading depth measure from the newspaper
reading studies in our lab. It shows that a longer text is not only read less deeply, but reader
comprehension is also better for shorter texts.

11.5 Pupil diameter

Target question	*How large is the pupil?*
Input representation	*Raw data*
Output	*Pupil diameter or area (mm, camera pixels, mm^2, or pixels^2)*

Pupil diameter ('dilation', 'size') is raw data provided as samples (in sample frequency).
Values are typically given in pixels of the eye camera. Some eye-trackers can also report pupil
diameter in millimetres after a simple calibration routine. When considering this measure as
a property of eye position, it is important to point out that although in terms of the eye camera
data points are recorded giving the pupil diameter when fixating a certain position, changes in
pupil diameter may occur as a function of what has just been looked at, not what is presently
being fixated (i.e. there may be some latency, see page 434). For the purposes of this chapter
however, we deal with pupil diameter as it relates to the current position being looked at in
space, as per the data recorded.

Operational definitions of pupil size

The recording software implements one of three different operational definitions. The simplest is to use the horizontal pupil diameter. The reason for measuring the horizontal diameter
is that the vertical diameter is too sensitive to eyelid closure. With extreme gaze directions,
however, the optical perspective may cause the horizontal diameter calculation to underestimate pupil diameter. Fitting an oval to the pupil image of the eye video and calculating the
largest diameter, irrespective of direction, somewhat remedies the error due to gaze direction,

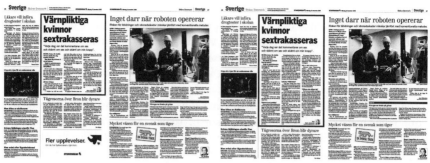

(a) Two identical newspaper folds, except that one article is shorter in the leftside version, and an advertisement fills the remaining space.

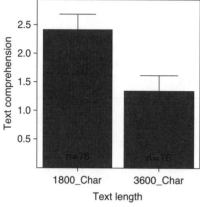

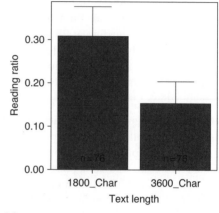

(b) Text comprehension is significantly better for shorter newspaper articles.

(c) Reading depth (ratio) is significantly lower for longer newspaper articles.

Fig. 11.19 In newspaper reading, article length influences both reading ratio (in this case number of fixations per word in the AOI) and text comprehension. Recorded using a head-mounted eye-tracker at 50 Hz with Polhemus head-tracking, and 40 participants on authentic but manipulated newspapers.

but this is more sensitive to eyelid closure. Calculating the area of the pupil is sensitive to both eyelid closure and gaze direction. These errors are known, but their magnitudes not systematically investigated (Klingner, Kumar, & Hanrahan, 2008; Pomplun & Sunkara, 2003).

Analysing pupil diameter in data recorded from a remote system may also introduce artefacts, since motion of the head closer to and further away from the camera also changes the pixel size of the pupil in the camera image. Measuring the camera–eye distance and applying some trigonometry can remedy this problem, but any noise or latencies that you have in the measured distance will be inherited in your pupil dilation measure. Therefore, pupil dilation is best recorded with a system that has a fixed distance between camera and eye. Beware of systems with automatic zoom in the camera, which can in itself cause large variations in recorded pupil dilation. Also, if your participant moves so much that now and then, part of the pupil is outside the eye camera image, data will not be valid.

Pupil size and luminance

When using pupil diameter as a measure of cognitive or emotional states, it is important to remember that the cognitive and emotional effects on pupil diameter are small and easily drown in the large changes due to variation in light intensity. Varying brightness of the stimulus (screen) may easily introduce artefacts into the data. It is necessary to produce stimulus slides with comparable brightness and contrast. A form of baseline can be achieved by letting each actual stimulus image be preceded for a period of 2–5 seconds with a slide with the same luminosity, either a homogeneous tint or a randomly scrambled version of the pixels in the following actual stimulus. In human factors studies with participants in situations with a natural variation in luminance, for instance aeroplane pilots, or when using web pages for stimuli, not to mention authentic advertisement videos, this is particularly difficult and data may have to be abandoned when luminance is not constant (Dehais, Causse, & Pastor, 2008).

Absolute pupil diameter is highly idiosyncratic; the correlation value, $r \in [0.811, 0.944]$, between the four conditions in the data of case study 2 on page 5 illustrate this. All pupil dilation values of a participant should be compared against an established baseline formed by fixating a blank screen for a longer period of time. Beatty and Lucero-Wagoner (2000) point out that normalized pupil diameter in % is inflated when the baseline pupil diameter is small, and recommend the absolute difference measure in millimetres.

Algorithms that compensate for changes in luminance have appeared, which analyse the variation in light on the stimulus monitor, using wavelets (Marshall, 2007) and principal component analysis (Oliveira, Aula, & Russell, 2009). Pupil dilation depends more on the light absorbed by the fovea, than on light hitting the peripheral parts of the retina (Piccoli, Soci, Zambelli, & Pisaniello, 2004), which could be used for further compensation.

Interpretations of the pupil diameter

The measure *can* be used to study a variety of cognitive and emotional states; note however that some commercial eye-tracking providers heavily over-estimate this possibility, and underestimate the difficulties involved (Bartels, 2009). Changes in pupil dilation are triggered by a variety of factors, which calls for a tight experimental design, if you want to make certain that the effect in pupil dilation is caused by one specific factor.

Mental workload increases pupil diameter Hess and Polt (1964) concluded that "changes in pupil size during the solving of simple multiplication problems can be used as a direct measure of mental activity". Pupil dilation increased about twice as much (22 versus 11 per cent) when participants calculated 16 times 23, compared to 7 times 8. This general finding was replicated by Ahern and Beatty (1979), who found diameter changes of 0.1–0.5 mm (also page 436). Hyönä, Tommola, and Alaja (1995) showed that pupil diameters for three different types of translating vary as a function of the level of effort (4.20 mm – listening; 4.72 mm – shadowing; 5.22 – interpreting). Just and Carpenter (1993) found that sentences of varying syntactic complexity gave different pupil diameters when read. Kahneman and Beatty (1966) found larger pupillary responses when participants memorized more digits (0.1 mm versus 0.55 mm for 3 versus 7 digits). In the human factors field, pupil dilation is one in a family of measures used to examine mental workload and cognitive processing. Pupil diameter is often combined with blink rate and duration, fixation durations, saccadic extent, fixation rate, and dwell time, to estimate the cognitive requirements of different tasks (Brookings, Wilson, & Swain, 1996; Van Orden et al., 2000, 2001). Although effects have been unclear when averaging over whole trials, data for the various phases of a task are clear: While blink rate, blink duration, and fixation duration all tend to decline as a function of increased workload (Van Orden et al., 2000; Veltman & Gaillard, 1998), pupil dilation instead increases (Iqbal, Zheng, & Bailey, 2004; Van Orden et al., 2000). Van Gerven, Paas, Van Merriënboer, and Schmidt (2002) found that mean pupil dilation is a useful event-related measure of cognitive load in research on education and learning, especially for young adults.Lying increases the pupil dilation, and attempts have been made to use the pupillary response as a lie-detector (Janisse & Bradley, 1980; Lubow

& Fein, 1996). The question remains, however, whether the pupil increases because of lying or because of a higher cognitive workload or stronger emotions in that measure situation. Dionisio, Granholm, Hillix, and Perrine (2001) concluded that "try[ing] to make their lies as believable as possible" was a more cognitively demanding task than truth-telling.

Emotion and anticipation increase pupil diameter Emotional and sexual arousal increase pupil dilation of the viewing participants in both males and females (Hess & Polt, 1960; Aboyoun & Dabbs, 1998). Partala and Surakka (2003) found larger average pupil diameter when participants listened to affect sounds, such as baby laughing and baby crying, compared to neutral sounds (office noise). Females responded more strongly to positive sounds, and males more strongly to negative ones. When anticipating to see answers to trivia questions that the participant reports being curious about, pupil dilation is larger if the participant was more curious about the answer (Kang et al., 2009). We also appear to react to pupil sizes of others. For instance, pictures of women are rated as more attractive, by post-pubertal males, when their pupils are larger; this does not hold when women make the ratings (Bull & Shead, 1979). Of course, this was known centuries ago by women who used extracts from the highly toxic plant belladonna (meaning 'beautiful lady') to enlarge their pupils and increase their attractiveness. Harrison, Wilson, and Critchley (2007) show that a diminished pupil in faces causes participants who watch those faces to judge them as sadder, although not as expressing more fear, surprise, or disgust; also, diminished pupil promotes more empathy towards the faces. Not only has pupil size been found to be associated with emotional judgment, it is also a social signal that influences the pupil size of others—termed 'pupil dilation mirroring' or 'pupillary contagion' (Harrison, Singer, Rotshtein, Dolan, & Critchley, 2006).

Drowsiness and fatigue decrease pupil diameter This effect was found by Lowenstein and Lowenfeld (1962) and Yoss, Moyer, and Hollenhorst (1970), but not by Beatty (1982), who all used visual and auditory vigilance tasks. It is likely that the studies varied with respect to participant workload.

Diabetes decreases pupil diameter Patients with diabetes tend to have small pupil size, possibly because their pupillary sympathetic pathway is affected (Cahill, Eustace, & de Jesus, 2001).

Age decreases pupil diameter The resting pupil diameter was found to be smaller in the elderly group (mean age 69) at all three illumination levels, compared to younger (mean age 19) (Bitsios et al., 1996).

Pain increases pupil diameter C. R. Chapman, Oka, Bradshaw, Jacobson, and Donaldson (1999) found that peak dilation increased significantly as pain intensity increased. Female participants show a greater increase at higher pain levels (Ellermeier & Westphal, 1995).

Drugs increase pupil diameter A large number of legal and illegal drugs increase pupil diameter, and pupil size is regularly used as a field indicator for drug intoxication.

11.6 Position data and confounding factors

A large variety of factors affect what positions in your stimuli your participants are likely to look at. As always, if you do not watch out for them, they may turn up as confounds in your experiment, but if you systematically utilize these factors, you may make new discoveries.

Table 11.1 Some participant factors that influence the positions they look at.

Factor	Likely effect	Sample reference
Alcohol	Missed event, tunnel vision	Buikhuisen and Jongman (1972)
Medication	Fixation dispersion, and saccade and smooth pursuit parameters	O'Driscoll and Callahan (2008)
Schizophrenia	Restricted dispersion	Loughland et al. (2002)
Autism	Eye and face avoidance	Klin, Jones, Schultz, Volkmar, and Cohen (2002).
Phobias	Avoidance	Pflugshaupt et al. (2007).
Eating disorder	More looks at their own unappealing body parts	Jansen, Nederkoorn, and Mulkens (2005).
Obesity	Look more at food when fasted	Castellanos et al. (2009); Nijs, Muris, Euser, and Franken (2009).
Sexuality	Looks at body parts of either gender	Rupp and Wallen (2007); Tsujimura et al. (2009)

Take alcohol as an example. The drug influences many parts of the brain and causes participants to miss task-important events, reduces their functional visual field, and induces tunnel vision (Buikhuisen & Jongman, 1972). If you have no control over blood alcohol levels with your participants, you have a confound that may overturn your results. But you may also control alcohol levels, and make a systematic comparison between levels or to sober participants.
In this section, we briefly point out a number of possibly confounding factors for position results in eye-tracking-based research: the participant himself, and the drugs and medication he uses, his cultural background, the task given to him, and the experiences he has, as well as the central bias effect with monitor-based, and research on features of the stimulus itself.

11.6.1 Participant brainware and substances

Participants vary in their brainware and in what substances they consumed before arriving in your lab. This not only makes eye tracking very interesting in the study of clinical groups, it also makes medication a possible confounding factor in many studies. Table 11.1 lists a number of participant factors.

11.6.2 Participant cultural background

The participant's *cultural background* would appear to be another possible confounding factor for experiments that use position measures. Chua, Boland, and Nisbett (2005) showed that participants from an American culture tend to look more at focal objects, and participants from a Chinese culture more at the background, when both are shown the same pictures with a focal object and a complex background. However, this result could not be replicated by Rayner, Castelhano, and Yang (2009); Evans, Rotello, Li, and Rayner (2009); Rayner, Li, et al. (2007).

However, Blais, Jack, Scheepers, Fiset, and Caldara (2008), and Miellet, Lingnan, Matthew, Rodger, and Caldara (2009) found that East Asians looking at faces look more at the nose than Western Caucasians, and that this was *not* due to a larger functional visual field. Also, McCarthy, Lee, Itakura, and Muir (2006) found that Canadians and Trinidadians who think about the answer to a question from an interlocutor tend to look up, while Japanese partici-

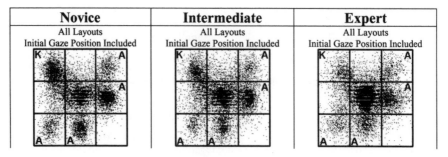

Fig. 11.20 Raw data sample from participants with varying levels of proficiency in chess, as they evaluate chess board with attackers (A) and a king (K). The figure suggests a lower dispersion of experts. Reprinted from Eyal M. Reingold, Neil Charness, Marc Pomplun, and Dave M. Stampe, *Psychological Science, 12*(1), copyright © 2001 by SAGE Publications. Reprinted by Permission of SAGE Publications.

pants look down. Canadians but not Japanese altered their gaze behaviour when knowing that they were observed (McCarthy, Lee, Itakura, & Muir, 2008).

11.6.3 Participant experience and anticipation

Another possibly confounding factor for position measures that may need to be controlled for is the participant's *experience* with the task. A host of studies show that expertise gives rise not only to a more task efficient selection of gaze positions, but also to a superior perceptual processing from a larger functional visual field, stretching further out from the fixation point, than it does for novices (although not overriding the physiological restrictions at the retina, visual pathway and visual cortex). Such effects of experience has been shown for painters (Vogt & Magnussen, 2007; Nodine et al., 1993; Antes & Kristjanson, 1991), drivers (Mourant & Rockwell, 1972), during the diagnoses of electrical circuits (Van Gog, Paas, & Van Merriënboer, 2005), of dental and mammography X-rays (Van Der Stelt-Schouten, 1995; Krupinski, 1996), chess (Reingold et al., 2001; Reingold & Charness, 2005) and basketball players (Memmert, 2006). As part of *training*, for instance in sign language or to drive, gaze positions gradually change (Emmorey, Thompson, & Colvin, 2008; Mourant & Rockwell, 1970; Mourant et al., 1969).

Why is experience so important? Gaze is generally anticipatory, reflecting the participant's probabilistic model of the world. For instance, if you meet a pedestrian coming from the other direction, and you judge her to be collision-prone, you will look earlier and more at her than if you feel safe with that person (Jovancevic-Misic & Hayhoe, 2009). In ball sports, the experts look at the bounce point 100–200 ms before the ball reaches it (Land & McLeod, 2000; Ripoll, Fleurance, & Cazeneuve, 1987), giving them time to confirm their prognosis for the continued trajectory, which in turn they need for quick action. Expert goalkeepers facing a penalty shot look at the legs and face of the kicker (Savelsbergh et al., 2002) as part of their preparation.

11.6.4 Communication, imagination, and problem solving

Not controlling *what is said to participants* is very likely to alter the position data you collect from them, as shown already by Yarbus (1967) in the example with the unexpected visitor. Both speaking and listening heavily influences the position of fixations (Holsanova, 2008; Griffin & Bock, 2000; Tanenhaus et al., 1995).

Other people's gaze will also alter the positions to which your participants will look. In general, people are well aware of other people's gaze direction, and it affects where they look themselves. In a series of studies on gesture perception, Gullberg and Holmqvist (2006, 1999) showed that speakers who fixate their own gestures attract significantly more gazes from the listener to these gestures, and this effect is used by magicians to govern the audience gazes (G. Kuhn & Tatler, 2005). Communication between two people becomes easier and mutual problem solving is quicker if they can see each other's gaze positions (Velichkovsky, Pomplun, Rieser, & Ritter, 1996).

An increased *mental workload during speech planning* or actively recalling a memory often causes participants to look away from their interlocutor, computer monitor etc. This is known as 'gaze aversion'. Doherty-Sneddon, Bruce, Bonner, Longbotham, and Doyle (2002) showed that 5-year old school children inconsistently avert gaze, but that it increases dramatically during the first years of primary education, reaching adult levels by 8-years of age. Glenberg, Schroeder, and Robertson (1998) showed that the amount of time spent looking away from an interlocutor increases with task difficulty, and that participants gave more correct answers when averting their gaze. Together, this indicates that gaze aversion may be functional.

Speech affects eye movement even if objects spoken about and looked at just represent the mental images produced by the participants (Polunin, Holmqvist, & Johansson, 2008; Loetscher, Bockisch, & Brugger, 2007; Zangemeister & Liman, 2007; Johansson et al., 2006; Laeng & Teodorescu, 2002; Brandt & Stark, 1997). When solving geometrical and graphical problems, the ability to imagine the functional role of part objects in the solution depends on where participants look, as shown by Grant and Spivey (2003); Yoon and Narayanan (2004b). In a study on ambiguous pictures, including the Necker cube, Pomplun et al. (1996) show that gaze position coincides with the interpretations participants subjectively experience.

11.6.5 Central bias

The vast majority of eye-tracking research, even if it purports to generalize to all visual activities, is made using stimuli presented on single monitors. With most stimuli—text being the large exception—participants show a marked tendency to fixate the centre of the screen more than any other part. Tatler (2007) attributes this observation to one of three possibilities:

> First, the center of the screen may be an optimal location for early information processing of the scene. Second, it may simply be that the center of the screen is a convenient location from which to start oculomotor exploration of the scene. Third, it may be that the central bias reflects a tendency to re-center the eye in its orbit.

Fehd and Seiffert (2010) point out that looking steadily at the centre of scenes allows a participant to keep a better overview of the multiple objects in it compared to looking around. Interestingly, monkeys appear to have less central bias (D. J. Berg et al., 2009), which suggests that specific human expectations and experiences cause it.

Researchers unaware of the central bias effect may erroneously generalize a result from monitors to real-life behaviour.

11.6.6 The stimulus

Elements in the stimulus itself may inadvertently attract participant gaze and become a confound in studies. For instance, accidentally having people or faces on a stimulus picture where the research question refers to the other visual elements (in a park, for instance) is very likely to alter results, because people and faces attract participant gaze. The 'visual search' paradigm has attempted to systematically investigate what other so-called 'bottom-up features' (colour, motion, orientation, for instance) in a picture attract visual attention, or in other words make an object 'pop out'. Wolfe and Horowitz (2004) review a large number of visual features that may or may not attract participant attention.

Some eye-tracking studies have indeed given support to the idea that bottom-up features are important to human choices of gaze positions. Reinagel and Zador (1999) and Parkhurst and Niebur (2003) report a higher luminance contrast around fixation than in randomly chosen regions, while Baddeley and Tatler (2006) conclude that high-frequency edges are good predictors of fixation locations.

The Itti and Koch (2000) saliency model is a hotly debated computational model of some of the assumed neurological principles that employ bottom-up (pre-attentive) features to select fixation targets. Implementations are available on several web pages and in some of the dedicated analysis softwares for eye-movement data. Competing but less known models include the target acquisition model (TAM) (Zelinsky, 2008), the gaze-attentive fixation finding engine (GAFFE) (Rajashekar et al., 2008), the contextual guidance model (Torralba, Oliva, Castelhano, & Henderson, 2006), and the neurodynamical cortical model (Deco & Rolls, 2004). None of these are as well investigated as the saliency model, but Nyström (2008) shows that the GAFFE model does somewhat better than the salience model in comparison to human data. Itti (2005) demonstrates a better than chance similarity between human eye-movement data and the output of the saliency model, however.

Models can be seen as useful and necessary steps in the evolution of our scientific understanding of what people look at, but the cost for false negatives could be very large in some specific applications. For instance, radiologists scanning X-ray images appear to use other features compared to those emphasized in the visual search paradigm (Krupinski, Berger, Dallas, & Roehrig, 2003).

Also, the dominance of bottom-up features is not supported by X. Chen and Zelinsky (2006) who show that top-down guidance of eye movements in a search task always prevails over bottom-up saliency features (colour coding of singular elements among grey-scale objects). Similarly, by blurring some parts of stimulus pictures and increasing contrast in others, Einhäuser et al. (2008, 15) show that "a visual search task can override and actively countermand sensory-driven saliency in naturalistic visual stimuli". Also J. M. Henderson, Brockmole, Castelhano, and Mack (2007) argue that Itti's bottom-up models of saliency do not account for human eye movements, while others have shown that central (Tatler, 2007) and oculomotor biases (Tatler & Vincent, 2009) can explain eye-movement data better than the saliency model.

12 Numerosity Measures

Maybe the most straightforward method to quantify eye-movement events is simply to count them, either in absolute numbers, in proportion to the total number of events, or as a rate over time. Indeed, event-counting measures appeared very early in eye-movement research. For instance, Dodge and Cline (1901, p. 154) analysed reading data from three participants and noted "a little less than five reading pauses per line, making an average of a little less than four movements to the right for every movement to the left."

In Part II of the book, over 25 events were defined. Many of them are counted in research, some of them very often (like number of fixations), and some very seldom (like number of look-aheads). Not only are events counted, however, but also the number of participants and trials that fulfil some given criterion. For example, it may be of interest to count the number of participants that looked at a specific area of interest. This chapter deals with the *number, proportion* and *rate* of such countable entities in eye-movement research. It differs from all other measure chapters, which are only about single events or representations.

Countable entities	How researchers count them	Page
Saccades	*Number, proportion and rate*	403
Glissades	*Proportion*	405
Microsaccades	*Rate*	406
Square-wave jerks	*Rate*	407
Smooth pursuits	*Rate*	408
Blinks	*Rate*	410
Fixations	*Number, proportion and rate*	412
Dwells	*Number, proportion and rate*	417
Participants, areas of interest and trials	*Number and proportion*	419
Transitions	*Number, proportion and rate*	422
Regressions, backtracks, look-backs, and look-aheads	*Number and rate*	425

What are number, proportion, and rate?

In Figures 12.1 and 12.2, we exemplify the three types of counting which are done with events and other entities in eye-tracking experiments. The *number of* (*N*) is a unit that simply represents how many occurrences of something there are, for example 12 saccades as in Figure 12.1.

Proportion is a fraction between a part and a whole, having values between 0 and 1, but is typically reported as %. In Figure 12.2(b), the proportion of glissadic saccades, seen as small notches directly after the large saccadic peaks, is 42%, and in Figure 12.2(c), we calculate the proportion of saccades with peak velocities above 75°/s to be 50%. Since two quantities with the same unit are divided, proportion is dimensionless.

Rate is the ratio between a number and the extension of the temporal range over which that number was counted. The example in Figure 12.2(d) is saccadic rate, which counts 12

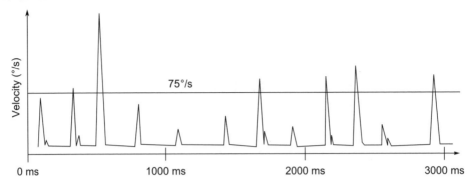

Fig. 12.1 Velocity-over-time diagram for a 3 second trial of synthetic data.

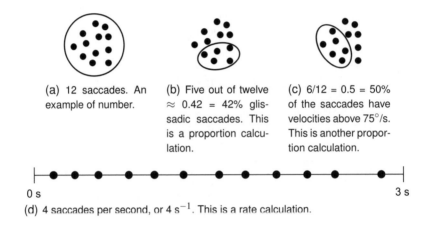

(a) 12 saccades. An example of number.

(b) Five out of twelve ≈ 0.42 = 42% glis-sadic saccades. This is a proportion calculation.

(c) 6/12 = 0.5 = 50% of the saccades have velocities above 75°/s. This is another proportion calculation.

(d) 4 saccades per second, or 4 s⁻¹. This is a rate calculation.

Fig. 12.2 Examples of number, proportion, and rate calculations for the data in Figure 12.1.

saccades over 3 seconds, equalling an average of 4 per second (or 4 s^{-1}).

All three types of counting are also used with the term 'frequency': in the terminology of the statistical analysis software SPSS, for instance, number is called 'absolute frequency', while 'relative frequency' covers both rate, proportion and various normalizations. These terms sift through to eye-tracking literature as well: Gilchrist and Harvey (2006) write 'frequency of saccades' when referring to number of saccades, and Foulsham and Kingstone (2010) use 'relative frequency' to denote proportion values, just to take two examples.

The term 'number of saccades' is about five times as common on Google Scholar as 'frequency of saccades' (January 2011). In this book, we reserve 'frequency' for the rate of regular repetitions per unit time, such as sampling frequency, and use the unit Hz for it. The term frequency will not be used with eye-movement data for other types of counting.

From an event-detection perspective, 'counting measures' are the least demanding. To count an event, it only needs to be detected, and no additional information about the event itself is needed: we only need to know that there is a saccade, but not its direction, velocity, duration, or skewness. Thus, event counting requires detection, but silently circumvents calculating values for event properties, and remains unaffected by the various noise this can introduce (Chapter 5).

However, as all events of a type are treated as equal when counting them (i.e. a 2° saccade equals a 25° saccade, and a 50 ms fixation is indistinguishable from a 1500 ms fixation) another type of noise, in the form of information reduction, is introduced. Although it may seem as though the events behind a count value are all equal, they very seldom are.

Grouping and limiting the counting range

There is often little point in calculating the total number of saccades or any other event in the whole recorded data. Instead, most researchers limit the counting process in a number of ways to extract count values that correspond to conditions in their experimental design. Data range restrictions can be imposed on the input to other measures also, but for counting measures this range is an integral part which defines the scope in which counting will be carried out.

A *spatial* division of data means, for instance, counting the number of fixations in each area of interest, as is common in scene perception research (p. 412).

A division of data into *temporal* portions can involve counting the event only in a limited temporal range: select to count in a single time period, for instance, the number of blinks during the three seconds before the participant clicks to end the trial, or the number of microsaccades during the first 250 milliseconds after fixation onset.

Some events can form temporal counting restrictions for other events. For instance, the number of microsaccades per fixation (Otero-Millan et al., 2008) involves counting how many microsaccades (events) there are in each fixation (temporal counting range).

Limiting the counting process to *conditions in the experimental design* means, for example, counting the number of first skips of the word 'of' in an easy text condition of a reading experiment (perhaps including only the data collected from a group of 12-year old readers). This example illustrates the counting processes for one condition of the experimental design to familiarize the reader with the principle, but usually however the required events will be counted across *all* conditions of the experiment, and counted in relation to each of the independent variables you manipulate.

Multiple counting ranges: histograms

If we select to count in multiple time periods, each of these portions of time can be divided into a bin, and the count in each bin can be used to make a histogram, such as the number of microsaccades for each 250 ms bin. Counting data from multiple areas of interest can also be made into a histogram. This is possible with other measures as well, but the selection of both single and multiple counting ranges is particularly emphasized in the case of counting measures.

The implicit presuppositions to event counting

Some events can only exist in the presence of other events or when certain conditions are fulfilled, and this affects how they are counted. For instance, while fixations can be counted in their own right, glissades always co-exist with saccades. Therefore, glissades are counted as a proportion per saccade, and never in absolute numbers or rates per second. Microsaccades, when occurring during long fixations, can be counted per second, however. Table 12.1 summarizes the presuppositions that events have. Dwells, transitions, skips, and returns are always counted with reference to one or more specific areas of interest.

Measures and other ways to count

Table 12.2 summarizes what we have said above about how to construct a multitude of counting measures; not all of the many possibilities to count events have actually been utilized in research however. As always, the vast freedom we have to build measures does not mean we *should* build and calculate values for all of them. In fact, the selection of precise counting restrictions is an essential part of designing the experiment where you plan to use the counting

Table 12.1 Groups of events in eye-movement data: glissades can only co-exist with saccades, for instance, and dwells can exist only when areas of interest have been set up. These dependencies affect how the events are counted.

Events	Presupposition—required data parsing	Chapter
Saccades, fixations, smooth pursuits, blinks, nystagmuses, and artefacts	Event detection	5
Drifts, microsaccades, inter-microsaccadic intervals, square-wave jerks, glissades, catch-up-, back-up-, and leading saccades	Fixation, saccade or smooth pursuit	5
Area of interest hits, dwells, transitions, total skips, first skips, entries, and returns	Area of interest division of stimulus	6
Backtracks, regressions, look-backs, and look-aheads	Scanpath	8

Table 12.2 The five steps of forming counting measure.

1 Select restriction/range in space, time, and data
2 Select what event to count
3 Select absolute number, proportion, or rate
4 Count
5 Optionally form averages or normalize

measures, and as such they are part of your hypotheses.

Counting measures are very prevalent in research, for instance "number of saccades" gives roughly the same number of hits on Google Scholar as "saccade [saccadic] amplitude" and "dwell time". However, the effects studied with some counting measures vary much more than for other measures. In this chapter, we present a selection of existing counting measures sorted by the events they count, address operational definitions and methodological issues, and in most cases give examples of common effects that the measure has been used to study.

Notable measures that involve counting but have nevertheless been left out of this chapter are those based on transition matrices and proportion over time representations. The transition matrix counts transitions to investigate overall eye-*movement* behaviour, and measures using it are found in Chapter 10. Proportion over time representations count participants, but they are used to measure latency, and are therefore in Chapter 13.

Counting participants and trials

Participants are counted using restriction criteria such as having had to look at a specified area of interest, which allows us to count the number of participants who met this requirement. Using thresholding, unlimited forms of criteria can be applied to participant counting: for instance, the number of participants who had a peak saccadic velocity larger than 600°/s in more than 30% of the saccades. Apart from its use as measures, participant counts are reported as numbers of data quality, for instance if 23% of participants had to be removed from data analysis because of inadequate precision (p. 181).

Data quality is often the reason for counting (excluded) trials, but trials can also be counted using restriction criteria such as the number of trials with fewer than 20 saccades, or the number of trials with four or more dwells. Researchers also count number of correct trials, where 'correct' refers to the participant succeeding in performing a task as per the experimental design.

Averaging and normalizing count data

Count data lend themselves excellently to averaging and normalizing. Proportion and rate measures in this chapter are forms of normalization, with respect to the whole or the duration. Other measures rely on normalization against other properties on the counting context. For example, the measure 'fixation density' [number/cm^2] counts the number of fixations and divides it by the area within which the fixations were counted. Fixation density pertains more to the location of fixations in space, hence we include it as measure of position (see p. 390).

Counting and statistics

When analysing count data, there are at least two issues to be wary about from a statistical standpoint. The first is that count data are not inherently normally distributed (Gaussian), but are best described by a Poisson or a binomial distribution. The solution is either to use a statistical model that can handle Poisson-distributed data, which is the proper solution, or, approximate the distribution with a Gaussian distribution. The latter is done when the expected count (typically denoted as λ in a Poisson distribution) is sufficiently large, typically when $\lambda > 10$.

The second issue concerns proportions. Proportions are, as previously described, the ratio between a part to the whole, and as such constitute a number between 0 and 1. They typically suffer from a restricted range, i.e. a tail of the distribution is truncated and the variance becomes restricted the further we go to either extreme point. This issue is mainly a problem if the scores occur outside of 0.3–0.7. This issue and its possible solutions were discussed earlier (pp. 87–90).

12.1 Saccades: number, proportion, and rate

Target question	*How many saccades?*
Input representation	*Event-processed data*
Output	*The amount of saccades in number, proportion, or rate (s^{-1})*

The chosen event detection algorithm operationalizes, detects, calculates, and outputs the saccades in a trial. They are then counted in absolute number, in proportion to something, or as a rate. Saccades may be distinguished based on different saccadic properties (see Table 12.3).

For still images, the number of saccades should be equal or ± 1 to the number of fixations. An increase in the number of saccades over a fixed trial duration equals a decrease in the average fixation duration. When there is motion and smooth pursuit, catch-up saccades may increase the number of saccades to be larger than that of fixations.

With reference to a well-known neurological patient, Land (2006) points out that people may often make more saccades than needed for the tasks at hand. A.I. is a participant with a condition called oculomotor apraxia in which saccades cannot be initiated; A.I instead makes saccadic-like head movements. In spite of this disorder A.I is, nevertheless, able to execute tasks with normal speed and competence, making only one third as many head saccades as controls make eye saccades. Thus, the implication is that we make more saccades than are strictly necessary.

Table 12.3 Common saccadic properties, and example criteria for proportion of saccade calculations from published research.

Saccadic property	Examples where proportion of saccades is commonly calculated
Direction towards locations	Saccades to each distractor type; saccades that ultimately end up in the target location; saccades that were captured by the onset; saccades that were directed at same-coloured targets or in the direction of the mouth in a face image
Direction, angular	Saccades in the correct direction; saccades where the direction changes relative to the previous saccade
Amplitude	Saccades with amplitudes smaller than $X°$; saccades that landed outside a specified $2°$ ring, for example
Latency	Saccades at a zero latency; saccades triggered after a certain time delay
Onset	Saccades launched during set timebands, of 500 ms for instance.

12.1.1   Number of saccades

The *absolute number of saccades* is calculated by using one of two operational definitions. The first counts saccades along *a distance with a constant length*, for instance the same line of text, or with sinusoidal smooth pursuit stimuli where the lengths are identical. The second definition instead uses *a fixed trial duration*, and counts the number of saccades from trial start to trial end. Both these operational definitions assure that count data are comparable between participants, trials, and conditions. It goes without saying that different stimuli evoke different numbers of saccades.

There are several sub-events to saccades that can be counted, for instance the number of large regressive saccades, or the number and extent of backtracking regressions, just to mention a few. The studies reviewed by O'Driscoll and Callahan (2008) use cyclic stimuli, and tend to show that participants with schizophrenia have significantly more saccades during smooth pursuit, both catch-up and leading saccades. Studies with higher proportions of medicated patients show smaller effect sizes for leading saccades and larger effect sizes for catch-up saccades.

12.1.2   Proportion of saccades

The proportion of saccades is counted by dividing the counted number of saccades in a subgroup by the number in the whole group. The subgroup and main group selected varies, and can depend on conditions in the experimental design and particular paradigm used. Nevertheless, when studies report the proportion of saccades, very often the subgroup is defined by saccadic properties that we recognize from other chapters.

Again, the specific subevents of saccades also form proportions, such as the proportion of saccades that were revisits, or the percentage of forward saccades from word N which skip word $N + 1$. These are just two examples of many which can be derived.

12.1.3   Saccadic rate

Saccadic rate is measured as the number of saccades per second (s^{-1}), and is also known as 'number of saccadic movements per unit time' (Ohtani, 1971), 'eye transition frequency' (Wierwille & Connor, 1983), and 'eye-movement rate' (Bergstrom & Hiscock, 1988). For still picture stimuli, the saccadic rate should be identical to the fixation rate, and thus also correlate closely to fixation duration. For stimuli that elicit only smooth pursuit, the saccadic rate would be a measure of the prevalence of catch-up saccades. For mixed stimuli, like standard video films or the real world (i.e. which contain both static and dynamic items), the saccadic rate is not the same as fixation rate, and it remains unclear exactly what it signifies.

In the following examples from research, we select only studies that explicitly report saccadic rate, but a comparison to studies reporting fixation duration is advisable.

Mental workload, arousal and fatigue Saccadic rate decreases when task difficulty or mental workload increases (Nakayama, Takahashi, & Shimizu, 2002). This interpretation is utilized in several applied studies, for instance Pan et al. (2004), who found a difference in saccadic rate between two types of web pages. Also, arousal increases (Morris & Miller, 1996) and higher fatigue levels reduce saccadic rate (Van Orden et al., 2000).

Visual imagery A task that requires visual imagery involving up/down or right/left movements increases saccadic rate significantly compared to visual imagery of inside/out (Demarais & Cohen, 1998), because the inside/out dimensions do not map as easily to stimulus space as up/down and right/left.

Disorders During smooth pursuit saccadic rate is higher for many psychiatric and neurological disorders, such as psychosis (Van Tricht et al., 2010), and schizophrenia in general O'Driscoll and Callahan (2008).

The neural sites responsible for saccade programming have also been examined by taking saccadic rate measurements. For instance, Paus, Marrett, Worsley, and Evans (1995) found that with increasing saccadic rate, cerebral blood flow also increased in the frontal eye fields, the superior colliculus, and the cerebellar vermis.

12.2 Glissadic proportion

Target question	*How many glissades per saccade?*
Input representation	*Event-processed data*
Output	*The proportion of glissades*

Glissades are always counted in proportion to the saccades which precede them. Although operational definitions measuring glissades differ considerably in the literature, and some authors and algorithms have even considered glissades to be measurement errors (p. 183), glissades are nevertheless real; moreover, they are also quite common (between 20 and 50% of all saccades end in a glissade (Nyström & Holmqvist, 2010; L. Wang, 1998)).

Studies have interpreted glissadic proportion in relation to:

Vigilance L. Wang (1998) interprets an increase in the percentage of glissadic saccades within anticipatory and return saccades (over time-on-task) as a possible index of vigilance decrement, and a similar interpretation is given by Ciuffreda and Tannen (1995).

Neurological diseases In the 1970s, glissades were used as an aid in diagnosing multiple sclerosis and vascular lesions (Bahill, Hsu, & Stark, 1978), and such neurological interpretations are reiterated by Ciuffreda and Tannen (1995, p. 39).

Saccade direction and amplitude Kapoula et al. (1986) found glissades to be overrepresented in the abducting eye, they also observed an over-representation of glissades in populations of saccades with short amplitude. In their much larger data set, with text and pictorial stimuli, Nyström and Holmqvist (2010) found no support for such a relation, neither in reading nor in scene perception.

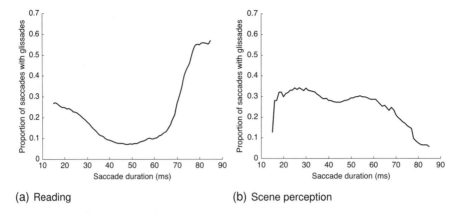

(a) Reading   (b) Scene perception

Fig. 12.3 Proportion of glissades for saccades made during reading and during scene perception, adapted from Nyström and Holmqvist (2010). Reprinted with kind permission from Springer Science + Business Media: *Behaviour Research Methods*, An adaptive algorithm for fixation, saccade, and glissade detection, *42*(1), 2010, Marcus Nyström and Kenneth Holmqvist.

Saccadic amplitude in reading Interestingly however, in reading data, the long (return sweep) saccades have a much higher percentage of glissades than equally long saccades during scene perception (see Figure 12.3). Nyström and Holmqvist (2010) speculate that this may be evidence that the oculomotor system adapts to the low velocities of the short saccades necessary when reading a line of text, but this adaptation does not spread to the programming of higher velocity return sweeps in reading. Conversely, in scene perception, where saccadic velocities are not bimodally distributed and much more random, the effect is rather the reverse.

12.3 Microsaccadic rate

Target question	*How often do microsaccades occur?*
Input representation	*Event-processed data*
Output	*Rate (s⁻¹)*

Microsaccadic rate, or 'frequency' as referred to by Martinez-Conde and Macknik (2007), is defined as the number of microsaccades per second, and has the unit s^{-1} (Engbert & Kliegl, 2003). When calculating the value, only divide the number of microsaccades by the period spent in fixations. Dividing by the trial duration means including saccadic duration and underestimates the rate values. Note that detection algorithms for microsaccades may also detect square-wave jerks as microsaccades, and that—in some studies—a distinction may have to be made between the two types of events.

Although microsaccades occur during fixations only, they are virtually never counted in relation to fixations (i.e. microsaccades per fixation), the exception being Otero-Millan et al. (2008), who counted the number of microsaccades per fixation in order to plot the prevalence of microsaccades in connection with fixation duration.

Reported microsaccade rate values tend to range from 0.2–3 s^{-1}. Microsaccadic rate is one of the major measures in the research field which investigates the role of microsaccades in visual perception. Studies with this measure have focused on:

Rate over time Microsaccades have systematically been shown to have a *minimum* rate approximately 150 ms after cue onset, known as 'microsaccade inhibition'. The *maximum* rate of microsaccades occurs approximately 350 ms after presentation of the cue, known as the 'rebound effect' (see Engbert & Kliegl, 2003, and Rolfs et al., 2005). In a task where participants scanned pictures, Otero-Millan et al. (2008) show that microsaccadic rate increases rapidly after around 300 ms; this is not the case when a blank screen is presented, however.

Visual illusions When a peripherally attended ring fades during maintained fixation due to neural adaptation (Troxler fading), this corresponds to a decrease in microsaccadic rate from around 3 to over 5 s^{-1} (Martinez-Conde, Macknik, Troncoso, & Dyar, 2006). The microsaccadic rate decrease precedes the subjective experience of perceptual fading, and rate increases again just before the peripheral ring is once again visible. This highlights a functional role of microsaccades during fixation, in that they enable a stable perception. Another finding is that subjective experience of illusory motion in what is known as the Enigma painting coincides with an increase of microsaccadic rate (Troncoso, Macknik, Otero-Millan, & Martinez-Conde, 2008).

Intermediate trajectories Engbert and Mergenthaler (2006) propose that the individual microsaccadic rate can be predicted by what is known as the fractal dimension (Theiler, 1990) of the intermediary trajectories, known as inter-microsaccadic intervals (IMSIs), between microsaccades.

Manual response preparation Microsaccadic rates appear to be affected by (manual) response preparation processes as part of target discrimination (Betta & Turatto, 2006).

Much of microsaccade research is neurologically motivated, with the goal of revealing the function(s) of microsaccades in vision and brain areas which subserve visual perception.

12.4   Square-wave jerk rate

Target question	How often do square-wave jerks occur?
Input representation	Event-processed data
Output	The number of square-wave jerks per minute (min^{-1})

Square-wave jerk rate (SWJ-r), also known as 'saccadic intrusion rate' and 'multiple saccadic wave intrusion rate' (MSWI), is defined as the number of square-wave jerk pairs per minute, resulting in the unit min^{-1} (see p. 183 for a reminder of the square-wave jerk event).

Most studies report that the range for square-wave jerk rate is around 1–40 min^{-1}, with an average of around 10 min^{-1}, in healthy adult participants (Abadi & Gowen, 2004). Many studies report that all participants tested exhibit SWJs, although rates vary between individuals. Sixty per cent of the participants in Abadi and Gowen exhibited SWJ rates up to 20 min^{-1}, even though clinical textbooks such as Wong (2008) consider rates above 15 min^{-1} as pathological. As pointed out by Salman, Sharpe, Lillakas, and Steinbach (2008): "The prevalence and frequency of square-wave jerks in normal adults vary between studies, largely because of variations in the recording sensitivity, alertness, and arbitrarily selected saccade-amplitude threshold or duration for definition or detection of square-wave jerks, and also because of the varied periods of fixation sampled" (p. 18).

The three less known varieties, the biphasic square wave, the intrusion single saccadic pulse, and the double saccadic pulse, have frequencies of 0.5–5 min^{-1} (Abadi & Gowen, 2004). Since the threshold for detection is variable across studies, frequencies also vary.

The following factors have been shown to increase square-wave jerk rate:

Disorders Increased square-wave jerk rates are seen in a wide variety of disorders. This includes progressive supranuclear palsy (Troost & Daroff, 1977), strabismus (Ciuffreda, Kenyon, & Stark, 1979), multiple sclerosis (Doslak, Dell'Osso, & Daroff, 1983), Parkinsons (Rascol et al., 1991), Friedrich's ataxia (Fahey et al., 2008), and many more. According to clinician Wong (2008), square-wave jerks can also result from basal ganglia and cerebral cortical diseases. When square-wave jerks occur continuously, they are symptomatic of Parkinson's disease, alcoholic cerebral degeneration, and some forms of palsy.

Age Although all participant have some square-wave jerks, they are particularly common with elderly people. For instance, Herishanu and Sharpe (1981) found that the mean rate was 4.7 min^{-1} for young people (mean age 32), compared to a mean rate value of 27.0 min^{-1} for elderly people (mean age 71).

Increased catch-up saccade amplitude There is possibly a relationship between the amplitudes of catch-up saccades during smooth pursuit and the rate of square-wave jerks, according to L. Friedman, Jesberger, Abel, and Meltzer (1992), who speculate that programming both types of eye movements simultaneously taxes the saccade system heavily.

Tobacco and other drugs During the first 5 minutes after smoking one cigarette, the participants of Sibony, Evinger, and Manning (1988) exhibited an increased rate of square-wave jerks on both vertical and horizontal smooth pursuit. The effect is found both in schizophrenic patients and healthy controls (Thaker, Ellsberry, Moran, & Lahti, 1991). Drugs such as L-tryptophan (Baloh, Dietz, & Spooner, 1982), and intravenous opioids (Rottach, Wohlgemuth, Dzaja, Eggert, & Straube, 2002), have also been found to increase square-wave jerk rate.

Lower visual task demands Shaffer, Krisky, and Sweeney (2003) found significantly lower square-wave jerk rates when observers fixated remembered target locations compared to visual targets which were present. Smooth pursuit tracking of faster-moving and less predictable targets also reduced square-wave jerk rate.

A high square-wave jerk rate may jeopardize accuracy in data, as a square-wave jerk that occurs when a participant looks at a calibration point will cause miscalibration at that location (see p. 130).

12.5 Smooth pursuit rate

Target question	*How often do smooth pursuits occur?*
Input representation	*Event-processed data*
Output	*The number of smooth pursuits or catch-up saccades per second* (s^{-1})

There are very few studies which count smooth pursuits, simply because of the lack of algorithms which detect the smooth pursuit event. Indeed, this gap in the event detection domain means that smooth pursuit has a very uncertain status as an event per se. Often, instead of smooth pursuit, the complimentary measure number of catch-up saccades is used. With commonly used sinusoidal velocity stimuli, the number of catch-up saccades is approximately equal to the number of smooth pursuits minus one, as exemplified in Figure 12.4 and Table 12.4. Either way, rate (or 'frequency') measures are preferred to simply counting the number of occurrences. With stimuli like motion pictures or the real world, it is very likely that smooth

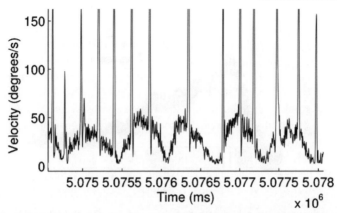

Fig. 12.4 Data collected from a person viewing a pendulum movement using a head-mounted 500 Hz system. A number of catch-up saccades interrupt the low-speed smooth pursuit. Values for relevant measures can be found in Table 12.4.

Table 12.4 Measurement values resulting from the data in Figure 12.4

Measure	Value
Number of catch-up saccades	14
Number of glissadic catch-up saccades	1
Number of smooth pursuits	15
Duration of this trial	3.6 seconds
Smooth pursuit rate	4.17 s^{-1}
Rate of catch-up saccades	3.89 s^{-1}

pursuits will not correspond to any other occulomotor event in terms of number (hence, using catch-up saccades to indirectly count smooth pursuits is unlikely to be a tenable alternative). This highlights the need for an algorithm which captures smooth pursuits in raw data samples for a variety of stimulus types.

The reader should also be aware that the rate of saccades within smooth pursuit (catch-up, back-up etc.) increases when the velocity of the stimulus target increases. Typical stimulus point velocities range from 10–40°/s.

Kremenitzer et al. (1979) measured the number of smooth pursuit segments per second on infants tracking smoothly moving targets, and found values of 0.07–0.38 s^{-1}. Smooth pursuits were counted by manual inspection. In this study, the number of smooth pursuits per second is a measure of the ability to keep tracking smoothly and continuously.

Measuring the rate of catch-up and back-up saccades during continuous smooth pursuit, Radant and Hommer (1992) found values of 0.62 s^{-1} for catch-up saccades, 0.16 s^{-1} for back-up saccades, and 1.04 s^{-1} for all forward-going saccades (these data come from their control group of "normal" participants). This rate measure is also frequently used in the study of schizophrenia, depression, and various other clinical disorders. Moreover, it is used to investigate the effects of medication and substance abuse, which tends to increase the rate.

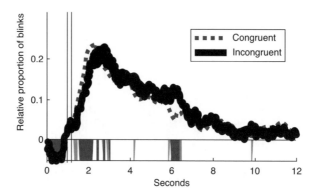

Fig. 12.5 A continuous measure of blink rate, also known as 'Relative proportion of blinks'. Vertical bars signify the onset of Stroop test trials, which could either be congruent or incongruent. The bar below the x-axis shows significance calculations between the congruent and incongruent trial types. Reprinted from Siegle et al. (2008) with kind permission from John Wiley and Sons: *Psychophysiology*, Blink before you think: Blinks occur prior to and following cognitive load indexed by pupillary responses, *45*(5), 2008, Greg J. Siegle, Naho Ichikawa, and Stuart Steinhauer, pp. 679–687.

12.6 Blink rate

Target question	How many blinks?
Input representation	Event-processed data
Output	The number of blinks per minute (min^{-1})

Blink rate ('frequency') is defined as the number of blinks per second or minute. Some researchers in ophthalmology prefer to use the inverse of blink rate, which may be called the 'inter-blink interval', which is defined as the duration between blinks in seconds (Montes-Mico, Alio, & Charman, 2005). Blink rate is a measure known to laypersons, who may ask "do people with lenses blink less?" and "do people blink more in front of a computer?".

Because blink rate only requires detecting the blink event, not measuring its amplitude, duration, and other properties, blink rate may appear the easiest blink measure to record with a video-oculographic eye-tracker. However, coverage of the pupil by reflection in glasses, and motion of the participant when using a remote eye-tracker causes a loss of pupil detection which many event detection algorithms may misinterpret as blinks. Such artefacts may be very common, as examplified by the histogram on page 325.

There appears to be a considerable variation in blink rate both between and within partici-pants (Doughty & Naase, 2006), as well as over time for individual participants. For instance, Zaman and Doughty (1997) showed that participants exhibit large fluctuations in blink rate over time during a five minute recording. Clearly this can have important consequences for your results because the calculation of blink rate depends on *when* the data was recorded with respect to the length of the experiment. Moreover, the distribution of data may often be non-Gaussian; thus, alternative statistical methods may be necessary.

Blinks do not easily provide a continuous measure comparable to pupil dilation or pro-portion over time graphs, but Siegle, Ichikawa, and Steinhauer (2008) describe a method to calculate blink rate over time by comparing a short moving window of samples marked as belonging to a blink (or not) against a prerecorded baseline sample of individual blink rate. From this one can then produce graphs such as Figure 12.5.

The first studies of blink rate were conducted in the 1890s. Most authors, including those mentioned in the excellent overview of blink rate research from Stern et al. (1994), conclude that blink rate is a robust measure that increase with time-on-task and fatigue. Blink rate exhibits average values of 3–7 blinks per minute during reading and 15–30 during most non-reading tasks. The following effects on blink rate can be found in the literature:

Dry eyes Montes-Mico et al. (2005) conclude that the need to moisten the eyeball is not a major determinant of blinking. However, Montes-Mico et al. (2005), amongst others, report that " the typical inter-blink interval in normal patients is approximately 4 to 5 seconds and in those with dry eyes is approximately 1 to 2 seconds in normal conditions" (p. 1618). It is intuitive that a function of blinking is to keep the eyeball moist, and the results of the latter authors support this.

Air pollutants Air particulates, such as those resulting from cigarette smoking, increase blink rate (Stern et al., 1994).

Contact lenses Blink rates initially increase when wearing lenses, but may return to base values following long-term wear (Collins, Seeto, Campbell, & Ross, 1989).

Monitors In normal healthy participants, blink rate drops on average by 20% during use of monitors (Patel, Henderson, Bradley, Galloway, & Hunter, 1991).

Time on task The vast majority of earlier studies (before 1990) were conducted using prolonged reading tasks, which could be up to six hours in length. Blink rate generally increases with time on task (i.e. length of time of reading), but intermediate pauses with comprehension questions eradicate this effect.

Time of day Blink rate appears to be higher during late afternoon than during morning (Stern et al., 1994).

Mental workload Several studies associate the rate of blinks with mental workload (Wolkoff et al., 2005). In a study where car drivers had simultaneous auditory tasks, Y. F. Tsai, Viirre, Strychacz, Chase, and Jung (2007) found an increase in blink rate compared to the driving-only task. Van Orden et al. (2000) found that blink rate increased as a function of tracking error in a human factors tracking task. Brookings et al. (1996) showed that blink rate positively correlates with mental workload in air traffic controllers. However, Veltman and Gaillard (1996) conclude that blinking is independent of mental workload. This conclusion is based on physiological observations from a flight simulator study, where participants experienced in aviation had a concurrent auditory memory task, as well as the primary task of controlling and landing the simulated aircraft. Veltman and Gaillard (1996) found that during landing, when pilots had to process more visual information, the number and duration of blinks decreased, irrespective of the demands of the auditory task. The authors suggest this decrease reflects a strategy to maximize the time available for visual processing when visual demands are highest. It is possible the differences in findings for blink rate and mental/visual workload reflect the different types of task. One can easily envisage, for example, a situation where blinks are infrequent owing to maintained concentration when visual (and cognitive) demands are high. However when the requirements of the task exceed available cognitive resources, concentration may falter, and blink rate may increase due to mental workload.

Saccade amplitude Blinks are more likely to co-occur with large-amplitude than with small-amplitude saccades. Evinger et al. (1994) observed that activation of the lid-closing muscle occurred with 97% of saccadic gaze shifts larger than 33°.

Age Young children blink significantly less frequently than adults. When younger than two months, infants have almost no blinks at all (Stern et al., 1994).

Psychoticism Participants with higher scores on the psychoticism scale showed higher blink rates (Colzato, Slagter, Van Den Wildenberg, & Hommel, 2009).

Individual differences Using a cluster analysis, Doughty and Naase (2006) group their participants into two groups: normal blinkers, with around 10 blinks per second, and frequent blinkers, with more than 20 blinks per second.

12.7 Fixations: number, proportion, and rate

Target question	*How many fixations?*
Input representation	*Event-processed data*
Output	*The amount of fixations in number, proportion or rate (s^{-1})*

Fixations are detected and their properties calculated by an event-detection algorithm. Fixations are then counted in the selected space, time, or portion of data. In practice, the number of fixations often refers implicitly to an entire trial (such as reading one page, or looking at an image), and in some cases to the number of fixations in an area of interest (AOI) during a trial. When comparing two numbers of fixations, it is important that space, time etc. are of equal size—if not, consider using fixation rate.

With still images, and if the event-detection algorithm is good enough, the number of fixations should equal the number of saccades ± 1. With animated stimuli, smooth pursuit may occur, and the number of fixations may be lower than the number of saccades. Also, slow smooth pursuit may be taken to be fixations and artificially increase their number.

There is also an inverse relationship between number of fixations and fixation durations when the trial duration is constant: the more fixations, the lower the durations, and vice versa, as exemplified in Figure 12.6. There are also several other relationships between number of fixations and other measures, illustrated in Figure 12.6.

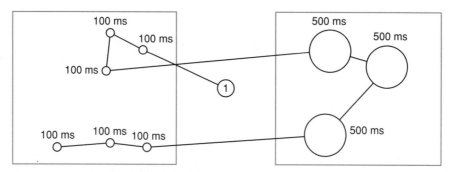

Fig. 12.6 Two areas of interest, left and right, and one scanpath starting at the central fixation (1). Trial duration is 2450 ms, of which saccades make up 300 ms and the initial central fixation is split so that 50 ms falls into this trial. Small fixation rings represent 100 ms fixations, and large rings 500 ms fixations. Measure values can be found in Table 12.5.

12.7.1 Number of fixations

When inside an area of interest, the number of fixations has also been called 'fixation density' (J. M. Henderson et al., 1999). When counted over the whole of the stimulus, another term has been 'fixation frequency'—not to be confused with the measure fixation rate (p. 416) which sometimes goes under the same name. Number of fixations can also be counted per area unit, as an operational definition of reading depth (pp. 390–391). Number of fixations from onset until task completion or object detection is a latency measure (pp. 437–438).

Table 12.5 Values for a variety of duration and counting measures, derived from the synthetic data in Figure 12.6. The 'target' in post-target fixations is the selected area of interest. Stars indicate measures included within this chapter.

	Left AOI	Right AOI
Total dwell time (incl. saccades)	772 ms	1582 ms
Proportion of total dwell time	31.5%	64.5%
Number of fixations*	6	3
Proportion of fixations*	67%	33%
Number of dwells*	2	1
Number of fixations per dwell*	3	3
Number of post-target fixations*	6	3
Number of returns*	1	0
Fixation rate*	2.4 s^{-1}	1.22 s^{-1}
Dwell rate*	0.83 s^{-1}	0.41 s^{-1}

The number of fixations in an area of interest is a very general measure. It is correlated to total dwell time (p. 389), but is not the same, since number of fixations ignores fixation durations. The difference between dwell time and number of fixations will be particularly apparent if a number of short fixations in one area of interest (such as a text) is compared to a smaller number of long fixations in another area of interest (such as a face image). This is illustrated in Figure 12.6. Number of fixations is one of the most used metrics in usability research, according to the review in Jacob and Karn (2003), and it often appears in scene perception research, and in different forms in reading research.

Number of fixations has been used as an indication of the following:

Semantic importance Buswell (1935) and Yarbus (1967) present many scanpath visualizations which give the impression that the semantic importance of a region within a picture affects the number of fixations on that region. Many usability researchers (e.g. Poole et al., 2004, Jacob & Karn, 2003, Fitts et al., 1950) argue that the general importance or noticeability of an object increases the number of fixations in the area of interest allocated to that object. In later scene perception research, J. M. Henderson et al. (1999) and Loftus and Mackworth (1978), found that significantly more fixations landed on semantically informative areas.

Search efficiency and difficulty The number of fixations overall is thought to be negatively correlated with search efficiency (see, for example, Goldberg & Kotval, 1999, who identify a number of measures for assessing usability). Rötting (2001) posits that a low number of fixations could mean either that the task goal has been reached, that the participant is experienced, or that the search task is (too) simple. A high number of fixations would then be indicative of difficulty in interpreting the fixated information or layout. This interpretation is supported by Ehmke and Wilson (2007). In a survey by Jacob and Karn (2003) covering early usability studies and the measures they used, the number of fixations measure was found to be the most common, used in 11 out of 24 studies.

Experience A large number of studies employing various tasks report that experts have fewer fixations in their domain of experience (and sometimes this also transfers to other areas of visual skill). Here follows a few pertinent examples. More accurate circuit chip inspectors required fewer fixations to complete an inspection cycle (Schoonahd, Gould, & Miller, 1973). More experienced tin can inspectors have fewer fixations because they omit fixations on irrelevant parts of the tin can (Megaw & Richardson, 1979). In chess, it has been argued that experts have a larger visual span, therefore make fewer fixations than their less experienced counterparts (Reingold et al., 2001). Fewer fixations is also true of reading skill, where proficient readers make fewer fixations than beginners, as well as other tasks where experts have faster processing of information conveyed in the form of high-resolution detail. However, there are some exceptions to this general rule: Kasarskis, Stehwien, Hickox, Aretz, and Wickens (2001) report that expert pilots have significantly more fixations than novices on all cockpit instruments, and A. M. Williams, Davids, Burwitz, and Williams (1994) found that experienced soccer players exhibit more fixations of shorter duration. This pattern of results is not contradictory however if one considers that an expert's fixations are more efficient. In Kasarskis et al. (2001), although more fixations were observed for experienced pilots, their dwell times were shorter than novices, suggesting that with greater experience information uptake is enhanced, and search optimally directed to relevant areas. This interpretation also holds for soccer players, and is supported in the literature on expertise differences in eye-movements more generally. Clearly however, the interaction between task and experience is important for the number of fixations measure, also explaining differences in results: beginning tennis players show more fixations towards the head of their opponent than do experts (R. N. Singer, Cauraugh, Chen, Steinberg, & Frehlich, 1996); and in golf putting, Vickers (1992) found that a low handicap group directed more fixations to the ball, whereas a high handicap group directed more fixations to the club.

Memory build-up For every new fixation upon an object in a room, memory for the position of that object will improve (Tatler, Gilchrist, & Land, 2005). This has the implication that fewer fixations will be required to locate objects once they have been encoded and a memory representation accumulated through multiple fixations.

Word properties in reading In reading, the number of fixations is used as a measure of morphological complexity, word frequency, and familiarity (Clifton et al., 2007). For example, an area of interest containing a long composite word, or an unfamiliar word, receives more fixations.

Dysfunctions It has been frequently reported that dyslexic readers as a group tend to make more fixations than control readers. Participants with peripheral visual field defects make significantly more fixations than controls (Coeckelbergh, Cornelissen, Brouwer, & Kooijman, 2002). Macular pathology, the loss of foveal vision, also increases the number of fixations, at least during reading (Rohrschneider et al., 1996). During oral reading, stutterers evidence more fixations and regressions per line than do non-stutterers (Brutten & Janssen, 1979). Phobias can result in fewer fixations on anxiety-inducing stimuli (such as spiders). This may reflect an avoidance coping strategy, particular to some phobic participants but not others (Pflugshaupt et al., 2007). Hori, Fukuzako, Sugimoto, and Takigawa (2002) found that schizophrenic patients made a smaller number of fixations (as well as a smaller number of fixated areas) when looking at Rorschach pictures—these are some of the most well known ink-blot pictures used in assessment of personality and schizophrenia.

Age Older participants make significantly more fixations when scanning driving scenes (Ho, Scialfa, Caird, & Graw, 2001), although when their participants made passing manoeuvres in a simulator, Lavallière, Tremblay, Cantin, Simoneau, and Teasdale (2006) found the reverse effect: elderly drivers made fewer fixations.

Spectacles with progressive lenses When reading with progressive lenses, participants exhibit impaired reading in a number of measures, including an increase in the number of fixations (Han et al., 2003). These multi-focal lenses have a gradient for people who are both near-sighted (Myopia) and far-sighted (Hyperopia). The gradient begins at the top of the lens, correcting for viewing objects in the distance, and progresses downwards to correct for close viewing, commonly reading. As a result the wearer is forced to find the best gaze direction through the variable glass, and if failing to do so, may have blurred vision where they read, and with more fixations and regressions as a result.

Sex Both sexes direct more fixations at female rather than male targets (Locher, Unger, Sociedade, & Wahl, 1993), which could explain the domination of female faces on the front pages of gossip magazines, which need to be seen to be sold.

Calculating the measure variety *number of fixations per dwell in each area of interest* (Figure 12.6), Gajewski and Henderson (2005), using a copy task where source and copy are the two areas of interest, argue that a small number of objects fixated per dwell in combination with frequent transitions from one area of interest to another indicates a strategy to minimize the use of visual working memory to one object at a time.

The *number of post-target fixations* for an area of interest is the number of fixations on other areas of interest, from the first entry of the area of interest until the end of the trial. Goldberg and Kotval (1999) who define the measure, speculate that it "can indicate the target's meaningfulness to a user. High values of non-target checking, following initial target capture indicate target representations with poor meaningfulness or visibility" (p. 643). After it was stated, this speculation has been repeated, but the measure itself has hardly been used. In fact, post-target duration (from leaving the area of interest the last time until the end of trial), or alternatively the number of post-target dwells, would probably be a better measure of how much a participant attends (or rather ignores) an area of interest.

12.7.2 Proportion of fixations

Proportion of fixations have been operationalized in one out of two ways.

The *first group* of operarationalizations compare number of fixations between areas of interest and between experimental groups. For instance, Adolphs et al. (2005) calculate the number of fixations on eyes in a face picture, divided by the total number of fixations made in the face. Behrmann, Watt, Black, and Barton (1997) found a significantly higher proportion of fixations on the ipsilesional right side of space for patients with unilateral neglect.

Other operational definitions commonly found in literature include a higher proportion of fixations 'on objects of the specified color' (of many colours), 'on salient regions' (rather than unsalient), 'on relevant pieces' (for the chess task), 'to the critical region' (in a nuclear control room), 'on the face' (in stimuli with people) etc. The areas of interest in focus can be given meaning by an uncontrolled action from the participant, as in the operational definition 'the proportion of fixations on the chosen alternative'. When comparing between areas of interest, the measure has also been called 'the ratio of on-target versus all-target fixations' by Goldberg and Kotval (1999).

Comparisons between participants involve examples such as finding the proportion of fixations made by the clinical group (53%) versus control participants (47%), over fixed trial durations. Commonly, studies use a combined experimental design where both participants and areas of interest are taken into account in the calculation of fixation proportion. Among many results, we find that "The larger visual span of experts in this [chess] task results in fewer fixations per trial, and a greater proportion of fixations between individual pieces, rather than on pieces" (Reingold et al., 2001, p. 54).

The *second type* of operational definition utilizes the fact that fixations have properties that allow us to divide them into groups. The proportion of fixations with durations greater than 150 ms, for instance, or the proportion of fixations whose durations fall between 50 ms and 70 ms, and upward in 20 ms bins. Different fixation durations are argued to convey different cognitive processes (p. 377), which was used as a counting criterion by Schleicher, Galley, Briest, and Galley (2008), who argue that: "the proportion of fixations with a duration between 150 and 900 ms is associated with cognitive processing, while the remaining percentage of fixations are interpreted as express and overlong staring" (p. 15).

Dividing up fixations by their function, Land and Hayhoe (2001) reported that the majority of fixations (more than 50%) in studies on sandwich making, had task-relevant functions. There are many other examples where the *function* of fixations is used as a criterion.

The binocular disparity between fixations of each eye can be thresholded by the distance between characters in reading (and in principle other spatial cutoffs), and so Liversedge, White, et al. (2006) report that 47% of fixations have a disparity greater than one character space.

Other subgroups for dividing fixations into categories so that they can be counted and proportionalized include first fixations, such as the first ones in an area of interest, and ambient versus focal fixations. In reading literature, it is common to attribute saccadic properties to fixations, such as 'the proportion of fixations that were regressive', which should be read as 'the proportions of fixations following a saccade going in the opposite direction to the text'.

12.7.3 Fixation rate

Fixation rate ('fixation frequency', 'gazing time') is the number of fixations divided by a period such as the duration of a trial in seconds, giving the unit per second s^{-1}. The number of fixations in a period of time is roughly proportional to the inverse of the average fixation duration, but differs in two ways: first, fixation rate indirectly includes saccade and blink durations, smooth pursuit, and various other noise. Second, in recordings where there are a few very long and otherwise mostly short fixations, the fixation rate may be much lower than would be expected from the average fixation duration of the same data, as is the case in the study of a painter's eye-movements by Miall and Tchalenko (2001). This is because a small number of long fixations biases the mean fixation duration upwards, thus affecting the approximately inverse relationship between fixation duration and fixation rate.

Fixation rate values can also be divided into areas of interest. For instance, Colvin, Dodhia, and Dismukes (2005) compare pilots scanning in the cockpit, and find large differences in fixation rate within the different areas of interest, with some instruments very regularly hit by fixations, and others much more seldom.

Fixation rate is mostly used by reading, human factors, and usability researchers. Below are a few examples where fixation rate has been explicitly used as a measure in its own right.

Time on task Fixation rate is reported by McGregor and Stern (1996) and Morris and Miller (1996) to decline with time on task.

Task difficulty Fixation rate was found to be negatively correlated to task difficulty by Nakayama et al. (2002).

Performance quality McGregor and Stern (1996) found that fixation rate was correlated with performance only in the flight manoeuvre portion of their experiment, during which participants needed to focus attention on a greater number of cockpit displays than in the straight-and-level flight segments. Van Orden et al. (2001) found fixation rate to be variably correlated to tracking performance across participants, and showed that fixation rate is predictive of target density in a surveillance task, and that it could therefore be used as a measure of mental workload.

In reading research, fixation rate is a central measure used in the operational definition of reading speed (p. 330).

12.8   Dwells: number, proportion, and rate

Target question	*How many dwells?*
Input representation	*Area of interest-processed data*
Output	*The number, proportion, or rate (s^{-1}) of dwells*

The number of dwells is one measure in a whole family, some of which are illustrated in Figure 12.6 on page 412. Dwells are of course a different kind of events from fixations, so bear in mind that these measures refer to dwells.

12.8.1   Number of dwells (entries) in an area of interest

The number of dwells ('gazes', 'glances', 'visits', or 'transitions into and out of the area of interest') is counted over a limited time period which is usually a trial, but can also be a period ended with a participant action like selection or recognition. Precise counting criteria vary somewhat: most definitions allow for a new dwell (entry into an area of interest) to start directly after the previous dwell ended (gaze exited the area of interest). However, in their standard for car-driving research, ISO/TS 15007-1 (2002) require each new dwell in an area of interest to be separated by at least one dwell to a different area of interest. The two definitions only differ when there is whitespace in the stimulus, which is often the case in car-driving studies.

Figure 12.6 shows two areas of interest with whitespace in between. The left area of interest contains two dwells and the right area of interest one dwell. Table 12.5 shows measure values for these data and AOIs. As each dwell requires exactly one entry, the *number of dwells* and the *number of entries* are identical. Both of these are one more than the *number of returns* into an area of interest, that is

$$N_{dwells} = N_{entries} = N_{returns} + 1 \tag{12.1}$$

Number of dwells is a common measure in human factors and driving studies, which are often published in less accessible reports, PhD theses and conference papers. The measure has been given the following interpretations:

Semantic informativeness Although entering an area many times is a different behaviour compared to making many fixations in it, both are sensitive to semantic informativeness (Loftus & Mackworth, 1978; J. M. Henderson et al., 1999).

Difficulty of instruments Presenting car drivers with the task of operating a simple and a difficult MP3 player, Chisholm, Caird, and Lockhart (2008) found many more dwells on the difficult player. The correlation to task completion time was high, see Figure 12.7. The safety limit used by several car manufacturers, based on the study by Zwahlen et al. (1988), is to design in-car instruments so that maximum three dwells are required until task completion. Above that level, the danger of drifting between lanes when driving increases rapidly.

Practice When submitted to a training programme in airport security screening, participants improved from originally on average 1.24 dwells on the target (a knife etc.) before recognizing it, to 1.08 dwells after four training sessions (McCarley, Kramer, Wickens, Vidoni, & Boot, 2004).

Animation Car drivers make a significantly lower number of dwells towards passive road-side advertisement signs (0.64 dwells per participant and sign) compared to animated signs (1.31 dwells per participant and sign) (Beijer, Smiley, & Eizenman, 2004).

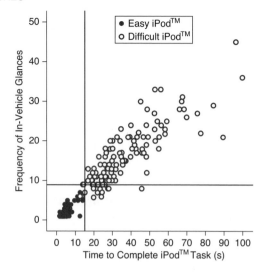

Fig. 12.7 Number (here called 'Frequency') of in-car dwells ('glances') towards an easy to manipulate MP3 player (iPod™) and difficult one during car driving. Reprinted from *Accident Analysis & Prevention*, S.L. Chisholm, and J.K. Caird, J. Lockhart, 704–713, Copyright (2008) with permission from Elsevier.

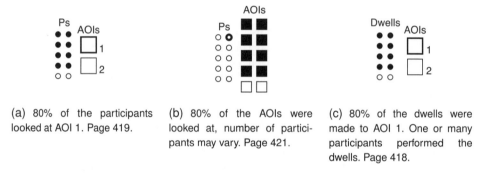

(a) 80% of the participants looked at AOI 1. Page 419.

(b) 80% of the AOIs were looked at, number of participants may vary. Page 421.

(c) 80% of the dwells were made to AOI 1. One or many participants performed the dwells. Page 418.

Fig. 12.8 Proportion calculations with participants (Ps), dwells, and AOIs. Note the variation not only in what is counted, but also whether participants, AOIs, and trial extent is specified or all-including.

Simulator versus real situation The number of dwells to in-car instruments is larger in field driving than in simulator driving, Y. Wang et al. (2010) find in a validation study.

12.8.2 Proportion of dwells to an area of interest

The proportion of dwells tells us, for a single participant, or as an average over all participants, what percentage of the dwells made were directed at a specific area of interest; for example in Figure 12.8(c).

When the proportion of dwells to an area of interest is zero for a participant, the area of interest is considered totally skipped (see pages 192 and 419).

This measure is used infrequently in research, typically appearing in real-world studies with head-mounted eye-trackers, where dwells are calculated rather than fixations. G. Kuhn, Tatler, and Cole (2009) use this measure to show that when a magician looks away from the point in space where the trick takes place, participants follow the gaze of the magician and fail to see the trick.

12.8.3 Dwell rate

Dwell rate is the number of entries into a specific area of interest per minute. It is also known as 'gaze rate' (Fitts et al., 1950). In particular when social and interactional scientists observe and estimate gaze of interlocutors without the use of eye-trackers (Vigil, 2009; Shrout & Fiske, 1981), 'gaze rate' is the most common term.

In the context of usability and human factors research, Jacob and Karn (2003) point out that the proportion of dwell time at a particular area of interest may indeed reflect the importance of the underlying area, but also that researchers using this metric should be careful to note that proportion of time confounds the rate of looking at an area of interest with the duration of those dwells. They quote Fitts et al. (1950) in that dwell rate and dwell time should be treated as separate metrics, with dwell time reflecting difficulty of information extraction, and dwell rate reflecting the importance of that area to the task.

Note that dwell rate is not equal to transition rate. While dwell rate is calculated *per area of interest*, transitions rate is often an overall measure *for two or more areas of interest*, and sometimes a measure counting *pairwise transitions between two areas of interest*.

The dwell rate measure is remarkably little used in eye-tracking research. These are two examples:

Drugs When driving, alcohol but not marijuana leads to decreased dwell rate to critical areas (Moskowitz et al., 1976).

Preference task: Selecting a photo among many based on subjective preferences ('Do I like it?') requires fewer dwells per minute on average than selecting the photo on the basis of subjective recency ('Is it recently taken?') (Glaholt & Reingold, 2009).

12.9 Participant, area of interest, and trial proportion

Target question	*What proportion of participants, areas of interest, or trials fulfil a certain criterion?*
Input representation	*Data from multiple participants and trials*
Output	*The proportion of participants, areas of interest, or trials that fulfil a specified criterion*

Participants, areas of interest, and trials are not events, and should not have to be counted using the same principles as counting eye-movement data. Researchers do know how many participants and trials they have recorded, how many areas of interest they have specified etc, as it is defined in their experimental design (Chapter 3). Thus, these are not dependent variables that we wish to find out the number of.

Nevertheless, many researchers count both participants, areas of interest, and trials as part of their data analysis. This is because *it can be revealing to quantify the number of times a particular criterion is fulfilled* with respect to the experimental design in question and the eye-movement data it produces.

12.9.1 Participant looking and skipping proportions

As researchers know how many participants they have recorded, the absolute number is not of much interest. Instead we calculate the proportion of participants that fulfil a criterion which usually relates to a specific area of interest (Figure 12.8(a)). We might find, for instance, that 25% of the participants looked at the brand logo in an advertisement, or 94.5% skipped

the high frequency word 'of'. More complex counting criteria are the proportion of participants that leave a target word with a regression back to prior text, and the probability that a
participant will make more than two fixations on a specified word (see Pollatsek & Hyönä,
2005).

The *proportion of participants that look at an area of interest* is a very different measure
from number of dwells and dwell time. A 100% proportion of participants for an area of
interest only means that every participant must have looked at the area of interest once, but
says nothing about how long, since a very short dwell time is enough to be included within
the proportion calculation. Other areas of interest may have received many dwells or long
dwell times from only some of the participants, which make them high in number of dwells
and dwell time, but low in proportion of participants.

Percentage of participants fixating on areas of interest is interpreted by Albert (2002) and
Jacob and Karn (2003) as a sign of attention-grabbing properties of an interface element. This
interpretation was picked up very early in advertisement studies such as Treistman and Gregg
(1979), who quantify the proportion of participants noting each primary ad element. Poole
and Ball (2005) add that if a low proportion of participants is fixating an area that is important
to the task, it may need to be highlighted or moved.

Participant *skipping proportion* is, for a selected area of interest, the proportion of all
participants who never looked at the area of interest (total skipping proportion), or the proportion of readers who skipped the word area of interest when first encountering it (first
skipping proportion).

In reading research, skipping proportion is often called 'skipping rate'. Skipping rate
is one of eight selected reading measures in the review by Inhoff and Radach (1998), and
many other reading researchers point out its importance. The reported skipping proportion
for words in sentences constructed for experiments ranges from 0–80%. The important theoretical questions revolve around whether words are skipped because they were identified
parafoveally during the previous fixation, and the extent to which lexical identification of the
skipped word can be achieved from that previous fixation position. Four factors have been
investigated:

High versus low frequency Several studies have used identical sentence pairs with a high-
frequency word in one and a low-frequency in the other. For instance, Rayner and
Fischer (1996) compared sentences like "He invested his money to build a store and
was soon bankrupt" with sentences like "He invested his money to build a wharf
and was soon bankrupt". Schilling, Rayner, and Chumbley (1998) report that a low-
frequency word (1–10 occurrences per million—opm) has a 10% probability of being
first skipped, while a high-frequency word (more than 10,000 opm) will be skipped
67% of the time.

Word length The shorter a word is, the more often it will be skipped (Inhoff & Radach,
1998).

Contextual predictability Given the sentence "The man decided to shave his ____", participants are much more likely to fill in "beard" (83%) than "chest" (8%) (Rayner & Well,
1996). When reading such sentences with the contextually predictable word filled in,
that word is also more likely to be skipped than a contextually unpredictable word in
the same sentence.

Writing system In Chinese, skipping proportion of a single character is reported to be between 40–80% (H. M. Yang & McConkie, 1999). Readers of Chinese even skip two or
three characters, although the skipping proportion is then lower.

12.9.2   Proportion of areas of interest looked at

The area of interest proportion measure tells us by reviewing all the areas of interest shown to a single participant, how many of the areas of interest were looked at (Figure 12.8(b)), or for that matter how many were skipped. This is a measure used in traffic research, where drivers are shown videos of more or less hazardous situations, and researchers then count the percentage of pedestrians, cyclists, grandmothers with baby carriages, and other potentially dangerous things outside the vehicle (even a suddenly appearing moose has been used as a hazard in such studies!) which were fixated. The fixated proportion can then be related to the position, type, or movement direction of the target, or to the level of blood alcohol of the driver.

For instance, Underwood, Chapman, Berger, and Crundall (2003) found that 83.1% of central hazardous events were looked at, but only 66.8% of central non-hazardous events. Further comparisons reveal that central events were looked at more often (74.9%) than 'incidental events' (49.8%), and that dynamic events (69.2%) were looked at more often than static hazards (55.6%). Measuring how much drivers later recall objects in these scenes, (Underwood, Chapman, Berger, & Crundall, 2003) found that "fixated objects were recalled on around 50% of occasions, but details about non-fixated objects were recalled approximately 20% of the time." (p. 301)

Researchers using this proportion measure often warn against interpreting non-fixated as non-processed. In addition to driving research, the same observation has been made in psycholinguistic research, where for instance Griffin and Spieler (2006) point out that people often speak about objects in a scene although the objects were not fixated, and are able to include detail such as agency (actor versus receiver), relative humanness (human versus other primate), and animacy (animate versus inanimate).

12.9.3   Proportion of trials

Trials are counted like participants: each trial is identified using a criterion from the eye-movement data within it, for example, how many saccades are made during the trial, or how many transitions are made, etc.

Reingold et al. (2001) counted the proportion of trials where participants could evaluate the positions on a chess board without making any eye movements, reporting 15.9% of trials for experts, 2.6% for intermediate players, and 1.6% for novices. Using data from a visual search task, Gilchrist and Harvey (2000) first counted the number of saccades in each trial; then for each such number of saccades, the number of trials with that number were counted. The resulting histogram in Figure 12.9 shows that there were more trials with many saccades in which the target was absent compared to when the target was present.

In their problem solving task, Peebles and Cheng (2002) divide trials on the basis of the number of transitions between question and graph areas of interest. 37.1% of the trials involved only one transition from the question to the graph, 48% involved two such transitions, 11.9% involved three transitions and 2.8% involved four or more transitions. The one-, two-, three-, and four-transition(s) trials did not differ in how long participants took to read the elements in the question, but the strategies used did differ: "in the 1 transition trials, participants took approximately 2.28 s to scan the graph before entering an answer, whereas in the other trials, participants looked at the graph for a shorter time before looking again at the question for approximately 300 ms. In the two- and three-transition trials, participants then looked at the graph again for over a second before entering an answer or looking for a third time at the question, respectively. Participants in the three-transition trials scanned the graph for a third time before entering an answer". (p. 82)

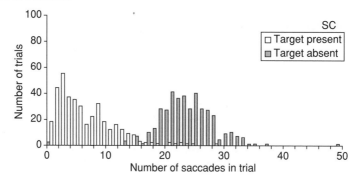

Fig. 12.9 Number of trials as a function of the number of saccades made in the trial. Data from a single participant (SC) who performed visual search trials with the target either present or absent. Reprinted from *Current Biology, 10*(19), Iain D Gilchrist and Monika Harvey, Refixation frequency and memory mechanisms in visual search, 1209–1212, Copyright (2000), with permission from Elsevier.

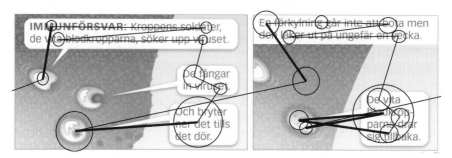

Fig. 12.10 A participant reading a piece of information graphics describing an attack of viruses inside the nose, and the response of the immune system. Bold saccades are *integrative* in the sense of bringing the reader between content-identical visual and textual information. Recorded 2005 with a 50 Hz head-mounted system with magnetic headtracking. Events are counted in Table 12.6. Data are described in Holsanova et al. (2008).

12.10 Transition number, proportion, and rate

Target question	*How many transitions?*
Input representation	*Area of interest-processed data*
Output	*The number of transitions, their proportion or their rate* (s^{-1})

Transitions are movements between areas of interest, and are counted for pairs of areas of interest, for instance the number of transitions from the mouth to the eyes in a face stimulus. Transition matrix measures are used to study overall transition behaviour and longer sequences of transitions (p. 339). The number of transitions measure concerns counting and comparing transitions in small numbers of pairs.

12.10.1 Number of transitions

The number of transitions between two areas has been used as a measure to evaluate the following:

Design Holsanova et al. (2008) compared reading of identical information graphics material in a radial versus a serial design, finding that the serial design resulted in a larger num-

Table 12.6 Number of integrative and non-integrative saccades shown in Figure 12.10.

	Left box	Right box
Number of saccades	10	12
Number of integrative saccades	2	4

ber of transitions between content-identical text and graphics areas of interest. Stolk and Brok (1999) report that the number of transitions between text and picture is related to the complexity of their stimulus material. Hannus and Hyönä (1999) often found only one transition from text to visualization at the end of school textbook reading, and that high-ability children were better at utilizing the relationship between text and visualization.

Expertise Expert pilots make a larger number of transitions between the runway and the airspeed indicator compared to novices, which indicates that expert pilots are following their training and making more of the runway, Kasarskis et al. (2001) note. Kramer and McCarley (2003) suggest that instruments with a large number of transitions between them should be located in close proximity. Studying computer menu search, Card (1982) argues that *conceptual chunking* of menu items can be seen in eye-movement data as sequences of short-amplitude transitions to spatially neighbouring menu items, interrupted by longer transitions.

Importance of an area When an area is so important that it must be more or less continuously monitored, transitions rates drop. Thus Vatikiotis-Bateson et al. (1998) found that the number of transitions between eye and mouth areas of the face is decreased in the presence of noise during a speech task, while dwell time on the mouth is increased.

12.10.2 Number of returns to an area of interest

Returns ('refixations', 'rechecks') are a specific type of transition into an area of interest. To count as a return it is required that there has been at least one previous dwell in the area of interest. In Figure 12.10, the only returns are made to the text at the bottom right, and to the white blood cell that it points to. Note that the number of returns to an area of interest always equals the number of dwells in the area of interest minus one (Figure 12.6). There is at least one proportion variety of this measure: Mannan et al. (2005) defined 're-fixation proportion' for each participant as the total number of re-fixations divided by the total number of targets fixated. A number of effects on this measure have been observed in the literature:

Semantically informative areas Returns are interesting for the same reason as number of dwells: they show that the area is semantically informative. The results that semantically informative and interesting areas are often looked at (many dwells) largely results from many returns in those areas.

Memory Amnesia patients make fewer returns to manipulated areas in a scene, compared to controls, which J. D. Ryan, Althoff, Whitlow, and Cohen (2000) take to indicate a deficit in relational (declarative) memory processing.

Need to confirm In eye tracking on radiological images, the number of returns to a lesion is taken as a measure of confirmatory scanning before the final judgement as to whether it is a malign structure or not (Mello-Thoms et al., 2005).

Age In a change detection task with simple visual patterns, older participants made more returns to already visited areas. Veiel, Storandt, and Abrams (2006) speculate that more

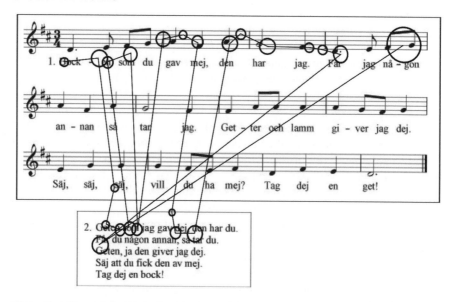

Fig. 12.11 Transition rate in prima vista singing; participants had not seen scores or lyrics before, and had to start singing directly. The division of lyrics at the bottom and music score at the top forces the singer to move up and down in regular intervals, giving a transition rate of 1.48 s^{-1} on average. Recorded 2001 with the an older remote system.

returns indicate a need to refresh visual working memory more often. Gilchrist, North, and Hood (2001) find that the number of returns to an area of interest is much lower if the cost for returning is increased, which increases memory load.

12.10.3 Transition rate

Transition rate is defined as the number of area of interest transitions—movements from one area of interest to another—per second. Transition rate can be calculated *for single pairs of areas of interest over all participants*, in which case transition rate equals dwell rate for the areas of interest. As there are often more than two areas of interest in a stimulus, there can be different transition rates for different pairs of areas of interest. A transition rate matrix has rate values in the cells rather than count values, and can be easily constructed by dividing all transition matrix values by the trial duration. Alternatively, transition rate can be calculated *for participant groups or conditions over all areas of interest*.

Nobody has purported a general interpretation of a high transition rate, but the measure has been used in two broad types of studies:

Working memory capacity Berséus (2002) use transition rate, in combination with dwell time, to study memory buffers of singers who have music and text information separate. Figure 12.11 shows typical data. Results showed that these choir singers had to make 1.48 transitions per second to perform smoothly. Thus, transition rate could be a measure of the demand on (visual) working memory buffers in repetitive tasks. Similarly, Miall and Tchalenko (2001) recorded the eye (and hand) movements of a portrait artist making a pencil sketch of a model. The regular alternation between sitter and drawing gave a transition rate of about 0.5–0.7 s^{-1}.

Integration between modalities There is no consensus that a higher transition rate between two modalities implies better integration between the two information sources. Yet the transition rate measure has often shown effects in studies with multimodal stimuli. For instance, Schmidt-Weigand, Kohnert, and Glowalla (2010) computed the transition rate between text and visualization, after initial instructions varying between fast, medium, and slow pace. Learners in medium and slow instruction pace exhibited more transitions per second between text and visualization compared to the fast instruction pace. Bartels and Marshall (2006) used the measure in a study of the effect of colour codings in displays used by air traffic controllers.

12.11   Number and rate of regressions, backtracks, look-backs, and look-aheads

Target question	*How many regressions?*
Input representation	*Event- or area of interest-processed data*
Output	*The number of regressions, backtracks, look-backs, or look-aheads*

There are hundreds of journal papers that have investigated reading processes by counting the number of regressions. There are two recurring themes: first, dyslexia leads to an increase in regressions. Second, 'garden-path' (leading) sentences and other sentences which require search for an antecedent are common stimuli used with the regression measure.

Compared to regressions, backtracks, look-backs and look-aheads are much more seldom counted in published research.

12.11.1   Number of regressions in and between areas of interest

As we have noted on pages 263–264, the regressions *inside words* are thought to reflect *lexical activation processes* (understanding the word), while regressions *between words* reflect *sentence integration processes* (understanding how several words relate). See Chapters 4 and 5 in Underwood (1998) for further discussion of this difference.

When studying reading of texts longer than one sentence, what is known as the sentence wrap-up effect may cause more regressions near sentence borders.

Spelling errors Zola (1984) found that introducing spelling errors into text resulted in an increase in the number of regressions (in addition to an increase in the fixation duration at the error). When S. N. Yang and McConkie (2001) showed even more deteriorated texts, where letters are replaced with various non-text patterns, the number of regressions greatly increased.

Reader proficiency It has been argued that better readers have a spatial coding of the text that allows them to resolve anaphoric expression by executing a single long saccade to the antecedent (Murray & Kennedy, 1988). Readers without such a spatial coding instead must search for the antecedent using backtracking.

Visual disorders Several visual disorders increase the number of regressions, for instance macular pathology (Trauzettel-Klosinski, Teschner, Tornow, & Zrenner, 1994; Rohrschneider et al., 1996). Training may help in some cases, as Reinhard et al. (2005) show by giving participants with homonymous visual field defects visual restitution training.

Other disorders Many studies have found that readers with dyslexia have more regressions (Elterman, Abel, Daroff, Dell'Osso, & Bornstein, 1980; Rayner, 1985). Also

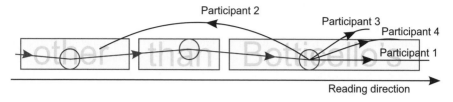

Fig. 12.12 The definition of regression-out is exemplified by these four participants reading. After the fixation of 'Botticello's', there is a 25% regression-out proportion, provided by participant 2.

Alzheimer patients make more regressions compared to controls (K. L. Lueck et al., 2000), and the number of regressions in patients with Broca's and Wernicke's aphasia has been found to be approximately two or threefold the mean value in a normal group (Klingelhöfer & Conrad, 1984).

Age Throughout the primary school years reading skills improve, and the number of regressions continue to decrease up to late university years. However, Rayner, Reichle, Stroud, Williams, and Pollatsek (2006) claim to have found that higher age again increases the number of regressions.

12.11.2 Number of regressions out of and into an area of interest

The reading measure *regression-out* is the proportion of exits from a [word] area of interest that go backward in the reading direction, relative to all exits. This measure is particularly used in first-pass reading (Clifton et al., 2007). Figure 12.12 shows how three participants leave the word area of interest "Botticello's" in the reading direction, while one participant makes a regression-out. The proportion of regression-out is therefore 25%. The regressions-out measure is indicative of both early and late processing.

The *regression-in* measure is for an area of interest the proportion of participants that have regressed to that area of interest, or the proportion of trials where regressions happened. Pollatsek and Hyönä (2005) use the terms 'probability of refixating target word', and 'probability of refixating target word at least twice'.

Both these reading measures are used in branches of reading research. For instance, Pollatsek and Hyönä (2005) compared sentences with fully opaque compounds such as "humbug" (where the meaning of neither constituent is related to the meaning of the compound) to sentences with fully transparent ("milkbottle") and partially opaque compounds such as "strawberry" (where the meaning of one of the constituents is related to the meaning of the compound). The number of regressions from opaque words was almost double the number of regressions from transparent words.

12.11.3 Regression rate

Regression rate is counted as the number of regressions per second, per 100 words, per line, sentence, or paragraph. The measure is used to compare reading processes between conditions such as blood alcohol levels, paragraph width, and type of glasses. For instance, Han et al. (2003) found that using progressive spectacles when reading results in a higher regression rate than single-vision spectacles. Beymer et al. (2005) found regression rate values of 0.54 s^{-1} for text with paragraph width 9 inches, while it was only 0.39 s^{-1} for paragraph width 4.5 inches.

12.11.4   Number of backtracks

Backtracks are notoriously ambiguous events, as explained on pages 262–264. Count values in the literature rely on varying operational definitions, and cannot be easily compared.

Nevertheless, the number of backtracks was found by Goldberg and Kotval (1999) to be one of the best predictors of usability. However the studies that use this measure (and different operational definitions of backtracks) to investigate webpage use, appear not to have been able to replicate this finding.

12.11.5   Number of look-aheads

Look-ahead fixations tend to cluster around 3 s ahead of the action, which is taken as support for the view that they are anticipatory and preparatory for the upcoming action.

Mennie et al. (2007) compute number of look-aheads in a grasping task. Look-aheads prove to be much less common than guiding fixations, and the look-ahead fixation is also shorter in duration. Finding no decrease in the number of look-aheads over the one hour sessions, Mennie et al. conclude that look-aheads are not influenced by familiarity with the scene layout.

13   Latency and Distance Measures

Although latencies and distances are central metrics in the vast majority of eye-tracking measures covered thus far in this book, we reserve this chapter for 'time' and 'space' specifically as it pertains to unitary eye-tracking events *in relation to other events*.

Latency is a measure of time delay, that is the time from the on- or offset of one event to the on- or offset of another (p. 286). Eye–voice latency, for instance, is the time between looking at a word or picture and saying it. Several of the latency measures can be used as reaction time measures.

Distance measures return the distance from one point to another (for instance gaze and mouse cursor) at one and the same time, either as a single value (e.g. saccadic gain) or as a continuous measure (e.g. smooth pursuit gain). These distance measures differ from saccadic amplitude for example, where the distance refers to the movement of *one single point* over a period of time.

Both latencies and distances are often called 'spans', and eye–voice span is identical to eye–voice latency. Spatial distance and temporal latency are tightly coupled aspects of relative motion between the two events. Because of this, latency and distance are often used interchangeably: eye–voice latency can either be measured in the temporal domain (milliseconds), or the spatial domain (number of words, or pixels). Measures that are predominantly 'time-based' have been put in the latency section of this chapter, while measures that are more 'space-based' are found in the distances section.

Because they have a true zero-point, namely the zero milliseconds latency when both events are simultaneous, all latency measures are of the ratio type, which allows for the usage of a wide variety of parametric tests for statistical calculations (p. 90). The exception is the complex latency of the proportion over time measures, for which we present a separate statistical section.

Be aware that these latencies are dependent measures, and not sources of error like the system latencies on page 43. However, for values of latency measures to be correctly measured, it is crucial that your stimulus program and recording system are temporally accurate; if the flash or new stimulus picture is shown 48 ms later than the mark shows in your eye-tracking data file, due to slow loading and rendering, your latency value will be 48 ms too high. Also, your *detection algorithm* must calculate the onset of the eye-movement event correctly, which is easier for fast saccades and more difficult for slow smooth pursuit. In addition to these hidden and variable errors in the stimulus software and detection algorithms, the *sampling frequency* on average causes a constant error of half a sample (e.g. 1 ms for a 500 Hz eye-tracker) for all latency measures. Also note that using a stimulus monitor with, for instance, an 8 ms refresh time will reduce the efficient speed to 125 Hz for these measures, even if a much faster eye-tracker is being used. Historically, cathode ray tube (CRT) monitors have lower latencies and refresh times than the more modern thin film transistor (TFT) monitors. Measuring your monitor with a photodiode is the only way to make sure that it does not buffer the image, and shows it more seldom and later than your experiment presumes. In the remainder of this chapter, it is assumed that all these technical issues have been addressed or can be neglected, and therefore do not add additional system latencies to the collected data.

In eye-tracking research, there are many latency and distance measures, summarized in the following two tables.

Latency measure	Target question	Page
Saccadic latency	How soon after target onset does the saccade start?	430
Smooth pursuit latency	How soon after target motion onset does smooth pursuit start?	432
Latency of the reflex blink	How soon after onset of an event which causes blink does the blink commence?	434
Pupil dilation latency	How soon after onset of an event which causes dilation does the pupil start to dilate?	434
Eye fixation related potential (EFRP)	How soon after the eye started looking at X does the ERP component show?	436
Entry time	How soon after onset is the AOI entered?	437
TX: Thresholded entry time	How soon after onset have X % of participants visited the AOI?	438
Proportion of participants over time	What proportion of the participants look or have looked at an AOI at a specific point in time?	440
Eye–voice latency	How soon after the eye started looking at X does the participant verbalize X?	442
Eye–hand span	How soon after the eye looked at X does the hand perform the corresponding action?	445
The eye–eye span (cross-recurrence analysis)	How soon, on average, does a listener look where the speaker looks?	447

Distance measure	Target question	Page
Eye–mouse distance	What is the distance between the point of gaze and the mouse position?	448
Disparity	What is the distance between the points of gaze of left and right eye?	449
Smooth pursuit gain	What is the velocity ratio between point of gaze and the target?	450
Smooth pursuit phase	How far behind or ahead is the eye with respect to the target?	451
Saccadic gain	What is the distance between saccadic ending point and target?	452

13.1 Latency measures

Latencies measure the difference in *time* between two events, for instance from the onset of a stimulus until the onset of the first saccade. The majority of latency measures operate with absolute time in milliseconds, but some of the longer-duration measures—for instance entry time—alternatively count time in units of number of fixations or number of unique AOIs.

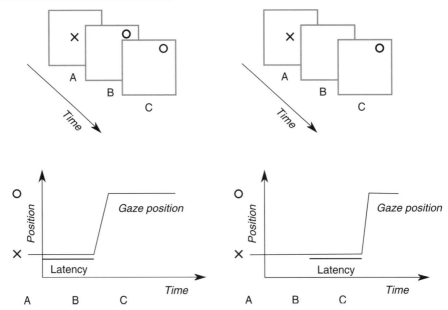

Fig. 13.1 On the left side, the *principle of saccadic latency*: A fixation point (X) holds the participant's gaze until onset of target point (O) between time A and B. In the *gap* condition to the right, the fixation point (X) is removed some time before the target point (O) is onset, and for a period called the gap, there is no item that could lock the participant's attention.

13.1.1 Saccadic latency

Target question	*How soon after onset does the saccade start?*
Input representation	*A saccade and an onset time of the stimulus*
Output	*Latency (ms)*

Saccadic latency is a measure of reaction time to stimuli. It is defined as the time it takes for the brain to program and launch the saccade to the onset target point. Since saccades have very sharp and easily pinpointed onsets, it is relatively easy to calculate the latency accurately.

The specific event that triggers the saccade is known as the 'onset' of a stimulus. The onset can be a sudden flash in the periphery, or a complete change of a stimulus picture. Saccadic latency is a widely used measure, and there are several named experimental paradigms that differ in how stimuli are presented. The most well known is the 'gap' paradigm (see also p. 68) in which visual attention is released for a short while (the gap) between the offset of a fixation point and the onset of a saccade target; commonly an empty white screen is presented within this interval. Figure 13.1 illustrates both the basic and 'gap' conditions. Saccadic latencies are also regularly reported from studies in the *anti-saccade paradigm* described on pages 305–307.

Simultaneously flashing two scenes with animals or distractors for 20 ms, Rousselet, Fabre-Thorpe, and Thorpe (2002) showed that human participants can reliably make saccades to the side containing an animal within 120 ms (Kirchner & Thorpe, 2006). For comparison, the differential ERP effect starts at 150 ms, while manual button pressing has latencies starting at 180 ms for visual stimuli (Welford & Brebner, 1980).

Saccadic latencies have repeatedly been shown to have a *bimodal distribution*. In monkeys, for instance, there are an abundance of saccades with a latency of 80 ms and also many

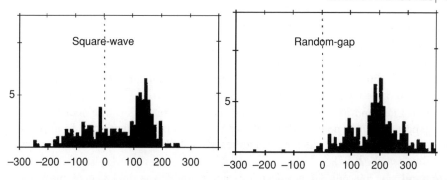

Fig. 13.2 On the right side, saccadic latency histogram for a (random) gap paradigm with one participant. Note the tendency for a bimodal distribution with two peaks. On the left side a predictable square wave stimulus where a large part of the latencies are negative. Bin size 10 ms. With kind permission from Springer Science+Business Media: *Experimental Brain Research*, A short-latency transition of visually-guided and predictive saccades, *76*(1), 1989, A.C. Smit.

saccades with a latency of 120 ms, but only few saccades with a 100 ms latency (Fischer & Boch, 1983). The faster saccades in the first peak of this distribution have been named 'express saccades' while the slower ones are thought to be regular saccades. If the superior colliculus, a brain area important to saccades, is damaged, express saccades disappear from the latency distribution. Because of this, express saccades became important in the study of the neural structures that drive rapid oculomotor responses (Schiller & Tehovnik, 2001).

When designing your experiment or interpreting results, take into account the existing research on what makes an upcoming saccadic latency short:

Releasing attention Removal of the fixated point—and hence *releasing attention* to it— before onsetting the peripheral target reduces saccadic reaction times from the typical 200 ms down to 120–150 ms. This is known as the 'gap effect', because of the temporal gap between the removal of the fixated object and the onset of the target (see Figure 13.1). The opposite is sustained attention to the fixated point by showing it even after the target has been onset, which prolongs latencies.

Distractors When the stimulus image contains a simultaneous distractor, saccadic latencies will increase by 20–40 ms compared to trials where no distractor is present. If the distractor is instead flashed as little as 50–100 ms before the target, latencies are reduced. The distractor then works as a facilitating warning signal (Born & Kerzel, 2008).

Splitting attention Directing a saccade to one hemifield (i.e. one half of the visual field) and performing a manual reaction to an object in the opposite hemifield—*splitting attention* in two directions—results in prolonged saccade latencies as well as manual reaction times (Shepherd, Findlay, & Hockey, 1986).

Anticipation When the task is sufficiently predictable that it allows the participant to anticipate the direction and amplitude of the next saccade, the latency may be negative, i.e. the saccade shifts the eye before the target appears (Smit & Van Gisbergen, 1989).

Type of stimulus Natural stimuli elicit much lower saccadic latencies than classical lab stimuli consisting of a black background with a few white dots (Trottier & Pratt, 2005; White, Stritzke, & Gegenfurtner, 2008). This suggests that the second latency peak in the bimodal distribution, at 180–200 ms, may be a laboratory artefact, and the 'express saccades' with a latency of 120–150 ms the natural latencies that occur with everyday stimuli and environments.

The target point Saccade latencies to Gabor patches, a wavy luminance pattern, decrease as a function of contrast at the target point, and increase with the spatial frequency of the waves (Ludwig, Gilchrist, & McSorley, 2004).

The task instruction When asked to react quickly, participants respond with a decreased saccadic latency (Kapoula, 1984).

Expertise Land and McLeod (2000) found that in cricket batsmen, a short latency to the expected bounce point of the ball after bowling, distinguishes good from poorer batsmen. Also, elite shooters have a significantly shorter saccadic latency than controls (Di Russo et al., 2003).

Participant age Saccadic latency decreases significantly by around 25 to 60 ms when participant age increases from 8 to 19 years (Salman, Sharpe, Eizenman, et al., 2006). Saccadic gain, however, and peak velocity, remain constant. As participants grow older, latency increases once more (Moschner & Baloh, 1994).

Impaired processing *Increased* saccadic latencies appear with a large number of impairing factors, such as schizophrenia, melancholic depression, alcohol levels above 0.5‰ and total sleep deprivation (Bocca & Denise, 2006; Winograd-Gurvich et al., 2006; Buser, Lachenmayr, Priemer, Langnau, & Gilg, 1996), just to mention a few. Some drugs (e.g. nicotine, amphetamine) appear to *decrease* these increased latencies, but never below the original baseline.

Transcranial magnetic stimulation A number of studies have shown that saccadic latencies are prolonged by transcranial magnetic stimulation of the frontal and parietal areas of the brain, which are thought to regulate the control of eye movements. The combined technique then became important in testing neurological models for eye-movement generation (Müri, Hess, & Pierrot-Deseilligny, 2005; Kapoula et al., 2001; Muri, Vermersch, Rivaud, Gaymard, & Pierrot-Deseilligny, 1996; Zangemeister, Canavan, & Hoemberg, 1995; Priori, Bertolasi, Rothwell, Day, & Marsden, 1993).

In other words, to be sure of 'typical' saccadic latencies, your participants' attention should not be unduly locked to a fixation point, the stimulus should be natural and the target salient. He should be around 20 years of age, be well practiced in the task, know that he has to be quick, and not be impaired by neurological deficiencies, transcranial magnetic stimulation, alcohol, drugs, or sleep deprivation.

Release of attention from a target is also studied using the non-eye-tracking paradigm 'attentional blink': Rapidly showing e.g. letters with ~100 ms interval between them, participants are asked to identify a subset of the letters and at the same time report if there is an X in the subsequent 12 letters (Hari, Valta, & Uutela, 1999). As the identification of the first letter locks participants' attention for 200–600 ms, X:s that appear in that period are seldom identified even when appearing in the foveal projection of the participant.

13.1.2 Smooth pursuit latency

Target question	How soon after onset does smooth pursuit start?
Input representation	Onset time of smooth pursuit and stimulus
Output	Latency (ms)

Smooth pursuit latency (also known as 'latency of pursuit initiation') is a measure of reaction time, where the triggering event is the onset of a smoothly moving target object. Be aware that smooth pursuit initiation consists of two parts: the earliest 100 ms phase in smooth pursuit, so-called 'open loop pursuit', is considered to be a ballistic acceleration towards the estimated target direction. The second phase, 'closed-loop pursuit', starts before 300 ms after stimulus onset. The target moving away from the gaze point, known as 'retinal slip' owing to target motion, is continuously and much more accurately compensated for in the second phase (Wallace, Stone, & Masson, 2005). There is also an offset latency in smooth pursuit, measuring the time from offset of target movement until the eye starts to decelerate, but this variety is rarely utilized.

Both gap and no-gap paradigms are used. In the gap condition, to release the participants' visual attention, the target disappears for a short period, then reappears, and starts to move.

While the precise onset of a saccade is possible to calculate even with a fairly simple detection algorithm, detecting smooth pursuit onset is much more difficult and latencies have often been calculated by manual inspection: "Latencies for smooth eye movements were estimated visually from the eye velocity records for individual trials" (Lisberger & Westbrook, 1985). Beginning in the mid 1990s, several detection algorithms for smooth pursuit onset appeared, that calculate them slightly differently (p. 178).

Latencies for smooth pursuit onset are around 100–200 ms when the direction and velocity of the target motion are unpredictable to the participant, but as soon as the participant has a possibility to predict the upcoming target motion, latencies may drop to under 0 ms; that is the smooth pursuit motion starts before the target motion (Burke & Barnes, 2006) in an anticipatory manner. Offset latency of smooth pursuit is in the same range as onset latency (Becker & Fuchs, 1985).

The following factors are known to influence smooth pursuit latency:

Anticipation When the visual system has information on the future direction of smooth pursuit, latencies are not only shorter, but even negative, i.e. the eye starts to move before the target does (De Hemptinne, Lefevre, & Missal, 2006; Burke & Barnes, 2006).

Chromatic isoluminant stimuli Latencies of pursuit initiation are prolonged by 50 ms when the stimulus is isoluminant—that is, luminance of the background equals that of the moving target—and hence appears to move more slowly (Braun et al., 2008).

Single distractors When there was a distractor moving in the opposite direction, smooth pursuit latency of rhesus monkeys was prolonged by about 150 ms, Ferrera and Lisberger (1995) found when empirically testing a neurological model for smooth pursuit. However, distractors only affected the latency, not the continued tracking.

Moving stimulus background A dotted background—a whole field of distractors—moving in the same direction as the target decreases smooth pursuit latency, and increases it if moving in the opposite direction (Spering & Gegenfurtner, 2007).

Schizophrenia Some studies report shorter smooth pursuit latencies in schizophrenia patients, although this effect is debatable and other studies have found the reverse (O'Driscoll & Callahan, 2008).

Participant age J. A. Sharpe and Sylvester (1978) report longer latencies for older participants (mean 67 years of age) than for younger ones (mean 42), which make age an important factor to take into account when selecting participants and analysing data. Morrow and Sharpe (1993) used a variety of unpredictable smooth pursuit initiations, and noticed an age-related degeneration in smooth pursuit acceleration.

Many studies that use the smooth pursuit latency measure are designed with the explicit goal of understanding the neurological underpinnings of smooth pursuit, and the extent to which they differ from the systems that drive saccades.

Table 13.1 Data from an early investigation on blink latencies (Rushworth, 1962). Latency values refer to the first reaction recorded with needle electrodes in the orbicularis oculi muscles.

Stimulus	First peak	Second peak
Glabella tap	12–18 ms	25–45 ms
Electrical stimulation of supraorbital nerve	10–13 ms	25–38 ms
Corneal irritation	-	25–40 ms
Loud click next to ear	-	23–33 ms
Bright flash close to eye	30–58 ms	60–90 ms

13.1.3 Latency of the reflex blink

Target question	*How soon after onset does the eye blink?*
Input representation	*Onset of blink and stimulus*
Output	*Latency (ms)*

The *latency of the reflex blink* is the time from stimulation onset until eye blink onset, or in some varieties until maximum eyelid closure. Eye blinks occur after a variety of stimulations: bright flashes, auditory beeps, puffs of air, tapping on the glabella (the space between the eyebrows and above the nose), irritation of the cornea, etc. Stimulation of one eye causes blink reflexes in both eyes.

The reflex blink is a reflex and not a reaction, because the initiation of the blink takes place without any involvement of cognitive or deliberate action. The reflex blinks can therefore be much shorter than reaction times such as saccadic latency.

As blinks are movements with a rapid acceleration, detection of blink onset has never been considered difficult. Note however that pupil and corneal reflection eye-trackers detect onset of blink only when part of the pupil is covered, rather than at onset of eyelid movement. Blink measurements have previously been made with needle electrodes in the blink muscles, and with electromagnetic sensors placed on the eyelid.

The reflex blink has a bimodal distribution, and the precise values vary with the type of stimulation. The very low values indicate that the neurological route between stimulation and reaction is short and does not involve cognitive decisions. Table 13.1 summarizes results from the seminal investigation by Rushworth (1962).

Factors influencing the blink reflex latency often relate to basic alertness states. For example, Grillon, Ameli, Woods, Merikangas, and Davis (1991) found that when participants were feeling anxious about the risk of sudden electrical shock, their blink reflex latencies (to acoustic stimuli) were shorter compared to when they felt safe.

13.1.4 Pupil dilation latency

Target question	*How soon after onset does the pupil start to dilate?*
Input representation	*Onset of pupil dilation and stimulus*
Output	*Latency (ms)*

Pupil dilation latency is defined as the time elapsing between the onset of increased luminance (or other stimulus) and the beginning of pupil dilation. In addition to high sampling frequency and few or no system latencies, pupil dilation latency measurements are benefitted from the use of a high-resolution eye camera with a fixed distance to the eye, a uniformly luminous stimulus and—if the task allows it—a fixation point that the participant must look at (p. 392)

It has been known since the late 19th century that pupil dilation varies with both light variation and sensory, cognitive, and emotional events (Beatty & Lucero-Wagoner, 2000). Furthermore, the magnitude of change is large with light stimuli, but quite small when the change is due to internal events, down to 0.01 mm. Note that cognitive and affective pupil reactions *are only indirectly linked* to the stimulus or internal state, and the connection is not necessarily causal (Beatty & Lucero-Wagoner, 2000, p. 143). More precisely, small movements due to mental effort and arousal are superimposed onto two larger effects from the light reflex and the accommodation of the lens. To detect these small movements in pupil size—given the much larger sensory movements—it is necessary to average over many trials to reliably tell whether the effect is indeed present. Since pupil size is individual and sensitive to the environment, pupil size is measured against a baseline obtained during some interval prior to onset (Van Gerven, Paas, Van Merriënboer, & Schmidt, 2004). If the pupil is already involved in a dilation movement, latencies are longer (220–385 ms) than if it is stabilized before onset (about 180 ms) (F. A. Young & Biersdorf, 1954). Therefore always allow time to stabilize the pupil before latency measurements.

Changes in pupil dilation are comparatively slow with respect to onset, and as with smooth pursuit latency, difficult to pinpoint exactly. Small-magnitude changes are less easy to detect than the large ones owing to changes in light. Detection by manual inspection of the pupil dilation curve was the only available alternative until the mid 1900s. F. A. Young and Biersdorf (1954); R. E. Lee, Cohen, and Boynton (1969) used curve-fitting techniques to model the dilation curve, and defined the latency as the time delay giving the most accurate fit. Later studies define the moment of onset as the time when *pupil acceleration is maximally negative*. Onset is only looked for *inside a finite time window* of for instance 200–450 ms after stimulus onset, so that variations other than the reflex are excluded. According to Bergamin, Zimmerman, and Kardon (2003) "This time window is also very easy to define with software analysis ... and also showed greater diagnostic power than the most commonly used contraction" (p. 110).

The following summary of reported latencies to different stimuli describes the overall trend:

Light Latencies to light are about 150–400 ms for control participants. Age, several illnesses, personality disorders and drug abuse strongly alter the latency, and hence much clinical research as well as practical diagnosis use pupil dilation latency as one diagnostic criterion.

Auditory signals Pupil dilation latency is around 600 ms when judging single tones (Beatty, 1982).

Pain C. R. Chapman et al. (1999) found that pupil dilation responses to pain begin at 330 ms, and peak at 1.25 seconds after stimulus onset.

Mental multiplication When Ahern and Beatty (1979) presented spoken integers to be multiplied, the pupil reacted within less than 300 ms, and the reaction was stronger for more difficult multiplications and also stronger for students weaker in mathematics, as shown in Figure 13.3.

Social stimuli Latencies reach 600–800 ms when control participants react to the emotional state—and in particular the pupil—of another person (Harrison et al., 2006).

Bearing the above findings in mind when working with pupil dilation latency, also note that inter-eye asymmetry in control participants may range between 8 and 35 ms (Bergamin, Schoetzau, Sugimoto, & Zulauf, 1998).

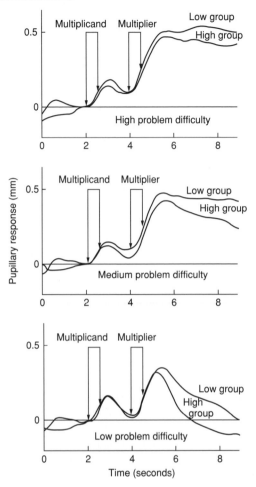

Fig. 13.3 The pupillary response to spoken integers that were to be multiplied by the participant, the on- and offset of which are shown. Three levels of difficulty were used, the most difficult task at the top. The two groups of participants are either high or low in psychometric measures of intelligence. Overall latencies from onset of multiplicands and multipliers to pupil response are around 300 ms. Reprinted from Ahern and Beatty (1979) with kind permission from the AAAS (American Association for the Advancement of Science).

13.1.5 EFRPs—eye fixation related potentials

Target question	How soon after the eye started looking at X does the ERP component show?
Input representation	Onset of fixation and ERP event
Output	Latency (ms)

Eye-fixation related potential simply means that the ERP component in question is *related to the onset of an eye-fixation* (the EF in the acronym) rather than to the onset of the stimulus per se (p. 288).

This is a relatively new measure that arises from the combination of technologies for eye tracking and measuring brain activity. Apart from the distinction in onset, an EFRP-latency is just like any other ERP latency, and thus not really an eye-movement measure. Simola,

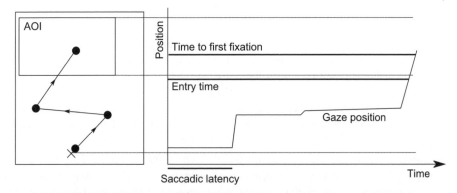

Fig. 13.4 Saccadic latency, entry time, and time to first fixation. Entry into the AOI is reached only during the third saccade–left. Saccadic latency is the time until the first saccade is launched–right. Time to first fixation in AOI is always longer than entry time.

Holmqvist, and Lindgren (2009) measured EFRPs to investigate parafoveal preview benefit, and observed a right visual field advantage associated with an occipital EFRP component which differentiated between processing words and non words.

13.1.6 Entry time in AOI

Target question	*How soon after onset is the AOI entered?*
Input representation	*Gaze samples or fixations, AOI location, and onset time of stimulus*
Output	*Entry time in AOI (ms) or number of events until AOI entry*

The term *entry time* is closely related to, but not synonymous with 'search time' in Rötting (2001), 'time to first hit' in Krupinski et al. (2003), 'distraction time' in Casey and Richards (1988), and 'time to first fixation on target area of interest' in Jacob and Karn (2003). Entry time is defined as the duration from onset of stimulus until the AOI is first entered, whether entry is made via a saccade or via smooth pursuit. Time to first fixation includes the time period from entering the AOI until the first fixation is made, and is therefore always somewhat longer (Figure 13.4).

As time can be represented either at sample level, or as given by the sequence of a selected event, the precise operational definition of the duration from trial start to first entry has three varieties, each of which can be absolute or relative:

1. *Time in milliseconds* was used by Giorgetti, D'Amato, Pagani, Cavarzeran, and Tagliabracci (2007) for studying the effects of alcohol. The entry time value can also be made relative to the trial duration.

2. *Number of fixations* from trial start until first entry, used by Bojko (2006) for studying web page design, and Kundel and La Follette Jr (1972) in studying experience of radiologists. The number of fixations until entry can also be divided by the total number of fixations in the trial to give a relative value.

3. *Number of unique AOIs* visited before first entry, or this absolute number divided by the total number of unique AOIs visited during the trial. The latter method thus results in a relative value.

Entry time is a latency measure, that can be used in reaction time studies, but it differs from the other latency measures, for instance saccadic latency, in a number of ways. First, while saccadic latency only concerns the onset of the first saccade, entry time runs until the AOI is first visited, irrespective of how many saccades are needed en route. Second, while entry time measures the duration until entry into the AOI, saccadic latency measures only up until the start of the saccade (not until the entry into the target AOI). Also, entry time is a valid measure for all AOIs, not only for one selected target.

Irrespective of how the measure is operationalized, it is generally considered that a short entry time to a target AOI reflects higher efficiency in locating for the stimulus in question. The following factors have been found to affect the entry time measure:

Visual saliency In the low-level sense of Itti and Koch (2000), visual saliency (i.e. discontinuities in colour, intensity, and orientation) appears *not* to attract early fixations *when the participant has a specific purpose* when inspecting an image (Underwood, Foulsham, Van Loon, Humphreys, & Bloyce, 2006). These authors' conclusions are based on the fixation count definition of the entry time measure. In fact, there is evidence that saliency does a poor job of attracting early attention even during more neutral tasks when there is no specific purpose in mind (Nyström & Holmqvist, 2008).

Out of context objects Objects that violate the 'gist' of a scene, that is they have a low probability of appearing in this context, are likely to attract early fixations (Loftus & Mackworth, 1978). However, this finding has been disputed in later work (De Graef et al., 1990).

General conspicuity When the target AOI is made to stand out this leads to shorter entry times. For instance, changing the warning labels on cigarette advertisements to be more visible and direct decreases entry time significantly (Krugman, Foxer, Fletcher, Fischer, & Rojas, 1994). Also, redesigning a web page to highlight important elements can lead to significantly shorter entry time to target links (Bojko, 2006).

A preview or memory of the scene Previews lead to faster target fixation (short entry times in target AOIs), according to Hollingworth (2009), even for short preview presentations of 500 ms during which the target is absent.

Alcohol Ethanol consumption slows down entry time for at least 150 minutes after intake, compared to controls (Giorgetti et al., 2007).

Expertise Experts in quickly and accurately identifying pathologies in radiological images can be identified by their lower entry times (Krupinski, 1996; Nodine, Kundel, Lauver, & Toto, 1996). Higher age, often correlated with less experience with user interfaces leads to longer entry times for the interface in question, in comparison to the shorter entry times of younger users with more experience (Obrist, Bernhaupt, Beck, & Tscheligi, 2007).

Spoken language Hearing speech very often leads the listener to earlier entries into the corresponding semantic element to which the speech refers. First utilized by Eberhard et al. (1995) to measure point-of-disambiguation effects, this use of the entry time measure has now developed into proportion over time-curves (pp. 197–205 and p. 440).

13.1.7   Thresholded entry time

Target question	*How soon after onset have X% of the participants looked at the AOI?*
Input representation	*Gaze samples or fixations, AOI location, and onset time of stimulus*
Output	*Latency (ms)*

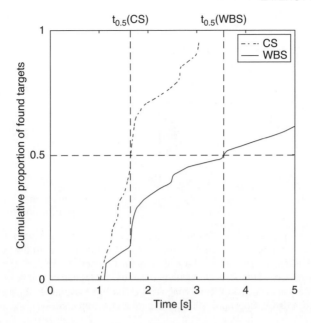

Fig. 13.5 Cumulative proportion of targets found for two groups, one group with Williams Beuren syndrome and a control group. With a 5 second trial time, only 67% of the WBS participants found the target, but 99% of the CS participants. T50 are shown for both curves. Reprinted from *Neuropsychologia, 45*(5), Montfoort, I,. *et al,* Visual search deficits in Williams-Beuren syndrome, 931–938, Copyright (2007), with permission from Elsevier.

While previous latency measures concerned single events, the *thresholded entry time* is the time (in milliseconds) until a specified proportion (X) of all participants have looked at a particular AOI. The T50, for instance, is the time that it takes until *50%* of the participants have looked at an AOI. The X, thus, signifies the threshold, and can be adjusted according to the purpose of the study.

The originators of the measure, Montfoort, Frens, Hooge, Lagers-Van Haselen, and Van Der Geest (2007), point out, however, that calculating average entry time on data where not all participants actually found the target can be misleading. For the data in Figure 13.5, the average entry times for both sets would be very similar. This is why it is advisable to use the median rather than the mean, and thus compensate for incomplete data sets within trials.

When a single participant does many trials, T50 is a better measure than average entry time for the trials where the participant found the AOI, because T50 yields performance (percentage correct) and timing in one number. When multiple participants do a single trial, T50 is equivalent to a cumulative proportion over time graph (p. 197 and below), as it uses a curve delineating the cumulative proportion of AOIs inspected within a fixed time period.

As Figure 13.5 illustrates, the T50 method has been used to identify the visual search processes underlying inefficient visual scanning in Williams Beuren syndrome (Montfoort et al., 2007).

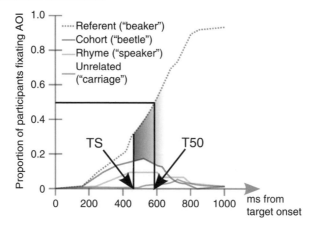

Fig. 13.6 Two common types of latencies in a momentous proportion over time graph: T50 is the time when 50% of the participants look at the AOI 'Referent'. TS is the time when the curves for 'Referent' and 'Cohort' are significantly different for the first time since onset of stimulus. Modified from *Journal of Memory and Language, 38*(4), Paul D. Allopenna, James S. Magnuson, and Michael K. Tanenhaus, Tracking the Time Course of Spoken Word Recognition Using Eye Movements: Evidence for Continuous Mapping Models, pp. 413–39, Copyright (1998), with permission from Elsevier.

13.1.8   Latency of the proportion of participants over time

Target question	*At what time has a specific proportion of the participants looked at an AOI?*
Input representation	*Proportion over time graphs*
Output	*Latency (ms)*

A proportion over time graph (pp. 197–205) visualizes how the proportion of participants that look at each AOI develops over time. It is used as a measure of the timing and development of cognitive processes over time. It is a relatively complex measure, but also an intuitive visualization. It is often a very sensitive measure, which can be exploited to the researcher's benefit. Typically, this takes the form of a presentation of the visual stimuli, and then introduces some task-critical information which causes the participant to start allocating attention in a new pattern and thus changing the proportion over time curve. We now have a gaze pattern before the critical information bit as a baseline, and we can contrast this to the gaze following the introduction of the critical information. The researcher now has both baseline and treatment data for every unique trial.

Different properties of this curve change can then be extracted and used as predicting variables, but as Figure 13.6 illustrates, it is typically the latency—the time from onset to when a given amplitude is reached (T50 in Figure 13.6), or until a significant difference between two AOIs or two conditions are reached (TS in Figure 13.6)—that is focused on.

Statistical analysis of proportion over time curves

The analysis typically starts with some form of preprocessing of the data. Often the continuous time line gets divided up into several 'bins' which will then be used as a predictor, depending on the particular analysis method. There are two reasons for this binning of time. The first is that the data become more manageable with only a few bins rather than raw data samples. This may also be a requirement by some statistical tests where time cannot be used as a continuous predictor. The second reason is for fulfilling any assumptions of independence. A particular raw data sample at point t_1 is very likely to have similar properties to a gaze sample at point t_2. By binning and treating many data samples as a whole, we are more likely to have samples that are independent of each other. A rule of thumb would be to have bins of at least 200 ms, as this is the typical programming time of a saccade. So, with 200 ms or more, we can be more confident that the participant has had a chance to reallocate his attention if he wanted to, i.e. independence in this setting. (See Barr, 2008 for a discussion of this and more).

The second 'preprocessing' we need to do is to determine the window of analysis. Most often we already know the onset of the manipulation, and we know that we need at least a window before the onset point to provide the baseline data, and a window after the onset point to provide the treatment data. However, we need to know how long our expected effect is to capture it in an analysis window. If we select a too small window, the effect may peak after the window and we may miss the effect, resulting in a false negative. Contrarily, if we select too large a window, the effect will have dissipated before the window ends, and we include more noise than necessary, also risking a false negative as a result. The approach most commonly encountered involves two parts. The first part is selecting a very large baseline window and a very large treatment window. Then, the data from these curves are collapsed and a proportion over time curve for this grand average is plotted. As both baseline data and treatment data are included in this curve and the researcher does not know which hump in the line comes from what data, it is assumed to be safe to visually inspect the curve and determine window intervals from this. Additionally, it is common to divide up the treatment window into several bins, for example one bin covering the onset of the critical manipulation, a bin to cover the growth of the effect, and a bin to cover the peak of the effect. If the decline or dissipation of the effect is also of interest, then further bins can be used after the peak of the effect.

In the past, ANOVA has been used for the analysis of proportion over time curves. In short, this analysis consists of calculating for each bin whether there is a significant difference between the average proportions of participants who looked at, for instance, the target AOI, and the proportion of participants who looked elsewhere. However, there are several reasons why this analysis is not optimal for this design. The choice of bin size, for instance, is an arbitrary choice, but smaller bins imply more analyses, thereby affecting the experiment-wise error rate (p. 94). Furthermore, proportions are bound by the limits of 0 and 1, which may result in violation of the underlying assumptions of the ANOVA. By definition, proportion over time curves imply that the dependent variable is a dichotomous variable: the participant either looked at an AOI or not. Furthermore, the independent variable is time, which is a continuous predictor. This design makes an ANOVA not well suited for the analysis, since it is assumed for the ANOVA that the dependent variable is continuous, and the independent variables are nominal. Here we briefly describe an alternative method that can be used for the analysis of proportion over time curves: multilevel logistic regression.

The most promising analysis method today for analysing AOI proportions over time, is multilevel logistic regression. Logistic regression is well suited, because it is assumed that the dependent variable is a dichotomous variable, and because it allows predictors to be continuous as well as categorical. The multilevel analysis allows control of variation that is due to random factors: participant variation and item variation. Furthermore, the multilevel model allows the error to be auto-correlated (J. Singer & Willett, 2003), which eliminates the problem of dependent measurements. A final advantage of multilevel modelling is that the shape of the development over time may be included in the model by using time as a continuous predictor. In other words, it is possible to evaluate whether change over time is linear or curvilinear, avoiding the need divide up data into bins (except for problematic cases with much zero data). For illustrations of the use of multilevel modelling for the analysis of proportion over time curves, we refer to Barr (2008) and Mirman, Dixon, and Magnuson

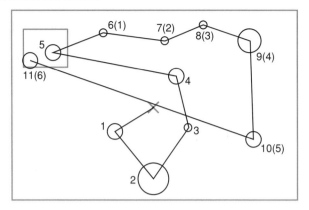

Fig. 13.7 Two operational definitions of return time using index number of fixations. The fixation sequence starts at the fixation cross in the middle. Fixations are numbered from the start of the trial, and in parentheses, from the end of the last dwell in the AOI. Return time could therefore be fixation 11 or 6 respectively, depending on the definition used. Larger circles signify longer fixation durations.

(2008).

13.1.9 Return time

Target question	How soon after onset, or after the previous dwell to an AOI does the eye return to it?
Input representation	Gaze samples or fixations, onset of change, and location of the AOI
Output	Return time (ms)

The *return time* is the time it takes until a participant returns to an AOI already looked at. J. D. Ryan and Cohen (2004) operationalize this duration as the index number of the first returning fixation to the AOI. Another possible, but apparently unused operational definition, is to count the number of fixations since the last dwell on an AOI until a return to the same AOI takes place. For both these operational definitions, time can be calculated as the number of fixations, or as real time, which would take into account the processing duration, and not only sequential order.

Independently of definition, this measure is particularly important when the AOI is manipulated or changed during a trial, but is also very revealing when returns to an AOI are a fundamental part of a diagnostic or problem solving task, where return time can serve as a measure of working memory.

13.1.10 Eye–voice latencies

Target question	How soon after the eye started looking at X does the participant verbalize X?
Input representation	Gaze samples or fixations, location of X, and onset time of verbalization
Output	Latency (ms), number of words, letters, or notes

Eye–voice latency is an umbrella term for a whole family of measures, which all measure the duration between onset of speech and entry into an AOI. Figure 13.8 (a) and (b) shows the

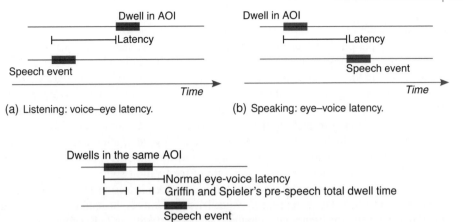

Fig. 13.8 In (a) and (b), the two basic eye–voice latencies. In both cases the speech event is semantically equivalent in meaning to the AOI in which the dwell is made. In (c), a variety of eye–voice latencies based on total dwell time.

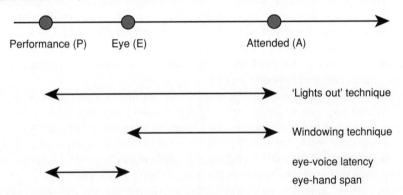

Fig. 13.9 Eye–voice latency is the time (or distance) from the eye (E) until the performance (P). The lights-out technique measures a much larger span, from performance at the time of lights-out, until the further end of what has been attended (A), or what is known as the perceptual span. For comparison, the moving window technique measures the size from the eye (E) until (A) (see page 50 for a full description of the moving window technique).

two basic measures, of which one is used to study listening to speech and the other to study verbalising pictorial material or written text, respectively. Other common terms for the same measure are 'eye–voice span' (A. S. Meyer & Lethaus, 2004) and 'first fixation time [relative to noun phrase onset]' (Brown-Schmidt & Tanenhaus, 2006).

In the majority of studies, latency is counted from onset to onset. Of course, latencies are positive when participants are speaking, and tend to be negative when they are listening to speech. There is one notable alternative operational definition, however: Griffin and Spieler (2006) only count the total dwell time on the AOI, not including the time looking at other objects. This 'pre-speech total dwell time' variety of eye–voice latency, exemplified in Figure 13.8(c), focuses on the *amount of processing* of the AOI before speech starts, while classical eye–voice latency measures *the overall time elapsed* until speech is produced.

Beware that some studies of eye–voice latencies (and eye–hand span, covered next) do not use eye-movement recordings at all, but rely on what is known as the 'lights-out' technique (Levin & Kaplan, 1970). Here, turning out the light unexpectedly while participants are reading, singing, or playing a musical instrument from sheet music, allows the researcher to gauge how far ahead they had read before the light was turned out. Participants are instructed to continue to speak, sing or play without light, for as long as they can, and without guessing. The lights-out method returns the duration from lights-out until the participant ceases to verbalize (or stops singing or playing if the study is concerned with music reading). Thus, this technique gives an indirect measure of the latency between reading and speaking. It is another type of eye–voice span, related to what is known as the perceptual span in reading research, which measures visual intake to the right of the fixation point (see Figure 13.9 for comparison). It should be noted that different techniques for measuring eye–voice latencies yield very different result. For instance, eye–voice latency during sight-reading is seven notes for skilled readers using the lights-out technique (Sloboda, 1985), while it is four notes when using eye tracking (Jacobsen, 1941; Goolsby, 1994).

The unit of the eye–voice latency measure varies between applications: latencies in milliseconds are the default unit with pictorial stimuli for eye–voice and voice–eye studies, while with text and music stimuli, latencies are also measured in number of words, letters or notes. In a few studies, latencies are reported in pixels within the stimulus.

When participants *read texts aloud*, the main finding is that eye–voice latencies hover around 800 ms. More experienced, better readers, have *larger spans* (Buswell, 1920). Buswell found that the eye–voice latency of high-school students is approximately 0.79 s, corresponding to an eye–voice distance of 13 letters, while 5th graders exhibited an eye–voice latency of 0.91 s and 11 letters. Correspondingly, good readers have an eye–voice latency of about 4–5 letters larger compared to poorer readers.

When studying *singing*, most of the studies have looked at either *skill* or *the musical structure*. Skilled singers have an eye–voice span of around four notes, while unskilled show a latency of on average two notes, when sight-singing to melodies (Jacobsen, 1941). Goolsby (1994) finds the same result, but adds the observation that "skilled music readers look farther ahead in the notation and then back to the point of performance" (p. 77), a strategy to refresh working memory that is also known from the picture viewing literature.

Sloboda (1985), using the 'lights-out' technique, found that the eye–voice latency coincides with *musical phrasing*. More precisely, "a boundary just beyond the average span 'stretches' the span, and a boundary just before the average 'contracts' it" (p. 72). Musical boundary is the point at which the melody changes. Experienced musicians can cope with larger boundaries, and as this boundary is extended so to is the perceptual span. Good readers, Sloboda found, maintain a larger span size (up to seven notes) than do poor readers (up to four notes).

When singing prima vista to notes only, the eye–voice latency is around 500 ms, but the latency increases significantly to 750 ms when text is added to the notes (Berséus, 2002). This difference may be a linguistic effect since we are more accustomed to text, and can therefore retain more in our visual buffer, but it is also likely that it reflects the greater importance of the vertical dimension in eye movements to notes only.

The largest variation in eye–voice latencies has been found in studies of *spoken descriptions of pictures*. Griffin and Bock (2000) conclude that eye–voice latency when describing pictures is around 800–900 ms, while Brown-Schmidt and Tanenhaus (2006) found latencies as low as 600 ms. Both these studies used fairly simple utterances and stimuli consisting of distinct, but visually sparse line-drawings. When using naturalistic stimuli and free discourse, Holsanova (2008) found latencies up to 2500 ms and frequent refixations to the point of performance (speech). In a series of studies of imagery, where participants are looking into empty space, latencies were up to 5 seconds (Johansson et al., 2006). This variation most likely reflects the complexity of the tasks.

A further complication with eye–voice latencies in naturalistic tasks, pointed out by Holsanova (2008), is that the eye–voice relationships are seldom as simplistic as the upper part of Figure 13.8 suggests. For instance, it often happens that a participant looks twice or more at an AOI before making an utterance referring to it (as exemplified on page 259). The uncertainty over which of the two fixations to select for the calculation points to the need for additional requirements and more refined operational definitions of the measure.

According to Chafe (1994), conscious ideas are constantly activated and deactivated during speech. If the eye is a bit ahead of speech, pushing to activate new conscious ideas from vision, it may happen that ideas that were about to be spoken have already been deactivated ("forgotten") before they have been spoken. This would appear in data as scanpath patterns where sudden regressions occurred back to the entity in the picture that was just about to be spoken. Such patterns were exactly what Holsanova (2008, 2001) and Goolsby (1994) found.

Bock, Irwin, Davidson, and Levelt (2003) showed analogue and digital clocks and asked participants to tell the time, finding longer latencies for analogue than for digital clocks, reflecting the difference in processing each of the two formats to language. More interestingly, they showed the clocks with two trial durations, 100 ms and 3000 ms, finding that the time and accuracy of the subsequent expression is not different between a 100 ms and a 3000 ms trial, which they argue have implications for models of language production.

13.1.11   Eye–hand span

Target question	How soon after the eye looked at X does the hand perform the corresponding action?
Input representation	Gaze samples or fixations, location of hand, and onset time of action
Output	Latency (ms) between look at X and action, distance (pixels), or number of beats

The eye–hand span is a relative of the eye–voice span. It has been frequently utilized in studies of piano players, but also in studying how participants look ahead when following a walkway. For studies of eye–hand coordination, the eye–hand span is a crucial measure.

Formally, the eye–hand span is defined as the duration from the start of a fixation on an item until the hand (or other effector) performs the action associated with the item; such as pressing the correct piano key. Other terms include 'eye–hand latency', 'eye–hand lead time' and 'latency of the hand movement relative to the eye'. The unit of the eye–hand span measures also varies. Although time in milliseconds is the most common, eye–hand span is often expressed in number of notes or other task-specific units.

Weaver (1943) found a considerable variation in eye–hand spans during piano playing; a variation of up to eight chords. Distributions from piano players (Truitt, Clifton, Pollatsek, & Rayner, 1997) and typists (Inhoff & Gordon, 1997) show small variation and appear statistically very well-behaved (see Figure 13.10).

Recorded eye–hand spans vary from about −3 to around 1.5 seconds, but the averages depend on a variety of factors:

Task requirements Wilmut et al. (2006) had participants point at one object after another, and they report eye–hand lead times of approximately 200 ms. With the task requirement to point at sudden onset LED lights, Binsted, Chua, Helsen, and Elliott (2001) report latencies of 300 ms. Patla and Vickers (2003) required their participants to step on a series of irregularly spaced 'footprints' over a 10 metre walkway. They found that

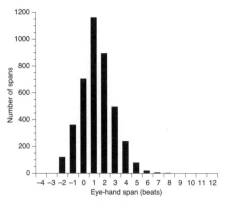

(a) A histogram of eye–hand latencies during piano playing. From Truitt et al. (1997), and reproduced with kind permission from Psychological Press.

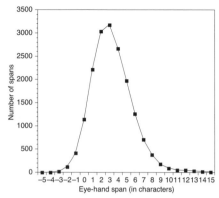

(b) A histogram of eye–hand latencies when copy typing. From Inhoff and Gordon (1997), and reproduced with kind permission from Blackwell Publishing.

Fig. 13.10 Distributions of eye–hand latencies (spans) in two different tasks.

participants fixated the footprints on average two steps ahead, or 0.8–1 s in time. When playing the piano, eye–hand spans of 3.1 notes (0.78 s) (Weaver, 1943), a single beat or 450 ms (Truitt et al., 1997), and up to 1.3 seconds (Furneaux & Land, 1999) have been reported in the literature. When playing the violin, the eye–hand span is around 1 second (3–6 notes), with a larger variance for a sonata by Telemann than a sonata by Correlli (Wurtz et al., 2009), again highlighing the influence of task *even within a task*. When typing, Butsch (1932) found that typists of all skill levels have an eye–hand span of about 1 second or around five characters.

Skill Already Jacobsen (1941) found a difference in skill, with eye–hand spans during piano playing ranging from zero up to four notes. Later studies have found that skill in piano playing increases eye–hand span when measured in number of notes, but not in terms of time (Furneaux & Land, 1999), which would mean that although processing time is the same, throughput rate differs. This means that more information is processed in a fixed time interval—the span is increased, but the time remains the same, therefore greater efficiency.

Repetition Epelboim et al. (1995) showed a substantial reduction in eye–hand spans when participants repeated the task of tapping a sequence of lights.

Non-repeated whole-body tasks Land et al. (1999) found eye–hand latencies of about 530 ms (ranging from 430 to 680 ms) when participants were engaged in the everyday task of making a pot of tea.

Musical tempo A slower tempo increases the eye–hand span in piano playing to 1.3 s, while fast tempos reduce it to 0.7 s (Furneaux & Land, 1999).

Target visibility When the target is continuously visible, eye–hand latencies are reduced (Abrams, Meyer, & Kornblum, 1990).

Allocation of attention Frens and Erkelens (1991) showed that eye–hand coordination is disrupted by auditory distractors presented at the initiation of the reaching movement. This result has been interpreted as evidence for a single central attentional control of both movements.

Look-ahead fixations Following a look-ahead fixation, the eye departs earlier relative to the hand, increasing the eye–hand latency from on average 2.7 to 3.1 seconds (Mennie et al., 2007).

A theoretical interpretation of the eye–hand span is that its size reflects a continuous 'push–pull' relationship between two forces: one, the need for material to be held in *working memory* long enough to be processed into musculoskeletal commands, and second, the need to limit the demand on span size and therefore the workload in the memory system. For most readers, the need to limit the workload of the memory system prevails, and this results in the very small spans that are mostly found in studies of eye movements in reading (Rayner & Pollatsek, 1997).

13.1.12 The eye–eye span (cross-recurrence analysis)

Target question	*How soon does a listener look where the speaker looks?*
Input representation	*Gaze samples or fixations from listener and speaker AOI*
Output	*Latency (ms) or distance (pixels)*

Only scattered studies have looked at collaborative tasks or face-to-face communication where both participants have been eye-tracked. In such studies, there is a need to measure the duration or distance between the two gaze points. Hadelich and Crocker (2006) suggest the term 'eye–eye span' for this latency, finding a span of 1400 ms during production of referring expressions. The Euclidean distance between two participants' gaze at a frame on a video stimulus is an alternative variety of eye–eye span (p. 370). Reported values in literature vary. In a collaborative building task, Velichkovsky et al. (1996) note a lag of only 500 ms. In a collaborative web-based task, Cherubini, Nüssli, and Dillenbourg (2008) find that utterances not followed by a repair act (such as "I did not understand that last thing you said") resulted in an average eye–eye distance of 85.65 pixels, while messages followed by a repair act with an average distance of 231.37 pixels.

Cross-recurrence analysis is a mathematical method to investigate the overall latency by visualising and quantifying recurrent patterns of states between two time series (essentially two eye movement data files). This type of analysis was introduced into eye-movement research by Richardson and Dale (2005), who found that a listener follows the gaze of a speaker with a latency (or lag) of around 2 seconds on average. Figure 13.11 shows the principle for calculating this latency. In short, the eye–eye latency calculated from a cross-recurrence analysis is the speaker's eye–voice latency plus the listener's voice–eye latency, of which there can indeed be several. The strength of this method is that it allows us to estimate the latency with the best overall fit.

Success in communication is reflected in the co-alignment of gaze between speaker and listener, Richardson and Dale argue, after showing that listener comprehension varies with the listeners ability to align with speaker gaze.

13.2 Distances

Distance measures compare the simultaneous spatial positions of two separate entities, for instance eye to stimulus point, left eye to right eye, or eye to mouse position. We have already seen how the same measure can have both time and space for units, for instance the eye–hand span. Under this heading, we present measures that are predominantly spatial.

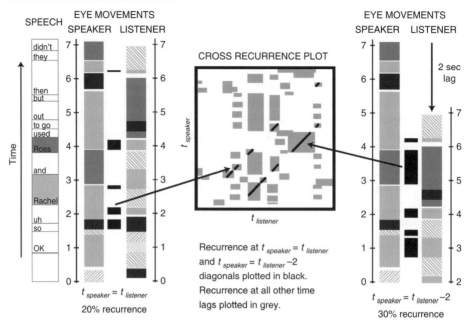

Fig. 13.11 Calculation of cross-recurrence plots and associated latencies may appear complex, but are actually fairly intuitive. To the left, speech and speaker and listener eye-movements as scarf plots in real time. We can recognize the eye–voice latencies in the speaker eye-movements and speech, for instance 'Rachel' is mentioned around 400 ms after the speaker looks at her. The listener in turn looks at the 'Rachel' AOI some 500 ms later. As the speaker dwells on the Rachel AOI for some time, it will overlap with listener dwell on the same AOI. Overlaps are marked as black in between the scarf plots. The cross-recurrence plot is produced by placing the scarf plots of speaker and listener on the x- and y-dimensions (called $t_{speaker}$ and $t_{listener}$), and each (x,y) on the surface is marked grey if both speaker and listener look at the same AOI. Now, diagonals in the plot correspond to alignment over time. One of the black-marked diagonals correspond to the overlaps between speaker and listener in real time. The other marked diagonal corresponds to a shift of the listener data in time by two seconds, corresponding to the scarf plots on the right side of the figure. The shift in time—the 'lag'—producing the longest diagonal is the eye–eye latency with the best overall fit. With kind permission from The Cognitive Science Society, John Wiley and Sons:*Cognitive Science*, Looking To Understand: The Coupling Between Speakers' and Listeners' Eye Movements and Its Relationship to Discourse Comprehension, *29*(6), 2005, Daniel C. Richardson and Rick Dale, pp. 1045-60.

13.2.1   Eye–mouse distance

Target question	What is the distance between the point of gaze and the mouse position?
Input representation	Gaze and mouse position
Output	Distance (pixels)

Eye–mouse distance measures Euclidean distance in number of pixels or visual degrees between the position of the mouse cursor (in a computer monitor) and the gaze position. Rodden and Fu (2007) present a histogram of eye–mouse latencies from a variety of Google search tasks (Figure 13.12). Some of the mouse–eye research has attempted to show that recording mouse movements provides comparable data to recording eye movements (e.g. Granka, Feusner, & Lorigo, 2008); however, these studies have varying results, finding only some coarse correlations.

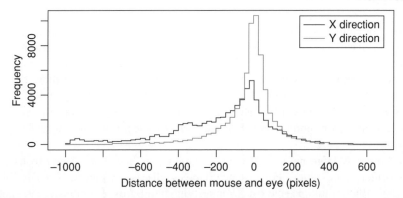

Fig. 13.12 Horizontal and vertical eye–mouse distances. Although both are centred around zero, there is a large spread, in particular in the horizontal direction. Reproduced from Rodden and Fu (2007).

Of the very few studies that report eye–mouse distance, many include alternative operational definitions. For instance, after finding that eye–mouse distance varies from 0.1 to over 1000 pixels (on average 290), M. C. Chen, Anderson, and Sohn (2001) decide to make an AOI-based analysis of dwell time for mouse and eye, and finding a fair correlation of 0.58 between the two.

Overall, it does not seem likely that recording of mouse movements can replace eye tracking. Rather, the potential with eye–mouse distance is to investigate the dynamics in the interplay between eye and mouse. Rodden and Fu (2007) argue to have found three strategies that influence the eye–mouse distance. One, keeping the mouse still while reading; two, using the mouse as a reading aid with the cursor to help guide the eye; and three, using the mouse to indicate interesting points to return to. Visually marking an area on a web page that might be interesting to return to, by placing the mouse cursor on it, is a strategy that has repeatedly been found (Ballard, Hayhoe, & Pelz, 1995; Cox & Silva, 2006), as this is the most cost-efficient use of working memory. B. A. Smith, Ho, Ark, and Zhai (2000) found three different eye–mouse behaviours when users select a target. One, eye gaze following the cursor to the target; two, eye gaze leading the cursor to the target; and three, eye gaze switching between the cursor and the target until the target is reached. Each of these give different eye–mouse distances over time.

13.2.2 Disparities

Target question	What is the distance between the points of gaze of left and right eye?
Input representation	Binocular gaze position
Output	Distance (pixels)

Binocular disparity is the distance between the gaze positions of the left and the right eye.

Note that the values calculated for this distance measure *may* be invalid if the participant's eyes are not calibrated separately (Liversedge, White, et al., 2006, but see Nuthmann & Kliegl, 2009 for counter arguments). Accuracy and precision of the equipment are also of extreme importance when measuring the small distances between the gaze points of the two eyes.

Another line of research investigates variability in disparities between different participant populations:

Children For children, the disparity between eyes is much higher than for adults, and this inverse linear relationship holds in early childhood, the youngest children presenting greater disparity. (Fioravanti, Inchingolo, Pensiero, & Spanio, 1995). This reflects the development of dual eye control, but it also tells us it may make more sense to use binocular eye tracking when studying children than when studying adults.

Dyslexia Bucci, Brémond-Gignac, and Kapoula (2008) found that dyslexic children have poorer binocular coordination (larger disparity values) following saccadic eye movements.

Clinical groups A large number of clinical populations have been found to have poorer binocular coordination. For instance, Graves' disease (Wouters, Van Den Bosch, & Lemij, 1998), multiple sclerosis (Ventre, Vighetto, Bailly, & Prablanc, 1991), cerebellar disease (Versino, Hurko, & Zee, 1996), and deep amblyopia (passive eye) (Maxwell, Lemij, & Collewijn, 1995) can all lead to an impaired ability to direct both eyes equivalently.

Reading research has recently focused on reliably measuring and quantifying disparity; whether the eyes show alignment, crossed or uncrossed disparity. The following factors have been investigated:

Linguistic and higher-level processing There is little evidence that binocular coordination can be modulated by higher-level cognitive processing (Kirkby, Blythe, Benson, & Liversedge, 2009; Juhasz, Liversedge, White, & Rayner, 2006; Bucci & Kapoula, 2006).

Gaze crossing Some studies have found crossed disparities to be prevalent (e.g. Kliegl et al., 2006 and Nuthmann & Kliegl, 2009), while others have obtained a majority of uncrossed disparities (e.g. Blythe et al., 2006; Juhasz et al., 2006; Liversedge, Rayner, White, Findlay, & McSorley, 2006; Liversedge, White, et al., 2006).

The distance between the two eyes when reading was reported by Heller and Radach (1999) to be 1–2 characters.

13.2.3 Smooth pursuit gain

Target question	*What is the velocity ratio between point of gaze and target?*
Input representation	*Gaze and target positions/velocity*
Output	*Gain*

In smooth pursuit research, closed-loop *smooth pursuit gain* is almost always defined as the ratio of eye velocity to target velocity. Thus, a 1.0 value indicates a perfect match, while lower values mean that the eye falls behind, and an increasing number of catch-up saccades are made to compensate for the slowness of the smooth pursuit system. Gain values are typically slightly below 1.0, and tend to fall off at higher target velocities.

However, when using sine wave stimuli, smooth pursuit gain is often measured only at the peak of eye velocity: *Peak gain* is then defined as the ratio of peak eye velocity to target velocity. A third operational definition of smooth pursuit gain is to count the rate of catch-up saccades.

Furthermore, the root mean square (RMS) error quantifies gain as the cumulative distance between the eye and the target during smooth pursuit. Assume that at each recorded data sample n, θ_n is a measure of the distance between the position of gaze and the position of the target. Then RMS error is defined as:

$$\theta_{RMSE} = \sqrt{\frac{1}{n}\sum_{i=1}^{n}\theta_i^2} = \sqrt{\frac{\theta_1^2 + \theta_2^2 + \cdots + \theta_n^2}{n}}. \tag{13.1}$$

In a meta-analysis of schizophrenia research, O'Driscoll and Callahan (2008) find RMS values to be atypical in schizophrenic patients. RMS values also correlate strongly with both previous subjective quality ratings of pursuit, and with smooth pursuit gain (Gooding, Iacono, & Beiser, 1994).

The following influences on smooth pursuit gain have been investigated:

Inattention and distraction Conditions designed to distract attention, or to produce declining arousal and attention, produced reduced smooth pursuit gain (Brezinova & Kendell, 1977).

Motion direction For predictable target motions, most participants exhibit higher gain values during horizontal than during vertical smooth pursuit movements (Rottach et al., 1996).

Age Smooth pursuit gain is on average 0.7–0.8 for 8–19 year olds and increases significantly with age (Salman, Sharpe, Lillakas, Dennis, & Steinbach, 2006).

Schizophrenia A large number of studies have found that participants with schizophrenia have a poorer than normal smooth pursuit gain (O'Driscoll & Callahan, 2008).

Nicotine Nicotine intake appears to help the smooth pursuit system of schizophrenic patients: directly after smoking, smooth pursuit gain increases and the number of catch-up saccades decreases significantly (Olincy, Ross, Young, Roath, & Freedman, 1998).

Alcohol Smooth-pursuit eye-movements are significantly disturbed by increasing blood alcohol levels, as measured by smooth pursuit gain (Wilkinson, Kime, & Purnell, 1974), even if the participant reports not feeling sedated (Holdstock & De Wit, 2006).

Barbiturates and benzodiazepines Smooth pursuit gain decreases and the number of catch-up saccades increase with increasing doses of the drug (Bittencourt, Wade, Smith, & Richens, 1983).

13.2.4 Smooth pursuit phase

Target question	*How far behind or ahead is the eye?*
Input representation	*Raw data samples and synchronized movement data for the stimulus.*
Output	*Phase (ms or degrees).*

When presenting participants with sinusoidal stimulus points (such as when tracking the motion of a pendulum), smooth pursuit performance is in addition to gain often evaluated with *phase*. Phase is a "measure of the temporal synchrony between the target and the eye" (Leigh & Zee, 2006). It can be defined either in terms of a spatial (angular) *shift* which measures the difference in phase between the target and eye traces, or in terms of a temporal *lag* which reflects the amount of time the eye is lagging behind the target. Figure 13.13 illustrates these two varieties of phase.

Phase shift and lag are often used interchangeably, and terminology and operational definitions vary across publications. The meta-analytic overview by O'Driscoll and Callahan (2008, p. 361) uses an overarching term lag, which has one spatial variety "phase lag, which quantifies the difference in phase between the eye trace and the target trace" and one temporal variety "temporal lag, which can be quantified as the interval between the moment the target reverses direction and the moment the eye reverses direction".

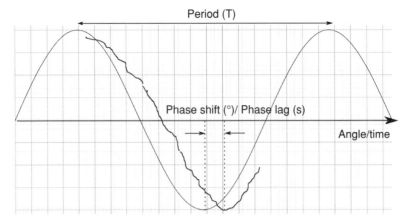

Fig. 13.13 The thin sinusoidal curve indicates the motion of a stimulus point, while the thick line superimposed represents fictitious data of a participant following this point. Phase *shift* and *lag* represent respectively the spatial (angular) and temporal difference between the position of the eye and the position of the target.

Phase has been an important measure of tracking accuracy when studying the visual processes involved in smooth pursuit. In short, phase shift has been reported to stay below 5° but to increase with increasing frequencies (Collewijn & Tamminga, 1984, p. 223). With predictable stimuli, phase shift may disappear although gain remains smaller than one (accounted for due to the presence of catch-up saccades). With unpredictable stimuli, phase lag can increase further (Collewijn & Tamminga, 1984; Goldreich, Krauzlis, & Lisberger, 1992).

Phase measures are also employed in clinical and neurophysiological research. For instance, a significantly larger phase lag compared to controls has been observed in patients with Parkinson's disease (Bronstein & Kennard, 1985) and unilateral frontal lobe lesions (Morrow & Sharpe, 1995), which could tell us about the role of these brain areas to the predictive component in smooth pursuit.

13.2.5 Saccadic gain

Target question	*What is the distance between saccadic ending point and target?*
Input representation	*Saccadic landing position and target position*
Output	*Gain*

Saccadic gain, which is also called 'saccadic accuracy', is mostly defined as the initial saccadic amplitude divided by the target amplitude, as exemplified by Figure 13.14. Initial means that we measure only the first saccade to the target, not additional corrections, to which correction saccades count but rarely glissades. Target amplitude is the distance from the saccade starting point to the intended saccadic goal. The saccadic gain unit is %, so less than 100% is sometimes called undershoot (or hypometric), while more than 100% is overshoot (or hypermetric). In an alternative operational definition, saccadic accuracy is instead measured as the Euclidean distance between saccadic endpoint and target.

Note that if the saccade is curved, and saccadic amplitude is calculated as the length along the curve (p. 311), but the distance from origin to target as the straight Euclidean distance, then saccadic gain values will be miscalculated. A perfect hit would be counted as an overshoot, for instance.

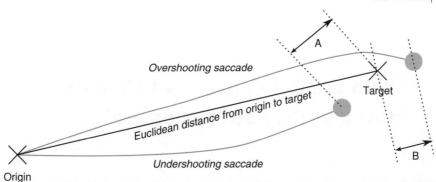

Origin

Fig. 13.14 The principle for saccadic gain/accuracy. An overshoot (top saccade) and an undershoot (bottom saccade). Gain is calculated as the amplitude of the saccade divided by the Euclidean distance from origin to target. A and B are the differences in landing point with respect to the target, so-called endpoint deviations.

Nummenmaa et al. (2008) define the very related 'endpoint deviation' as the size of the saccadic error: the Euclidean distance from the observed landing position to the intended location, A in Figure 13.14.

Saccadic gain is a measure frequently used in neurological studies of saccadic and movement control. The number of papers using the saccadic gain measure in neurology is very large, and the measure seems to be virtually unknown outside of that field. Ettinger et al. (2002) show that the volume of the cerebellar vermis (a brain area thought important in directing saccades) predicts saccadic gain. Saccadic accuracy appears to be unaffected by age (Q. Yang & Kapoula, 2008). Both eye and hand movements typically undershoot the target position, requiring a second corrective movement, or in the case of the eyes, a saccade, bringing the effector to rest on the target (Binsted et al., 2001). In a human factors study, S. Green and Farnborough (1986) found that severe sleep deprivation reduces saccadic accuracy.

14 What are Eye-Movement Measures and How can they be Harnessed?

Previous chapters have described four large groups of measures which can be derived from the data produced by eye-trackers. We have also covered in detail the many ways these measures can be operationalized. Eye tracking as a research tool is particular in providing its users with well over a hundred different measures. Manual reaction time, EEG and fMRI measures come only in a handful. Why is eye tracking so different? Does this abundance of possibilities make eye-trackers particularly versatile and useful, or does it reflect some deep internal difficulty in working with eye-movement data that other biometric measurement instruments are not hampered by?

In this chapter, we investigate the concept of measures, and relate this to the methods for calculating events and representations. This allows us to propose a general model for existing measures, as well as a schema for building new ones. The chapter is divided into five short sections.

- Section 14.1 (p. 454) attempts an explanation to why there are so many measures, and why it is that researchers so often have trouble finding appropriate measures for their studies.
- The important difference between a measure concept and how it is operationalized is scrutinized in Section 14.2 (p. 456). We question the ambiguity surrounding whether the concept is referred to as a measure, or whether the operational definition itself is referred to as a measure.
- In Section 14.3 (p. 458), we more precisely relate measures to the preceding calculation of events and representations, and propose a general model for measures, based on data transformation, events, representations, and operational definitions.
- In Section 14.4 (p. 463), we argue for the division of measures into categories as outlined in the measure chapters in Part III of this book. We compare this taxonomy to other alternatives that we dismissed.
- In Section 14.5 (p. 465), we discuss different ways of enriching research with new eye-movement measures, but draw caution to the fact that developing new measures without considering those that are available already may not be a useful exercise.

14.1 Eye-movement measures: plentiful but poorly accessible

In this book, we list around 120 measures for eye-movement data. Why are there so many, and do they have to be that many? The first answer can be found in the data themselves: eye-tracking data are very versatile; rich in information in both the spatial and the temporal domains. They can be recorded in a large variety of application fields, with many types of stimuli and in combination with many other technical systems. The methods in Part II that form events and representations allow complex layers of analysis to be built.

The second reason that there are so many measures is that it is relatively easy to build new ones. Eye-movement data are very tangible, computationally easy to work with, and rich enough to generate new ideas. If a researcher is trained in mathematics or computer science, measure development and implementation is not too difficult, and may appear an intellectual challenge of the right magnitude.

While some subject areas are prone to experimentation with new measures, others can be fairly rigid. These people rely on the measures that others in their field have always used, without considering the vast range of options available to them. This may be because of lack of interdisciplinary collaboration, or a lack of proficiency in calculating new measures themselves, or simply because they work inside a paradigm or line of research where a few measures are well-examined and their effects known and trusted.

Nevertheless, current research practices allow any author of a journal paper or book chapter to define her own measure by simply writing, for instance, "In this paper, we define fixation depth to mean...". As it is much easier to define a new measure than it is to evaluate it, and because most scholarly journals put much more emphasis on the theoretical question being addressed than the measure being used to address it, journal editors and reviewers are not always expected to delve too deep into the properties of measures developed by authors. In particular, if the new measure uses mathematics that the reviewer is not acquainted with, errors in calculation and interpretation can slip under the radar. One may suspect that this is true of many new measures and the conclusions that have been drawn from their use.

Many many eye-tracking measures exist, more than we have listed in this book. Omissions are owing to two main reasons: we considered some measures not sufficiently developed to be included, and also because, despite our best efforts, it is quite likely that we have not found all of the measures that have been used.

In fact, many measures are specific to certain application fields, and only appear in their journals. Sometimes a measure is limited to a single PhD thesis, with little availability to the entire community of eye-tracking users. The fact that eye-tracking publications are so fragmented make it very difficult to find the best methods and measures. Say that you are an educational psychologist or a marketing researcher. Would you ever come across a publication in a medical imaging journal that just happens to have the measure that you need for the experiment you are in the midst of planning? You probably would not browse through all the journals where eye-tracking studies are published, because there are hundreds of them, and most are way outside your scope of theoretical interest. Search engines could do the job for you, were it not for the highly divergent terminology between the different fields of research.

Thus, somewhat paradoxically, despite there being a multitude of measures, many researchers do not find the ones that are relevant to them—sometimes it is not even apparent that a measure is relevant even when it is found. The authors of this book have many times witnessed how a researcher is unhappy with not finding the right measures for her eye-tracking experiment, and very exited when she has found a candidate. Finding the right measure is often the most difficult thing when designing an experiment, particularly for someone who is not trained in mathematics, computer science, or experimental psychology, or who is working outside established eye-tracking paradigms.

Part of the problem is that no dedicated and widely known journals exist for eye-movement methodology (as opposed to theoretical journals). No one performs benchmarking tests of eye-tracker hard- and software systems, and no standardization committees exist for hardware and data quality measurements. There is a need for systematic evaluation of the programming routines developed by the providers of eye-tracking systems: methods for filtering, detecting, and calculating fixations, saccades, and other events should be agreed upon in the industry, in collaboration with researchers. Precise operational definitions for each measure should be standardized and stated in software manuals and help functions.

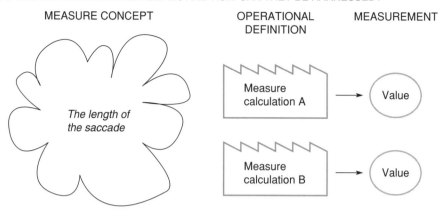

Fig. 14.1 A less precise or ambiguous measure concept, *The length of the saccade*, has two precise operational definitions that calculate the actual measure values. eye-tracking measures at their core consist of one concept and one or many operational definitions, which can produce measurement values when fed with data.

For a beginning researcher using eye tracking, the de facto authority when it comes to methods and measures has lately been the manufacturers of eye-trackers. Manufacturer terminology and the operationalizations built into their software end up in journal papers, and are often accepted without question although they should be scrutinized more.

14.2   Measure concepts and operationalizing them

Differentiating between *the measure concept, the way the concept is operationalized,* and the resulting *measurement values* is of great importance to understanding why we have the measures we have. A measure concept consists of the idea and name which are known in the literature and theories. Take saccadic amplitude as an example. Loosely speaking, it is the length of the saccade, which equals the distance between fixations. That is the measure concept, which is illustrated as a disconnected bubble in Figure 14.1, to highlight that the concept is mostly vague in literature as well as throughout the design of the experiment. Saccades were called "movements", and saccadic amplitude "arc of the movement" by Dodge and Cline (1901, p. 154), and it was implicitly assumed that it moved along a straight line. This implicit 'straight line' assumption about saccadic amplitudes grew into literature for many decades, and was later implemented as a calculation along the Euclidean distance between the start and end point of the saccade. Only much later were curved saccades focused upon in research, and slowly the saccadic amplitude measure became less vague but instead ambiguous. Now, in addition to the Euclidean calculation, there was an amplitude calculation given as saccade duration multiplied by average velocity (p. 311). These two methods to calculate saccadic amplitude values are the two operational definitions, and each results in its own value, which we may call the measurement. In practice, a researcher may calculate saccadic amplitude values using the operational definition implemented in her software without even reflecting that there is another one.

Even when a measure appears conceptually and operationally clear-cut, like the well-known fixation duration (p. 377) and its counterpart saccadic amplitude (p. 312), the many little known event calculation algorithms of Chapter 5 nevertheless produce fixations and saccades according to very different methods, and often this can result in differing measurement values.

A strong measure concept tends to hide variation in the way the measure is operationalized, and hence journal papers do not use labels for event detection algorithms such as 'I-DT fixation durations' or 'Eyelink fixation durations' (the operational definitions) for calculated values, but just call them 'fixation durations' (the measure concept)—although if one pays careful attention to the method section of journal papers the information about the precise calculation is sometimes provided. Few if any studies make multiple calculations of fixation durations with different event detection algorithms to validate the results they present.

When the measure concept is more vague, such as 'position similarity' (p. 359), researchers tend to produce a range of ways to operationalize it. It is not uncommon for these operational definitions to be labelled with a name and given measure status, such as the 'Mannan similarity index' or 'the Kullback-Leibler distance measure', in papers which often do not quote other operational definitions of the same measure concept. With a measure concept as weak as position similarity, we forget the overarching measure concept and are confused into believing that Kullback-Leibler distance is on par with fixation duration. In reality, the Mannan similarity index and the Kullback-Leibler distance are both operational definitions of position similarity. Just like we compare different calculations of fixation duration to one another, we should remember to compare the different calculations of position dispersion, and not let ourselves think that they are measure concepts whose importance in theory relieves us of the need to evaluate them.

The misalignment between measure concepts and their operational definitions that characterizes parts of eye-tracker-based research is a consequence of how the different measures were developed, and where they originate from. When the measure is a concept with many synonymous operationalizations (like fixation duration), it typically originates from theory in a broad sense. When precise operational definitions are marketed as measures, they are often mathematically exact solutions to specific problems in a particular line of research, and the overarching measure concept is largely anonymous. The Mannan similarity index and Kullback-Leibler distance are both examples of this.

The distinction between the theoretical measure *concept*, the *process* of performing a calculation (i.e. the operational definition) and the *value this process results in* (i.e. the measurement) is an important one because some operationalizations have been used for multiple purposes. This is true of the Mannan similarity index, a measure of position similarity which has been used to compare scanpaths, but which will tell you nothing about the temporal order of fixations, a fundamental property of a scanpath. If one is not clear on what the operational definition actually measures, i.e. what the measure concept is, much confusion can ensue and more appropriate alternatives can be overlooked.

In the choice between presenting concepts as measures or rather their precise operational definitions as measures, the authors of this book have decided to choose that which is more established. The sections of this book therefore reflect the fact that fixation duration is an established concept with several different operational definitions, while scanpath similarity, position dispersion, and position similarity are little known, and not well-established concepts in their own right. Therefore, these over-arching concepts have a set of very precisely defined 'measures' which each operationalize the concept in its own way, and which should be regarded as operational definitions.

Note that our term 'measurement' differs from 'measurement' in the sense of the totality of operations needed to establish a value, according to psychometrics and measurement theory. An eye-tracking measure has come to mean only the final calculation of, for instance saccadic amplitude, not the entire measurement completed by an eye-tracker of a specific technical build, and inclusive of all data filtering and the detection of saccades using a specific algorithm and its corresponding settings. In research with eye-tracking data, the measurement and computational history of a measure are typically forgotten, possibly because the measure

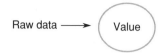

Raw data ⟶ (Value)

Fig. 14.2 A few measures equal a value in the raw data samples. Pupil diameter, for instance, just reads the values from the samples.

description would otherwise be too complex.

Also, the term 'operational definitions' used here differs somewhat from psychometrics and other branches of psychology. In this book operational definition is used to refer to the precise, unambiguous calculation of a value for a given measure. It thus differs from operationalization in the sense of an experimental design which utilizes an eye-tracking measure to quantify some other concept, be it fatigue, mental workload, or something else we wish to use eye tracking to investigate. For example, we could 'operationalize' fixation durations over 300 ms to indicate general interest; this is not however how the term is used to refer to eye-tracking measures in this book. 'Interest' is a possible interpretation of high fixation durations amongst others, but the operational definitions—the very calculations—of fixation duration themselves are independent of any such interpretation.

14.3   Proposed model of eye-tracking measures

By definition, every eye-tracking measure presumes a recording that produces raw data samples. Only a few measures have values that equal a value in the raw data stream, for instance the x coordinate or pupil diameter. Figure 14.2 illustrates the very simple copying of values that make up the pupil diameter measure.

Part II of this book describes methods to build events and representations by transforming the data. In Figure 14.3, we have made the method of oculomotor event detection (Chapter 5) look like a little factory to signify that it is a complex process, not unlike an industry, to take raw data of varying quality and make a refined product such as lists of fixations, saccades, and the other events. The product are events and representations, filled with more or less correct values, depending on the proficiency of the algorithms in the transformation factory.

A measure such as saccadic amplitude uses values in the events and representations, not in the raw data. Quantification of this measure requires small calculations, which we call the operational definitions of the measure. If you work with a particular operational definition you should report your measurement values according to that operational definition. There are two of them for saccadic amplitude, because this measure can and has been calculated in two different ways. These measure calculations are generally much smaller than the algorithms that transform data into events and representations. For saccadic amplitude, for instance, one operational definition consist of a multiplication of duration by average velocity, and the other of a Euclidean distance calculation between the endpoints of the saccade.

In the scanpath comparison measures, there are three levels of transformations before the measure calculation can be done. As Figure 14.4 shows, we first have oculomotor event detection, then dwell and transition detection, followed by scanpath simplification. Only after all this is done can the actual measure calculation takes place.

Based on the previous section and Figures 14.2–14.4, we can define the following:

1. An eye-tracking measure consist of a concept and one or many operational definitions. Both exist without data, like a business concept and the associated production site exist without raw material. Like any other factories, the operational definitions—implemented with algorithms—take data and refine them according to their criteria.

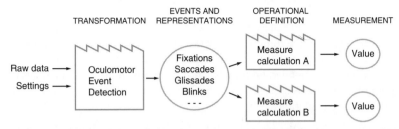

Fig. 14.3 How a measurement value for saccadic amplitude is produced from raw data and settings. The operational definition presumes a transformation of data that we know as oculomotor event detection, and which is performed using one from a variety of algorithms, using appropriate settings as secondary input (not shown). The transformation produces events and representations. The second set of algorithms (factories) are the operational definitions belonging to the measure itself, in our case the two ways of calculating saccadic amplitude, each producing its own measurement value.

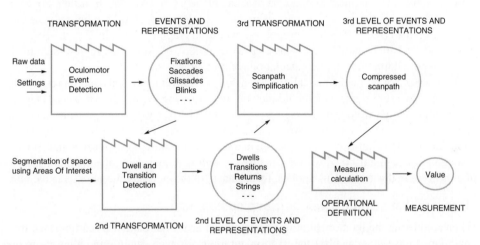

Fig. 14.4 Several of the scanpath comparison measures use repeated transformations of data before reaching the level of actual measure calculation.

2. The measure concept is expressed in words such as 'saccadic amplitude' or 'scanpath similarity' during the development of the experimental design for a study, and may have many conceptual ties to theories and previous studies. But like a business concept, the measure concept is often vague or ambiguous.

3. The value produced is called the 'measurement', and it is a product of operational definitions of the measure.

4. There are many competing algorithms (factories) on each level. In fact, choosing the right event detection algorithm for a scanpath comparison task is much like being a purchasing manager in a production site for scanpath similarity values and choosing among competing subcontractors. If you want to produce a good measurement value scanpath similarity, chose a proficient subcontractor for fixations and another for AOI strings.

5. The long calculation path shown in Figures 14.3 and 14.4 up until before the operational definition is not part of the measure. These subcontractors have to do a good job calculating fixations, saccades, and strings of AOIs, because otherwise the calculation of the value will suffer and the measurement quality will be low.

6. In general, eye-tracking measures are not taken to operationalize interest, fatigue, degree of dyslexia, or anything else. Operationalizations in this psychometric sense are taken care of by the experimental design, and are therefore specific to each experiment and must be founded on previous results in which the same interpretation of the measure was used. In contrast, eye-tracking measures are operationalized by precise mathematical calculations.

From the perspective of the researcher developing a measure, all transformation methods (subcontractors) are available simultaneously. All their products form more than 20 events and a handful of representations which can be manipulated at the operationalization stage to form a new measure. In principle therefore, any measure can be formed by combining the output from any method or combination of methods. In particular, the calculation of fixations, saccades, and other oculomotor events is *not* a prerequisite to producing other measures, which is sometimes claimed; raw sample data can in theory be taken much further. For example, you do not have to parse raw data using an event detection algorithm before generating an attention map (see p. 233) or a proportion over time graph (p. 197). In fact, the collection of methods in Part II should be seen as a growing toolbox of events and representations that can be imported into the simpler calculations of measures.

Of course, not all mathematical operations on eye-movement events and representations are granted measure status, nor should they be. Just counting the number of saccades is only a way of counting. Moreover, averaging is also so trivial that we do not consider this alone sufficient to form a new measure: average fixation duration is not a different measure than fixation duration, but simply puts the measure in a statistical context. Only when a mathematical operation has been attributed with *a measure concept* is it considered the operationalization of a measure in this book. This applies, for instance, to the counting measure saccadic rate.

Measures that include a pair or group comparison

When comparing the fixation durations between two groups of data files (participants, trials, conditions...), we first calculate the fixation durations for each data file in either group (e.g. Figure 3.2). These fixation duration data are then imported into a statistics software, still in two groups of lists of fixation duration values. We tell the statistics software to make the relevant statistical comparison, which it can do, because data include all fixation duration values needed for variance calculations. Figure 14.5(a) illustrates this standard method for statistical comparisons. It gives the researcher a p-value and a df-value that can be reported in papers, and which is necessary to compute in order to estimate the likelihood that between-group effects differ from chance.

However, suppose that instead you were to compare the distribution of position values in the two data files. Here you may take the two fundamental position coordinates, (x, y), from all fixations in each group, and generate two attention maps. When comparing the two attention maps you calculate a single value which reflects the difference between them (p. 372). Neither p-value, nor df-value applies in this case. All variance information is lost. Figure 14.5(b) illustrates this.

Measures that make pair-wise comparisons are a particular case where group comparisons can be made with variance estimations. The Levenshtein string-edit measure, for instance, returns a single value representing the similarity between two AOI strings (p. 348). Again, no p-value is reported. However, when comparing AOI strings for two groups of participants using systematic multiple pair-wise comparisons between these scanpath representations, this gives a set of values that can be used to calculate significance levels (i.e. including variance information) (Feusner & Lukoff, 2008).

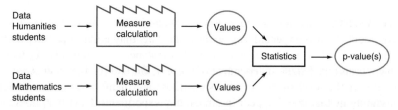

(a) Most measures calculate a large set of values for each condition in the experiment. These values are imported into a statistics calculation to give one or more p-values, representing the probability that we are wrong when we claim the conditions to be different.

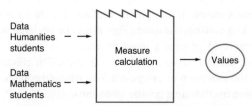

(b) The comparison is inherent in position and scan-path similarity measures. A single value is output, reflecting the similarity between two representations.

Fig. 14.5 When two groups of data files are input to a measure, some measures both calculate and compare (b). Most measures do not include a comparison (a), which allows for a comparison in a statistics package, with p-values as output.

Validity, reliability, and other requirements of measures

Building eye-tracking methods and measures is not only a matter of computation. Measures that aspire to generality must be more than just specific methods for how to calculate some values. A number of requirements can be identified for new measures:

Usefulness First and foremost, a measure must be useful. This includes generating data which can help answer the researcher's particular question. This criterion is given. Usefulness is best proven by at least one, but preferably more experiments in a series (compare to *replication* in research methodology texts). Employing a variety of newly developed eye-tracking measures, Goldberg and Kotval (1999) highlighted which ones are appropriate for identifying differences between poor and good computer interface design. Further comparisons of measures between conditions should be encouraged. Meta-analyses, moreover, provide insights into the usefulness of measures. Meta-analyses often focus on the validity and reliability of specific interpretations of measures. For example, O'Driscoll and Callahan (2008) in schizophrenia research, Clifton et al. (2007) in reading research and Jacob and Karn (2003) in usability research.

Uniqueness A new measure should differentiate from earlier ones in a relevant way, in the way it deals with the data, reduces the information, and summarizes it. There is little point in having yet another measure which provides values for something we can already measure perfectly well given already existing measures. Uniqueness has been difficult to demonstrate due to the fragmentation of eye-tracker-based research. For instance, the many position dispersion measures were often proposed without any demonstration of uniqueness. As alluded to before, this fragmentation stems from a lack of clarity in what is actually being measured.

Reliability A reliable measure is one that is consistent in its measurement of the same effect in contexts it is expected to generalize to. This may entail reliability across time, participants, and/or experimental designs. For instance, saccadic velocity may be a reliable measure of fatigue independent of context, but fixation duration is *not* a reliable measure of the level of processing, since there are many other causes of long fixation durations that could appear in almost any experiment. Note that an eye-tracking measure can be reliable within only *one specific paradigm or type of experiment*. In standard reading research, for example, first fixation duration appears to be a reliable measure of lexical processing because this has been established over many experiments. By contrast, if we go to a completely different branch of research in reading with much different material, e.g. poetry reading, it is not obvious that first fixation duration would be a reliable measure. This could be so because poetry reading does not necessarily strive to process a word as quickly as possible and then proceed, as there is an added value in lingering on the text units. The reliability of a measure can be thought of as the precision of an eye-tracker, where the same measurement value is produced over time for the same position/conditions.

Validity A valid measure is one that measures what it is intended to measure. What we intend to measure, however, usually boils down to two things. First, a measure can be valid with regard to the oculomotor event it measures. For example, the fact that a fixation duration actually measures the durations of an objectively determined event known as a fixation. Secondly, a measure can be valid with regard to the cognitive process we believe is involved in generating this eye-movement. For example, that the duration of a fixation on a text unit actually reflects the processing difficulty for the reader. Eye-tracking measures may or may not be open to interpretation within specific paradigms and experiments, and the interpretation may or may not be valid. The validity of implementing a measure for a specific purpose can be assessed in a number of ways. Concurrent and predictive validity can be established by correlating the proposed measure with a criterion measure which is known to be valid. For instance, one could correlate a psychiatric diagnosis of schizophrenia with various smooth pursuit measures. Content validity refers to the degree to which a measure covers all variation of the effect (i.e. is the number of catch-up saccades in smooth pursuit higher for all varieties of schizophrenia?). We can think of validity as the accuracy of the eye-tracker: we may still have reliable measurements over time (precision), but indicating the wrong position (invalid). Getting the correct position corresponds to us having a valid measure to answer our research questions.

When referring to validity and reliability in the last two points, we do so in the sense of what the measure can be used for, irrespective of eye-tracking terminology. Of course, there is also the question of whether the measure encapsulates the concept properly, the *concept validity*. The *internal validity* of an eye-tracking measure could be taken as an index of, for example, how well operational definitions of saccadic rate or scanpath similarity actually quantify the frequency of saccades, or the degree of resemblance between eye-movement sequences, respectively. Other types of validity also exist that do not exclusively relate to measures themselves. For instance *ecological validity*, which refers to the ability to generalize the result; that is, how similar the whole experimental situation and procedure is to all other situations that the study purports to shed light upon. What do results from a car simulator study tell us about real car driving, for instance. Figure 14.6 illustrates the different types of validity against a dimmed background of Figure 14.1.

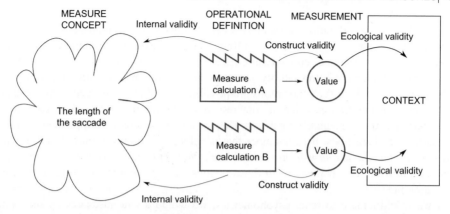

Fig. 14.6 *Internal* validity refers to whether the operational definition actually measures the concept, for instance does your measure of saccadic amplitude actually measure saccadic amplitude? Internal validity is more important for more complex measures. *Construct* validity concerns whether the operational definition actually measures the intended behaviour, such as, does your measure of saccadic rate actually measure tiredness? *Ecological* validity is whether the operational definition and measurement value obtained in the recording scenario generalizes to the real world. Is it a valid measure in other contexts outside the Lab or wherever else the test was carried out?

14.4   Classification of eye-movement measures

In journal papers and book chapters, on the internet, and in some dissertations, it is possible to find lists of eye-movement measures and accompanying interpretations. There have been very few attempts however to classify measures of eye-movements across research fields according to a broad taxonomy. The nature of measures becomes even clearer when we compare different classification systems.

In this book, we have used a principle of categorization built upon *operational definitions*. Take the measures of latency in Chapter 13 as an example: any measure that is defined as a duration between two separate events will be found in the latency chapter, whether the two events are the stimulus onset and the start of the saccade, the time it takes the eye to reach an area referred to in speech, after speech has commenced, or the duration between a puff of air on the eyeball and a resulting blink. We considered that using operational definitions from published research as a guiding principle to build measures into a classification system was the optimal approach. We hope that readers in that stage of an eye-tracking study where operational definitions are key, and measure selection is crucial, will see the benefit of structuring measures in this way. The semi-encyclopedic nature of Part III means that we assume that anyone reading about a particular measure is interested in using it. We do not explain *when* or *why* it is important to consider latency measures; we assume that the reader can decide that for themselves, comparing the information provided along with each measure to the needs of their own experimental design.

One tempting and common suggestion is to divide measures by *application field*. Comprehensive lists and meta-studies have been made of 'human factors measures' (Rötting, 2001), 'car driving measures' (ISO/TS 15007-1, 2002; ISO/TS 15007-2, 2001), 'usability measures' (Jacob & Karn, 2003), 'reading measures' (Clifton et al., 2007), and 'schizophrenia research measures' (O'Driscoll & Callahan, 2008) etc. Some measures have indeed been tightly associated with a particular paradigm in a particular field of research. Proportion over time graphs are mostly found in psycholinguistic research, anti-saccade measures in neuropsychological studies, and first pass regression scanpaths are mainly limited to papers on reading. However, measures are more closely related and relevant *between* fields than researchers think. Whilst it is clear that fixation duration is ubiquitous between disciplines, other measures are being adopted more and more by people with different areas of expertise, for example, the Levenstein string-edit technique. This measure has its roots in mental imagery research, but has subsequently appeared in both usability and scene perception investigations. There are many more examples of where such transitions are possible: do not feel restricted to use measures just because it is common practice in your research field, but use this book to shop around for alternative and more suitable measures. There is a lot of potential in implementing different measures and methods, but remember that novelty alone does not make good research; *your choice of methods and measures should be tailored to your research question and experimental design* (see Chapter 3). For these reasons we chose not to categorize methods by application field.

If we would adhere to strict psychometrics, we would divide measures by their *interpretation*. A psychometric division would give categories of 'early processing measures', 'prefrontal control measures', 'emotional reaction measures', 'interest measures', 'workload measures' etc. However desirable such a division might seem, there are serious problems with it. As interpretations of measures vary between paradigms, measures would appear in more than one category, and have no single natural place in the system. Moreover, eye-tracking data do not have straightforward interpretations outside of the context of the experiment where they were recorded. Thus we could not say conclusively for instance, that longer fixation durations *always* mean that the fixated region has been processed to a greater extent. Furthermore, interpretations of lesser known measures are far from validated; some have appeared in only one journal paper and never been used again. The recent commercialization of eye-tracker-based studies has led to dubious interpretations of eye-tracking measures to say the least. Meaning is attributed to some measures in a manner which appears purely subjective—heat maps (p. 239) and pupil diameter (p. 391) in particular, are often taken to indicate constructs such as 'informativeness' and 'mental work load' respectively, where more likely causes of the effect have not been accounted for. Categorizing measures by their interpretation may thus inadvertently support an overly simplistic view of eye-movements and what they actually reveal insights into. Also, new research revises and finds additional interpretations all the time, so such a division would soon be outdated.

The precise calculation of measures depends on the computation of events and representations in Part II of this book. One alternative means of measure classification would be to create a taxonomy based on this, i.e. *the preceding calculations of events and representations*. This would give us categories such as 'fixation measures', 'AOI-measures', and 'scanpath measures'. However, although many measures indeed take only one type of event as input, many others combine two or three events, or even make use of representations to build a measure: number of fixations in AOIs for instance, the main sequence measure, and transition matrix measures. Moreover, an event-based division would also obscure the large similarity between some measures, such as fixation duration and dwell time, which would end up in different chapters according to an event-and-representation-based classification system.

A similar idea would be to categorize measures according to *how many steps need to be taken with data* to reach the measure? Karn, Ellis, and Juliano (1999) propose a categorization of all measures into four levels, similar to that shown in Figures 14.2–14.4 on pages 458–459 above. Pupil dilation comes right out of the gaze estimation algorithm, while fixation durations require additional filtering and event calculation. Heat maps add a layer of Gaussian calculations, and the Levenshtein string-edit measure adds AOI segmentation of the stimulus, and data alignment. Every measure has a calculation path from raw data to measure value, but how informative is it to the reader to have chapters entitled 'Measures that can be directly used from raw data', 'Measures that require event detection', and 'Measures that require AOIs'? Again, measures with large similarities would end up in different categories, according to this structure.

Lastly, one could potentially classify measures by *mathematical principles*; this would emphasize the crucial calculations behind measures, the very foundations of the numerical values we report as scientific results. More mathematical and information theoretic tools are gradually diffusing into eye-tracking research, and the space for mathematically tractable measures will slowly be filled by new research to the extent that it is needed. A categorization of chapters according to mathematical principles would require chapter titles such as, 'Measures that require trigonometry' and 'Measures that are based on correlational analysis'. Whilst this could doubtless further the detailed understanding of measures, such a book would be less accessible to many eye-tracker users, as hard-core mathematics can be intimidating to some.

These principles for classification of measures all describe important properties across all measures, but for the reader who uses the book to find methods and measures at the point in time when designing an experiment, we consider a classification system based on operationalizations to be the most efficient—this is how Part III is organized.

14.5   How to construct even more measures

Eye-tracking data have a structure that lends itself to many types of data analysis, which is one reason why we find so many measures. Suppose that we want to enrich eye-tracker-based research with even more measures—how should we go about this?

First of all, it is important to realize that *analysing eye-movement data is always a matter of reducing the amount of information in the data*, and through that reduction one achieves overviews and summaries at a new level of information. Reducing and selecting information is what the data transformation methods of Part II do for us. A recording, with its raw data samples and stimulus images is so full of unstructured information it is virtually impossible to make sense of without some form of reduction and re-representation; conversely, a transition matrix with its simple summary does not retain very much of the original information from a recording. Hence, devising a new measure is largely a matter of actively deciding what information *not* to keep, rather than just what summary to produce. This can be a fine balance.

Of course, it is the research question and the experimental design that you are working on which decide what summary of data your new measure should produce. If your hypothesis is that fixation stability is better for professional elite shooters, then you need to worry about what to do with the raw data samples inside fixations. Is the size of a boundary box a good enough summary, or does your experimental design require that you quantify each minute intra-fixational eye movement for you to prove that your hypothesis is correct? The choice of precise operationalization depends on the counter-arguments you can expect to your conclusions, and this depends on the theory and earlier studies on fixational eye-movements that you would have to consider. From this perspective, Viviani (1990) was correct when concluding that eye-movement data can only be interpreted within a specific theoretical framework.

It should however be emphasized that it is equally possible to construct measures from fictitious data alone, using the existing events and representations, without having a particular experiment or theory in mind. For instance, take the measure we called angle between dwell map vectors (p. 374). It compares two dwell maps, that is the dwell time values in the cells of two gridded AOI matrices, and tells us how similarly distributed they are. Now, transition matrices also consist of values in the cells of a matrix. Mathematically, one can use the procedure from the measure 'angle between dwell map vectors' to compare two transition matrices rather than two dwell maps. This is perfectly valid in mathematical terms. The output value would tell you how similar two transition matrices are with respect to which types of transition are common. In other words, we can indeed interpret this new measure—which we may call 'the angle between transition matrix vectors'—without ever designing or conducting an experiment, or thinking about a particular theory.

The following list presents six examples of how new and useful measures can be invented:

Detect a new event in the raw data samples Microsaccades and glissades are examples of events that have only become detectable relatively recently, owing to the advancement of event detection algorithms and faster sampling frequency of eye-trackers with better accuracy and precision. It may seem that there is not much room for further events in the raw data stream, but this is clearly not the case. Take the multi-step saccades on page 327 as an example. Detecting and accurately measuring these could yield a variety of velocity and counting measures. Another possibility would be to use thresholding on pupil data, for instance to identify all increases in pupil diameter lasting for at least 100 ms, with a total increase of at least 0.3 mm, and no intermediary decrease larger than 0.05 mm, and count the number of such occurrences in your trials.

Define new events from AOI strings and scanpath representations In-word and between-word regressions, and first pass regression scanpaths are only a few of the full possibilities of events which could be constructed from scanpath or AOI-based representations. Hyönä et al. (2003) propose several innovative events for the analysis of reading data according to such principles. Mathematically there is an infinite number of scanpath forms, and more than a handful could be expected to be generally useful. There is a great need for such measures in several of the applied fields; usability and educational psychology, to mention a few.

Re-use representational forms across types of data The similarity of dwell maps to transition matrices allows us to reuse the angle between dwell map vectors measure for transition matrices. Seeing similarities, breaking hidden assumptions, and generalizing a measure can make it applicable to new types of data. As another example, take the AOI dwell string. All measures assume that these are strings of AOI names, but from a computational viewpoint, a string of fixation durations or a string of saccadic amplitudes makes just as much sense, and such strings could easily be processed using the AOI string and scanpath measures we describe on page 339.

Import mathematical constructs Mathematical constructs can be imported that are similar to representations in eye movement data. There are many previous examples: string-editing stems from methods for comparing gene sequences, which were seen as similar to sequences of dwells. Scanpaths are similar to sequences of vectors and graphs. Gridded AOIs are matrices covering space. Mathematics is large in scope however, and there are many untried candidates. Time series has obvious similarities with both raw data and all sequence and over-time data. Knot theory deals with graphs that have a great similarity to scanpaths.

Plot a single-value measure over time If a measure can be calculated to give a value per data sample, or per fixation or any other chronometric unit, then it can be plotted over time, and the growth and decline of this measure can be modelled. Both the magnitude and the time course of the effect driving the measure can be examined. In fact, a large number of the measures in earlier chapters can be made into a value-over-time measures, when restricted into a time window and used across many participants, stimuli, or trials (according to the experimental design). For instance, the value-over-time measure 'Average fixation duration over time' is produced by selecting a time window of, say 500 ms, and for all participants and/or stimuli, averaging the durations of all fixations starting in each interval. This will give a curve showing how the average fixation duration changes over a trial. The measure 'Dwell time over dwell order' for each dwell, in order from one and up, sums the dwell times across participants, stimuli, or trials. The measure 'Number of returns over time' counts number of returns to AOIs already seen in successive windows of size 1 second, and could be expected to vary during decision processes, for instance in supermarket shopping (see Gidlöf et al., in progress). These value-over-time graphs are easy to produce, and if the data files are not too long, they can even be calculated in a spreadsheet program such as OpenOffice Calc.

Replace or reverse space and time By replacing spatial dimensions with feature dimensions (p. 215), many measures can be revived in new forms. Reversing and binning time (p. 205) allows for a whole array of measure variants.

Amalgamate measure concepts In the context of some experiments one or either measure that you choose as a tool to tackle your research question, may not be sufficient in its own right. In such cases it is theoretically possible to merge measures. For instance, suppose you expect participants to 'look for longer' on a particular AOI in one condition of your experiment compared to another. Although this prediction is imprecise it poses a genuine problem in that the number of fixations and their duration might confound each other with respect to your hypothesis. If one condition has a larger number of fixations on the AOI than another, in the predicted direction, but the duration of fixations between conditions is comparable, it is not possible to conclude that people 'look for longer' only that they 'look more often', since conventional statistical tests rely on the calculation of means and variance. The mean fixation duration on the AOI will be comparable between conditions, but fewer data points will contribute to it in one condition. The latter conclusion, 'look more often', thus relates only to frequency, despite the fact that the sum total of fixation durations is longer in the condition that you predicted it would be. Dwell time is not useful since some trials contain no fixations at all on the AOI in question. Again this is in line with the hypothesis, but not captured by your two measures (number of fixations in an AOI, and mean fixation duration in an AOI). One possible solution therefore, is to combine the two measures and take an average of fixation duration for each condition, *including trials in which no fixation occurred* (Dewhurst & Crundall, 2008; Dewhurst, 2009). The resulting value will be an amalgamation of number of fixations and fixation duration, and should be higher in line with your prediction. This issue relates to missing data, and the calculation of measures with respect to the experimental design and how eye-movement data is collapsed across trials and conditions (p. 78). The principle of merging measures in this way however, could be applied to a range of different events and representations, where the field of mathematics is open to you.

On the one hand, a systematic investigation into the full possibilities of developing measures for eye-movement data would be of great theoretical interest. It must be properly grounded in the needs of actual research, however, so that measures devised can actually come to good use. So far the mathematics used within measures is somewhat dichotomous: many measures rely on simple event counting, AOI region inclusion calculations, and possibly some trigonometry; others involve advanced filtering, probability density functions, Markov models, multidimensional vector spaces, and skewness and entropy calculations. This gives the impression that one half of the measures are only for mathematically advanced researchers. This is particularly paradoxical, in view of the fact that many applied researchers are in need of more mathematically advanced measures, while many researchers in neurological and vision research fields are satisfied with event counting and region inclusion calculations.

It is necessary to draw caution to the development of new measures without considering those that are available already, however. This may not be a useful exercise. A vast choice of measures are packaged and ready to go, being well grounded in theory and empirical investigation. Developing a new measure should really only be a consequence of encountering a specific problem, and even then you should be sure that you know the implications of your new calculation for your results. For the inexperienced researcher a likely reason for wanting to calculate a new measure could be that the experimental design is not tight enough, or some aspect was overlooked. Moreover, if we calculate too many measures, the fragmentation between research fields will increase exponentially, raising more of the problems already addressed in this chapter, most importantly the difficulty in deciphering what the measure actually measures.

14.6 Summary

There are so many eye-tracking measures, because eye-tracking is so versatile, and it is easy and fun to construct new measures. Easier, perhaps, than to find an already existing measure in the highly fragmented channels for publication of eye-tracker-based studies. In fact, the number of methods and measures for eye-tracking grows much faster than the validation of their interpretations. Awaiting enough empirical evidence, the responsibility for using measures correctly therefore rests upon authors and reviewers. Standardization of existing measures with respect to terminology and precise operationalizations is of essence to support them.

References

Aaltonen, A., Hyrskykari, A., & Räihä, K.-J. (1998). 101 spots, or how do users read menus? In C.-M. Karat, A. Lund, J. Coutaz, & J. Karat (Eds.), *Proceedings of the SIGCHI Conference on Human Factors in Computing Systems* (pp. 132–139). New York: ACM Press.

Abadi, R. V., & Gowen, E. (2004). Characteristics of saccadic intrusions. *Vision Research*, *44*(23), 2675–2690.

Abbott, T. S., Nataupsky, M., & Steinmetz, G. G. (1987). *Effects of combining vertical and horizontal information into a primary flight display* (Tech. Rep. No. 2873). NASA.

Abel, L. A., & Hertle, R. W. (1988). Effects of psychoactive drugs on ocular motor behavior. In C. W. Johnston & F. J. Pirozzolo (Eds.), *Neuropsychology of Eye Movements* (pp. 81–114). Mahwah NJ: Lawrence Erlbaum Associates.

Abel, L. A., Troost, B. T., & Dell'Osso, L. F. (1983). The effects of age on normal saccadic characteristics and their variability. *Vision Research*, *23*(1), 33–37.

Abernethy, B. (1990). Expertise, visual search, and information pick-up in squash. *Perception*, *19*(1), 63–77.

Abernethy, B., & Russell, D. G. (1987). The relationship between expertise and visual search strategy in a racquet sport. *Human Movement Science*, *6*(4), 283–319.

Aboyoun, D. C., & Dabbs, J. M. (1998). The Hess pupil dilation findings: Sex or novelty. *Social Behavior and Personality: An International Journal*, *26*(4), 415–419.

Abrams, R. A., Meyer, D. E., & Kornblum, S. (1990). Eye-hand coordination: Oculomotor control in rapid aimed limb movements. *Journal of Experimental Psychology: Human Perception and Performance*, *16*(2), 248–267.

Abrams, R. A., Pratt, J., & Chasteen, A. L. (1998). Aging and movement: Variability of force pulses for saccadic eye movements. *Psychology and Aging*, *13*(3), 387–395.

Adolphs, R., Gosselin, F., Buchanan, T. W., Tranel, D., Schyns, P. G., & Damasio, A. R. (2005). A mechanism for impaired fear recognition after amygdala damage. *Nature*, *433*(7021), 68–72.

Agustin, J. S. (2010). *Off-the-Shelf Gaze Interaction*. Unpublished doctoral dissertation, IT University of Copenhagen.

Ahern, S., & Beatty, J. (1979). Pupillary responses during information processing vary with Scholastic Aptitude Test scores. *Science*, *205*(4412), 1289–1292.

Ahlstrom, U., & Friedman-Berg, F. J. (2006). *Controller scan-path behavior during severe weather avoidance* (Tech. Rep. No. DOT/FAA/TC-06/07). Federal Aviation Administration, William J. Hughes Technical Center, Atlantic City International Airport.

Aizawa, H., & Wurtz, R. H. (1998). Reversible inactivation of monkey superior colliculus. I. Curvature of saccadic trajectory. *Journal of Neurophysiology*, *79*(4), 2082–2096.

Alamargot, D., Chesnet, D., Dansac, C., & Ros, C. (2006). Eye and Pen: A new device for studying reading during writing. *Behavior Research Methods*, *38*(2), 287–299.

Albert, W. (2002). Do web users actually look at ads? A case study of banner ads and eye-tracking technology. In *Proceedings of the 11th Annual Conference of the Usability Professionals' Association*.

Allopenna, P. D., Magnuson, J. S., & Tanenhaus, M. K. (1998). Tracking the time course of spoken word recognition using eye movements: Evidence for continuous mapping models. *Journal of Memory and Language, 38*(4), 419–439.

Altmann, G., & Kamide, Y. (2007). The real-time mediation of visual attention by language and world knowledge: Linking anticipatory (and other) eye movements to linguistic processing. *Journal of Memory and Language, 57*(4), 502–518.

Andersson, B., Dahl, J., Holmqvist, K., Holsanova, J., Johansson, V., Karlsson, H., et al. (2006). Combining keystroke logging with eye-tracking. In L. Van Waes, M. Leijten, & C. M. Neuwirth (Eds.), *Writing and Digital Media* (pp. 166–172). Amsterdam: Elsevier.

Andersson, R., Henderson, J. M., & Ferreira, F. (2011). I see what you're saying: The integration of complex speech and scenes during language comprehension. *Acta Psychologica, 137*(2), 208–216.

Andersson, R., Nyström, M., & Holmqvist, K. (2010). Sampling frequency and eye-tracking measures: How speed affects durations, latencies, and more. *Journal of Eye Movement Research, 3*(6), 1–12.

Andrews, T. J., & Coppola, D. M. (1999). Idiosyncratic characteristics of saccadic eye movements when viewing different visual environments. *Vision Research, 39*(17), 2947–2953.

Anliker, J. (1976). Eye movements: On-line measurement, analysis, and control. In R. A. Monty & J. Senders (Eds.), *Eye Movements and Psychological Processes* (pp. 185–199). New York: John Wiley & Sons.

Antes, J. R., & Kristjanson, A. F. (1991). Discriminating artists from nonartists by their eye-fixation patterns. *Perceptual and Motor Skills, 73*(1), 893–894.

Applied Science Laboratories. (2001). Eyenal (Eye-Analysis) Manual Version 1.0 (Windows) for use with ASL Series 5000 [Computer software manual]. 175 Middlesex Turnpike Bedford, MA 01730.

Applied Science Laboratories. (2011). *Information brochure.* (Version accessed January 2011.)

Aserinsky, E., Joan, A. L., Mack, M. E., Tzankoff, S. P., & Hurn, E. (1985). Comparison of eye motion in wakefulness and REM sleep. *Psychophysiology, 22*(1), 1–10.

Avila, M. T., Hong, L. E., Moates, A., Turano, K. A., & Thaker, G. K. (2006). Role of anticipation in schizophrenia-related pursuit initiation deficits. *Journal of Neurophysiology, 95*(2), 593–601.

Baccino, T., & Manunta, Y. (2005). Eye-fixation-related potentials: Insight into parafoveal processing. *Journal of Psychophysiology, 19*(3), 204–215.

Baddeley, R. J., & Tatler, B. W. (2006). High frequency edges (but not contrast) predict where we fixate: A Bayesian system identification analysis. *Vision Research, 46*(18), 2824–2833.

Bahill, A. T., Brockenbrough, A., & Troost, B. T. (1981). Variability and development of a normative data base for saccadic eye movements. *Investigative Ophthalmology & Visual Science, 21*(1), 116–125.

Bahill, A. T., Clark, M. R., & Stark, L. (1975a). Glissades–eye movements generated by mismatched components of the saccadic motoneuronal control signal. *Mathematical Biosciences, 26*(3-4), 303–318.

Bahill, A. T., Clark, M. R., & Stark, L. (1975b). The main sequence, a tool for studying human eye movements. *Mathematical Biosciences, 24*(3-4), 191–204.

Bahill, A. T., Hsu, F. K., & Stark, L. (1978). Glissadic overshoots are due to pulse width errors. *Archives of Neurology, 35*(3), 138–142.

Bahill, A. T., & LaRitz, T. (1984). Why can't batters keep their eyes on the ball? *American Scientist, 72*(3), 249–253.

Bakeman, R., & Gottman, J. M. (1997). *Observing Interaction: An Introduction to Sequential Analysis*. Cambridge: Cambridge University Press.

Ball, L. J., Eger, N., Stevens, R., & Dodd, J. (2006). Applying the post-experience eye-tracked protocol (PEEP) method in usability testing. *Interfaces, 67*, 15–19.

Ballard, D. H., Hayhoe, M. M., Li, F., Whitehead, S. D., Frisby, J. P., Taylor, J. G., et al. (1992). Hand-eye coordination during sequential tasks [and discussion]. *Philosophical Transactions of the Royal Society of London. Series B: Biological Sciences, 337*(1281), pp. 331–339.

Ballard, D. H., Hayhoe, M. M., & Pelz, J. B. (1995). Memory representations in natural tasks. *Journal of Cognitive Neuroscience, 7*(1), 66–80.

Baloh, R. W., Dietz, J., & Spooner, J. W. (1982). Myoclonus and ocular oscillations induced by L-tryptophan. *Annals of Neurology, 11*(1), 95–97.

Banks, M. S., Sekuler, A. B., & Anderson, S. J. (1991). Peripheral spatial vision: Limits imposed by optics, photoreceptors, and receptor pooling. *Journal of the Optical Society of America, 8*(11), 1775–1787.

Barr, D. (2008). Analyzing 'visual world' eyetracking data using multilevel logistic regression. *Journal of Memory and Language, 59*(4), 457–474.

Bartels, M. (2009). *The proof is in the pupil.* (Electronic publication distributed by Quirk's Marketing Research Review (www.quirk.com), accessed February 2011.)

Bartels, M., & Marshall, S. P. (2006). Eye tracking insights into cognitive modeling. In *Proceedings of the 2006 Symposium on Eye-Tracking Research & Applications* (pp. 141–147). New York: ACM.

Batschelet, E. (1981). *Circular Statistics in Biology*. London: Academic Press.

Beatty, J. (1982). Task-evoked pupillary responses, processing load, and the structure of processing resources. *Psychological Bulletin, 91*(2), 276–292.

Beatty, J., & Lucero-Wagoner, B. (2000). The pupillary system. In J. T. Cacioppo, G. Berntson, & L. G. Tassinary (Eds.), *Handbook of Psychophysiology* (Vol. 2, pp. 142–162). Cambridge: Cambridge University Press.

Becker, W., & Fuchs, A. F. (1969). Further properties of the human saccadic system: Eye movements and correction saccades with and without visual fixation points. *Vision Research, 9*(10), 1247–1258.

Becker, W., & Fuchs, A. F. (1985). Prediction in the oculomotor system: Smooth pursuit during transient disappearance of a visual target. *Experimental Brain Research, 57*(3), 562–575.

Becker, W., Hoehne, O., Iwase, K., & Kornhuber, H. H. (1972). Bereitschaftspotential, prämotorische Positivierung und andere Hirnpotentiale bei sakkadischen Augenbewegungen. *Vision Research, 12*(3), 421–436.

Becker, W., & Jürgens, R. (1979). An analysis of the saccadic system by means of double step stimuli. *Vision Research, 19*(9), 967–983.

Becker, W., & Jürgens, R. (1990). Human oblique saccades: Quantitative analysis of the relation between horizontal and vertical components. *Vision Research, 30*(6), 893–920.

Behrens, F., MacKeben, M., & Schröder-Preikschat, W. (2010). An improved algorithm for automatic detection of saccades in eye movement data and for calculating saccade parameters. *Behavior Research Methods, 42*(3), 701–708.

Behrens, F., & Weiss, L. R. (1992). An algorithm separating saccadic from nonsaccadic eye movements automatically by use of the acceleration signal. *Vision Research, 32*(5), 889–893.

Behrmann, M., Watt, S., Black, S. E., & Barton, J. J. S. (1997). Impaired visual search in patients with unilateral neglect: An oculographic analysis. *Neuropsychologia, 35*(11),

1445–1458.

Beijer, D., Smiley, A., & Eizenman, M. (2004). Observed driver glance behavior at roadside advertising signs. *Transportation Research Record*, *1899*, 96–103.

Beintema, J. A., Van Loon, E. M., & Van Den Berg, A. V. (2005). Manipulating saccadic decision-rate distributions in visual search. *Journal of Vision*, *5*(3), 150–164.

Benson, P. J., Leonards, U., Lothian, R. M., St Clair, D. M., & Merlo, M. C. G. (2007). Visual scan paths in first-episode schizophrenia and cannabis-induced psychosis. *Journal of Psychiatry & Neuroscience*, *32*(4), 267–74.

Berg, D. J., Boehnke, S. E., Marino, R. A., Munoz, D. P., & Itti, L. (2009). Free viewing of dynamic stimuli by humans and monkeys. *Journal of Vision*, *9*(5), 1–15.

Berg, P., & Scherg, M. (1994). A multiple source approach to the correction of eye artifacts. *Electroencephalography & Clinical Neurophysiology*, *90*(3), 229–241.

Bergamin, O., Schoetzau, A., Sugimoto, K., & Zulauf, M. (1998). The influence of iris color on the pupillary light reflex. *Graefe's Archive for Clinical and Experimental Ophthalmology*, *236*(8), 567–570.

Bergamin, O., Zimmerman, M. B., & Kardon, R. H. (2003). Pupil light reflex in normal and diseased eyes: Diagnosis of visual dysfunction using waveform partitioning. *Ophthalmology*, *110*(1), 106–114.

Bergstrom, K. J., & Hiscock, M. (1988). Factors influencing ocular motility during the performance of cognitive tasks. *Canadian Journal of Psychology*, *42*(1), 1–23.

Bergström, P. (2003). *Eye-Movement Controlled Image Coding*. Unpublished doctoral dissertation, Lund University.

Berséus, P. (2002). *Eye Movement in Prima Vista Singing and Vocal Text Reading*. Unpublished master's thesis, Lund University.

Bestelmeyer, P. E. G., Tatler, B. W., Phillips, L. H., Fraser, G., Benson, P. J., & St Clair, D. M. (2006). Global visual scanning abnormalities in schizophrenia and bipolar disorder. *Schizophrenia Research*, *87*(1-3), 212–222.

Betta, E., & Turatto, M. (2006). Are you ready? I can tell by looking at your microsaccades. *Neuroreport*, *17*(10), 1001–1004.

Beymer, D., Russell, D. M., & Orton, P. Z. (2005). Wide vs. narrow paragraphs: An eye tracking analysis. In M. F. Costabile & F. Paternò (Eds.), *Proceedings of Human-Computer Interaction – INTERACT 2005* (pp. 741–752). New York: Springer-Verlag.

Biederman, I., Rabinowitz, J. C., Glass, A. L., & Stacy, E. W. (1974). On the information extracted from a glance at a scene. *Journal of Experimental Psychology*, *103*(3), 597–600.

Binsted, G., Chua, R., Helsen, W., & Elliott, D. (2001). Eye-hand coordination in goal-directed aiming. *Human Movement Science*, *20*(4-5), 563–585.

Birmingham, E., Bischof, W., & Kingstone, A. (2009). Get real! Resolving the debate about equivalent social stimuli. *Visual Cognition*, *6*(7), 904–924.

Bitsios, P., Prettyman, R., & Szabadi, E. (1996). Changes in autonomic function with age: A study of pupillary kinetics in healthy young and old people. *Age and Ageing*, *25*(6), 432–438.

Bittencourt, P. R. M., Wade, P., Smith, A. T., & Richens, A. (1983). Benzodiazepines impair smooth pursuit eye movements. *British Journal of Clinical Pharmacology*, *15*(2), 259–262.

Black, J. L. (1984). Eye movement analysis: Reading and moving target pursuit. *International Journal of Bio-Medical Computing*, *15*(3), 199–217.

Blais, C., Jack, R. E., Scheepers, C., Fiset, D., & Caldara, R. (2008). Culture shapes how we look at faces. *PLoS ONE*, *3*(8), 3022–3022.

Blignaut, P. (2009). Fixation identification: The optimum threshold for a dispersion algorithm. *Attention, Perception & Psychophysics, 71*(4), 881–895.

Blignaut, P. (2010). Visual span and other parameters for the generation of heatmaps. In *Proceedings of the 2010 Symposium on Eye-Tracking Research & Applications* (pp. 125–128). New York: ACM.

Blignaut, P., & Beelders, T. (2009). The effect of fixational eye movements on fixation identification with a dispersion-based fixation detection algorithm. *Journal of Eye Movement Research, 2(5)*(4), 1–14.

Blythe, H. I., Liversedge, S. P., Joseph, H. S. S. L., White, S. J., Findlay, J. M., & Rayner, K. (2006). The binocular coordination of eye movements during reading in children and adults. *Vision Research, 46*(22), 3898–3908.

Bocca, M. L., & Denise, P. (2006). Total sleep deprivation effect on disengagement of spatial attention as assessed by saccadic eye movements. *Clinical Neurophysiology, 117*(4), 894–899.

Boccignone, G., Caggiano, V., Marcelli, A., Napoletano, P., & Di Fiore, G. (2005). An architectural model for combining spatial-based and object-based information for attentive video analysis. In *IEEE Proceedings of the Seventh International Workshop on Computer Architecture for Machine Perception* (pp. 116–121).

Bock, K., Irwin, D. E., Davidson, D. J., & Levelt, W. J. M. (2003). Minding the clock. *Journal of Memory and Language, 48*(4), 653–685.

Boff, K. R., & Lincoln, J. E. (1988). *Engineering Data Compendium: Human Perception and Performance.* Harry G. Armstrong Aerospace.

Bojko, A. A. (2006). Using eye tracking to compare web page designs: A case study. *Journal of Usability Studies, 1*(3), 112–120.

Bojko, A. A. (2009). Informative or misleading? Heatmaps deconstructed. In J. A. Jacko (Ed.), *Proceedings of the 13th International Conference on Human-Computer Interaction* (pp. 30–39).

Bonifacci, P., Ricciardelli, P., Lugli, L., & Pellicano, A. (2008). Emotional attention: Effects of emotion and gaze direction on overt orienting of visual attention. *Cognitive Processing, 9*(2), 127–135.

Boren, T., & Ramey, J. (2000). Thinking aloud: Reconciling theory and practice. *IEEE Transactions on Professional Communication, 43*(3), 261–278.

Born, S., & Kerzel, D. (2008). Influence of target and distractor contrast on the remote distractor effect. *Vision Research, 48*(28), 2805–2816.

Brainard, D. H. (1997). The psychophysics toolbox. *Spatial Vision, 10*(4), 433–436.

Brandt, S. A., & Stark, L. (1997). Spontaneous eye movements during visual imagery reflect the content of the visual scene. *Journal of Cognitive Neuroscience, 9*(1), 27–38.

Brasel, S. A., & Gips, J. (2008). Points of view: Where do we look when we watch TV? *Perception, 37*(12), 1890–1894.

Braun, D. I., Mennie, N., Rasche, C., Schutz, A. C., Hawken, M. J., & Gegenfurtner, K. R. (2008). Smooth pursuit eye movements to isoluminant targets. *Journal of Neurophysiology, 100*(3), 1287–1300.

Brezinova, V., & Kendell, R. E. (1977). Smooth pursuit eye movements of schizophrenics and normal people under stress. *The British Journal of Psychiatry, 130*(1), 59–63.

Bronstein, A. M., & Kennard, C. (1985). Predictive ocular motor control in Parkinson's disease. *Brain, 108*(4), 925–940.

Bronstein, A. M., & Kennard, C. (1987). Predictive eye saccades are different from visually triggered saccades. *Vision Research, 27*(4), 517–520.

Brookings, J. B., Wilson, G. F., & Swain, C. R. (1996). Psychophysiological responses to changes in workload during simulated air traffic control. *Biological Psychology, 42*(3),

361–377.

Brouwer, G. J., Van Ee, R., & Schwarzbach, J. (2005). Activation in visual cortex correlates with the awareness of stereoscopic depth. *Journal of Neuroscience, 25*(45), 10403–10413.

Brown-Schmidt, S., & Tanenhaus, M. K. (2006). Watching the eyes when talking about size: An investigation of message formulation and utterance planning. *Journal of Memory and Language, 54*(4), 592–609.

Brutten, G. J., & Janssen, P. (1979). An eye-marking investigation of anticipated and observed stuttering. *Journal of Speech and Hearing Research, 22*(1), 20–28.

Bryman, A. (1984). The debate about quantitative and qualitative research: A question of method or epistemology? *British Journal of Sociology, 35*(1), 75–92.

Bucci, M. P., Brémond-Gignac, D., & Kapoula, Z. A. A. (2008). Poor binocular coordination of saccades in dyslexic children. *Graefe's Archive for Clinical and Experimental Ophthalmology, 246*(3), 417–428.

Bucci, M. P., & Kapoula, Z. A. A. (2006). Binocular coordination of saccades in 7 years old children in single word reading and target fixation. *Vision Research, 46*(4), 457–466.

Buikhuisen, W., & Jongman, R. W. (1972). Traffic perception under the influence of alcohol. *Quarterly Journal of Studies on Alcohol, 33*(3), 800–806.

Bull, R., & Shead, G. (1979). Pupil dilation, sex of stimulus, and age and sex of observer. *Perceptual and Motor Skills, 49*(1), 27–30.

Bullimore, M. A., & Bailey, I. L. (1995). Reading and eye movements in age-related maculopathy. *Optometry & Vision Science, 72*(2), 125–138.

Burke, M. R., & Barnes, G. R. (2006). Quantitative differences in smooth pursuit and saccadic eye movements. *Experimental Brain Research, 175*(4), 596–608.

Burmester, M., & Mast, M. (2010). Repeated web page visits and the scanpath theory: A recurrent pattern detection approach. *Journal of Eye Movement Research, 3*(4), 1–20.

Buscher, G., Cutrell, E., & Morris, M. R. (2009). What do you see when you're surfing? Using eye tracking to predict salient regions of web pages. In *Proceedings of the 27th International Conference on Human Factors in Computing Systems* (pp. 21–30).

Buscher, G., & Dengel, A. (2009). *Gaze-based filtering of relevant document segments.* (Paper presented at Workshop on Web Search Result Summarization and Presentation, Madrid, Spain.)

Buser, A., Lachenmayr, B., Priemer, F., Langnau, A., & Gilg, T. (1996). Effect of low alcohol concentrations on visual attention in street traffic. *Der Ophthalmologe: Zeitschrift der Deutschen Ophthalmologischen Gesellschaft, 93*(4), 371–376.

Buswell, G. T. (1920). *An Experimental Study of the Eye-Voice Span in Reading.* Chicago: University of Chicago Press.

Buswell, G. T. (1935). *How People Look at Pictures.* Chicago: University of Chicago Press.

Butsch, R. L. C. (1932). Eye movements and the eye-hand span in typewriting. *Journal of Educational Psychology, 23*(2), 104–121.

Cahill, M., Eustace, P., & de Jesus, V. (2001). Pupillary autonomic denervation with increasing duration of diabetes mellitus. *British Journal of Ophthalmology, 85*(10), 1225–1230.

Camblin, C., Gordon, P., & Swaab, T. (2007). The interplay of discourse congruence and lexical association during sentence processing: Evidence from ERPs and eye tracking. *Journal of Memory and Language, 56*(1), 103–128.

Camilli, M., Terenzi, M., & Nocera, F. D. (2008). Effects of temporal and spatial demands on the distribution of eye fixations. In *Proceedings of the 52nd Annual Meeting of the Human Factors and Ergonomics Society* (pp. 1248–1251).

Campbell, C. S., & Maglio, P. P. (2001). A robust algorithm for reading detection. In *Proceedings of the 2001 Workshop on Perceptive User Interfaces* (pp. 1–7).

Canham, M., & Hegarty, M. (2010). Effects of knowledge and display design on comprehension of complex graphics. *Learning and Instruction, 20,* 155–166.

Card, S. K. (1982). User perceptual mechanisms in the search of computer command menus. In *Proceedings of the 1982 Conference on Human Factors in Computing Systems* (pp. 190–196).

Carney, L. G., & Hill, R. M. (1982). The nature of normal blinking patterns. *Acta Ophthalmologica, 60*(3), 427–433.

Carpenter, R. H. S. (1988). *Movements of the Eyes.* London: Pion.

Casey, B. J., & Richards, J. E. (1988). Sustained visual attention in young infants measured with an adapted version of the visual preference paradigm. *Child Development, 59*(6), 1514–1521.

Castelhano, M. S., & Henderson, J. M. (2007). Initial scene representations facilitate eye movement guidance in visual search. *Journal of Experimental Psychology, 33*(4), 753–763.

Castellanos, E. H., Charboneau, E., Dietrich, M. S., Park, S., Bradley, B. P., Mogg, K., et al. (2009). Obese adults have visual attention bias for food cue images: Evidence for altered reward system function. *International Journal of Obesity, 33*(9), 1063–1073.

Catrambone, R. (1998). The subgoal learning model: Creating better examples so that students can solve novel problems. *Journal of Experimental Psychology: General, 127*(4), 355–376.

Ceder, A. (1977). Drivers' eye movements as related to attention in simulated traffic flow conditions. *Human Factors, 19*(6), 571–581.

Cerbone, A., Sautter, F. J., Manguno-Mire, G., Evans, W. E., Tomlin, H., Schwartz, B., et al. (2003). Differences in smooth pursuit eye movement between posttraumatic stress disorder with secondary psychotic symptoms and schizophrenia. *Schizophrenia Research, 63*(1-2), 59–62.

Cerf, M., Harel, J., Huth, A., Einhäuser, W., & Koch, C. (2009). Decoding what people see from where they look: Predicting visual stimuli from scanpaths. *Lecture Notes in Artificial Intelligence, 5395,* 15–26.

Chafe, W. L. (1994). *Discourse, Consciousness, and Time: The Flow and Displacement of Conscious Experience in Speaking and Writing.* Chicago: University of Chicago Press.

Chapman, C. R., Oka, S., Bradshaw, D. H., Jacobson, R. C., & Donaldson, G. W. (1999). Phasic pupil dilation response to noxious stimulation in normal volunteers: Relationship to brain evoked potentials and pain report. *Psychophysiology, 36,* 44–52.

Chapman, P., & Underwood, G. M. (1998). Visual search of driving situations: Danger and experience. *Perception, 27*(8), 951–964.

Charness, N., Reingold, E. M., Pomplun, M., & Stampe, D. M. (2001). The perceptual aspect of skilled performance in chess: Evidence from eye movements. *Memory and Cognition, 29,* 1146–1152.

Chen, M. C., Anderson, J. R., & Sohn, M. H. (2001). What can a mouse cursor tell us more? Correlation of eye/mouse movements on web browsing. In *CHI '01 Extended Abstracts on Human Factors in Computing Systems* (pp. 281–282). New York: ACM.

Chen, X., & Zelinsky, G. J. (2006). Real-world visual search is dominated by top-down guidance. *Vision Research, 46*(24), 4118–4133.

Chenna, R., Sugawara, H., Koike, T., Lopez, R., Gibson, T. J., Higgins, D. G., et al. (2003). Multiple sequence alignment with the Clustal series of programs. *Nucleic Acids Research, 31*(13), 3497–3500.

Cherubini, M., Nüssli, M. A., & Dillenbourg, P. (2008). Deixis and gaze in collaborative work at a distance (over a shared map): A computational model to detect misunderstandings. In *Proceedings of the 2008 Symposium on Eye-Tracking Research & Applications* (pp. 173–180).

Chi, C. F., & Lin, F. T. (1997). A new method for describing search patterns and quantifying visual load using eye movement data. *International Journal of Industrial Ergonomics*, *19*(3), 249–257.

Chi, M. T. H. (1997). Quantifying qualitative analyses of verbal data: A practical guide. *Journal of Learning Sciences*, *6*(3), 271–315.

Chi, M. T. H. (2006). Laboratory methods for assessing experts' and novices' knowledge. In K. A. Ericsson, N. Charness, P. J. Feltovich, & R. R. Hoffman (Eds.), *The Cambridge Handbook of Expertise and Expert Performance* (pp. 167–184). Cambridge: Cambridge University Press.

Chi, M. T. H., De Leeuw, N., Chiu, M.-H., & LaVancher, C. (1994). Eliciting self-explanations improves understanding. *Cognitive Science*, *18*(3), 439–477.

Chisholm, S. L., Caird, J. K., & Lockhart, J. (2008). The effects of practice with MP3 players on driving performance. *Accident Analysis & Prevention*, *40*(2), 704–713.

Choi, Y. S., Mosley, A. D., & Stark, L. (1995). 'Starkfest' vision and clinic science special issue: String editing analysis of human visual search. *Optometry & Vision Science*, *72*(7), 439–451.

Chua, H. F., Boland, J. E., & Nisbett, R. E. (2005). Cultural variation in eye movements during scene perception. *Proceedings of the National Academy of Sciences*, *102*(35), 12629–12633.

Ciuffreda, K. J., Kenyon, R. V., & Stark, L. (1979). Saccadic intrusions in strabismus. *Archives of Ophthalmology*, *97*(9), 1673–1679.

Ciuffreda, K. J., & Tannen, B. (1995). *Eye Movement Basics for the Clinician*. St Louis: Mosby.

Claparède, E. (1934). La genèse de l'hypothèse. *Archives de Psychologie*, *24*(93-94), 1–155.

Clifton, C., Staub, A., & Rayner, K. (2007). Eye movements in reading words and sentences. In R. Van Gompel, M. Fischer, W. S. Murray, & R. L. Hill (Eds.), *Eye Movements: A Window on Mind and Brain* (pp. 341–372). Amsterdam: Elsevier.

Coeckelbergh, T. R. M., Cornelissen, F. W., Brouwer, W. H., & Kooijman, A. C. (2002). The effect of visual field defects on eye movements and practical fitness to drive. *Vision Research*, *42*(5), 669–677.

Cohen, P., Cohen, J., West, S. G., & Aiken, L. S. (2002). *Applied Multiple Regression / Correlation Analysis for the Behavioral Sciences* (third ed.). Mahwah NJ: Lawrence Erlbaum Associates.

Collewijn, H. (1998). Eye movement recording. In R. H. S. Carpenter & J. G. Robson (Eds.), *Vision Research: A Practical Guide to Laboratory Methods* (pp. 245–285). Oxford: Oxford University Press.

Collewijn, H., Erkelens, C. J., & Steinman, R. M. (1988). Binocular co-ordination of human horizontal saccadic eye movements. *Journal of Physiology*, *404*(1), 157–182.

Collewijn, H., & Tamminga, E. P. (1984). Human smooth and saccadic eye movements during voluntary pursuit of different target motions on different backgrounds. *The Journal of Physiology*, *351*(1), 217–250.

Collewijn, H., Van Der Steen, J., & Steinman, R. M. (1985). Human eye movements associated with blinks and prolonged eyelid closure. *Journal of Neurophysiology*, *54*(1), 11–27.

Collins, M., Seeto, R., Campbell, L., & Ross, M. (1989). Blinking and corneal sensitivity. *Acta Ophthalmologica*, *67*(5), 525–531.

Colombo, J., & Frick, J. E. (1999). Recent advances and issues in the study of preverbal intelligence. In M. Anderson (Ed.), *The Development of Intelligence* (pp. 43–71). East Sussex UK: Psychology Press.

Colvin, K., Dodhia, R., & Dismukes, R. K. (2005). Is pilots' visual scanning adequate to avoid mid-air collisions? In *Proceedings of the 13th International Symposium on Aviation Psychology* (pp. 104–109).

Colzato, L. S., Slagter, H. A., Van Den Wildenberg, W. P. M., & Hommel, B. (2009). Closing one's eyes to reality: Evidence for a dopaminergic basis of psychoticism from spontaneous eye blink rates. *Personality and Individual Differences, 46*(3), 377–380.

Cook, M., Wiebe, E. N., & Carter, G. (2008). The influence of prior knowledge on viewing and interpreting graphics with macroscopic and molecular representations. *Science Education, 92*(5), 848–867.

Cornell, E. D., MacDougall, H. G., Predebon, J., & Curthoys, I. S. (2003). Errors of binocular fixation are common in normal subjects during natural conditions. *Optometry and Vision Science, 80*(11), 764–771.

Cover, T. M., & Thomas, J. A. (1991). *Elements of Information Theory.* New York: John Wiley & Sons.

Cowen, L., Ball, L. J., & Delin, J. (2002). An eye movement analysis of web page usability. In X. Faulkner, J. Finlay, & F. Détienne (Eds.), *Proceedings of the HCI02 Conference on People and Computers XVI* (pp. 317–336). New York: Springer-Verlag.

Cox, A. L., & Silva, M. M. (2006). The role of mouse movements in interactive search. In R. Sun & N. Miyake (Eds.), *Proceedings of the 28th Annual Meeting of the Cognitive Science Society* (pp. 26–29). Mahwah NJ: Lawrence Erlbaum Associates.

Craik, F. I. M., & Lockhart, R. S. (1972). Levels of processing: A framework for memory research. *Journal of Verbal Learning & Verbal Behavior, 11*(6), 671–684.

Crane, H. D., & Steele, C. M. (1985, Feb). Generation-V dual-Purkinje-image eyetracker. *Applied Optics, 24*(4), 527–537.

Crawley, M. (2005). *Statistics: An Introduction Using R.* New York: John Wiley & Sons.

Cristino, F., Mathôt, S., Theeuwes, J., & Gilchrist, I. D. (2010). ScanMatch: A novel method for comparing fixation sequences. *Behavior Research Methods, 42*(3), 692–700.

Crossland, M. D., & Rubin, G. S. (2002). The use of an infrared eyetracker to measure fixation stability. *Optometry & Vision Science, 79*(11), 735–739.

Crossland, M. D., Sims, M., Galbraith, R. F., & Rubin, G. S. (2004). Evaluation of a new quantitative technique to assess the number and extent of preferred retinal loci in macular disease. *Vision Research, 44*(13), 1537–1546.

Crundall, D., & Underwood, G. M. (1998). Effects of experience and processing demands on visual information acquisition in drivers. *Ergonomics, 41*(4), 448–458.

Crundall, D., Underwood, G. M., & Chapman, P. (1999). Driving experience and the functional field of view. *Perception, 28*(9), 1075–1088.

Crundall, D., Underwood, G. M., & Chapman, P. (2002). Attending to the peripheral world while driving. *Applied Cognitive Psychology, 16*(4), 459–457.

Crutcher, R. J. (2007). CAPAS 2.0: A computer tool for coding transcribed and digitally recorded verbal reports. *Behavior Research Methods, 39*(2), 167–174.

Crystal, A., & Greenberg, J. (2006). Relevance criteria identified by health information users during Web searches. *Journal of the American Society for Information Science and Technology, 57*(10), 1368–1382.

Cui, Y., & Hondzinski, J. M. (2006). Gaze tracking accuracy in humans: Two eyes are better than one. *Neuroscience Letters, 396*(3), 257–262.

Dambacher, M., & Kliegl, R. (2007). Synchronizing timelines: Relations between fixation durations and N400 amplitudes during sentence reading. *Brain Research, 1155,* 147–

162.

Davies, S. P. (1995). Effects of concurrent verbalization on design problem solving. *Design Studies*, *16*(1), 102–116.

Day, R. F. (2010). Examining the validity of the Needleman-Wunsch algorithm in identifying decision strategy with eye-movement data. *Decision Support Systems*, *49*(4), 396–403.

De Graef, P., Christiaens, D., & D'Ydewalle, G. (1990). Perceptual effects of scene context on object identification. *Psychological Research*, *52*(4), 317–329.

De Groot, A. D. (1946/1978). *Thought and Choice and Chess*. The Hague, the Netherlands: Mouton.

De Hemptinne, C., Lefevre, P., & Missal, M. (2006). Influence of cognitive expectation on the initiation of anticipatory and visual pursuit eye movements in the rhesus monkey. *Journal of Neurophysiology*, *95*(6), 3770–3782.

De Valois, R. L., & De Valois, K. K. (1980). Spatial vision. *Annual Review of Psychology*, *31*(1), 309–341.

DeAngelus, M., & Pelz, J. B. (2009). Top-down control of eye movements: Yarbus revisited. *Visual Cognition*, *17*(6), 790–811.

Deco, G., & Rolls, E. T. (2004). A neurodynamical cortical model of visual attention and invariant object recognition. *Vision Research*, *44*(6), 621–642.

Dehais, F., Causse, M., & Pastor, J. (2008). *Embedded eye tracker in a real aircraft: New perspectives on pilot/aircraft interaction monitoring*. (Paper presented at the 3rd International Conference on Research in Air Transportation, Fairfax, Virginia.)

Delabarre, E. B. (1898). A method of recording eye movements. *American Journal of Psychology*, *9*(4), 572–574.

Demarais, A. M., & Cohen, B. H. (1998). Evidence for image-scanning eye movements during transitive inference. *Biological Psychology*, *49*(3), 229–247.

Dempere-Marco, L., Hu, X., Ellis, S. M., Hansell, D. M., & Yang, G. (2006). Analysis of visual search patterns with EMD metric in normalized anatomical space. *IEEE Transactions on Medical Imaging*, *25*(8), 1011–1021.

Dempere-Marco, L., Hu, X., & Yang, G. Z. (2011). A novel framework for the analysis of eye movements during visual search for knowledge gathering. *Cognitive Computation*, *3*(1), 206–222.

Denzin, N. K. (1970). *The Research Act in Sociology*. London: Butterworth.

De'Sperati, C., & Santandrea, E. (2005). Smooth pursuit-like eye movements during mental extrapolation of motion: The facilitatory effect of drowsiness. *Cognitive Brain Research*, *25*(1), 328–338.

De'Sperati, C., & Viviani, P. (1997). The relationship between curvature and velocity in two-dimensional smooth pursuit eye movements. *Journal of Neuroscience*, *17*(10), 3932–3945.

Deubel, H. (2008). The time course of presaccadic attention shifts. *Psychological Research*, *72*(6), 630–640.

Deubel, H., & Bridgeman, B. (1995). Perceptual consequences of ocular lens overshoot during saccadic eye movements. *Vision Research*, *35*(20), 2897–2902.

Deubel, H., & Schneider, W. X. (1996). Saccade target selection and object recognition: Evidence for a common attentional mechanism. *Vision Research*, *36*(12), 1827–1837.

Dewhurst, R. (2009). *Evaluating Strategies for Visual Search and Stimulus Discrimination: Implications for Training Eye-Movements*. Unpublished doctoral dissertation, University of Nottingham.

Dewhurst, R., & Crundall, D. (2008). Training eye movements: Can training people where to look hinder the processing of fixated objects? *Perception*, *37*(11), 1729–1744.

Di Nocera, F., Terenzi, M., & Camilli, M. (2006). Another look at scanpath: Distance to nearest neighbour as a measure of mental workload. In D. De Waard, K. Brookhuis, & A. Toffetti (Eds.), *Developments in Human Factors in Transportation, Design, and Evaluation* (pp. 295–303). Maastricht, the Netherlands: Shaker Publishing.

Di Russo, F., Pitzalis, S., & Spinelli, D. (2003). Fixation stability and saccadic latency in elite shooters. *Vision Research, 43*(17), 1837–1845.

Dickinson, C. A., & Zelinsky, G. J. (2007). Memory for the search path: Evidence for a high-capacity representation of search history. *Vision Research, 47*(13), 1745–1755.

Diderichsen, P. (2008). *One of a Kind—The Processing of Indefinite One-Anaphora in Spoken Danish.* Unpublished doctoral dissertation, Lund University.

Diefendorf, A. R., & Dodge, R. (1908). An experimental study of the ocular reactions of the insane from photographic records. *Brain, 31*(3), 451–489.

Dijkstra, E. W. (1959). A note on two problems in connexion with graphs. *Numerische Mathematik, 1*(1), 269–271.

Dionisio, D. P., Granholm, E., Hillix, W. A., & Perrine, W. F. (2001). Differentiation of deception using pupillary responses as an index of cognitive processing. *Psychophysiology, 38*(02), 205–211.

Ditchburn, R. W. (1973). *Eye Movements and Visual Perception.* Oxford: Oxford University Press.

Dodge, R. (1900). Visual perception during eye movement. *Psychological Review, 7*(5), 454–465.

Dodge, R., & Cline, T. S. (1901). The angle velocity of eye movements. *Psychological Review, 8*(2), 145–157.

Doherty, S., & O'Brien, S. (2009). Can MT output be evaluated through eye tracking? In *Proceedings of the Twelfth Machine Translation Summit* (pp. 214–221).

Doherty-Sneddon, G., Bruce, V., Bonner, L., Longbotham, S., & Doyle, C. (2002). Development of gaze aversion as disengagement from visual information. *Developmental Psychology, 38*(3), 438–445.

Dorr, M., Jarodzka, H., & Barth, E. (2010). Space-variant spatio-temporal filtering of video for gaze visualization and perceptual learning. In C. Morimoto & H. Instance (Eds.), *Proceedings of the 2010 Symposium on Eye Tracking Research & Applications* (pp. 307–314). New York: ACM.

Dorr, M., Vig, E., Gegenfurtner, K. R., Martinetz, T., & Barth, E. (2008). Eye movement modelling and gaze guidance. In *Proceedings of the Fourth International Workshop on Human-Computer Conversation.*

Doslak, M. J., Dell'Osso, L. F., & Daroff, R. B. (1983). Multiple double saccadic pulses occurring with other saccadic intrusions and oscillations. *Neuro-Ophthalmology, 3*(2), 109–116.

Doughty, M. J., & Naase, T. (2006). Further analysis of the human spontaneous eye blink rate by a cluster analysis-based approach to categorize individuals with 'normal' versus 'frequent' eye blink activity. *Eye & Contact Lens, 32*(6), 294–299.

Doyle, M., & Walker, R. (2001). Curved saccade trajectories: Voluntary and reflexive saccades curve away from irrelevant distractors. *Experimental Brain Research, 139*(3), 333–344.

Drew, T., & Doucet, S. (1991). Application of circular statistics to the study of neuronal discharge during locomotion. *Journal of Neuroscience Methods, 38*(2-3), 171–181.

Droege, D., & Paulus, D. (2009). Improved pupil center detection in low resolution images. In S. P. Liversedge (Ed.), *Proceedings of the 15th European Conference on Eye Movements.*

Duchowski, A. T. (2000). Acuity matching resolution degradation through wavelet coefficient scaling. *IEEE Transactions on Image Processing, 9*(8), 1437–1440.

Duchowski, A. T. (2007). *Eye tracking methodology: Theory and practice.* Secaucus, NJ, USA: Springer-Verlag New York, Inc. Available from http://portal.acm.org/citation.cfm?id=640601

Duncan, J. (1984). Selective attention and the organization of visual information. *Journal of Experimental Psychology: General, 113,* 501–517.

Duncker, K. (1945). On problem solving. *Psychological Monographs, 58*(270), 1–110.

Eberhard, K. M., Spivey-Knowlton, M. J., Sedivy, J. C., & Tanenhaus, M. K. (1995). Eye movements as a window into real-time spoken language comprehension in natural contexts. *Journal of Psycholinguistic Research, 24*(6), 409–436.

Ebisawa, Y., Minamitani, H., Mori, Y., & Takase, M. (1988). New methods for removing saccades in analysis of smooth pursuit eye movement. *Biological Cybernetics, 60*(2), 111–119.

Edelman, J. A., & Goldberg, M. E. (2001). Dependence of saccade-related activity in the primate superior colliculus on visual target presence. *Journal of Neurophysiology, 86*(2), 676–691.

Eenshuistra, R. M., Ridderinkhof, K. R., & Molen, M. W. (2004). Age-related changes in antisaccade task performance: Inhibitory control or working-memory engagement? *Brain and Cognition, 56*(2), 177–188.

Eger, N., Ball, L. J., Stevens, R., & Dodd, J. (2007). Cueing retrospective verbal reports in usability testing through eye-movement replay. In *Proceedings of the 21st British HCI Group Annual Conference on HCI* (Vol. 1, pp. 129–137).

Ehmke, C., & Wilson, C. (2007). Identifying web usability problems from eye tracking data. In *Proceedings of the 21st British HCI Group Annual Conference on HCI* (pp. 119–128).

Ehrmann, K., Ho, A., & Papas, E. (2005). A novel method for assessing variations in visual acuity after the blink. *Contact Lens and Anterior Eye, 28*(4), 157–162.

Einhäuser, W., Rutishauser, U., & Koch, C. (2008). Task-demands can immediately reverse the effects of sensory-driven saliency in complex visual stimuli. *Journal of Vision, 8*(2), 1–19.

Elias, G. S., Sherwin, G. W., & Wise, J. A. (1984). *Eye movements while viewing NTSC format television.* (SMPTE Psychophysics Subcommittee White Paper.)

Ellermeier, W., & Westphal, W. (1995). Gender differences in pain ratings and pupil reactions to painful pressure stimuli. *Pain, 61*(3), 435–439.

Ellis, C. J. (1981). The pupillary light reflex in normal subjects. *British Journal of Ophthalmology, 65*(11), 754–759.

Ellis, S. R., & Smith, J. D. (1985). Patterns of statistical dependency in visual scanning. In R. Groner, G. W. McConkie, & C. Menz (Eds.), *Eye Movements and Human Information Processing.* Amsterdam: Elsevier.

Ellis, S. R., & Stark, L. (1986). Statistical dependency in visual scanning. *Human Factors, 28*(4), 421–438.

Elterman, R. D., Abel, L. A., Daroff, R. B., Dell'Osso, L. F., & Bornstein, J. L. (1980). Eye movement patterns in dyslexic children. *Journal of Learning Disabilities, 13*(1), 16–21.

Emmorey, K., Thompson, R. L., & Colvin, R. (2008). Eye gaze during comprehension of American Sign Language by native and beginning signers. *Journal of Deaf Studies and Deaf Education, 14*(2), 237–243.

Engbert, R. (2006). Microsaccades: A microcosm for research on oculomotor control, attention, and visual perception. *Progress in Brain Research, 154,* 177–192.

Engbert, R., & Kliegl, R. (2003). Microsaccades uncover the orientation of covert attention. *Vision Research, 43*(9), 1035–1045.

Engbert, R., Longtin, A., & Kliegl, R. (2002). A dynamical model of saccade generation in reading based on spatially distributed lexical processing. *Vision Research, 42*(5), 621–636.

Engbert, R., & Mergenthaler, K. (2006). Microsaccades are triggered by low retinal image slip. *Proceedings of the National Academy of Sciences, 103*(18), 7192–7197.

Engbert, R., Nuthmann, A., Richter, E. M., & Kliegl, R. (2005). SWIFT: A dynamical model of saccade generation during reading. *Psychological Review, 112*(4), 777–813.

Engel, F. L. (1971). Visual conspicuity, directed attention and retinal locus. *Vision Research, 11*(6), 563–575.

Engel, F. L. (1977). Visual conspicuity, visual search and fixation tendencies of the eye. *Vision Research, 17*(1), 95–108.

Engmann, S., 't Hart, B. M., Sieren, T., Onat, S., König, P., & Einhäuser, W. (2009). Saliency on a natural scene background: Effects of color and luminance contrast add linearly. *Attention, Perception, & Psychophysics, 71*(6), 1337–1352.

Enright, J. T. (1998). Estimating peak velocity of rapid eye movements from video recordings. *Behavior Research Methods, Instruments, & Computers, 30*(2), 349–353.

Epelboim, J., Steinman, R. M., Kowler, E., Edwards, M., Pizlo, Z., Erkelens, C. J., et al. (1995). The function of visual search and memory in sequential looking tasks. *Vision Research, 35*(23-24), 3401–3422.

Epelboim, J., Steinman, R. M., Kowler, E., Pizlo, Z., Erkelens, C. J., & Collewijn, H. (1997). Gaze-shift dynamics in two kinds of sequential looking tasks. *Vision Research, 37*(18), 2597–2607.

Epelboim, J., & Suppes, P. (2001). A model of eye movements and visual working memory during problem solving in geometry. *Vision Research, 41*(12), 1561–1574.

Ericsson, K. A. (1988). Concurrent verbal reports on reading and text comprehension. *Text, 8*(4), 295–325.

Ericsson, K. A. (2006). Protocol analysis and expert thought: Concurrent verbalizations of thinking during experts' performance on representative tasks. In K. A. Ericsson, N. Charness, P. J. Feltovich, & R. R. Hoffman (Eds.), *The Cambridge Handbook of Expertise and Expert Performance* (pp. 223–241). Cambridge: Cambridge University Press.

Ericsson, K. A., & Lehmann, A. C. (1996). Expert and exceptional performance: Evidence of maximal adaption to task constraints. *Annual Reviews in Psychology, 47*, 273–305.

Ericsson, K. A., & Simon, H. A. (1980). Verbal reports as data. *Psychological Review, 87*(3), 215–251.

Ericsson, K. A., & Simon, H. A. (1993). *Protocol Analysis: Verbal Reports as Data.* Cambridge MA: MIT Press.

Eser, I., Durrie, D. S., Schwendeman, F., & Stahl, J. E. (2008). Association between ocular dominance and refraction. *Journal of Refractive Surgery, 24*(7), 685–689.

Ettinger, U., Kumari, V., Chitnis, X. A., Corr, P. J., Sumich, A. L., Rabe-Hesketh, S., et al. (2002). Relationship between brain structure and saccadic eye movements in healthy humans. *Neuroscience Letters, 328*(3), 225–228.

Ettinger, U., Kumari, V., Crawford, T. J., Davis, R. E., Sharma, T., & Corr, P. J. (2003). Reliability of smooth pursuit, fixation, and saccadic eye movements. *Psychophysiology, 40*(4), 620–628.

Evans, K., Rotello, C. M., Li, X., & Rayner, K. (2009). Scene perception and memory revealed by eye movements and receiver-operating characteristic analyses: Does a cultural difference truly exist? *The Quarterly Journal of Experimental Psychology, 62*(2), 276–285.

Everling, S., & Fischer, B. (1998). The antisaccade: A review of basic research and clinical studies. *Neuropsychologia, 36*(9), 885–899.

Evinger, C., Manning, K. A., Pellegrini, J. J., Basso, M. A., Powers, A. S., & Sibony, P. A. (1994). Not looking while leaping: The linkage of blinking and saccadic gaze shifts. *Experimental Brain Research, 100*(2), 337–344.

Fabrikant, S. I., Rebich-Hespanha, S., Andrienko, N., Andrienko, G., & Montello, D. R. (2008). Novel method to measure inference affordance in static small-multiple map displays representing dynamic processes. *The Cartographic Journal, 45*(3), 201–215.

Fahey, M. C., Cremer, P. D., Aw, S. T., Millist, L., Todd, M. J., White, O. B., et al. (2008). Vestibular, saccadic and fixation abnormalities in genetically confirmed Friedreich ataxia. *Brain, 131*(4), 1035–1045.

Fang, R., Chai, J. Y., & Ferreira, F. (2009). Between linguistic attention and gaze fixations in multimodal conversational interfaces. In *Proceedings of the 2009 International Conference on Multimodal Interfaces* (pp. 143–150).

Fehd, H. M., & Seiffert, A. E. (2010). Looking at the center of the targets helps multiple object tracking. *Journal of Vision, 10*(4), 1–13.

Feldon, S. E., & Langston, J. W. (1977). Square-wave jerks: A disorder of microsaccades? *Neurology, 27*(3), 278–281.

Ferrera, V. P. (2000). Task-dependent modulation of the sensorimotor transformation for smooth pursuit eye movements. *Journal of Neurophysiology, 84*(6), 2725–2738.

Ferrera, V. P., & Lisberger, S. G. (1995). Attention and target selection for smooth pursuit eye movements. *Journal of Neuroscience, 15*(11), 7472–7482.

Feusner, M., & Lukoff, B. (2008). Testing for statistically significant differences between groups of scan patterns. In *Proceedings of the 2008 Symposium on Eye-Tracking Research & Applications* (pp. 43–46). New York: ACM.

Findlay, J. M., & Brown, V. (2006). Eye scanning of multi-element displays: I. Scanpath planning. *Vision Research, 46*(1-2), 179–195.

Findlay, J. M., & Walker, R. (1999). A model of saccade generation based on parallel processing and competitive inhibition. *Behavioral and Brain Sciences, 22*(04), 661–674.

Fioravanti, F., Inchingolo, P., Pensiero, S., & Spanio, M. (1995). Saccadic eye movement conjugation in children. *Vision Research, 35*(23-24), 3217–3228.

Fischer, B., & Boch, R. (1983). Saccadic eye movements after extremely short reaction times in the monkey. *Brain Research, 260*(1), 21–26.

Fitts, P. M., Jones, R. E., & Milton, J. L. (1950). Eye movements of aircraft pilots during instrument-landing approaches. *Aeronautical Engineering Review, 9*(2), 24–29.

Fogarty, C., & Stern, J. A. (1989). Eye movements and blinks: Their relationship to higher cognitive processes. *International Journal of Psychophysiology, 8*(1), 35–42.

Ford, K. A., Goltz, H. C., Brown, M. R. G., & Everling, S. (2005). Neural processes associated with antisaccade task performance investigated with event-related fMRI. *Journal of Neurophysiology, 94*(1), 429–440.

Foulsham, T. (2008). *Saliency and Eye Movements in the Perception of Natural Scenes.* Unpublished doctoral dissertation, Nottingham University.

Foulsham, T. (2010). *EM Tools for scanpath comparison.* (Software available from the author's website (http://barlab.psych.ubc.ca/people/tom/programming), accessed February 2011.)

Foulsham, T., & Kingstone, A. (2010). Asymmetries in the direction of saccades during perception of scenes and fractals: Effects of image type and image features. *Vision*

Research, 50(8), 779–795.

Foulsham, T., Kingstone, A., & Underwood, G. M. (2008). Turning the world around: Patterns in saccade direction vary with picture orientation. *Vision Research, 48*(17), 1777–1790.

Foulsham, T., & Underwood, G. M. (2008). What can saliency models predict about eye movements? Spatial and sequential aspects of fixations during encoding and recognition. *Journal of Vision, 8*(2), 1–17.

Franck, M. C., & Kuhlo, W. (1970). Die Wirkung des Alkohols auf die raschen Blickzielbewegungen (Saccaden) beim Menschen. *European Archives of Psychiatry and Clinical Neuroscience, 213*(3), 238–245.

Frens, M. A., & Erkelens, C. J. (1991). Coordination of hand movements and saccades: Evidence for a common and a separate pathway. *Experimental Brain Research, 85*(3), 682–690.

Frens, M. A., & Van Der Geest, J. N. (2002). Scleral search coils influence saccade dynamics. *Journal of Neurophysiology, 88*(2), 692–698.

Friedman, A. (1979). Framing pictures: The role of knowledge in automatized encoding and memory for gist. *Journal of Experimental Psychology: General, 108*(3), 316–355.

Friedman, A., & Liebelt, L. S. (1981). On the time course of viewing pictures with a view towards remembering. In D. F. Fisher, R. A. Monty, & J. Senders (Eds.), *Eye Movements: Cognition and Visual Perception* (pp. 137–155). Hillsdale, NJ: Lawrence Erlbaum Associates.

Friedman, L., Jesberger, J. A., Abel, L. A., & Meltzer, H. Y. (1992). Catch-up saccade amplitude is related to square wave jerk rate. *Investigative Ophthalmology & Visual Science, 33*(1), 228–233.

Furneaux, S., & Land, M. F. (1999). The effects of skill on the eye-hand span during musical sight-reading. *Proceedings of the Royal Society B: Biological Sciences, 266*(1436), 2435–2440.

Gajewski, D., & Henderson, J. M. (2005). Minimal use of working memory in a scene comparison task. *Visual Cognition, 12*(6), 979–1002.

Galley, N. (1989). Saccadic eye movement velocity as an indicator of (de)activation. A review and some speculations. *Journal of Psychophysiology, 3*(3), 229–244.

Galley, N. (1993). The evaluation of the electrooculogram as a psychophysiological measuring instrument in the driver study of driver behaviour. *Ergonomics, 36*(9), 1063–1070.

Garcia, M. R., & Stark, P. (1988). Eye movements and coding of video sequences. In *SPIE Proceedings on Visual Communication and Image Processing* (Vol. 1001, pp. 398–405).

Gauthier, G. M., & Hofferer, J. M. (1976). Eye tracking of self-moved targets in the absence of vision. *Experimental Brain Research, 26*(2), 121–139.

Gbadamosi, J. (2000). *Visual Imagery und Mikro-Sakkaden bei Hemianopsie-Patienten.* Unpublished doctoral dissertation, Fachbereich Medizin der Universität Hamburg.

Gbadamosi, J., & Zangemeister, W. H. (2001). Visual imagery in hemianopic patients. *Journal of Cognitive Neuroscience, 13*(7), 855–866.

Geisler, W. S., & Perry, J. S. (1998). A real-time foveated multi-resolution system for low-bandwidth video communication. In B. E. Rogowitz & T. N. Pappas (Eds.), *SPIE Proceedings on Human Vision and Electronic Imaging III* (Vol. 3299, pp. 294–305).

Geng, J. J., Ruff, C. C., & Driver, J. (2009). Saccades to a remembered location elicit spatially specific activation in human retinotopic visual cortex. *Journal of Cognitive Neuroscience, 21*(2), 230–245.

Gerjets, P., Kammerer, Y., & Werner, B. (2011). Measuring spontaneous and instructed evaluation processes during web search: Integrating concurrent verbal protocols and eye tracking data. *Learning and Instruction, 21*(2), 220–231.

Ghent, L. (1956). Perception of overlapping and embedded figures by children of different ages. *The American Journal of Psychology, 69*(4), 575–587.

Gidlöf, K., Wallin, A., Dewhurst, R., & Holmqvist, K. (in progress). *Yarbus goes shopping - studying decision making in natural settings with eye tracking.* (Article submitted to the British Journal of Psychology.)

Gilchrist, I. D., & Harvey, M. (2000). Refixation frequency and memory mechanisms in visual search. *Current Biology, 10*(19), 1209–1212.

Gilchrist, I. D., & Harvey, M. (2006). Evidence for a systematic component within scan paths in visual search. *Visual Cognition, 14*(4), 704–715.

Gilchrist, I. D., North, A., & Hood, B. (2001). Is visual search really like foraging? *Perception, 30*(12), 1459–1464.

Gilland, J. (2004). *Age Differences in the Useful Field of View during Real World Driving.* Unpublished master's thesis, University of South Dakota.

Giorgetti, R., D'Amato, M., Pagani, S., Cavarzeran, F., & Tagliabracci, A. (2007). Automatic eye-tracking in study of visual function and attention capacity. In *Proceedings of the Annual Meetings of International Council on Alcohol, Drugs, and Traffic Safety.*

Girod, B. (1988). Eye movements and coding of video sequences. In T. R. Hsing (Ed.), *SPIE Proceedings on Visual Communication and Image Processing* (Vol. 1001, pp. 398–405).

Glaholt, M. G., & Reingold, E. M. (2009). The time course of gaze bias in visual decision tasks. *Visual Cognition, 17*(8), 1228–1243.

Glenberg, A. M., Schroeder, J. L., & Robertson, D. A. (1998). Averting the gaze disengages the environment and facilitates remembering. *Memory and Cognition, 26*(4), 651–658.

Godnig, E. C. (2003). Tunnel vision: Its causes and treatment strategies. *Journal of Behavioral Optometry, 14*(4), 95–99.

Goldberg, J. H., & Helfman, J. I. (2010). Scanpath clustering and aggregation. In *Proceedings of the 2010 Symposium on Eye-Tracking Research & Applications* (pp. 227–234). New York: ACM.

Goldberg, J. H., & Kotval, X. P. (1999). Computer interface evaluation using eye movements: Methods and construct. *International Journal of Industrial Ergonomics, 24*(6), 631–645.

Goldberg, J. H., & Schryver, J. C. (1995a). Eye-gaze contingent control of the computer interface: Methodology and example for zoom detection. *Behavior Research Methods, Instruments, & Computers, 27*(3), 338–350.

Goldberg, J. H., & Schryver, J. C. (1995b). Eye-gaze determination of user intent at the computer interface. In J. M. Findlay, R. Walker, & R. W. Kentridge (Eds.), *Eye Movement Research: Mechanisms, Processes and Applications* (pp. 491–502). New York: Elsevier Science.

Goldberg, J. H., Stimson, M. J., Lewenstein, M., Scott, N., & Wichansky, A. M. (2002). Eye tracking in web search tasks: Design implications. In *Proceedings of the 2002 Symposium on Eye-Tracking Research & Applications* (pp. 51–58). New York: ACM.

Goldberg, J. H., & Wichansky, A. M. (2003). Eye tracking in usability evaluation: A practitioner's guide. In J. Hyönä, R. Radach, & H. Deubel (Eds.), *The Mind's Eye: Cognitive and Applied Aspects of Eye Movement Research* (pp. 493–516). Oxford: Elsevier Science.

Goldreich, D., Krauzlis, R. J., & Lisberger, S. G. (1992). Effect of changing feedback delay on spontaneous oscillations in smooth pursuit eye movements of monkeys. *Journal of Neurophysiology, 67*(3), 625–638.

Gooding, D. C., Iacono, W. G., & Beiser, M. (1994). Temporal stability of smooth-pursuit eye tracking in first-episode psychosis. *Psychophysiology, 31*(1), 62–67.

Goolsby, T. W. (1994). Eye movement in music reading: Effects of reading ability, notational complexity, and encounters. *Music Perception, 12*, 77–96.

Gordon, P., & Moser, S. (2007). Insight into analogies: Evidence from eye movements. *Visual Cognition, 15*(16), 20–35.

Granka, L. A., Feusner, M., & Lorigo, L. (2008). Eye monitoring in online search. In R. I. Hammoud (Ed.), *Passive Eye Monitoring* (pp. 347–372). Heidelberg: Springer.

Granka, L. A., Hembrooke, H. A., Gay, G., & Feusner, M. (2008). *Correlates of visual salience and disconnect: An eye-tracking evaluation.* (Unpublished manuscript.)

Grant, E. R., & Spivey, M. J. (2003). Eye movements and problem solving: Guiding attention guides thought. *Psychological Science, 14*(5), 462–466.

Grauman, K., Betke, M., Gips, J., & Bradski, G. R. (2001). Communication via eye blinks-detection and duration analysis in real time. In *IEEE Proceedings of the Conference on Computer Vision and Pattern Recognition* (Vol. 1, pp. 1010–1017).

Gravetter, F. J., & Forzano, L. A. B. (2008). *Research Methods for the Behavioral Sciences.* Belmont CA: Wadsworth.

Green, A. J. F. (1998). *Using Verbal Protocols in Language Testing Research: A Handbook.* Cambridge: Cambridge University Press.

Green, M. J. (2006). *Facial Affect Processing in Delusion-Prone and Deluded Individuals: A Continuum Approach to the Study of Delusion Formation.* Unpublished doctoral dissertation, University of Sydney.

Green, M. J., Waldron, J. H., Simpson, I., & Coltheart, M. (2008). Visual processing of social context during mental state perception in schizophrenia. *Journal of Psychiatry & Neuroscience, 33*(1), 34–42.

Green, P. (2002). Where do drivers look while driving (and for how long)? In R. E. Dewar & P. L. Olson (Eds.), *Human Factors in Traffic Safety* (pp. 77–110). Tucson AZ: Lawyers and Judges Publishing Company.

Green, S., & Farnborough, H. (1986). Saccadic eye movement analysis as a measure of sleep loss effects on the central nervous system (CNS). In *Proceedings of the Annual International Industrial Ergonomics and Safety Conference* (pp. 379–387).

Greenacre, M. (2007). *Correspondence Analysis in Practice* (second ed.). London: Chapman Hall/CRC.

Griffin, Z. M. (2004). Why look? Reasons for eye movements related to language production. In J. M. Henderson & F. Ferreira (Eds.), *The Integration of Language, Vision, and Action: Eye Movements and the Visual World* (pp. 213–247). New York: Psychology Press.

Griffin, Z. M., & Bock, K. (2000). What the eyes say about speaking. *Psychological Science, 11*(4), 274–279.

Griffin, Z. M., & Spieler, D. H. (2006). Observing the what and when of language production for different age groups by monitoring speakers' eye movements. *Brain and Language, 99*(3), 272–288.

Griffiths, A. N., Marshall, R. W., & Richens, A. (1984). Saccadic eye movement analysis as a measure of drug effects on human psychomotor performance. *British Journal of Clinical Pharmacology, 18*(Suppl 1), 73S.

Grillon, C., Ameli, R., Woods, S. W., Merikangas, K., & Davis, M. (1991). Fear-potentiated startle in humans: Effects of anticipatory anxiety on the acoustic blink reflex. *Psychophysiology, 28*(5), 588–595.

Grindinger, T., Duchowski, A. T., & Sawyer, M. (2010). Group-wise similarity and classification of aggregate scanpaths. In *Proceedings of the 2010 Symposium on Eye-Tracking*

Research & Applications (pp. 101–104). New York: ACM.

Groner, R., Walder, F., & Groner, M. (1984). Looking at faces: Local and global aspects of scanpaths. In A. G. Gale & F. Johnson (Eds.), *Theoretical and Applied Aspects of Eye Movement Research* (pp. 523–533). Amsterdam: Elsevier.

Guan, Z., Lee, S., Cuddihy, E., & Ramey, J. (2006). The validity of the stimulated retrospective think-aloud method as measured by eye tracking. In *CHI 2006 Proceedings - Usability Methods* (pp. 1253–1262).

Guestrin, E. D., & Eizenman, M. (2006). General theory of remote gaze estimation using the pupil center and corneal reflections. *IEEE Transactions on Biomedical Engineering*, *53*(6), 1124–1133.

Gullberg, M., & Holmqvist, K. (1999). Keeping an eye on gestures: Visual perception of gestures in face-to-face communication. *Pragmatics and Cognition*, *7*(1), 35–63.

Gullberg, M., & Holmqvist, K. (2006). What speakers do and what addressees look at: Visual attention to gestures in human interaction live and on video. *Pragmatics and Cognition*, *14*(1), 53–82.

Hacisalihzade, S. S., Stark, W., & Allen, S. (2002). Visual perception and sequences of eye movement fixations: A stochastic modeling approach. *IEEE Transactions on Systems, Man, and Cybernetics*, *22*(3), 474–481.

Hadelich, K., & Crocker, M. W. (2006). Gaze alignment of interlocutors in conversational dialogues. In *Proceedings of the 2006 Symposium on Eye-Tracking Research & Applications* (pp. 38–38). New York: ACM.

Hafed, Z. M., & Clark, J. J. (2002). Microsaccades as an overt measure of covert attention shifts. *Vision Research*, *42*(22), 2533–2545.

Haider, H., & Frensch, P. A. (1999). Eye movement during skill acquisition: More evidence for the information-reduction hypothesis. *Journal of Experimental Psychology Learning Memory and Cognition*, *25*(1), 172–190.

Häkkänen, H., Summala, H., Partinen, M., Tiihonen, M., & Silvo, J. (1999). Blink duration as an indicator of driver sleepiness in professional bus drivers. *Sleep*, *22*(6), 798–802.

Hammoud, R. I. (2008). *Passive Eye Monitoring: Algorithms, Applications and Experiments.* New York: Springer-Verlag.

Han, Y., Ciuffreda, K. J., Selenow, A., Bauer, E., Ali, S. R., & Spencer, W. (2003). Static aspects of eye and head movements during reading in a simulated computer-based environment with single-vision and progressive lenses. *Investigative Ophthalmology & Visual Science*, *44*(1), 145–153.

Hannus, M., & Hyönä, J. (1999). Utilization of illustrations during learning of science textbook passages among low- and high-ability children. *Contemporary Educational Psychology*, *24*(2), 95–123.

Hansen, D. W., & Ji, Q. (2009). In the eye of the beholder: A survey of models for eyes and gaze. *IEEE Transactions on Pattern Analysis and Machine Intelligence*, *32*(3), 478–500.

Hansen, J. P. (1991). The use of eye mark recordings to support verbal retrospection in software testing. *Acta Psychologica*, *76*(1), 31–49.

Hansen, J. P. (1994). *Analyse af Læsernes Informationsprioritering.* (Unpublished Report, Kognitiv Systemgruppen, Forskningscenter Risø, Roskilde, Denmark.)

Hari, R., Valta, M., & Uutela, K. (1999). Prolonged attentional dwell time in dyslexic adults. *Neuroscience Letters*, *271*(3), 202–204.

Harris, C. M. (1993). On the reversibility of Markov scanning in free-viewing. In *Visual Search* (Vol. 2, pp. 123–136). New York: Taylor & Francis.

Harris, C. M., Hainline, L., Abramov, I., Lemerise, E., & Camenzuli, C. (1988). The distribution of fixation durations in infants and naive adults. *Vision Research*, *28*(3), 419–

432.

Harris, R. L., & Christhilf, D. M. (1980). What do pilots see in displays? In *Proceedings of the 24th Annual Meeting of the Human Factors and Ergonomics Society* (pp. 22–26).

Harris, R. L., Tole, J. R., Ephrath, A. R., & Stephens, A. T. (1982). How a new instrument affects pilots' mental workload. In *Proceedings of the 26th Annual Meeting of the Human Factors and Ergonomics Society* (pp. 1010–1013).

Harrison, N. A., Singer, T., Rotshtein, P., Dolan, R. J., & Critchley, H. D. (2006). Pupillary contagion: Central mechanisms engaged in sadness processing. *Social Cognitive and Affective Neuroscience, 1*(1), 5–17.

Harrison, N. A., Wilson, C. E., & Critchley, H. D. (2007). Processing of observed pupil size modulates perception of sadness and predicts empathy. *Emotion, 7*(4), 724–729.

Harwood, M. R., Mezey, L. E., & Harris, C. M. (1999). The spectral main sequence of human saccades. *Journal of Neuroscience, 19*(20), 9098–9106.

Hauland, G. (2002). *Measuring team situation awareness in training of en route air traffic control. Process oriented measures for experimental studies.* Unpublished doctoral dissertation, Risø Research Station and Aarhus University.

Hayhoe, M. M. (2000). Vision using routines: A functional account of vision. *Change Blindness and Visual Memory, 2000*(7), 43–64.

Hayhoe, M. M., & Ballard, D. H. (2005). Eye movements in natural behavior. *Trends in Cognitive Sciences, 9*(4), 188–194.

Heiman, G. (2006). *Basic Statistics for the Behavioral Sciences.* Boston: Houghton Mifflin Company.

Heller, D., & Radach, R. (1999). Eye movements in reading: Are two eyes better than one? In W. Becker, H. Deubel, & T. Mergner (Eds.), *Current Oculomotor Research: Physiological and Psychological Aspects* (pp. 341–348). Dordrecht, the Netherlands: Kluwer Academic Publishers.

Hembrooke, H. A., Feusner, M., & Gay, G. (2006). Averaging scan patterns and what they can tell us. In *Proceedings of the 2006 Symposium on Eye-Tracking Research & Applications* (p. 41). New York: ACM.

Henderson, J. M. (1992). Visual attention and eye movement control during reading and picture viewing. In K. Rayner (Ed.), *Eye Movements and Visual Cognition: Scene Perception and Reading* (pp. 260–283). New York: Springer-Verlag.

Henderson, J. M. (2003). Human gaze control during real-world scene perception. *Trends in Cognitive Sciences, 7*(11), 498–504.

Henderson, J. M., Brockmole, J. R., Castelhano, M. S., & Mack, M. (2007). Visual saliency does not account for eye movements during visual search in real-world scenes. In R. Van Gompel, M. Fischer, W. S. Murray, & R. L. Hill (Eds.), *Eye Movements: A Window on Mind and Brain* (pp. 537–562). Oxford: Elsevier.

Henderson, J. M., & Ferreira, F. (2004). Scene perception for psycholinguists. In J. M. Henderson & F. Ferreira (Eds.), *The Interface of Language, Vision, and Action: Eye Movements and the Visual World* (pp. 1–58). New York: Psychology Press.

Henderson, J. M., & Hollingworth, A. (1999). High-level scene perception. *Annual Review of Psychology, 50*(1), 243–271.

Henderson, J. M., & Pierce, G. L. (2008). Eye movements during scene viewing: Evidence for mixed control of fixation durations. *Psychonomic Bulletin & Review, 15*(3), 566–573.

Henderson, J. M., Weeks, P. A., & Hollingworth, A. (1999). The effects of semantic consistency on eye movements during complex scene viewing. *Journal of Experimental Psychology: Human Perception and Performance, 25*(1), 210–228.

Henderson, R. D., Smith, M. C., Podd, J., & Varela-Alvarez, H. (1995). A comparison of the four prominent user-based methods for evaluating the usability of computer software. *Ergonomics, 39*(10), 2030–2044.

Herishanu, Y. O., & Sharpe, J. A. (1981). Normal square wave jerks. *Investigative Ophthalmology & Visual Science, 20*(2), 268–272.

Hernandez, T. (2007). *Understanding eye tracking.* (Available at the Eyetools Website (http://eyetools.com), accessed February 2011.)

Hess, E. H., & Polt, J. M. (1960). Pupil size as related to interest value of visual stimuli. *Science, 132*(3423), 349–350.

Hess, E. H., & Polt, J. M. (1964). Pupil size in relation to mental activity during simple problem-solving. *Science, 143*(3611), 1190–1192.

Heywood, S., & Churcher, J. (1981). Saccades to step-ramp stimuli. *Vision Research, 21*(4), 479–490.

Hills, P., & Argyle, M. (2002). The Oxford Happiness Questionnaire: A compact scale for the measurement of psychological well-being. *Personality and Individual Differences, 33*(7), 1073–1082.

Hirose, Y., Kennedy, A., & Tatler, B. W. (2010). Perception and memory across viewpoint changes in moving images. *Journal of Vision, 10*(4), 1–20.

Ho, G., Scialfa, C. T., Caird, J. K., & Graw, T. (2001). Visual search for traffic signs: The effects of clutter, luminance, and aging. *Human Factors, 43*(2), 194–207.

Holdstock, L., & De Wit, H. (2006). Ethanol impairs saccadic and smooth pursuit eye movements without producing self-reports of sedation. *Alcoholism: Clinical and Experimental Research, 23*(4), 664–672.

Hollingworth, A. (2009). Two forms of scene memory guide visual search: Memory for scene context and memory for the binding of target object to scene location. *Visual Cognition, 17*(1-2), 273–291.

Holm, L. (2007). *Predictive Eyes Precede Retrieval: Visual Recognition as Hypothesis Testing.* Unpublished doctoral dissertation, Umeå University.

Holm, S. (1979). A simple sequentially rejective multiple test procedure. *Scandinavian Journal of Statistics, 6*(2), 65–70.

Holmberg, A. (2007). *Eye Tracking and Gaming Eye Movements in Quake III: Arena.* Unpublished master's thesis, Lund University.

Holmqvist, K., Andrà, C., Lindström, P., Arzarello, F., Ferrara, F., Robutti, O., et al. (2011, May). A method for quantifying focussed vs. overview behaviour in AOI sequences. *Behavior Research Methods,* 1–12.

Holmqvist, K., & Hanson, L. (1999). Are verbal retrospectives primed by eye-movements recordings a better method for evaluating interior design than retrospective from pure video priming? In A. Gale (Ed.), *Proceedings of the Eighth International Conference on Vision in Vehicles.* Amsterdam: Elsevier.

Holmqvist, K., Holsanova, J., Barthelson, M., & Lundqvist, D. (2003). Reading or scanning? A study of newspaper and net paper reading. In J. Hyönä, R. Radach, & H. Deubel (Eds.), *The Mind's Eye: Cognitive and Applied Aspects of Eye Movement Research* (pp. 657–670). Oxford: Elsevier Science.

Holmqvist, K., Nyström, M., & Andersson, R. (2011). *Participants know best: Influence of calibration method on accuracy.* (Poster presented at the 2011 Annual Meeting of the Vision Science Society.)

Holmqvist, K., & Wartenberg, C. (2005). *The role of local design factors for newspaper reading behaviour – an eye-tracking perspective.* (Working Papers, 127, Department of Cognitive Studies, Lund University.)

Holsanova, J. (2001). *Picture Viewing and Picture Description: Two Windows on the Mind.* Unpublished doctoral dissertation, Lund University.

Holsanova, J. (2006). Dynamics of picture viewing and picture description. In L. Albertazzi (Ed.), *Visual Thought. The Depictive Space of the Mind* (pp. 233–254). Amsterdam, Philadelphia: John Benjamins Publishing Company.

Holsanova, J. (2008). *Discourse, Vision, and Cognition.* Amsterdam, Philadelphia: John Benjamins Publishing Company.

Holsanova, J., Holmberg, N., & Holmqvist, K. (2008). Reading information graphics: The role of spatial contiguity and dual attentional guidance. *Applied Cognitive Psychology, 23*(9), 1215–1226.

Holsanova, J., Rahm, H., & Holmqvist, K. (2006). Entry points and reading paths on newspaper spreads: Comparing a semiotic analysis with eye-tracking measurements. *Visual Communication, 5*(1), 65–93.

Holzman, P. S., Proctor, L. R., & Hughes, D. W. (1973). Eye-tracking patterns in schizophrenia. *Science, 181*(95), 179–181.

Hooge, I. T. C., & Camps, G. (2009). *Entropy in scan paths obtained in natural images.* (Paper presented at the 15th European Conference on Eye Movements.)

Hooge, I. T. C., Vlaskamp, B. N. S., & Over, E. A. B. (2007). Saccadic search: On the duration of a fixation. In R. Van Gompel, M. Fischer, W. S. Murray, & R. W. Hill (Eds.), *Eye Movement Research: Insights into Mind and Brain* (pp. 581–595). Oxford: Elsevier.

Hori, Y., Fukuzako, H., Sugimoto, Y., & Takigawa, M. (2002). Eye movements during the Rorschach test in schizophrenia. *Psychiatry and Clinical Neurosciences, 56*(4), 409–418.

Horley, K., Williams, L. M., Gonsalvez, C., & Gordon, E. (2004). Face to face: Visual scanpath evidence for abnormal processing of facial expressions in social phobia. *Psychiatry Research, 127*(1-2), 43–53.

Hornof, A. (2007). Toward an integrated, comprehensive theory of visual search. In W. D. Gray (Ed.), *Integrated Models of Cognition Systems* (pp. 314–324). Oxford: Oxford University Press.

Hornof, A., & Halverson, T. (2002). Cleaning up systematic error in eye-tracking data by using required fixation locations. *Behavior Research Methods, Instruments, & Computers, 34*(4), 592–604.

Horowitz, T. S., Fine, E. M., Fencsik, D. E., Yurgenson, S., & Wolfe, J. M. (2007). Fixational eye movements are not an index of covert attention. *Psychological Science, 18*(4), 356–363.

Horowitz, T. S., & Wolfe, J. M. (2001). Search for multiple targets: Remember the targets, forget the search. *Perception & Psychophysics, 63*(2), 272–285.

Howell, D. C. (2007). *Statistical Methods for Psychology* (sixth ed.). Belmont CA: Wadsworth.

Hubel, D. H., & Wiesel, T. N. (1974). Uniformity of monkey striate cortex: A parallel relationship between field size, scatter, and magnification factor. *Journal of Comparative Neurology, 158*(3), 295–305.

Huettig, F., Rommers, J., & Meyer, A. S. (2011). Using the visual world paradigm to study language processing: A review and critical evaluation. *Acta Psychologica.* (Epub ahead of print.)

Huey, E. B. (1898). Preliminary experiments in the physiology and psychology of reading. *American Journal of Psychology, 9*, 575–586.

Hughes, J., & Parkes, S. (2003). Trends in the use of verbal protocol analysis in software engineering research. *Behaviour & Information Technology, 22*(2), 127–140.

Humphrey, K., & Underwood, G. M. (2008). Fixation sequences in imagery and in recognition during the processing of pictures of real-world scenes. *Journal of Eye Movement Research, 2*(2), 1–15.

Hutton, S. B., & Ettinger, U. (2006). The antisaccade task as a research tool in psychopathology: A critical review. *Psychophysiology, 43*(3), 302–313.

Hyönä, J., Lorch Jr, R. F., & Kaakinen, J. K. (2002). Individual differences in reading to summarize expository text: Evidence from eye fixation patterns. *Journal of Educational Psychology, 94*(1), 44–55.

Hyönä, J., Lorch Jr, R. F., & Rinck, M. (2003). Eye movement measures to study global text processing. In J. Hyönä, R. Radach, & H. Deubel (Eds.), *The Mind's Eye: Cognitive and Applied Aspects of Eye Movement Research* (pp. 313–334). Oxford: Elsevier Science.

Hyönä, J., Tommola, J., & Alaja, A. M. (1995). Pupil dilation as a measure of processing load in simultaneous interpretation and other language tasks. *The Quarterly Journal of Experimental Psychology, 48*(3), 598–612.

Hyrskykari, A. (2006). Utilizing eye movements: Overcoming inaccuracy while tracking the focus of attention during reading. *Computers in Human Behavior, 22*(4), 657–671.

Hyrskykari, A., Ovaska, S., Majaranta, P., Räihä, K.-J., & Lehtinen, M. (2008). Gaze path stimulation in retrospective think-aloud. *Journal of Eye Movement Research, 2*(4), 1–18.

Inamdar, I., & Pomplun, M. (2003). Comparative search reveals the tradeoff between eye movements and working memory use in visual tasks. In R. Alterman & D. Kirsh (Eds.), *Proceedings of the 25th Annual Meeting of the Cognitive Science Society* (pp. 599–604). Mahwah NJ: Lawrence Erlbaum Associates.

Inchingolo, P., & Spanio, M. (1985). On the identification and analysis of saccadic eye movements-A quantitative study of the processing procedures. *IEEE Transactions on Biomedical Engineering, 32*(9), 683–695.

Ingre, M., Åkerstedt, T., Peters, B., Anund, A., & Kecklund, G. (2006). Subjective sleepiness, simulated driving performance and blink duration: Examining individual differences. *Journal of Sleep Research, 15*(1), 47–54.

Inhoff, A. W., & Gordon, A. M. (1997). Eye movements and eye-hand coordination during typing. *Current Directions in Psychological Science, 6*(6), 153–157.

Inhoff, A. W., & Radach, R. (1998). Definition and computation of oculomotor measures in the study of cognitive processes. In G. M. Underwood (Ed.), *Eye Guidance in Reading and Scene Perception* (pp. 29–53). Oxford: Elsevier.

Iqbal, S. T., Zheng, X. S., & Bailey, B. P. (2004). Task-evoked pupillary response to mental workload in human-computer interaction. In *Extended Abstracts on Human Factors in Computing Systems* (pp. 1477–1480).

Irwin, D. E., & Brockmole, J. R. (2004). Suppressing Where but not What: The effect of saccades on dorsal- and ventral-stream visual processing. *Psychological Science, 15*(7), 467–473.

Irwin, H. J., Green, M. J., & Marsh, P. J. (1999). Dysfunction in smooth pursuit eye movements and history of childhood trauma. *Perceptual and Motor Skills, 89*(2), 1230–1236.

Ishizuka, K., Kashiwakura, M., & Oiji, A. (2007). Eye movements in patients with schizophrenia: Visual stimuli, semantic content and psychiatric symptoms. *Acta Psychiatrica Scandinavica, 97*(5), 364–373.

ISO/TS 15007-1. (2002). *Road Vehicles - Measurement of Driver Visual Behaviour with Respect to Transport Information and Control Systems - Part 1: Definitions and Parameters.* International standard, International Organization for Standardization.

ISO/TS 15007-2. (2001). *Road Vehicles - Measurement of Driver Visual Behaviour with Respect to Transport Information and Control Systems - Part 2: Equipment and Procedures.* Technical specification, International Organization for Standardization.

Itoh, K., Hansen, J. P., & Nielsen, F. R. (1998). Cognitive modelling of a ship navigator based on protocol and eye-movement analysis. *Le Travail Humain, 61*(2), 99–127.

Itti, L. (2004). Automatic foveation for video compression using a neurobiological model for visual attention. *IEEE Transactions on Image Processing, 13*(10), 1304–1318.

Itti, L. (2005). Quantifying the contribution of low-level saliency to human eye movements in dynamic scenes. *Visual Cognition, 12*(6), 1093–1123.

Itti, L. (2006). Quantitative modeling of perceptual salience at human eye position. *Visual Cognition, 14*(4-8), 959–984.

Itti, L., & Koch, C. (2000). A saliency-based search mechanism for overt and covert shifts of visual attention. *Vision Research, 40*(10-12), 1489–1506.

Itti, L., & Koch, C. (2001). Computational modelling of visual attention. *Nature Reviews Neuroscience, 2*, 194–203.

Jackson, S. L. (2008). *Research Methods and Statistics: A Critical Thinking Approach.* Belmont CA: Wadsworth.

Jacob, R. (1991). The use of eye movements in human-computer interaction techniques: What you look at is what you get. *ACM Transactions on Information Systems, 9*(2), 152–169.

Jacob, R., & Karn, K. S. (2003). Commentary on Section 4. Eye tracking in human-computer interaction and usability research: Ready to deliver the promises. In J. Hyönä, R. Radach, & H. Deubel (Eds.), *The Mind's Eye: Cognitive and Applied Aspects of Eye Movement Research* (pp. 573–605). Oxford: Elsevier Science.

Jacobsen, O. I. (1941). An analytical study of eye-movements in reading vocal and instrumental music. *Journal of Musicology, 3*(1), 3–32.

Jagla, F., Jergelová, M., & Riecanský, I. (2007). Saccadic eye movement related potentials. *Physiological Research, 56*(6), 707–713.

Jagla, F., Zikmund, V., & Kundrát, J. (1994). Differences in saccadic eye movement related potentials under regular and irregular intervals of visual stimulation. *Physiological Research, 43*(4), 229–232.

Jahnke, J. C. (1965). Primacy and recency effects in serial position curves of immediate recall. *Journal of Experimental Psychology, 70*(1), 130–132.

Jandziol, A. K., Prabhu, M., Carpenter, R. H. S., & Jones, J. G. (2006). Blink duration as a measure of low-level anaesthetic sedation. *European Journal of Anaesthesiology, 18*(7), 476–484.

Janisse, M. P., & Bradley, M. T. (1980). Deception, information and the pupillary response. *Perceptual and Motor Skills, 50*(3), 748–750.

Jansen, A., Nederkoorn, C., & Mulkens, S. (2005). Selective visual attention for ugly and beautiful body parts in eating disorders. *Behaviour Research and Therapy, 43*(2), 183–196.

Jarodzka, H., Balslev, T., Holmqvist, K., Nyström, M., Scheiter, K., Gerjets, P., et al. (2010). Learning perceptual aspects of diagnosis in medicine via eye movement modeling examples on patient video cases. In S. Ohlsson & R. Catrambone (Eds.), *Proceedings of the 32nd Annual Conference of the Cognitive Science Society* (pp. 1703–1708). Austin TX: Cognitive Science Society.

Jarodzka, H., Nyström, M., & Holmqvist, K. (2010). A vector-based, multidimensional scanpath similarity measure. In C. Morimoto & H. Instance (Eds.), *Proceedings of the 2010 Symposium on Eye-Tracking Research & Applications* (pp. 211–218). New York: ACM.

Jarodzka, H., Scheiter, K., Gerjets, P., & Van Gog, T. (2010). In the eyes of the beholder: How experts and novices interpret dynamic stimuli. *Journal of Learning and Instruction, 20*(2), 146–154.

Jarodzka, H., Van Gog, T., Dorr, M., Scheiter, K., & Gerjets, P. (forthcoming). *Guiding attentions guides thought, but what about learning? Eye movements in modeling examples.* (Manuscript submitted for publication.)

Johansson, R., Holmqvist, K., Mossberg, F., & Lindgren, M. (2011). Eye movements and reading comprehension while listening to preferred and non-preferred study music. *Psychology of Music.* (Epub ahead of print.)

Johansson, R., Holsanova, J., & Holmqvist, K. (2005). What do eye movements reveal about mental imagery? Evidence from visual and verbal elicitations. In B. G. Bara, L. Barsalou, & M. Bucciarelli (Eds.), *Proceedings of the 27th Annual Conference of the Cognitive Science Society* (pp. 1054–1059). Mahwah NJ: Lawrence Erlbaum Associates.

Johansson, R., Holsanova, J., & Holmqvist, K. (2006). Pictures and spoken descriptions elicit similar eye movements during mental imagery, both in light and in complete darkness. *Cognitive Science, 30*(6), 1053–1079.

Johansson, R., Johansson, V., Wengelin, Å., & Holmqvist, K. (2008). Reading during writing: Four groups of writers. In J. O. Svantesson (Ed.), *Lund Working Papers* (Vol. 53, pp. 43–59). Department of Linguistics, Lund University.

Johansson, R., Johansson, V., Wengelin, Å., & Holmqvist, K. (2010). Looking at the keyboard or the monitor: Relationship with text production processes. *Reading and Writing, 23*(7), 835–851.

Jordan, J., & Slater, M. (2009). An analysis of eye scanpath entropy in a progressively forming virtual environment. *Presence: Teleoperators and Virtual Environments, 18*(3), 185–199.

Josephson, S., & Holmes, M. E. (2002). Visual attention to repeated internet images: Testing the scanpath theory on the world wide web. In *Proceedings of the 2002 Symposium on Eye-Tracking Research & Applications* (pp. 43–49). New York: ACM.

Josephson, S., & Holmes, M. E. (2006). Clutter or content? How on-screen enhancements affect how TV viewers scan and what they learn. In *Proceedings of the 2006 Symposium on Eye-Tracking Research & Applications* (pp. 155–162). New York: ACM.

Jovancevic-Misic, J., & Hayhoe, M. M. (2009). Adaptive gaze control in natural environments. *Journal of Neuroscience, 29*(19), 6234–6238.

Juday, R. D., & Fisher, T. E. (1989). Geometric transformations for video compression and human teleoperator display. In H.-K. Liu (Ed.), *SPIE Proceedings on Optical Pattern Recognition* (Vol. 1053, pp. 116–123).

Juhasz, B. J., Liversedge, S. P., White, S. J., & Rayner, K. (2006). Binocular coordination of the eyes during reading: Word frequency and case alternation affect fixation duration but not fixation disparity. *The Quarterly Journal of Experimental Psychology, 59*(9), 1614–1625.

Juhola, M. (1988). Detection of nystagmus eye movements using a recursive digital filter. *IEEE Transactions on Biomedical Engineering, 35*(5), 389–395.

Juhola, M., Jäntti, V., & Pyykkö, I. (1985). Effect of sampling frequencies on computation of the maximum velocity of saccadic eye movements. *Biological Cybernetics, 53*(2), 67–72.

Jung, R., & Komhuber, H. H. (1964). Results of electro-nystagmography in man: The value of optokinetic, vestibular, and spontaneous nystagmus for neurologic diagnosis and research. In M. B. Bender (Ed.), *The Oculomotor System* (pp. 428–488). New York: Harper & Row.

Jung, T.-P., Makeig, S., Westerfield, M., Townsend, J., Courchesne, E., & Sejnowski, T. J. (2000). Removal of eye activity artifacts from visual event-related potentials in normal and clinical subjects. *Clinical Neurophysiology, 111*(10), 1745–1758.

Jürgens, R., Becker, W., & Kornhuber, H. H. (1981). Natural and drug-induced variations of velocity and duration of human saccadic eye movements: Evidence for a control of the neural pulse generator by local feedback. *Biological Cybernetics, 39*(2), 87–96.

Just, M. A., & Carpenter, P. A. (1980). A theory of reading: From eye fixations to comprehension. *Psychological Review, 87*(4), 329–354.

Just, M. A., & Carpenter, P. A. (1993). The intensity dimension of thought: Pupillometric indices of sentence processing. *Canadian Journal of Experimental Psychology, 47*(2), 310–339.

Kahneman, D., & Beatty, J. (1966). Pupil diameter and load on memory. *Science, 154*(3756), 1583–1585.

Kammerer, Y. (2009, May). How to overcome the inaccuracy of fixation data – the development and evaluation of an offset correction algorithm. In *The scandinavian workshop on applied eye-tracking (swaet)*. Stavanger, Norway.

Kammerer, Y., Bråten, I., Gerjets, P., & Strømsø, H. (2010). *Internet-specific epistemic beliefs predict users' source monitoring during web search*. Paper presented at the Meeting of the EARLI SIG2 Text and Graphics Comprehension. Tübingen.

Kane, M. J., Bleckley, M. K., Conway, A. R. A., & Engle, R. W. (2001). A controlled-attention view of working-memory capacity. *Journal of Experimental Psychology: General, 130*(2), 169–183.

Kang, M. J., Hsu, M., Krajbich, I. M., Loewenstein, G., McClure, S. M., Wang, J. T., et al. (2009). The Wick in the Candle of Learning. *Psychological Science, 20*(8), 963–973.

Kao, G. W., & Morrow, M. J. (1994). The relationship of anticipatory smooth eye movement to smooth pursuit initiation. *Vision Research, 34*(22), 3027–3036.

Kapoula, Z. A. A. (1984). Aiming precision and characteristics of saccades. *Advances in Psychology, 22*, 123–131.

Kapoula, Z. A. A., Isotalo, E., Elina, Müri, R. M., Bucci, M. P., & Rivaud-Péchoux, S. (2001). Effects of transcranial magnetic stimulation of the posterior parietal cortex on saccades and vergence. *Neuroreport, 12*(18), 4041–4046.

Kapoula, Z. A. A., Robinson, D. A., & Hain, T. C. (1986). Motion of the eye immediately after a saccade. *Experimental Brain Research, 61*(2), 386–394.

Karatekin, C., Marcus, D. J., & White, T. (2007). Oculomotor and manual indexes of incidental and intentional spatial sequence learning during middle childhood and adolescence. *Journal of Experimental Child Psychology, 96*(2), 107–130.

Karn, K. S., Ellis, S., & Juliano, C. (1999). The hunt for usability: Tracking eye movements. In *CHI'99 Extended Abstracts on Human Factors in Computing Systems* (p. 173).

Karpf, D. A. (1973). *Thinking aloud in human discrimination learning*. Unpublished doctoral dissertation, State University of New York.

Karsh, R., & Breitenbach, F. W. (1983). Looking at looking: The amorphous fixation measure. In R. Groner, C. Menz, D. F. Fisher, & R. A. Monty (Eds.), *Eye Movements and Psychological Functions: International Views* (pp. 53–64). Mahwah NJ: Lawrence Erlbaum Associates.

Kasarskis, P., Stehwien, J., Hickox, J. C., Aretz, A., & Wickens, C. D. (2001). Comparison of expert and novice scan behaviors during VFR flight. In *Proceedings of the 11th International Symposium on Aviation Psychology*.

Kenyon, R. V., Ciuffreda, K. J., & Stark, L. (1980). Unequal saccades during vergence. *American Journal of Optometry and Physiological Optics, 57*(9), 586–594.

Khan, S. A., Ford, K. A., Timney, B., & Everling, S. (2003). Effects of ethanol on anti-saccade task performance. *Experimental Brain Research*, *150*(1), 68–74.

Kingstone, A., & Klein, R. M. (1993). Visual offsets facilitate saccadic latency: Does predisengagement of visuospatial attention mediate this gap effect? *Journal of Experimental Psychology: Human Perception and Performance*, *19*(6), 1251–1265.

Kinsler, V., & Carpenter, R. H. S. (1995). Saccadic eye movements while reading music. *Vision Research*, *35*(10), 1447–1458.

Kirchner, H., & Thorpe, S. J. (2006). Ultra-rapid object detection with saccadic eye movements: Visual processing speed revisited. *Vision Research*, *46*(11), 1762–1776.

Kirk, E. P., & Ashcraft, M. H. (2001). Telling stories: The perils and promise of using verbal reports to study math strategies. *Journal of Experimental Psychology: Learning Memory and Cognition*, *27*(1), 157–175.

Kirkby, J. A., Blythe, H. I., Benson, V., & Liversedge, S. P. (2009). Binocular coordination during scanning of simple dot stimuli. *Vision Research*, *50*(2), 171–180.

Klein, R. M., & MacInnes, W. J. (1999). Inhibition of return is a foraging facilitator in visual search. *Psychological Science*, *10*(4), 346–352.

Kleiner, M., Brainard, D., & Pelli, D. (2007). What's new in Psychtoolbox-3? *Perception*, *36*. (ECVP Abstract Supplement.)

Kliegl, R., Nuthmann, A., & Engbert, R. (2006). Tracking the mind during reading: The influence of past, present, and future words on fixation durations. *Journal of Experimental Psychology: General*, *135*(1), 12–35.

Klin, A., Jones, W., Schultz, R., Volkmar, F., & Cohen, D. (2002). Defining and quantifying the social phenotype in autism. *American Journal of Psychiatry*, *159*(6), 895–908.

Klingelhöfer, J., & Conrad, B. (1984). Eye movements during reading in aphasics. *European Archives of Psychiatry and Clinical Neuroscience*, *234*(3), 175–183.

Klingner, J., Kumar, R., & Hanrahan, P. (2008). Measuring the task-evoked pupillary response with a remote eye tracker. In *Proceedings of the 2008 Symposium on Eye-Tracking Research & Applications* (pp. 69–72). New York: ACM.

Kluwe, R. H. (1988). Methoden der Psychologie zur Gewinnung von Daten über menschliches Wissen (Psychological methods for data acquisition on human knowledge). In H. Mandl & H. Spada (Eds.), *Wissenspsychologie* (pp. 359–385). München: Psychologie Verlags Union.

Knoblich, G., Ohlsson, S., & Raney, G. E. (2001). An eye movement study of insight problem solving. *Memory and Cognition*, *29*(7), 1000–1009.

Koga, K., & Groner, R. (1989). Intercultural experiments as a research tool in the study of cognitive skill acquisition: Japanese character recognition and eye movements in non-Japanese subjects. In H. Mandl & J. R. Levin (Eds.), *Knowledge Acquisition from Text and Pictures* (pp. 279–291). Amsterdam: Elsevier Science Publishers.

Koivunen, K., Kukkonen, S., Lahtinen, S., Rantala, H., & Sharmin, S. (2004). Towards deeper understanding of how people perceive design in products. In M. Agger Eriksen, L. Malmborg, & J. Nielsen (Eds.), *Proceedings of the Computers in Art and Design Education Conference*.

Kolakowski, S. M., & Pelz, J. B. (2006). Compensating for eye tracker camera movement. In *Proceedings of the 2006 Symposium on Eye-Tracking Research & Applications* (pp. 79–85). New York: ACM.

Kollmorgen, S., & Holmqvist, K. (2009). *Automatically detecting reading in eye tracking data.* (Working Papers, 144, Department of Cognitive Studies, Lund University.)

Komínková, B., Pedersen, M., Hardeberg, J. Y., & Kaplanová, M. (2008). Comparison of eye tracking devices used on printed images. In B. E. Rogowitz & T. N. Pappas

(Eds.), *SPIE Proceedings on Human Vision and Electronic Imaging XIII* (Vol. 6806, pp. 680611-1–680611-12).

Komogortsev, O. V., Gobert, D., Jayarathna, S., Koh, D. H., & Gowda, S. (2010). Standardization of automated analyses of oculomotor fixation and saccadic behaviors. *IEEE Transactions on Biomedical Engineering*, *57*(11), 2635–2645.

Komogortsev, O. V., & Khan, J. I. (2007). Kalman filtering in the design of eye-gaze-guided computer interfaces. In *Proceedings of the 12th International Conference on Human-Computer Interaction* (pp. 679–689).

Komogortsev, O. V., & Khan, J. I. (2008). Eye movement prediction by Kalman filter with integrated linear horizontal oculomotor plant mechanical model. In *Proceedings of the 2008 Symposium on Eye-Tracking Research & Applications* (pp. 229–236).

Kortum, P., & Geisler, W. S. (1996). Implementation of a foveated image coding system for image bandwidth reduction. In B. E. Rogowitz & J. P. Allebach (Eds.), *SPIE Proceedings on Human Vision and Electronic Imaging I* (Vol. 2657, pp. 350–360).

Kowler, E., & Steinman, R. M. (1977). The role of small saccades in counting. *Vision Research*, *17*(1), 141–146.

Kramer, A. F., & McCarley, J. S. (2003). Oculomotor behaviour as a reflection of attention and memory processes: Neural mechanisms and applications to human factors. *Theoretical Issues in Ergonomics Science*, *4*(1), 21–55.

Kremenitzer, J. P., Vaughan Jr, H. G., Kurtzberg, D., & Dowling, K. (1979). Smooth-pursuit eye movements in the newborn infant. *Child Development*, *50*(2), 442–448.

Krischer, C. C., & Zangemeister, W. H. (2007). Scanpaths in reading and picture viewing: Computer-assisted optimization of display conditions. *Computers in Biology and Medicine*, *37*(7), 947–956.

Krugman, D. M., Foxer, R. J., Fletcher, J. E., Fischer, P. M., & Rojas, T. H. (1994). Do adolescents attend to warnings in cigarette advertising? An eye-tracking approach. *Journal of Advertising Research*, *34*(6), 39–52.

Krupinski, E. A. (1996). Visual scanning patterns of radiologists searching mammograms. *Academic Radiology*, *3*(2), 137–144.

Krupinski, E. A., Berger, W. G., Dallas, W. J., & Roehrig, H. (2003). Searching for nodules: What features attract attention and influence detection? *Academic Radiology*, *10*(8), 861–868.

Krupinski, E. A., & Jiang, Y. (2008). Anniversary paper: Evaluation of medical imaging systems. *Medical Physics*, *35*(2), 645–659.

Kuhn, G., & Tatler, B. W. (2005). Magic and fixation: Now you don't see it, now you do. *Perception*, *34*(9), 1155–1161.

Kuhn, G., Tatler, B. W., & Cole, G. G. (2009). You look where I look! Effect of gaze cues on overt and covert attention in misdirection. *Visual Cognition*, *17*(6), 925–944.

Kuhn, H. W. (1955). The Hungarian method for the assignment problem. *Naval Research Logistics Quarterly*, *2*(1-2), 83–97.

Kumar, M., Klingner, J., Puranik, R., Winograd, T., & Paepcke, A. (2008). Improving the accuracy of gaze input for interaction. In *Proceedings of the 2008 Symposium on Eye-Tracking Research & Applications* (pp. 65–68). New York: ACM.

Kumari, V., & Postma, P. (2005). Nicotine use in schizophrenia: The self medication hypotheses. *Neuroscience & Biobehavioral Reviews*, *29*(6), 1021–1034.

Kundel, H. L., & La Follette Jr, P. S. (1972). Visual search patterns and experience with radiological images. *Radiology*, *103*(3), 523–528.

Kundel, H. L., Nodine, C. F., & Toto, L. C. (1991). Searching for lung nodules: The guidance of visual scanning. *Investigative Radiology*, *26*(9), 777–781.

Kuusela, H., & Paul, P. (2000). A comparison of concurrent and retrospective verbal protocol analysis. *The American Journal of Psychology*, *113*(3), 387–404.

Laeng, B., & Teodorescu, D.-S. (2002). Eye scanpaths during visual imagery reenact those of perception of the same visual scene. *Cognitive Science*, *26*(2), 207–231.

Lam, S. Y., Chau, A. W.-L., & Wong, T. J. (2007). Thumbnails as online product displays: How consumers process them. *Journal of Interactive Marketing*, *21*(1), 36–59.

Land, M. F. (2006). Eye movements and the control of actions in everyday life. *Progress in Retinal and Eye Research*, *25*(3), 296–324.

Land, M. F., & Hayhoe, M. M. (2001). In what ways do eye movements contribute to everyday activities? *Vision Research*, *41*(25-26), 3559–3565.

Land, M. F., & McLeod, P. (2000). From eye movements to actions: How batsmen hit the ball. *Nature Neuroscience*, *3*(12), 1340–1345.

Land, M. F., Mennie, N., & Rusted, J. (1999). The roles of vision and eye movements in the control of activities of daily living: Making a cup of tea. *Perception*, *28*(11), 1311–1328.

Land, M. F., & Tatler, B. W. (2009). *Looking and Acting: Vision and Eye Movements in Natural Behaviour*. Oxford: Oxford University Press.

Larsson, L. (2010). *Event Detection in Eye-Tracking Data*. Unpublished master's thesis, Lund University.

Lau, W. C., Goonetilleke, R. S., & Shih, H. M. (2001). Eye-scan patterns of Chinese when searching full screen menus. In C. Stephanidis (Ed.), *Universal Access in HCI – Towards an Information Society for All* (pp. 367–371). Mahwah NJ: Lawrence Erlbaum Associates.

Lavallière, M., Tremblay, M., Cantin, V., Simoneau, M., & Teasdale, N. (2006). Aging yields a smaller number of fixations and a reduced gaze amplitude when driving in a simulator. *Advances in Transportation Studies*, *special issue*, 21–30.

Laya, O. (1992). Eye movements in actual and simulated curve negotiation tasks. *IATSS Research*, *16*(1), 15–26.

Le, S., Raufaste, E., & Demonet, J.-F. (2003). Processing of normal, inverted, and scrambled faces in a patient with prosopagnosia: Behavioural and eye tracking data. *Cognitive Brain Research*, *17*(1), 26–35.

Lee, R. E., Cohen, G. H., & Boynton, R. M. (1969). Latency variation in human pupil contraction due to stimulus luminance and/or adaptation level. *Journal of the Optical Society of America*, *59*(1), 97–100.

Lee, S. P., Badler, J. B., & Badler, N. I. (2002). Eyes alive. *ACM Transactions on Graphics*, *21*(3), 637–644.

Lehtinen, I., Lang, A. H., Jäntti, V., & Keskinen, E. (1979). Acute effects of alcohol on saccadic eye movements. *Psychopharmacology*, *63*(1), 17–23.

Leigh, R. J., & Zee, D. S. (2006). *The Neurology of Eye Movements*. Oxford: Oxford University Press.

Levenshtein, V. I. (1966). Binary codes capable of correcting deletions, insertions and reversals. In *Soviet Physics Doklady* (Vol. 10, pp. 707–710).

Levin, H., & Kaplan, E. (1970). Grammatical structure and reading. In H. Levin & J. P. Williams (Eds.), *Basic Studies on Reading* (pp. 119–133). New York: Basic Books.

Levy, R., Bicknell, K., Slattery, T., & Rayner, K. (2009). Eye movement evidence that readers maintain and act on uncertainty about past linguistic input. *Proceedings of the National Academy of Sciences*, *106*(50), 21086–21090.

Lewalter, D. (2003). Cognitive strategies for learning from static and dynamic visuals. *Learning and Instruction*, *13*(2), 177–189.

Liao, K., Kumar, A. N., Han, Y. H., Grammer, V. A., Gedeon, B. T., & Leigh, R. J. (2006). Comparison of velocity waveforms of eye and head saccades. *Annals of the New York Academy of Sciences, 1039*, 477–479.

Lienert, G. A., & Raatz, U. (1998). *Testaufbau und Testanalyse*. Weinheim, Germany: Beltz PVU.

Linde, Y., Buzo, A., & Gray, R. (1980). An algorithm for vector quantizer design. *IEEE Transactions on Communications, 28*(1), 84–95.

Lipps, M., & Pelz, J. B. (2004). Yarbus revisited: Task-dependent oculomotor behavior. *Journal of Vision, 4*(8).

Lisberger, S. G., & Westbrook, L. E. (1985). Properties of visual inputs that initiate horizontal smooth pursuit eye movements in monkeys. *Journal of Neuroscience, 5*(6), 1662–1673.

Liu, A. (1998). What the driver's eye tells the car's brain. In G. M. Underwood (Ed.), *Eye Guidance in Reading and Scene Perception* (pp. 431–452). Oxford: Elsevier.

Liversedge, S. P., Paterson, K. B., & Pickering, M. J. (1998). Eye movements and measures of reading time. In G. M. Underwood (Ed.), *Eye Guidance in Reading and Scene Perception*. Oxford: Elsevier.

Liversedge, S. P., Rayner, K., White, S. J., Findlay, J. M., & McSorley, E. (2006). Binocular coordination of the eyes during reading. *Current Biology, 16*(17), 1726–1729.

Liversedge, S. P., White, S. J., Findlay, J. M., & Rayner, K. (2006). Binocular coordination of eye movements during reading. *Vision Research, 46*(15), 2363–2374.

Lobb, M. L., & Stern, J. A. (1986). Pattern of eyelid motion predictive of decision errors during drowsiness: Oculomotor indices of altered states. *International Journal of Neuroscience, 30*(1-2), 17–22.

Locher, P., Unger, R., Sociedade, P., & Wahl, J. (1993). At first glance: Accessibility of the physical attractiveness stereotype. *Sex Roles, 28*(11), 729–743.

Loetscher, T., Bockisch, C. J., & Brugger, P. (2007). Looking for the answer: The mind's eye in number space. *Neuroscience, 151*(3), 725–729.

Loftus, G. R., & Mackworth, N. H. (1978). Cognitive determinants of fixation location during picture viewing. *Journal of Experimental Psychology: Human Perception and Performance, 4*(4), 565–572.

Loomis, J. M. (1978). Lateral masking in foveal and eccentric vision. *Vision Research, 18*(3), 335–338.

Loschky, L. C., McConkie, G. W., Yang, J., & Miller, M. E. (2001). Perceptual effects of a gaze-contingent multi-resolution display based on a model of visual sensitivity. In P. N. Rose (Ed.), *Proceedings of the Fifth Annual Federated Laboratory Symposium on Advanced Displays and Interactive Displays* (pp. 53–58). College Park, MD: Army Research Laboratories.

Loschky, L. C., & Wolverton, G. S. (2007). How late can you update gaze-contingent multi-resolutional displays without detection? *ACM Transactions on Multimedia Computing, Communications and Applications, 3*(4), 1–10.

Loslever, P., Popieul, J. C., & Simon, P. (2007). Using correspondence analysis when the system description yields several transition matrices. Examples with simulated data and real driver-car-environment system data. *Cybernetics and Systems, 38*(1), 23–45.

Loughland, C. M., Williams, L. M., & Gordon, E. (2002). Visual scanpaths to positive and negative facial emotions in an outpatient schizophrenia sample. *Schizophrenia Research, 55*(1-2), 159–170.

Loughland, C. M., Williams, L. M., & Harris, A. W. (2004). Visual scanpath dysfunction in first-degree relatives of schizophrenia probands: Evidence for a vulnerability marker? *Schizophrenia Research, 67*(1), 11–21.

Lowe, R. K. (1999). Extracting information from an animation during complex visual learning. *European Journal of Psychology of Education*, *14*(2), 225–244.

Lowenstein, O., & Lowenfeld, I. E. (1962). The pupil. In H. Davson (Ed.), *The Eye: Vol. 3. Muscular Mechanisms* (pp. 256–329). New York: Academic Press.

Lubow, R. E., & Fein, O. (1996). Pupillary size in response to a visual guilty knowledge test: New technique for the detection of deception. *Journal of Experimental Psychology: Applied*, *2*(2), 164–177.

Luck, S. J. (2005). *An Introduction to the Event-Related Potential Technique*. Cambridge MA: MIT Press.

Luckiesh, M. (1947). Reading and the rate of blinking. *Journal of Experimental Psychology*, *37*(3), 266–268.

Ludwig, C. J. H., & Gilchrist, I. D. (2002). Measuring saccade curvature: A curve-fitting approach. *Behavior Research Methods, Instruments, & Computers*, *34*(4), 618–624.

Ludwig, C. J. H., Gilchrist, I. D., & McSorley, E. (2004). The influence of spatial frequency and contrast on saccade latencies. *Vision Research*, *44*(22), 2597–2604.

Lueck, C. J., Crawford, T. J., Hansen, H. C., & Kennard, C. (1991). Increase in saccadic peak velocity with increased frequency of saccades in man. *Vision Research*, *31*(7-8), 1439–1443.

Lueck, K. L., Mendez, M. F., & Perryman, K. M. (2000). Eye movement abnormalities during reading in patients with Alzheimer disease. *Cognitive and Behavioral Neurology*, *13*(2), 77–82.

Mackworth, N. H. (1965). Visual noise causes tunnel vision. *Psychonomic Science*, *3*(2), 67–68.

Mackworth, N. H., & Bruner, J. S. (1970). How adults and children search and recognize pictures. *Human Development*, *13*(3), 149–177.

Mackworth, N. H., & Morandi, A. J. (1967). The gaze selects informative details within pictures. *Perception & Psychophysics*, *2*(11), 547–552.

Mannan, S. K., Mort, D. J., Hodgson, T. L., Driver, J., Kennard, C., & Husain, M. (2005). Revisiting previously searched locations in visual neglect: Role of right parietal and frontal lesions in misjudging old locations as new. *Journal of Cognitive Neuroscience*, *17*(2), 340–354.

Mannan, S. K., Ruddock, K. H., & Wooding, D. S. (1995). Automatic control of saccadic eye movements made in visual inspection of briefly presented 2-D images. *Spatial Vision*, *9*(3), 363–386.

Mannan, S. K., Ruddock, K. H., & Wooding, D. S. (1996). The relationship between the locations of spatial features and those of fixations made during visual examination of briefly presented images. *Spatial Vision*, *10*(3), 165–188.

Mannan, S. K., Ruddock, K. H., & Wooding, D. S. (1997). Fixation sequences made during visual examination of briefly presented 2D images. *Spatial Vision*, *11*(2), 157–178.

Manor, B. R., & Gordon, E. (2003). Defining the temporal threshold for ocular fixation in free-viewing visuocognitive tasks. *Journal of Neuroscience Methods*, *128*(1-2), 85–93.

Marple-Horvat, D. E., Gilbey, S. L., & Hollands, M. A. (1996). A method for automatic identification of saccades from eye movement recordings. *Journal of Neuroscience Methods*, *67*(2), 191–195.

Marshall, S. (2007). Identifying cognitive state from eye metrics. *Aviation, space, and environmental medicine*, *78*(Supplement 1), B165–B175.

Martinez-Conde, S., & Macknik, S. L. (2007). Windows on the mind. *Scientific American Magazine*, *297*(2), 56–63.

Martinez-Conde, S., Macknik, S. L., & Hubel, D. H. (2000). Microsaccadic eye movements and firing of single cells in the striate cortex of macaque monkeys. *Nature Neuro-*

science, *3*(3), 251–258.

Martinez-Conde, S., Macknik, S. L., & Hubel, D. H. (2004). The role of fixational eye movements in visual perception. *Nature Reviews Neuroscience*, *5*(3), 229–240.

Martinez-Conde, S., Macknik, S. L., Troncoso, X. G., & Dyar, T. A. (2006). Microsaccades counteract visual fading during fixation. *Neuron*, *49*(2), 297–305.

Martinez-Conde, S., Macknik, S. L., Troncoso, X. G., & Hubel, D. H. (2009). Microsaccades: A neurophysiological analysis. *Trends in Neurosciences*, *32*(9), 463–475.

Mather, J. A., & Putchat, C. (1983). Motor control of schizophrenics–I. Oculomotor control of schizophrenics: A deficit in sensory processing, not strictly in motor control. *Journal of Psychiatric Research*, *17*(4), 343–360.

Maxwell, G. F., Lemij, H. G., & Collewijn, H. (1995). Conjugacy of saccades in deep amblyopia. *Investigative Ophthalmology & Visual Science*, *36*(12), 2514–2522.

May, J. G., Kennedy, R. S., Williams, M. C., Dunlap, W. P., & Brannan, J. R. (1990). Eye movement indices of mental workload. *Acta Psychologica*, *75*(1), 75–89.

McBurney, D., & White, T. L. (2007). *Research Methods*. Belmont CA: Wadsworth.

McCarley, J. S., Kramer, A. F., Wickens, C. D., Vidoni, E. D., & Boot, W. R. (2004). Visual skills in airport-security screening. *Psychological Science*, *15*(5), 302–306.

McCarthy, A., Lee, K., Itakura, S., & Muir, D. W. (2006). Cultural display rules drive eye gaze during thinking. *Journal of Cross-Cultural Psychology*, *37*(6), 717–722.

McCarthy, A., Lee, K., Itakura, S., & Muir, D. W. (2008). Gaze display when thinking depends on culture and context. *Journal of Cross-Cultural Psychology*, *39*(6), 716–729.

McConkie, G. (1981). Evaluating and reporting data quality in eye movement research. *Behavior Research Methods*, *13*(2), 97–106.

McConkie, G. W., Kerr, P. W., Reddix, M. D., & Zola, D. (1988). Eye movement control during reading: I. The location of initial eye fixations on words. *Vision Research*, *28*(10), 1107–1118.

McConkie, G. W., Kerr, P. W., Reddix, M. D., Zola, D., & Jacobs, A. M. (1989). Eye movement control during reading: II. Frequency of refixating a word. *Perception & Psychophysics*, *46*(3), 245–253.

McConkie, G. W., & Loschky, L. C. (2002). Perception onset time during fixations in free viewing. *Behavior Research Methods, Instruments, & Computers*, *34*(4), 481–490.

McConkie, G. W., & Rayner, K. (1975). The span of the effective stimulus during a fixation in reading. *Perception & Psychophysics*, *17*(6), 578–586.

McConkie, G. W., Reddix, M. D., & Zola, D. (1992). Perception and cognition in reading: Where is the meeting point? In V. Zikmund (Ed.), *Eye Movements and Visual Cognition: Scene Perception and Reading* (pp. 293–303). New York: Springer-Verlag.

McGregor, D. K., & Stern, J. A. (1996). Time on task and blink effects on saccade duration. *Ergonomics*, *39*(4), 649–660.

McLaughlin, S. C. (1967). Parametric adjustment in saccadic eye movements. *Perception & Psychophysics*, *2*(8), 359–362.

McNamara, D. S. (2004). SERT: Self-explanation reading training. *Discourse Processes*, *38*(1), 1–30.

McNamara, D. S., O'Reilly, T., Rowe, M., Boonthum, C., & Levinstein, I. B. (2007). iSTART: A web-based tutor that teaches self-explanation and metacognitive reading strategies. In D. S. McNamara (Ed.), *Reading Comprehension Strategies: Theories, Interventions, and Technologies* (pp. 397–421). Mahwah NJ: Lawrence Erlbaum Associates.

Megaw, E. D., & Richardson, J. (1979). Eye movements and industrial inspection. *Applied Ergonomics*, *10*(3), 145–154.

Mello-Thoms, C., Hardesty, L., Sumkin, J., Ganott, M., Hakim, C., Britton, C., et al. (2005). Effects of lesion conspicuity on visual search in mammogram reading. *Academic Radiology*, *12*(7), 830–840.

Memmert, D. (2006). The effects of eye movements, age, and expertise on inattentional blindness. *Consciousness and Cognition*, *15*(3), 620–627.

Mennie, N., Hayhoe, M. M., & Sullivan, B. T. (2007). Look-ahead fixations: Anticipatory eye movements in natural tasks. *Experimental Brain Research*, *179*(3), 427–442.

Meyer, A. S., & Lethaus, F. (2004). The use of eye tracking in studies of sentence generation. In J. M. Henderson & F. Ferreira (Eds.), *The Interface of Language, Vision, and Action: Eye Movements and the Visual World* (pp. 191–211). New York: Psychology Press.

Meyer, A. S., Sleiderink, A. M., & Levelt, W. J. M. (1998). Viewing and naming objects: Eye movements during noun phrase production. *Cognition*, *66*(2), B25–B33.

Meyer, C. H., Lasker, A. G., & Robinson, D. A. (1985). The upper limit of human smooth pursuit velocity. *Vision Research*, *25*(4), 561–563.

Miall, R. C., & Tchalenko, J. (2001). A painter's eye movements: A study of eye and hand movement during portrait drawing. *Leonardo*, *34*(1), 35–40.

Miellet, S., Lingnan, H., Matthew, P., Rodger, H., & Caldara, R. (2009). Investigating cultural diversity for extrafoveal information use in scenes. In S. P. Liversedge (Ed.), *Proceedings of the 15th European Conference on Eye Movements* (pp. 1–18).

Miles, W. R. (1929). Ocular dominance demonstrated by unconscious sighting. *Journal of Experimental Psychology*, *12*(2), 113–126.

Mirman, D., Dixon, J., & Magnuson, J. S. (2008). Statistical and computational models of the visual world paradigm: Growth curves and individual differences. *Journal of Memory and Language*, *59*(4), 475–494.

Miura, T. (1990). Active function of eye movement and useful field of view in a realistic setting. In R. Groner, G. D'Ydewalle, & R. Parham (Eds.), *From Eye to Mind: Information Acquisition in Perception, Search, and Reading* (pp. 119–127). Amsterdam: Elsevier Science Publishers.

Miura, T. (1992). Visual search in intersections. *IATSS Research*, *16*(1), 42–49.

Møller, F., Laursen, M., Tygesen, J., & Sjølie, A. (2002). Binocular quantification and characterization of microsaccades. *Graefe's Archive for Clinical and Experimental Ophthalmology*, *240*(9), 765–770.

Montes-Mico, R., Alio, J. L., & Charman, W. N. (2005). Dynamic changes in the tear film in dry eyes. *Investigative ophthalmology & visual science*, *46*(5), 1615–1619.

Montfoort, I., Frens, M. A., Hooge, I. T. C., Lagers-Van Haselen, G. C., & Van Der Geest, J. N. (2007). Visual search deficits in Williams-Beuren syndrome. *Neuropsychologia*, *45*(5), 931–938.

Moraal, J. (1975). The analysis of an inspection task in the steel industry. In C. G. Drury & J. G. Fox (Eds.), *Human Reliability in Quality Control* (pp. 217–230). London: Taylor & Francis.

Moray, N., & Rotenberg, I. (1989). Fault management in process control: Eye movements and action. *Ergonomics*, *32*(11), 1319–1342.

Morisita, M., & Yagi, T. (2001). The stability of human eye orientation during visual fixation and imagined fixation in three dimensions. *Auris Nasus Larynx*, *28*(4), 301–304.

Moriyama, T., Kanade, T., Cohn, J. F., Xiao, J., Ambadar, Z., Gao, J., et al. (2002). Automatic recognition of eye blinking in spontaneously occurring behavior. In *IEEE Proceedings of the 16th International Conference on Pattern Recognition* (pp. 78–81).

Moriyama, T., Xiao, J., Cohn, J. F., & Kanade, T. (2006). Meticulously detailed eye model and its application to analysis of facial image. *IEEE Transactions on Pattern Analysis and Machine Intelligence*, *28*(1), 738–752.

Morris, T. L. (1984). *Electrooculographic Measurement, Fatigue and Variability of Performance in Simulated Aircraft Flight.* Unpublished doctoral dissertation, Texas A&M University, College Station.

Morris, T. L., & Miller, J. C. (1996). Electrooculographic and performance indices of fatigue during simulated flight. *Biological Psychology, 42*(3), 343–360.

Morrison, J. G., Marshall, S. P., Kelly, R. T., & Moore, R. A. (1997). Eye tracking in tactical decision making environments: Implications for decision support evaluation. In *Proceedings of the Third International Command and Control Research and Technology Symposium* (pp. 355–364).

Morrow, M. J., & Sharpe, J. A. (1993). Smooth pursuit initiation in young and elderly subjects. *Vision Research, 33*(2), 203–210.

Morrow, M. J., & Sharpe, J. A. (1995). Deficits of smooth-pursuit eye movement after unilateral frontal lobe lesions. *Annals of Neurology, 37*(4), 443–451.

Mortimer, R. G., & Jorgeson, C. M. (1974). *Eye fixations of drivers in night driving with three headlight beams* (Tech. Rep. No. UM-HSRI-HF7-4-1). Highway Safety Research Institute, University of Michigan.

Morton, H. B., & Cobb, W. A. (1973). The effect of eye movements on visual evoked responses in man. In V. Zikmund (Ed.), *The Oculomotor System and Brain Functions* (pp. 105–115). London: Butterworths.

Moschner, C., & Baloh, R. W. (1994). Age-related changes in visual tracking. *The Journal of Gerontology, 49*(5), M235.

Moschner, C., Crawford, T. J., Heide, W., Trillenberg, P., Kompf, D., & Kennard, C. (1999). Deficits of smooth pursuit initiation in patients with degenerative cerebellar lesions. *Brain, 122*(11), 2147–2158.

Moser, A., Heide, W., & Kömpf, D. (1998). The effect of oral ethanol consumption on eye movements in healthy volunteers. *Journal of Neurology, 245*(8), 542–550.

Mosimann, U. P., Muri, R. M., Felblinger, J., & Radanov, B. P. (2000). Saccadic eye movement disturbances in whiplash patients with persistent complaints. *Brain, 123*(4), 828–835.

Moskowitz, H., Ziedman, K., & Sharma, S. (1976). Visual search behaviour while viewing driving scenes under the influence of alcohol and marijuana. *Human Factors, 18*(5), 417–432.

Mossfeldt, L., & Tillander, J. (2005). *Design and Implementation of a Region of Interest Analysis System for Eye-Tracking Studies.* Unpublished master's thesis, Lund University.

Motter, B. C., & Belky, E. J. (1998). The guidance of eye movements during active visual search. *Vision Research, 38*(12), 1805–1815.

Mourant, R. R., & Rockwell, T. H. (1970). Mapping eye-movement patterns to the visual scene in driving: An exploratory study. *Human Factors, 12*(1), 81–87.

Mourant, R. R., & Rockwell, T. H. (1972). Strategies of visual search by novice and experienced drivers. *Human Factors, 14*(4), 325–335.

Mourant, R. R., Rockwell, T. H., & Rackoff, N. J. (1969). Drivers' eye movements and visual workload. In *Highway Research Record* (Vol. 292). Washington DC: National Academy Press.

Mullin, J., Anderson, A. H., Smallwood, L., Jackson, M., & Katsavras, E. (2001). Eye-tracking explorations in multimedia communications. In A. Blandford, J. Vanderdonckt, & P. Gray (Eds.), *Proceedings of IHM/HCI 2001: People and Computers XV – Interaction without Frontiers* (pp. 367–382). Cambridge: Cambridge University Press.

Munn, S. M., Stefano, L., & Pelz, J. B. (2008). Fixation-identification in dynamic scenes: Comparing an automated algorithm to manual coding. In *Proceedings of the 5th Sym-*

posium on Applied Perception in Graphics and Visualization (pp. 33–42). New York: ACM.

Munoz, D. P., & Everling, S. (2004). Look away: The anti-saccade task and the voluntary control of eye movement. *Nature Reviews Neuroscience, 5*(3), 218–228.

Müri, R. M., Hess, C. W., & Pierrot-Deseilligny, C. (2005). Eye movements. In M. Hallett & S. Chokroverty (Eds.), *Magnetic Stimulation in Clinical Neurophysiology* (second ed., pp. 349–363). Philadelphia: Butterworth-Heinemann.

Muri, R. M., Vermersch, A. I., Rivaud, S., Gaymard, B., & Pierrot-Deseilligny, C. (1996). Effects of single-pulse transcranial magnetic stimulation over the prefrontal and posterior parietal cortices during memory-guided saccades in humans. *Journal of Neurophysiology, 76*(3), 2102–2106.

Murray, W. S., & Kennedy, A. (1988). Spatial coding in the processing of anaphor by good and poor readers: Evidence from eye movement analyses. *The Quarterly Journal of Experimental Psychology, 40*(4), 693–718.

Myers, C. W., & Schoelles, M. J. (2005). ProtoMatch: A tool for analyzing high-density, sequential eye gaze and cursor protocols. *Behavior Research Methods, 37*(2), 256–270.

Nakayama, M., Takahashi, K., & Shimizu, Y. (2002). The act of task difficulty and eye-movement frequency for the 'Oculo-motor indices'. In *Proceedings of the 2002 Symposium on Eye-Tracking Research & Applications* (pp. 37–42). New York: ACM.

Needleman, S. B., & Wunsch, C. D. (1970). A general method applicable to the search for similarities in the amino acid sequence of two proteins. *Journal of Molecular Biology, 48*(3), 443–453.

Neggers, S. F. W., Huijbers, W., Vrijlandt, C. M., Vlaskamp, B. N. S., Schutter, D. J. L. G., & Kenemans, J. L. (2007). TMS pulses on the frontal eye fields break coupling between visuo-spatial attention and eye movements. *Journal of Neurophysiology, 98*(5), 2765–2778.

Nelson, W. W., & Loftus, G. R. (1980). The functional visual field during picture viewing. *Journal of Experimental Psychology: Human Learning and Memory, 6*(4), 391–399.

Nevalainen, S., & Sajaniemi, J. (2004). Comparison of three eye tracking devices in psychology of programming research. In *Proceedings of the 16th Annual Workshop of the Psychology of Programming Interest Group* (pp. 151–158).

Newsham, D., Knox, P. C., & Cooke, R. W. I. (2007). Oculomotor control in children who were born very prematurely. *Investigative Ophthalmology & Visual Science, 48*(6), 2595–2601.

Nielsen, J. (2006). *F-shaped pattern for reading web content.* (Text available at the author's website (www.useit.com/alertbox/reading_pattern.html), accessed May 2011.)

Nielsen, J., Clemmensen, T., & Yssing, C. (2002). Getting access to what goes on in people's heads? Reflections on the think-aloud technique. In *Proceedings of the Second Nordic Conference on Human-Computer Interaction* (pp. 101–110). New York: ACM.

Niemenlehto, P. H. (2009). Constant false alarm rate detection of saccadic eye movements in electro-oculography. *Computer Methods and Programs in Biomedicine, 96*(2), 158–171.

Nijs, I. M. T., Muris, P., Euser, A. S., & Franken, I. H. A. (2009). Differences in attention to food and food intake between overweight/obese and normal-weight females under conditions of hunger and satiety. *Appetite, 54*(2), 243–254.

Nodine, C. F., Kundel, H. L., Lauver, S. C., & Toto, L. C. (1996). Nature of expertise in searching mammograms for breast masses. *Academic Radiology, 3*(12), 1000–1006.

Nodine, C. F., Locher, P., & Krupinski, E. A. (1993). The role of formal art training on perception and aesthetic judgment of art compositions. *Leonardo, 26*(3), 219–227.

Nordh, H. (2010). *Restorative Components of Small Urban Parks*. Unpublished doctoral dissertation, Norwegian University of Life Sciences.

Nordqvist, S. (1990). *Kackel i Grönsakslandet*. Bromma: Opal.

Noton, D., & Stark, L. (1971a). Scanpaths in eye movements during pattern perception. *Science*, *171*(3968), 308–311.

Noton, D., & Stark, L. (1971b). Scanpaths in saccadic eye movements while viewing and recognizing patterns. *Vision Research*, *11*(9), 929–942.

Nummenmaa, L., Hyönä, J., & Calvo, M. G. (2008). Do emotional scenes catch the eye? In K. Rayner, D. Shen, X. Bai, & G. Yan (Eds.), *Cognitive and Cultural Influences on Eye Movements*. New York: Psychology Press.

Nuthmann, A., & Kliegl, R. (2009). An examination of binocular reading fixations based on sentence corpus data. *Journal of Vision*, *9*(5), 1–28.

Nyström, M. (2008). *Offline Foveated Compression and Scene Perception: An Eye-Tracking Approach*. Unpublished doctoral dissertation, Lund University.

Nyström, M., & Holmqvist, K. (2008). Semantic override of low-level features in image viewing – both initially and overall. *Journal of Eye Movement Research*, *2*(2), 2:1–2:11.

Nyström, M., & Holmqvist, K. (2010). An adaptive algorithm for fixation, saccade, and glissade detection in eye-tracking data. *Behavior Research Methods*, *42*(1), 188–204.

Nyström, M., Novak, M., & Holmqvist, K. (2004). A novel approach to image coding using off-line foveation controlled by multiple eye-tracking measurements. In *Proceedings of the Picture Coding Symposium*.

O'Brien, S. (2006). *Investigating translation from an eye-tracking perspective*. (Paper presented at the Second Conference of the International Association for Translation and Intercultural Studies.)

Obrist, M., Bernhaupt, R., Beck, E., & Tscheligi, M. (2007). Focusing on elderly: An iTV usability evaluation study with eye-tracking. In P. Cesar, K. Chorianopoulos, & J. F. Jensen (Eds.), *Interactive TV: A Shared Experience* (pp. 66–75). Berlin, Heidelberg: Springer-Verlag.

O'Driscoll, G. A., & Callahan, B. L. (2008). Smooth pursuit in schizophrenia: A meta-analytic review of research since 1993. *Brain and Cognition*, *68*(3), 359–370.

Ohtani, A. (1971). An analysis of eye movements during a visual task. *Ergonomics*, *14*(1), 167–174.

Olincy, A., Ross, R. G., Young, D. A., Roath, M., & Freedman, R. (1998). Improvement in smooth pursuit eye movements after cigarette smoking in schizophrenic patients. *Neuropsychopharmacology*, *18*(3), 175–185.

Oliveira, F. T. P., Aula, A., & Russell, D. M. (2009). Discriminating the relevance of web search results with measures of pupil size. In *Proceedings of the 27th International Conference on Human Factors in Computing Systems* (pp. 2209–2212).

Olsson, P. (2007). *Real-time and offline filters for eye tracking*. Unpublished master's thesis, Royal Institute of Technology, Stockholm, Sweden.

Onat, S., Libertus, K., & König, P. (2007). Integrating audiovisual information for the control of overt attention. *Journal of Vision*, *7*(10), 1–16.

Oster, P. J., & Stern, J. A. (1980). Measurement of eye movement. In J. Martin & P. H. Venables (Eds.), *Techniques of Psychophysiology* (pp. 275–308). New York: John Wiley & Sons.

Otero-Millan, J., Troncoso, X. G., Macknik, S. L., Serrano-Pedraza, I., & Martinez-Conde, S. (2008). Saccades and microsaccades during visual fixation, exploration and search: Foundations for a common saccadic generator. *Journal of Vision*, *8*, 14–21.

Ottati, W. L., Hickox, J. C., & Richter, J. (1999). Eye scan patterns of experienced and novice pilots during visual flight rules (VFR) navigation. In *Proceedings of the 43rd Annual Meeting of the Human Factors and Ergonomics Society*.

Ouerhani, N., Von Wartburg, R., Hügli, H., & Müri, R. M. (2003). Empirical validation of the saliency-based model of visual attention. *Electronic Letters on Computer Vision and Image Analysis*, *3*(1), 13–24.

Over, E. A. B., Hooge, I. T. C., & Erkelens, C. J. (2006). A quantitative measure for the uniformity of fixation density: The Voronoi method. *Behavior Research Methods*, *38*(2), 251–261.

Over, E. A. B., Hooge, I. T. C., Vlaskamp, B. N. S., & Erkelens, C. J. (2007). Coarse-to-fine eye movement strategy in visual search. *Vision Research*, *47*(17), 2272–2280.

Pan, B., Hembrooke, H. A., Gay, G., Granka, L. A., Feusner, M., & Newman, J. K. (2004). The determinants of web page viewing behavior: An eye-tracking study. In *Proceedings of the 2004 Symposium on Eye-Tracking Research & Applications* (pp. 147–154). New York: ACM.

Papenmeier, F., & Huff, M. (2010). DynAOI – A tool for matching eye movement data with dynamic areas of interest in animations and movies. *Behavior Research Methods*, *42*(1), 179–187.

Parkhurst, D. J., & Niebur, E. (2002). Variable-resolution displays: A theoretical, practical, and behavioral evaluation. *Human Factors*, *44*(4), 611–629.

Parkhurst, D. J., & Niebur, E. (2003). Scene content selected by active vision. *Spatial Vision*, *16*(2), 125–154.

Partala, T., & Surakka, V. (2003). Pupil size variation as an indication of affective processing. *International Journal of Human-Computer Studies*, *59*(1-2), 185–198.

Patel, S., Henderson, R., Bradley, L., Galloway, B., & Hunter, L. (1991). Effect of visual display unit use on blink rate and tear stability. *Optometry & Vision Science*, *68*(11), 888–892.

Patla, A. E., & Vickers, J. N. (2003). How far ahead do we look when required to step on specific locations in the travel path during locomotion? *Experimental Brain Research*, *148*(1), 133–138.

Paus, T., Marrett, S., Worsley, K. J., & Evans, A. C. (1995). Extraretinal modulation of cerebral blood flow in the human visual cortex: Implications for saccadic suppression. *Journal of Neurophysiology*, *74*(5), 2179–2183.

Peebles, D., & Cheng, P. C.-H. (2002). Extending task analytic models of graph-based reasoning: A cognitive model of problem solving with Cartesian graphs in ACT-R/PM. *Cognitive Systems Research*, *3*(1), 77–86.

Peirce, J. W. (2007). PsychoPy - psychophysics software in Python. *Journal of Neuroscience Methods*, *162*(1-2), 8–13.

Pelli, D. G. (1997). The VideoToolbox software for visual psychophysics: Transforming numbers into movies. *Spatial Vision*, *10*(4), 437–442.

Pelz, J. B., & Canosa, R. (2001). Oculomotor behavior and perceptual strategies in complex tasks. *Vision Research*, *41*(25-26), 3587–3596.

Pelz, J. B., Canosa, R., Babcock, J., & Barber, J. (2001). Visual perception in familiar, complex tasks. In *Proceedings of the 2001 International Conference on Image Processing* (Vol. 2, pp. 12–15).

Pernice, K., & Nielsen, J. (2009). *Eyetracking methodology - how to conduct and evaluate usability studies using eyetracking*. Berkeley, CA: New Riders Press.

Peterson, M. S., Kramer, A. F., Wang, R. F., Irwin, D. E., & McCarley, J. S. (2001). Visual search has memory. *Psychological Science*, *12*(4), 287–292.

Petrie, H., & Harrison, C. (2009). Measuring users' emotional reactions to websites. In *Proceedings of the 27th International Conference Extended Abstracts on Human Factors in Computing Systems* (pp. 3847–3852).

Pflugshaupt, T., Mosimann, U. P., Schmitt, W. J., Von Wartburg, R., Wurtz, P., Lüthi, M., et al. (2007). To look or not to look at threat? Scanpath differences within a group of spider phobics. *Journal of Anxiety Disorders, 21*(3), 353–366.

Phillips, M. H., & Edelman, J. A. (2008). The dependence of visual scanning performance on search direction and difficulty. *Vision Research, 48*(21), 2184–2192.

Piccoli, B., Soci, G., Zambelli, P. L., & Pisaniello, D. (2004). Photometry in the workplace: The rationale for a new method. *Annals of Occupational Hygiene, 48*(1), 29–38.

Pieters, R., Rosbergen, E., & Hartog, M. (1996). Visual attention to advertising: The impact of motivation and repetition. *Advances in Consumer Research, 23*, 242–248.

Pieters, R., Rosbergen, E., & Wedel, M. (1999). Visual attention to repeated print advertising: A test of scanpath theory. *Journal of Marketing Research, 36*(4), 424–438.

Pieters, R., & Wedel, M. (2004). Attention capture and transfer in advertising: Brand, pictorial, and text-size effects. *Journal of Marketing, 68*(2), 36–50.

Poldrack, R. A. (2006). Can cognitive processes be inferred from neuroimaging data? *Trends in Cognitive Sciences, 10*(2), 59–63.

Pollatsek, A., & Hyönä, J. (2005). The role of semantic transparency in the processing of Finnish compound words. *Language and Cognitive Processes, 20*(1), 261–290.

Polunin, O., Holmqvist, K., & Johansson, R. (2008). The time line is mapped onto the visual field. *International Journal of Psychology, 43*(3-4), 610.

Pomplun, M., Ritter, H., & Velichkovsky, B. M. (1996). Disambiguating complex visual information: Towards communication of personal views of a scene. *Perception, 25*(8), 931–948.

Pomplun, M., & Sunkara, S. (2003). Pupil dilation as an indicator of cognitive workload in human-computer interaction. In V. D. D. Harris, M. Smith, & C. Stephanidis (Eds.), *Proceedings of the 10th International Conference on Human-Computer Interaction* (pp. 542–546).

Ponsoda, V., Scott, D., & Findlay, J. M. (1995). A probability vector and transition matrix analysis of eye movements during visual search. *Acta Psychologica, 88*(2), 167–185.

Poole, A. (2003). *Issues of Saliency and Recognition in the Search for Web Page Bookmarks.* Unpublished master's thesis, Lancaster University.

Poole, A., & Ball, L. J. (2005). Eye tracking in human-computer interaction and usability research: Current status and future prospects. In C. Gahoui (Ed.), *Encyclopedia of Human-Computer Interaction.* Hersey PA: Idea Group Reference.

Poole, A., Ball, L. J., & Phillips, P. (2004). In search of salience: A response time and eye movement analysis of bookmark recognition. In S. Fincher, P. Markopolous, D. Moore, & R. Ruddle (Eds.), *Proceedings of HCI conference on People and Computers XVIII* (pp. 19–26). London: Springer-Verlag.

Port, N. L., & Wurtz, R. H. (2003). Sequential activity of simultaneously recorded neurons in the superior colliculus during curved saccades. *Journal of Neurophysiology, 90*(3), 1887–1903.

Posner, M. I. (1980). Orienting of attention. *The Quarterly Journal of Experimental Psychology, 32*(1), 3–25.

Posner, M. I., & Cohen, Y. (1984). Components of visual orienting. In H. Bouma & D. Bouwhuis (Eds.), *Attention and Performance X: Control of Language Processes* (pp. 531–556). Mahwah NJ: Lawrence Erlbaum Associates.

Posner, M. I., Rafal, R. D., Choate, L. S., & Vaughan, J. (1985). Inhibition of return: Neural basis and function. *Cognitive Neuropsychology, 2*(3), 211–228.

Preparata, F. P., & Hong, S. J. (1977). Convex hulls of finite sets of points in two and three dimensions. *Communications of the ACM, 20*(2), 87–93.

Pressley, M., & Afflerbach, P. (1995). *Verbal Protocols of Reading: The Nature of Constructively Responsive Reading*. Hillsdale, NJ: Lawrence Erlbaum Associates.

Priori, A., Bertolasi, L., Rothwell, J. C., Day, B. L., & Marsden, C. D. (1993). Some saccadic eye movements can be delayed by transcranial magnetic stimulation of the cerebral cortex in man. *Brain, 116*(2), 355–367.

Privitera, C. M. (2006). The scanpath theory: Its definition and later developments. In B. E. Rogowitz, T. N. Pappas, & S. Daly (Eds.), *SPIE Proceedings on Human Vision and Electronic Imaging XI* (Vol. 6057, pp. 87–91).

Privitera, C. M., & Stark, L. (2000). Algorithms for defining visual regions of interest: Comparison with eye fixations. *IEEE Transactions on Pattern Analysis and Machine Intelligence, 22*(9), 970–982.

Radant, A. D., & Hommer, D. (1992). A quantitative analysis of saccades and smooth pursuit during visual pursuit tracking: A comparison of schizophrenics with normals and substance abusing controls. *Schizophrenia Research, 6*(3), 225–235.

Rajashekar, U., Cormack, L. K., & Bovik, A. C. (2004). Point of gaze analysis reveals visual search strategies. In B. E. Rogowitz & T. N. Pappas (Eds.), *SPIE Proceedings on Human Vision and Electronic Imaging IX* (Vol. 5292, pp. 296–306).

Rajashekar, U., Van Der Linde, I., Bovik, A. C., & Cormack, L. K. (2008). GAFFE: A gaze-attentive fixation finding engine. *IEEE Transactions on Image Processing, 17*(4), 564–573.

Rambold, H., Sprenger, A., & Helmchen, C. (2002). Effects of voluntary blinks on saccades, vergence eye movements, and saccade-vergence interactions in humans. *Journal of Neurophysiology, 88*(3), 1220–1233.

Rantanen, E. M., & Goldberg, J. H. (1999). The effect of mental workload on the visual field size and shape. *Ergonomics, 42*(6), 816–834.

Rao, R. P. N., Zelinsky, G. J., Hayhoe, M. M., & Ballard, D. H. (2002). Eye movements in iconic visual search. *Vision Research, 42*(11), 1447–1463.

Rascol, O., Sabatini, U., Simonetta-Moreau, M., Montastruc, J. L., Rascol, A., & Clanet, M. (1991). Square wave jerks in Parkinsonian syndromes. *British Medical Journal, 54*(7), 599–602.

Rayner, K. (1978). Eye movements in reading and information processing. *Psychological Bulletin, 85*(3), 618–660.

Rayner, K. (1985). Do faulty eye movements cause dyslexia? *Developmental Neuropsychology, 1*(1), 3–15.

Rayner, K. (1998). Eye movements in reading and information processing: 20 years of research. *Psychological Bulletin, 124*(3), 372–422.

Rayner, K., Castelhano, M. S., & Yang, J. (2009). Eye movements when looking at unusual/weird scenes: Are there cultural differences? *Journal of Experimental Psychology: Learning, Memory and Cognition, 35*(1), 254–259.

Rayner, K., & Fischer, M. (1996). Mindless reading revisited: Eye movements during reading and scanning are different. *Perception & Psychophysics, 58*(5), 734–747.

Rayner, K., Li, X., Williams, C. C., Cave, K. R., & Well, A. D. (2007). Eye movements during information processing tasks: Individual differences and cultural effects. *Vision Research, 47*(21), 2714–2726.

Rayner, K., & Pollatsek, A. (1989). *The Psychology of Reading*. Englewood Cliffs, NJ: Prentice Hall.

Rayner, K., & Pollatsek, A. (1997). Eye movements, the eye-hand span, and the perceptual span during sight-reading of music. *Current Directions in Psychological Science, 6*(2),

49–53.

Rayner, K., Pollatsek, A., Drieghe, D., Slattery, T. J., & Reichle, E. D. (2007). Tracking the mind during reading via eye movements: Comments on Kliegl, Nuthmann, and Engbert (2006). *Journal of Experimental Psychology: General*, *136*(3), 520–529.

Rayner, K., Reichle, E. D., Stroud, M. J., Williams, C. C., & Pollatsek, A. (2006). The effect of word frequency, word predictability, and font difficulty on the eye movements of young and older readers. *Psychology and Aging*, *21*(3), 448–465.

Rayner, K., & Well, A. D. (1996). Effects of contextual constraint on eye movements in reading: A further examination. *Psychonomic Bulletin & Review*, *3*(4), 504–509.

Recarte, M. A., & Nunes, L. M. (2000). Effects of verbal and spatial imagery tasks on eye fixations while driving. *Journal of Experimental Psychology: Applied*, *6*, 31–43.

Recarte, M. A., & Nunes, L. M. (2003). Mental workload while driving: Effects on visual search, discrimination, and decision making. *Journal of Experimental Psychology: Applied*, *9*(2), 119–137.

Reder, S. M. (1973). On-line monitoring of eye position signals in contingent and noncontingent paradigms. *Behavior Research Methods & Instrumentation*, *5*, 218–228.

Reichle, E. D., Rayner, K., & Pollatsek, A. (2004). The EZ Reader model of eye-movement control in reading: Comparisons to other models. *Behavioral and Brain Sciences*, *26*(4), 445–476.

Reinagel, P., & Zador, A. M. (1999). Natural scene statistics at the centre of gaze. *Computation in Neural Systems*, *10*(4), 341–350.

Reingold, E. M., & Charness, N. (2005). Perception in chess: Evidence from eye movements. In G. M. Underwood (Ed.), *Cognitive Processes in Eye Guidance* (pp. 325–354). Oxford: Oxford University Press.

Reingold, E. M., Charness, N., Pomplun, M., & Stampe, D. M. (2001). Visual span in expert chess players: Evidence from eye movements. *Psychological Science*, *12*(1), 48–55.

Reinhard, J., Schreiber, A., Schiefer, U., Kasten, E., Sabel, B. A., Kenkel, S., et al. (2005). Does visual restitution training change absolute homonymous visual field defects? A fundus controlled study. *British Journal of Ophthalmology*, *89*(1), 30–35.

Reisen, N., Hoffrage, U., & Mast, F. W. (2008). Identifying decision strategies in a consumer choice situation. *Judgment and Decision Making*, *3*(8), 641–658.

Renkl, A. (1997). Learning from worked-out examples: A study in individual differences. *Cognitive Science*, *21*(1), 1–29.

Renkl, A., & Atkinson, R. K. (2003). Structuring the transition from example study to problem solving in cognitive skill acquisition: A cognitive load perspective. *Educational Psychologist*, *38*(1), 15–22.

Renkl, A., Stark, R., Gruber, H., & Mandl, H. (1998). Learning from worked-out examples: The effects of example variability and elicited self-explanations. *Contemporary Educational Psychology*, *23*(1), 90–108.

Renshaw, J. A., Finlay, J. E., Tyfa, D., & Ward, R. D. (2003). Designing for visual influence: An eye tracking study of the usability of graphical management information. In M. Rauterberg, M. Menozzi, & J. Wesson (Eds.), *Proceedings of Human-Computer Interaction – INTERACT 2003* (pp. 144–152). Amsterdam: IOS Press.

Renshaw, J. A., Finlay, J. E., Tyfa, D., & Ward, R. D. (2004). Regressions re-visited: A new definition for the visual display paradigm. In *CHI '04 Extended Abstracts on Human Factors in Computing Systems* (pp. 1437–1440). New York: ACM.

Richardson, D. C., & Dale, R. (2005). Looking to understand: The coupling between speakers' and listeners' eye movements and its relationship to discourse comprehension. *Cognitive Science*, *29*(6), 1045–1060.

Ridder III, W. H., & Tomlinson, A. (1995). Spectral characteristics of blink suppression in normal observers. *Vision Research*, *35*(18), 2569–2578.

Rieh, S. Y. (2002). Judgment of information quality and cognitive authority in the Web. *Journal of the American Society for Information Science and Technology*, *53*(2), 145–161.

Ripoll, H., Fleurance, P., & Cazeneuve, D. (1987). Analysis of visual patterns of table tennis players. In J. K. O'Regan & A. Levy-Schoen (Eds.), *Eye Movements: From Physiology to Cognition* (pp. 616–617). Amsterdam: Elsevier Science Publishers.

Robinson, G. H., Erickson, D. J., Thurston, G. L., & Clark, R. L. (1972). Visual search by automobile drivers. *Human Factors: The Journal of the Human Factors and Ergonomics Society*, *14*(4), 315–323.

Rockwell, T. H. (1988). Spare visual capacity in driving-revisited. In *Vision in Vehicles–II: Proceedings of the Second International Conference on Vision in Vehicles* (pp. 317–324). Amsterdam: Elsevier.

Rodden, K., & Fu, X. (2007). Exploring how mouse movements relate to eye movements on web search results pages. In *Proceedings of ACM SIGIR 2007 Workshop on Web Information Seeking and Interaction* (pp. 29–32).

Rohrschneider, K., Bethke-Jaenicke, C., Becker, M., Kruse, F. E., Blankenagel, A., & Völcker, H. E. (1996). Fundus-controlled examination of reading in eyes with macular pathology. *German Journal of Ophthalmology*, *5*(5), 300–307.

Rolfs, M., Engbert, R., & Kliegl, R. (2005). Crossmodal coupling of oculomotor control and spatial attention in vision and audition. *Experimental Brain Research*, *166*(3), 427–439.

Rolfs, M., Kliegl, R., & Engbert, R. (2008). Toward a model of microsaccade generation: The case of microsaccadic inhibition. *Journal of Vision*, *8*(11), 1–23.

Ross, J., Morrone, M. C., & Burr, D. C. (1997). Compression of visual space before saccades. *Nature*, *386*(6625), 598–601.

Ross, R. G., Olincy, A., Harris, J. G., Radant, A. D., Adler, L. E., Compagnon, N., et al. (1999). The effects of age on a smooth pursuit tracking task in adults with schizophrenia and normal subjects. *Biological Psychiatry*, *46*(3), 383–391.

Rothkopf, C. A., Ballard, D. H., & Hayhoe, M. M. (2007). Task and context determine where you look. *Journal of Vision*, *7*(14), 1–20.

Rothkopf, C. A., & Pelz, J. B. (2004). Head movement estimation for wearable eye tracker. In *Proceedings of the 2004 Symposium on Eye-Tracking Research & Applications* (pp. 123–129). New York: ACM.

Rottach, K. G., Das, V. E., Wohlgemuth, W. A., Zivotofsky, A. Z., & Leigh, J. R. (1998). Properties of horizontal saccades accompanied by blinks. *Journal of Neurophysiology*, *79*(6), 2895–2902.

Rottach, K. G., Wohlgemuth, W. A., Dzaja, A. E., Eggert, T., & Straube, A. (2002). Effects of intravenous opioids on eye movements in humans: Possible mechanisms. *Journal of Neurology*, *249*(9), 1200–1205.

Rottach, K. G., Zivotofsky, A. Z., Das, V. E., Averbuch-Heller, L., Discenna, A. O., Poonyathalang, A., et al. (1996). Comparison of horizontal, vertical and diagonal smooth pursuit eye movements in normal human subjects. *Vision Research*, *36*(14), 2189–2195.

Rötting, M. (2001). *Parametersystematik der Augen- und Blickbewegungen für arbeitswissenschaftliche Untersuchungen*. Unpublished doctoral dissertation, RWTH Aachen.

Rousselet, G. A., Fabre-Thorpe, M., & Thorpe, S. J. (2002). Parallel processing in high-level categorization of natural images. *Nature Neuroscience*, *5*, 629–630.

Rucker, J. C., Shapiro, B. E., Han, Y. H., Kumar, A. N., Garbutt, S., Keller, E. L., et al. (2004). Neuro-ophthalmology of late-onset Tay-Sachs disease (LOTS). *Neurology, 63*(10), 1918–1926.

Rupp, H. A., & Wallen, K. (2007). Sex differences in viewing sexual stimuli: An eye-tracking study in men and women. *Hormones and Behavior, 51*(4), 524–533.

Rushworth, G. (1962). Observations on blink reflexes. *Journal of Neurology, Neurosurgery, and Psychiatry, 25*(2), 93–108.

Russo, M., Thomas, M., Thorne, D., Sing, H., Redmond, D., Rowland, L., et al. (2003). Oculomotor impairment during chronic partial sleep deprivation. *Clinical neurophysiology, 114*(4), 723–736.

Ryan, B., & Haslegrave, C. M. (2007). Use of concurrent and retrospective verbal protocols to investigate workers' thoughts during a manual-handling task. *Applied Ergonomics, 38*(2), 177–190.

Ryan, J. D., Althoff, R. R., Whitlow, S., & Cohen, N. J. (2000). Amnesia is a deficit in relational memory. *Psychological Science, 11*(6), 454–461.

Ryan, J. D., & Cohen, N. J. (2004). The nature of change detection and online representations of scenes. *Journal of Experimental Psychology: Human Perception and Performance, 30*(5), 988–1015.

Saida, S., & Ikeda, M. (1979). Useful visual field size for pattern perception. *Perception & Psychophysics, 25*(2), 119–125.

Saito, S. (1992). Does fatigue exist in a quantitative measurement of eye movements? *Ergonomics, 35*(5), 607–615.

Salman, M. S., Sharpe, J. A., Eizenman, M., Lillakas, L., Westall, C., To, T., et al. (2006). Saccades in children. *Vision Research, 46*(8-9), 1432–1439.

Salman, M. S., Sharpe, J. A., Lillakas, L., Dennis, M., & Steinbach, M. J. (2006). Smooth pursuit eye movements in children. *Experimental Brain Research, 169*(1), 139–143.

Salman, M. S., Sharpe, J. A., Lillakas, L., & Steinbach, M. J. (2008). Square wave jerks in children and adolescents. *Pediatric Neurology, 38*(1), 16–19.

Salvucci, D. (1999). Inferring intent in eye-based interfaces: Tracing eye movements with process models. In *CHI '99: Proceedings of the SIGCHI Conference on Human Factors in Computing Systems* (pp. 254–261). New York: ACM.

Salvucci, D., & Goldberg, J. H. (2000). Identifying fixations and saccades in eyetracking protocols. In *Proceedings of the 2002 Symposium on Eye-Tracking Research & Applications* (pp. 71–78). New York: ACM.

Sandberg, H., Gidlöf, K., & Holmberg, N. (2011). Children's exposure to and perceptions of online advertising. *International Journal of Communication, 5*, 21–50.

Santella, A., & DeCarlo, D. (2004). Robust clustering of eye movement recordings for quantification of visual interest. In *Proceedings of the 2004 Symposium on Eye-Tracking Research & Applications* (pp. 27–34). New York: ACM.

Santini, F., Redner, G., Iovin, R., & Rucci, M. (2007). EyeRIS: A general-purpose system for eye-movement-contingent display control. *Behavior Research Methods, 39*(3), 350–364.

Sauter, D., Martin, B. J., Di Renzo, N., & Vomscheid, C. (1991). Analysis of eye tracking movements using innovations generated by a Kalman filter. *Medical and Biological Engineering and Computing, 29*(1), 63–69.

Savelsbergh, G. J. P., Williams, A. M., Van Der Kamp, J., & Ward, P. (2002). Visual search, anticipation and expertise in soccer goalkeepers. *Journal of Sports Sciences, 20*(3), 279–287.

Savolainen, R., & Kari, J. (2005). User-defined relevance criteria in web searching. *Journal of Documentation, 62*, 685–707.

Sawahata, Y., Khosla, R., Komine, K., Hiruma, N., Itou, T., Watanabe, S., et al. (2008). Determining comprehension and quality of TV programs using eye-gaze tracking. *Pattern Recognition, 41*(5), 1610–1626.

Schiller, P. H., & Tehovnik, E. J. (2001). Look and see: How the brain moves your eyes about. *Progress in Brain Research, 134*, 127–142.

Schilling, H. E. H., Rayner, K., & Chumbley, J. I. (1998). Comparing naming, lexical decision, and eye fixation times: Word frequency effects and individual differences. *Memory and Cognition, 26*(6), 1270–1281.

Schleicher, R., Galley, N., Briest, S., & Galley, L. (2008). Blinks and saccades as indicators of fatigue in sleepiness warnings: Looking tired? *Ergonomics, 51*(7), 982–1010.

Schmidt-Weigand, F., Kohnert, A., & Glowalla, U. (2010). A closer look at split visual attention in system-and self-paced instruction in multimedia learning. *Learning and Instruction, 20*(2), 100–110.

Schnipke, S. K., & Todd, M. W. (2000). Trials and tribulations of using an eye-tracking system. In *CHI'00 Extended Abstracts on Human Factors in Computing Systems* (pp. 273–274).

Schoonahd, J. W., Gould, J. D., & Miller, L. A. (1973). Studies of visual inspection. *Ergonomics, 16*(4), 365–379.

Shaffer, D. M., Krisky, C. M., & Sweeney, J. A. (2003). Frequency and metrics of square-wave jerks: Influences of task-demand characteristics. *Investigative Ophthalmology & Visual Science, 44*(3), 1082–1087.

Shannon, C. E. (1948). A mathematical theory of communication. *Bell System Technical Journal, 27*, 379–423, 623–656.

Sharpe, D., & Faye, C. (2009). A second look at debriefing practices: Madness in our method? *Ethics & Behavior, 19*(5), 432–447.

Sharpe, J. A., & Sylvester, T. O. (1978). Effect of aging on horizontal smooth pursuit. *Investigative Ophthalmology & Visual Science, 17*(5), 465–468.

Sheliga, B. M., Riggio, L., Craighero, L., & Rizzolatti, G. (1995). Spatial attention-determined modifications in saccade trajectories. *Neuroreport, 6*(3), 585–588.

Shepherd, M., Findlay, J. M., & Hockey, R. J. (1986). The relationship between eye movements and spatial attention. *The Quarterly Journal of Experimental Psychology, 38*(3), 475–491.

Shic, F., Chawarska, K., & Scassellati, B. (2008). Autism, eye-tracking, entropy. In *IEEE Proceedings of the 7th International Conference on Development and Learning* (pp. 73–78).

Shic, F., Scassellati, B., & Chawarska, K. (2008). The incomplete fixation measure. In *Proceedings of the 2008 Symposium on Eye-Tracking Research & Applications* (pp. 111–114). New York: ACM.

Shimojo, S., Simion, C., Shimojo, E., & Scheier, C. (2003). Gaze bias both reflects and influences preference. *Nature Neuroscience, 6*(12), 1317–1322.

Shinar, D., McDowell, E. D., & Rockwell, T. H. (1977). Eye movements in curve negotiation. *Human Factors, 19*(1), 63–71.

Shioiri, S., & Ikeda, M. (1989). Useful resolution for picture perception as a function of eccentricity. *Perception, 18*(3), 347–361.

Shrout, P. E., & Fiske, D. W. (1981). Nonverbal behaviors and social evaluation. *Journal of Personality, 49*(2), 115–128.

Sibony, P. A., Evinger, C., & Manning, K. A. (1988). The effects of tobacco smoking on smooth pursuit eye movements. *Annals of Neurology, 23*(3), 238–241.

Siegel, S., & Castellan, J. (1988). *Nonparametric Statistics for the Behavioral Sciences* (second ed.). New York: McGraw-Hill.

Siegle, G. J., Ichikawa, N., & Steinhauer, S. (2008). Blink before and after you think: Blinks occur prior to and following cognitive load indexed by pupillary responses. *Psychophysiology*, *45*(5), 679–687.

Simola, J., Holmqvist, K., & Lindgren, M. (2008). *Hemispheric differences in parafoveal processing: Evidence from eye-fixation related potentials.* (Poster presentation at BrainTalk: Discourse with and in the brain.)

Simola, J., Holmqvist, K., & Lindgren, M. (2009). Right visual field advantage in parafoveal processing: Evidence from eye-fixation related potentials. *Brain and Language*, *111*(2), 101–113.

Simola, J., Salojärvi, J., & Kojo, I. (2008). Using hidden Markov model to uncover processing states from eye movements in information search tasks. *Cognitive Systems Research*, *9*(4), 237–251.

Simola, J., Stenbacka, L., & Vanni, S. (2009). Topography of attention in the primary visual cortex. *European Journal of Neuroscience*, *29*(1), 188–196.

Simonin, J., Kieffer, S., & Carbonell, N. (2005). Effects of display layout on gaze activity during visual search. In M. F. Costabile & F. Paternò (Eds.), *Proceedings of Human-Computer Interaction - INTERACT 2005* (Vol. 3585, pp. 1054–1057). New York: Springer-Verlag.

Singer, J., & Willett, J. (2003). *Applied Longitudinal Data Analysis: Modeling Change and Event Occurrence* (first ed.). Oxford: Oxford University Press.

Singer, R. N., Cauraugh, J. H., Chen, D., Steinberg, G. M., & Frehlich, S. G. (1996). Visual search, anticipation, and reactive comparisons between highly-skilled and beginning tennis players. *Journal of Applied Sport Psychology*, *8*(1), 9–26.

Sloboda, J. A. (1985). *The Musical Mind*. Oxford: Clarendon Press.

Smeets, J. B., & Hooge, I. T. C. (2003). Nature of variability in saccades. *Journal of Neurophysiology*, *90*(1), 12–20.

SMI. (2007). *SMI BeGaze Event Detection*. (Technical Note.)

Smit, A. C., & Van Gisbergen, J. A. M. (1989). A short-latency transition in saccade dynamics during square-wave tracking and its significance for the differentiation of visually-guided and predictive saccades. *Experimental Brain Research*, *76*(1), 64–74.

Smit, A. C., & Van Gisbergen, J. A. M. (1990). An analysis of curvature in fast and slow human saccades. *Experimental Brain Research*, *81*(2), 335–345.

Smit, A. C., Van Gisbergen, J. A. M., & Cools, A. R. (1987). A parametric analysis of human saccades in different experimental paradigms. *Vision Research*, *27*(10), 1745–1762.

Smith, B. A., Ho, J., Ark, W., & Zhai, S. (2000). Hand eye coordination patterns in target selection. In *Proceedings of the 2000 Symposium on Eye-Tracking Research & Applications* (pp. 117–122). New York: ACM.

Smith, M. U., & Good, R. (1984). Problem solving and classical genetics: Successful versus unsuccessful performance. *Journal of Research in Science Teaching*, *21*(9), 895–912.

Smith, T. J., & Henderson, J. M. (2009). Facilitation of return during scene viewing. *Visual Cognition*, *17*(6-7), 1083–1108.

Snodderly, D. M., & Kurtz, D. (1985). Eye position during fixation tasks: Comparison of macaque and human. *Vision Research*, *25*(1), 83–98.

Snyder, L. H., Batista, A. P., & Andersen, R. A. (2000). Saccade-related activity in the parietal reach region. *Journal of Neurophysiology*, *83*(2), 1099–1102.

Soetedjo, R., Kaneko, C. R. S., & Fuchs, A. F. (2002). Evidence that the superior colliculus participates in the feedback control of saccadic eye movements. *Journal of Neurophysiology*, *87*(2), 679–695.

Spering, M., & Gegenfurtner, K. R. (2007). Contextual effects on smooth-pursuit eye movements. *Journal of Neurophysiology*, *97*(2), 1353–67.

Sporn, A., Greenstein, D., Gogtay, N., Sailer, F., Hommer, D., Rawlings, R., et al. (2005). Childhood-onset schizophrenia: Smooth pursuit eye-tracking dysfunction in family members. *Schizophrenia Research*, *73*, 243–252.

Sprenger, A., Lappe-Osthege, M., Talamo, S., Gais, S., Kimmig, H., & Helmchen, C. (2010). Eye movements during REM sleep and imagination of visual scenes. *Neuroreport*, *21*(1), 45–49.

SR Research. (2007). EyeLink User Manual 1.3.0 [Computer software manual]. Mississauga, Ontario, Canada.

Stager, P., & Angus, R. (1978). Locating crash sites in simulated air-to-ground visual search. *Human Factors: The Journal of the Human Factors and Ergonomics Society*, *20*(4), 453–466.

Stampe, D. M. (1993). Heuristic filtering and reliable calibration methods for video-based pupil tracking systems. *Behavior Research Methods, Instruments, & Computers*, *25*(2), 137–142.

Stelmach, L. B., & Tam, W. J. (1994). Processing image sequences based on eye movements. In B. E. Rogowitz & J. Allebach (Eds.), *SPIE Proceedings on Human Vision, Visual Processing and Digital Display* (Vol. 2179, pp. 90–98).

Stern, J. A., Boyer, D., & Schroeder, D. (1994). Blink rate: A possible measure of fatigue. *Human Factors: The Journal of the Human Factors and Ergonomics Society*, *36*(2), 285–297.

Stevenson, S. B., Volkmann, F. C., Kelly, J. P., & Riggs, L. A. (1986). Dependence of visual suppression on the amplitudes of saccades and blinks. *Vision Research*, *26*(11), 1815–1824.

Stolk, H., & Brok, E. (1999). A descriptive framework for analyzing eye movements during studying. In B. Den Brinker, P. Beek, A. Brand, F. Maarse, & L. Mulder (Eds.), *Cognitive Ergonomics, Clinical Assessment, and Computer-Assisted Learning* (pp. 22–34). Lisse, the Netherlands: Swets and Zeitlinger Publishers.

Straube, A., & Deubel, H. (1995). Rapid gain adaptation affects the dynamics of saccadic eye movements in humans. *Vision Research*, *35*(23-24), 3451–3458.

Sudman, S., Bradbrun, N. M., & Schwarz, N. (1996). *Thinking about Answers: The Application of Cognitive Processes to Survey Methodology*. San Francisco: Jossey-Bass.

Sullivan, B. T., Jovancevic, J., Hayhoe, M. M., & Sterns, G. (2005). Use of gaze in natural tasks in Stargardt's disease: A preferred retinal region. In *Vision 2005 - Proceedings of the International Congress* (Vol. 1282, pp. 608–612).

Suppes, P. (1990). Eye-movement models for arithmetic and reading performance. In E. Kowler (Ed.), *Eye Movements and their Role in Visual and Cognitive Processes* (pp. 455–477). Amsterdam: Elsevier.

Synder, J. J., & Kingstone, A. (2000). Inhibition of return and visual search: How many separate loci are inhibited? *Perception & Psychophysics*, *62*(3), 452–458.

't Hart, B. M., Vockeroth, J., Schumann, F., Bartl, K., Schneider, E., König, P., et al. (2009). Gaze allocation in natural stimuli: Comparing free exploration to head-fixed viewing conditions. *Visual Cognition*, *17*(6), 1132–1158.

Tabachnick, B. G., & Fidell, L. S. (2000). *Using Multivariate Statistics* (fourth ed.). Boston: Allyn & Bacon.

Takarae, Y., Minshew, N. J., Luna, B., Krisky, C. M., & Sweeney, J. A. (2004). Pursuit eye movement deficits in autism. *Brain*, *127*(12), 2584–2594.

Takeda, Y., Sugai, M., & Yagi, A. (2001). Eye fixation related potentials in a proof reading task. *International Journal of Psychophysiology*, *40*(3), 181–186.

Tall, M. (2008). *NEOVISUS - Gaze Interaction Interface Components*. Unpublished master's thesis, Lund University.

Tanenhaus, M. K., & Brown-Schmidt, S. (2008). Language processing in the natural world. *Philosophical Transactions of the Royal Society of London. Series B: Biological Sciences*, *363*, 1105–1122.

Tanenhaus, M. K., Spivey-Knowlton, M. J., Eberhard, K. M., & Sedivy, J. C. (1995). Integration of visual and linguistic information in spoken language comprehension. *Science*, *268*(5217), 1632–1634.

Tarita-Nistor, L., Gonzalez, E. G., Mandelcorn, M. S., Lillakas, L., & Steinbach, M. J. (2009). Fixation stability, fixation location, and visual acuity after successful macular hole surgery. *Investigative Ophthalmology & Visual Science*, *50*(1), 84–89.

Tatler, B. W. (2007). The central fixation bias in scene viewing: Selecting an optimal viewing position independently of motor biases and image feature distributions. *Journal of Vision*, *7*(14), 1–17.

Tatler, B. W., Baddeley, R. J., & Gilchrist, I. D. (2005). Visual correlates of fixation selection: Effects of scale and time. *Vision Research*, *45*(5), 643–659.

Tatler, B. W., Baddeley, R. J., & Vincent, B. T. (2006). The long and the short of it: Spatial statistics at fixation vary with saccade amplitude and task. *Vision Research*, *46*(12), 1857–1862.

Tatler, B. W., Gilchrist, I. D., & Land, M. F. (2005). Visual memory for objects in natural scenes: From fixations to object files. *The Quarterly Journal of Experimental Psychology*, *58*(5), 931–960.

Tatler, B. W., & Hutton, S. B. (2007). Trial by trial effects in the antisaccade task. *Experimental Brain Research*, *179*(3), 387–396.

Tatler, B. W., & Vincent, B. T. (2008). Systematic tendencies in scene viewing. *Journal of Eye Movement Research*, *2*(5), 1–18.

Tatler, B. W., & Vincent, B. T. (2009). The prominence of behavioural biases in eye guidance. *Visual Cognition*, *6*(7), 1029–1054.

Taylor, J. R., Elsworth, J. D., Lawrence, M. S., Sladek, J. R., Roth, R. H., & Redmond Jr, D. E. (1999). Spontaneous blink rates correlate with dopamine levels in the caudate nucleus of MPTP-treated monkeys. *Experimental Neurology*, *158*(1), 214–220.

Taylor, K. L., & Dionne, J. P. (2000). Accessing problem-solving strategy knowledge: The complementary use of concurrent verbal protocols and retrospective debriefing. *Journal of Educational Psychology*, *92*(3), 413–425.

Tedeschi, G., Bittencourt, P. R. M., Smith, A. T., & Richens, A. (1983). Effect of amphetamine on saccadic and smooth pursuit eye movements. *Psychopharmacology*, *79*(2), 190–192.

Teiwes, W. (1991). *Video-Okulographie–Registrierung von Augenbewegungen in drei Freiheitsgraden zur Erforschung und medizinischen Diagnostik des Gleichgewichtssystems*. Unpublished doctoral dissertation, Technische Universität Berlin.

Thaker, G. K., Ellsberry, R., Moran, M., & Lahti, A. (1991). Tobacco smoking increases square-wave jerks during pursuit eye movements. *Biological Psychiatry*, *29*(1), 82–88.

Theiler, J. (1990). Estimating fractal dimension. *Journal of the Optical Society of America A*, *7*(6), 1055–1073.

Thompson, J. D., Higgins, D. G., & Gibson, T. J. (1994). CLUSTAL W: Improving the sensitivity of progressive multiple sequence alignment through sequence weighting, position-specific gap penalties and weight matrix choice. *Nucleic Acids Research*, *22*(22), 4673–4680.

Tinker, M. A. (1945). Reliability of blinking frequency employed as a measure of readability. *Journal of Experimental Psychology*, *35*(5), 418–424.

Tole, J. R., & Young, L. R. (1981). Digital filters for saccade and fixation detection. In D. Fisher, R. A. Monty, & J. Senders (Eds.), *Eye movements: Cognition and Visual Perception* (pp. 247–256). Hillsdale, NJ: Lawrence Erlbaum Associates.

Tombros, A., Ruthven, I., & Jose, J. M. (2005). How users assess web pages for information-seeking. *Journal of the American Society for Information Science and Technology*, *56*, 327–344.

Torralba, A., Oliva, A., Castelhano, M. S., & Henderson, J. M. (2006). Contextual guidance of eye movements and attention in real-world scenes: The role of global features in object search. *Psychological Review*, *113*(4), 766–786.

Torstling, A. (2007). *The Mean Gaze Path: Information Reduction and Non-Intrusive Attention Detection for Eye Tracking*. Unpublished master's thesis, Stockholm Royal Institute of Technology.

Träisk, F., Bolzani, R., & Ygge, J. (2005). A comparison between the magnetic scleral search coil and infrared reflection methods for saccadic eye movement analysis. *Graefe's Archive for Clinical and Experimental Ophthalmology*, *243*(8), 791–797.

Trauzettel-Klosinski, S., Teschner, C., Tornow, R. P., & Zrenner, E. (1994). Reading strategies in normal subjects and in patients with macular scotoma-assessed by two new methods of registration. *Neuro-Ophthalmology*, *14*(1), 15–30.

Treisman, A. M., & Gelade, G. (1980). A feature-integration theory of attention. *Cognitive Psychology*, *12*(1), 97–136.

Treistman, J., & Gregg, J. P. (1979). Visual, verbal, and sales responses to print ads. *Journal of Advertising Research*, *19*(4), 41–47.

Triesch, J., Ballard, D. H., Hayhoe, M. M., & Sullivan, B. T. (2003). What you see is what you need. *Journal of Vision*, *3*(1), 86–94.

Trillenberg, P., Lencer, R., & Heide, W. (2004). Eye movements and psychiatric disease. *Current Opinion in Neurology*, *17*(1), 43–47.

Troncoso, X. G., Macknik, S. L., Otero-Millan, J., & Martinez-Conde, S. (2008). Micro-saccades drive illusory motion in the Enigma illusion. *Proceedings of the National Academy of Sciences*, *105*(41), 16033–16038.

Troost, B. T., & Daroff, R. B. (1977). The ocular motor defects in progressive supranuclear palsy. *Annals of Neurology*, *2*(5), 397–403.

Trottier, L., & Pratt, J. (2005). Visual processing of targets can reduce saccadic latencies. *Vision Research*, *45*(11), 1349–1354.

Troy, M., Chen, S. C., & Stern, J. A. (1972). Computer analysis of eye movement patterns during visual search. *Aerospace Medicine*, *43*(4), 390–394.

Truitt, F. E., Clifton, C., Pollatsek, A., & Rayner, K. (1997). The perceptual span and the eye-hand span in sight reading music. *Visual Cognition*, *4*(2), 143–161.

Tsai, C. H. (2010). *A C program for scanpath compression*. (Software available from the author's website (http://research.chtsai.org), accessed February 2011.)

Tsai, Y. F., Viirre, E., Strychacz, C., Chase, B., & Jung, T. P. (2007). Task performance and eye activity: Predicting behavior relating to cognitive workload. *Aviation, Space, and Environmental Medicine*, *78*(Supplement 1), B176–B185.

Tsujimura, A., Miyagawa, Y., Takada, S., Matsuoka, Y., Takao, T., Hirai, T., et al. (2009). Sex differences in visual attention to sexually explicit videos: A preliminary study. *The Journal of Sexual Medicine*, *6*(4), 1011–1017.

Turano, K. A., Geruschat, D. R., & Baker, F. H. (2002). Fixation behavior while walking: Persons with central visual field loss. *Vision Research*, *42*(23), 2635–2644.

Turano, K. A., Geruschat, D. R., & Baker, F. H. (2003). Oculomotor strategies for the direction of gaze tested with a real-world activity. *Vision Research*, *43*(3), 333–346.

Tweed, D., & Vilis, T. (1990). Geometric relations of eye position and velocity vectors during saccades. *Vision Research, 30*(1), 111–127.

Tzanidou, E., Minocha, S., & Petre, M. (2005). Applying eye tracking for usability evaluations of e-commerce sites. In *Proceedings of the Workshop on 'Commercial Uses of Eye Tracking' held at the 19th British HCI Group Annual Conference.*

Underwood, G. M. (1998). *Eye Guidance in Reading, Driving, and Scene Perception.* New York: Elsevier.

Underwood, G. M., Chapman, P., Berger, Z., & Crundall, D. (2003). Driving experience, attentional focusing, and the recall of recently inspected events. *Transportation Research Part F: Traffic Psychology and Behaviour, 6*(4), 289–304.

Underwood, G. M., Chapman, P., Brocklehurst, N., Underwood, J., & Crundall, D. (2003). Visual attention while driving: Sequences of eye fixations made by experienced and novice drivers. *Ergonomics, 46*(6), 629–646.

Underwood, G. M., Foulsham, T., & Humphrey, K. (2009). Saliency and scan patterns in the inspection of real-world scenes: Eye movements during encoding and recognition. *Visual Cognition, 17*(6-7), 812–834.

Underwood, G. M., Foulsham, T., Van Loon, E. M., Humphreys, L., & Bloyce, J. (2006). Eye movements during scene inspection: A test of the saliency map hypothesis. *European Journal of Cognitive Psychology, 18*(3), 321–342.

Underwood, G. M., Humphrey, K., & Foulsham, T. (2008a). Knowledge-based patterns of remembering: Eye movement scanpaths reflect domain experience. In A. Holzinger (Ed.), *Proceedings of the 4th Symposium of the Workgroup Human-Computer Interaction and Usability Engineering of the Austrian Computer Society on HCI and Usability for Education and Work* (Vol. 5298, pp. 125–144). New York: Springer-Verlag.

Underwood, G. M., Humphrey, K., & Foulsham, T. (2008b). Knowledge-based patterns of remembering: Eye movement scanpaths reflect domain experience. In *HCI and Usability for Education and Work* (Vol. 5298, pp. 125–144). Berlin, Heidelberg: Springer-Verlag.

Unema, P. J. A., Pannasch, S., Joos, M., & Velichkovsky, B. M. (2005). Time course of information processing during scene perception: The relationship between saccade amplitude and fixation duration. *Visual Cognition, 12*(3), 473–494.

Unema, P. J. A., & Rötting, M. (1990). Differences in eye movements and mental workload between experienced and inexperienced motor-vehicle drivers. In D. Brogan (Ed.), *Visual Search* (pp. 193–202). London: Taylor & Francis.

Urruty, T., Lew, S., Ihadaddene, N., & Simovici, D. A. (2007). Detecting eye fixations by projection clustering. *ACM Transactions on Multimedia Computing, Communications and Applications, 3*(4), 1–20.

Van Der Geest, J. N., & Frens, M. A. (2002). Recording eye movements with video-oculography and scleral search coils: A direct comparison of two methods. *Journal of Neuroscience Methods, 114*(2), 185–195.

Van Der Lans, R., Pieters, R., & Wedel, M. (2008). Eye-movement analysis of search effectiveness. *Journal of the American Statistical Association, 103*(482), 452–461.

Van Der Lans, R., Wedel, M., & Pieters, R. (2010). Defining eye-fixation sequences across individuals and tasks: the Binocular-Individual Threshold (BIT) algorithm. *Behavior Research Methods, 43*(1), 239–257.

Van Der Stelt-Schouten, E. (1995). The effect of expertise on the interpretation of dental radiographic images. *Nederlands Tijdschrift voor Tandheelkunde, 102*(12), 476–479.

Van Diepen, P. M. J. (2002). Foveal stimulus degradation during scene perception. In S. P. Shohov (Ed.), *Trends in Cognitive Psychology* (pp. 193–216). Hauppauge NY: Nova Science Publishers.

Van Diepen, P. M. J., De Graef, P., & D'Ydewalle, G. (1995). Chronometry of foveal information extraction during scene perception. In J. M. Findlay, R. Walker, & R. W. Kentridge (Eds.), *Eye Movement Research: Mechanisms, Processes and Applications* (pp. 349–362). Amsterdam: Elsevier.

Van Diepen, P. M. J., & D'Ydewalle, G. (2003). Early peripheral and foveal processing in fixations during scene perception. *Visual Cognition, 10*(1), 79–100.

Van Diepen, P. M. J., Wampers, M., & D'Ydewalle, G. (1998). Functional division of the visual field: Moving masks and moving windows. In G. M. Underwood (Ed.), *Eye Guidance in Reading and Scene Perception* (pp. 337–355). Oxford: Elsevier.

Van Gerven, P. W. M., Paas, F., Van Merriënboer, J. J. G., & Schmidt, H. G. (2002). Cognitive load theory and aging: Effects of worked examples on training efficiency. *Learning and Instruction, 12*(1), 87–105.

Van Gerven, P. W. M., Paas, F., Van Merriënboer, J. J. G., & Schmidt, H. G. (2004). Memory load and the cognitive pupillary response in aging. *Psychophysiology, 41*(2), 167–174.

Van Gog, T. (2006). *Uncovering the problem-solving process to design effective worked examples.* Unpublished doctoral dissertation, Heerlen, the Netherlands: Open University.

Van Gog, T., Paas, F., & Van Merriënboer, J. J. G. (2005). Uncovering expertise-related differences in troubleshooting performance: Combining eye movement and concurrent verbal protocol data. *Applied Cognitive Psychology, 19*(2), 205–221.

Van Gog, T., Paas, F., Van Merriënboer, J. J. G., & Witte, P. (2005). Uncovering the problem-solving process: Cued retrospective reporting versus concurrent and retrospective reporting. *Journal of Experimental Psychology: Applied, 11*(4), 237–244.

Van Meeuwen, L. W. (2008). *Tracking the Brain.* Unpublished master's thesis, Eindhoven University of Technology.

Van Opstal, A. J., & Van Gisbergen, J. A. M. (1987). Skewness of saccadic velocity profiles: A unifying parameter for normal and slow saccades. *Vision Research, 27*(5), 731–745.

Van Orden, K. F., Jung, T. P., & Makeig, S. (2000). Combined eye activity measures accurately estimate changes in sustained visual task performance. *Biological Psychology, 52*(3), 221–240.

Van Orden, K. F., Limbert, W., Makeig, S., & Jung, T. P. (2001). Eye activity correlates of workload during a visuospatial memory task. *Human Factors, 43*(1), 111–121.

Van Someren, M. W., Barnard, Y. F., & Sandberg, J. A. C. (1994). *The Think Aloud Method: A Practical Guide to Modelling Cognitive Processes.* Amsterdam: Academic Press.

Van Tricht, M. J., Nieman, D. H., Bour, L. J., Boerée, T., Koelman, J., De Haan, L., et al. (2010). Increased saccadic rate during smooth pursuit eye movements in patients at Ultra High Risk for developing a psychosis. *Brain and Cognition, 73*(3), 215–221.

Vatikiotis-Bateson, E., Eigsti, I. M., Yano, S., & Munhall, K. G. (1998). Eye movement of perceivers during audiovisual speech perception. *Perception & Psychophysics, 60*(6), 926–940.

Veiel, L. L., Storandt, M., & Abrams, R. A. (2006). Visual search for change in older adults. *Psychology and Aging, 21*(4), 754–762.

Velichkovsky, B. M., Dornhöfer, S. M., Pannasch, S., & Unema, P. J. A. (2000). Visual fixations and level of attentional processing. In *Proceedings of the 2000 Symposium on Eye-Tracking Research & Applications* (pp. 79–85). New York: ACM.

Velichkovsky, B. M., Pomplun, M., Rieser, J., & Ritter, H. (1996). Attention and communication: Eye-movement-based research paradigms. In W. H. Zangemeister, H. S. Stiehl, & C. Freksa (Eds.), *Visual Attention and Cognition* (Vol. 116, pp. 125–154). Amsterdam: Elsevier Science.

Velichkovsky, B. M., Rothert, A., Kopf, M., Dornhöfer, S. M., & Joos, M. (2002). Towards an express-diagnostics for level of processing and hazard perception. *Transportation Research Part F: Traffic Psychology and Behaviour*, 5(2), 145–156.

Veltman, J. A., & Gaillard, A. W. K. (1996). Physiological indices of workload in a simulated flight task. *Biological Psychology*, 42(3), 323–342.

Veltman, J. A., & Gaillard, A. W. K. (1998). Physiological workload reactions to increasing levels of task difficulty. *Ergonomics*, 41(5), 656–669.

Ventre, J., Vighetto, A., Bailly, G., & Prablanc, C. (1991). Saccade metrics in multiple sclerosis: Versional velocity disconjugacy as the best clue? *Journal of the Neurological Sciences*, 102(2), 144–149.

Versino, M., Hurko, O., & Zee, D. S. (1996). Disorders of binocular control of eye movements in patients with cerebellar dysfunction. *Brain*, 119(6), 1933–1950.

Vickers, J. N. (1992). Gaze control in putting. *Perception*, 21(1), 117–132.

Vigil, J. M. (2009). A sociorelational framework of sex differences in the expression of emotion. *Behavioral and Brain Sciences*, 32(5), 375–390.

Vikström, K. (2006). *Consumer Decision Making Adaptation to Differences in the Choice Environment*. Unpublished master's thesis, Lund University.

Vishwanath, D., & Kowler, E. (2004). Saccadic localization in the presence of cues to three-dimensional shape. *Journal of Vision*, 4(6), 445–458.

Viviani, P. (1990). Eye movements in visual search: Cognitive, perceptual and motor control aspects. In E. Kowler (Ed.), *Eye Movements and Their Role in Visual and Cognitive Processes* (pp. 353–393). Amsterdam: Elsevier.

Viviani, P., Berthoz, A., & Tracey, D. (1977). The curvature of oblique saccades. *Vision Research*, 17(5), 661–664.

Võ, M. L. H., & Henderson, J. M. (2010). The time course of initial scene processing for eye movement guidance in natural scene search. *Journal of Vision*, 10(3), 1–13.

Vogt, S., & Magnussen, S. (2007). Expertise in pictorial perception: Eye-movement patterns and visual memory in artists and laymen. *Perception*, 36(1), 91–100.

Volkmann, F. C. (1986). Human visual suppression. *Vision Research*, 26(9), 1401–1416.

Volkmann, F. C., Riggs, L. A., & Moore, R. K. (1980). Eyeblinks and visual suppression. *Science*, 207(4433), 900–902.

Von Wartburg, R., Wurtz, P., Pflugshaupt, T., Nyffeler, T., Lüthi, M., & Müri, R. M. (2007). Size matters: Saccades during scene perception. *Perception*, 36(3), 355–365.

Vosskuhler, A., Nordmeier, V., Kuchinke, L., & Jacobs, A. M. (2008). OGAMA (Open Gaze and Mouse Analyzer): Open-source software designed to analyze eye and mouse movements in slideshow study designs. *Behavior Research Methods*, 40(4), 1150–1162.

Vuori, T., Olkkonen, M., Pölönen, M., Siren, A., & Häkkinen, J. (2004). Can eye movements be quantitatively applied to image quality studies? In *Proceedings of the Third Nordic Conference on Human-computer Interaction* (pp. 335–338).

Wade, N. J., & Tatler, B. W. (2005). *'The Moving Tablet of the Eye': The Origins of Modern Eye Movement Research*. Oxford: Oxford University Press.

Walker, R., Deubel, H., Schneider, W. X., & Findlay, J. M. (1997). Effect of remote distractors on saccade programming: Evidence for an extended fixation zone. *Journal of Neurophysiology*, 78(2), 1108–1119.

Wallace, J. M., Stone, L. S., & Masson, G. S. (2005). Object motion computation for the initiation of smooth pursuit eye movements in humans. *Journal of Neurophysiology*, 93(4), 2279–2293.

Wang, L. (1998). Glissadic saccades: A possible measure of vigilance. *Ergonomics*, 41(5), 721–732.

Wang, Y., Mehler, B., Reimer, B., Lammers, V., D'Ambrosio, L. A., & Coughlin, J. F. (2010). The validity of driving simulation for assessing differences between in-vehicle informational interfaces: A comparison with field testing. *Ergonomics, 53*(3), 404–420.

Wang, Z., & Bovik, A. C. (2001). Embedded foveation image coding. *IEEE Transactions on Image Processing, 10*(10), 1397–1410.

Wang, Z., Lu, L., & Bovik, A. C. (2003). Foveation scalable video coding with automatic fixation selection. *IEEE Transactions on Image Processing, 12*(2), 243–254.

Watson, J. B. (1913). Psychology as the behaviorist views it. *Psychological Review, 20,* 158–177.

Watson, J. B. (1920). Is thinking merely the action of language mechanisms? *British Journal of Psychology, 11,* 87–104.

Weaver, H. E. (1943). A study of visual processes in reading differently constructed musical selections. *Psychological Monographs, 55*(1), 1–30.

Webb, E. J., Campbell, D. T., Schwartz, R. D., & Sechrest, L. (1966). *Unobtrusive Measures: Nonreactive Measures in the Social Sciences.* Chicago: Rand McNally.

Weber, R. B., & Daroff, R. B. (1972). Corrective movements following refixation saccades: Type and control system analysis. *Vision Research, 12*(3), 467–475.

Welchman, A. E., & Harris, J. M. (2003). Task demands and binocular eye movements. *Journal of Vision, 3*(11), 817–830.

Welford, A. T., & Brebner, J. M. T. (1980). *Reaction Times.* New York: Academic Press.

Wengelin, Å., Torrance, M., Holmqvist, K., Simpson, S., Galbraith, D., Johansson, V., et al. (2009). Combined eyetracking and keystroke-logging methods for studying cognitive processes in text production. *Behavior Research Methods, 41*(2), 337–351.

West, J. M., Haake, A. R., Rozanski, E. P., & Karn, K. S. (2006). eyePatterns: Software for identifying patterns and similarities across fixation sequences. In *Proceedings of the 2006 Symposium on Eye-Tracking Research & Applications* (pp. 149–154). New York: ACM.

Westerman, S. J., Sutherland, E. J., Robinson, L., Powell, H., & Tuck, G. (2007). A multi-method approach to the assessment of web page designs. *Lecture Notes in Computer Science, 4738,* 302–313.

White, B. J., Stritzke, M., & Gegenfurtner, K. R. (2008). Saccadic facilitation in natural backgrounds. *Current Biology, 18*(2), 124–128.

Whittaker, S. G., & Eaholtz, G. (1982). Learning patterns of eye motion for foveal pursuit. *Investigative Ophthalmology & Visual Science, 23*(3), 393–397.

Wiens, S., Moniri, F., Kerimi, N., & Juth, P. (2009). *Attention capture by faces: Ethnicity outweighs emotion.* (Paper presented at the 4th Scandinavian Workshop for Applied Eye Tracking. Stavanger, Norway.)

Wierts, R., Janssen, M. J. A., & Kingma, H. (2008). Measuring saccade peak velocity using a low-frequency sampling rate of 50 Hz. *IEEE Transactions on Biomedical Engineering, 55*(12), 2840–2842.

Wierwille, W. W., & Connor, S. A. (1983). Evaluation of 20 workload measures using a psychomotor task in a moving-base aircraft simulator. *Human Factors: The Journal of the Human Factors and Ergonomics Society, 25*(1), 1–16.

Wieser, M. J., Pauli, P., Alpers, G. W., & Mühlberger, A. (2009). Is eye to eye contact really threatening and avoided in social anxiety? An eye-tracking and psychophysiology study. *Journal of Anxiety Disorders, 23*(1), 93–103.

Wilkinson, I. M. S., Kime, R., & Purnell, M. (1974). Alcohol and human eye movement. *Brain, 97*(1), 785–792.

Williams, A. M., Davids, K., Burwitz, L., & Williams, J. G. (1994). Visual search strategies in experienced and inexperienced soccer players. *Research Quarterly for Exercise and*

Sport, *65*(2), 127–135.

Williams, L. J. (1988). Tunnel vision or general interference? Cognitive load and attentional bias are both important. *American Journal of Psychiatry*, *101*(2), 171–191.

Wilmut, K., Wann, J. P., & Brown, J. H. (2006). How active gaze informs the hand in sequential pointing movements. *Experimental Brain Research*, *175*(4), 654–666.

Wilson, C., Harvey, A., & Thompson, J. D. (1999). *ClustalG: Software for analysis of activities and sequential events.* (Paper presented at the Workshop on Longitudinal Research in Social Science: A Canadian focus.)

Wineburg, S. S. (1991). Historical problem solving: A study of the cognitive processes used in the evaluation of documentary and pictorial evidence. *Journal of Educational Psychology*, *83*(1), 73–87.

Winer, B. J., Brown, D. R., & Michels, K. M. (1991). *Statistical Principles in Experimental Design* (third ed.). New York: McGraw-Hill.

Winograd-Gurvich, C., Georgiou-Karistianis, N., Fitzgerald, P. B., Millist, L., & White, O. B. (2006). Ocular motor differences between melancholic and non-melancholic depression. *Journal of Affective Disorders*, *93*(1-3), 193–203.

Wolfe, J. M. (1998a). Visual search: A review. In H. Pashler (Ed.), *Attention*. London: University College London Press.

Wolfe, J. M. (1998b). What can 1 million trials tell us about visual search? *Psychological Science*, *9*(1), 33–39.

Wolfe, J. M., & Horowitz, T. S. (2004). What attributes guide the deployment of visual attention and how do they do it? *Nature Reviews Neuroscience*, *5*(6), 495–501.

Wolkoff, P., Nøjgaard, J., Troiano, P., & Piccoli, B. (2005). Eye complaints in the office environment: Precorneal tear film integrity influenced by eye blinking efficiency. *Occupational and Environmental Medicine*, *62*(1), 4–12.

Wong, A. M. F. (2008). *Eye Movement Disorders*. Oxford: Oxford University Press.

Wooding, D. S. (2002a). Eye movements of large populations: II. Deriving regions of interest, coverage, and similarity using fixation maps. *Behavior Research Methods, Instruments, & Computers*, *34*(4), 518–528.

Wooding, D. S. (2002b). Fixation maps: Quantifying eye-movement traces. In *Proceedings of the 2002 Symposium on Eye-Tracking Research & Applications* (pp. 31–36). New York: ACM.

Wooding, D. S., Mugglestone, M. D., Purdy, K. J., & Gale, A. G. (2002). Eye movements of large populations: I. Implementation and performance of an autonomous public eye tracker. *Behavior Research Methods, Instruments, & Computers*, *34*(4), 509–517.

Wouters, R. J., Van Den Bosch, W. A., & Lemij, H. G. (1998). Saccadic eye movements in Graves' disease. *Investigative Ophthalmology & Visual Science*, *39*(9), 1544–1550.

Wulff, A. (2007). Eyes Wide Shut. *International Journal of Public Information Systems*, *2007*(1), 1–12.

Wurtz, P., Müri, R. M., & Wiesendanger, M. (2009). Sight-reading of violinists: Eye movements anticipate the musical flow. *Experimental Brain Research*, *194*(3), 445–450.

Wyatt, H. J. (1998). Detecting saccades with jerk. *Vision Research*, *38*(14), 2147–2153.

Yang, H. M., & McConkie, G. W. (1999). Reading Chinese: Some basic eye-movement characteristics. In J. Wang, A. W. Inhoff, & H.-C. Chen (Eds.), *Reading Chinese Script: A Cognitive Analysis* (pp. 207–222). Mahwah NJ: Lawrence Erlbaum Associates.

Yang, Q., & Kapoula, Z. A. A. (2008). Aging does not affect the accuracy of vertical saccades nor the quality of their binocular coordination: A study of a special elderly group. *Neurobiology of Aging*, *29*(4), 622–638.

Yang, S. N., & McConkie, G. W. (2001). Eye movements during reading: A theory of saccade initiation times. *Vision Research*, *41*(25-26), 3567–3585.

Yarbus, A. L. (1967). *Eye Movements and Vision*. New York: Plenum Press.

Yoon, D., & Narayanan, N. H. (2004a). Mental imagery in problem solving: An eye tracking study. In *Proceedings of the 2004 Symposium on Eye-Tracking Research & Applications* (pp. 77–84). New York: ACM.

Yoon, D., & Narayanan, N. H. (2004b). Predictors of success in diagrammatic problem solving. *Lecture Notes in Computer Science, 2980*, 301–315.

Yoss, R. E., Moyer, N. J., & Hollenhorst, R. W. (1970). Pupil size and spontaneous pupillary waves associated with alertness, drowsiness, and sleep. *Neurology, 20*(6), 545–554.

Young, F. A., & Biersdorf, W. R. (1954). Pupillary contraction and dilation in light and darkness. *Journal of Comparative and Physiological Psychology, 47*(3), 264–268.

Young, L. R. (1971). Pursuit eye tracking movements. In P. Bach-y-Rita, C. C. Collins, & J. E. Hyde (Eds.), *The Control of Eye Movements* (pp. 429–443). New York: Academic Press.

Young, L. R., & Sheena, D. (1975). Survey of eye movement recording methods. *Behavior Research Methods & Instrumentation, 7*(5), 397–429.

Zaman, M. L., & Doughty, M. J. (1997). Some methodological issues in the assessment of the spontaneous eyeblink frequency in man. *Ophthalmic and Physiological Optics, 17*(5), 421–432.

Zangemeister, W. H., Canavan, A. G., & Hoemberg, V. (1995). Frontal and parietal transcranial magnetic stimulation (TMS) disturbs programming of saccadic eye movements. *Journal of the Neurological Sciences, 133*(1-2), 42–52.

Zangemeister, W. H., & Liman, T. (2007). Foveal versus parafoveal scanpaths of visual imagery in virtual hemianopic subjects. *Computers in Biology and Medicine, 37*(7), 975–982.

Zangemeister, W. H., Sherman, K., & Stark, L. (1995). Evidence for a global scanpath strategy in viewing abstract compared with realistic images. *Neuropsychologia, 33*(8), 1009–1025.

Zelinsky, G. J. (2008). A theory of eye movements during target acquisition. *Psychological Review, 115*(4), 787–835.

Zelinsky, G. J., & Sheinberg, D. L. (1997). Eye movements during parallel–serial visual search. *Journal of Experimental Psychology: Human Perception and Performance, 23*(1), 244–262.

Zingale, C. M., & Kowler, E. (1987). Planning sequences of saccades. *Vision Research, 27*(8), 1327–1341.

Zivotofsky, A. Z., Siman-Tov, T., Gadoth, N., & Gordon, C. R. (2006). A rare saccade velocity profile in stiff-person syndrome with cerebellar degeneration. *Brain Research, 1093*(1), 135–140.

Zola, D. (1984). Redundancy and word perception during reading. *Perception & Psychophysics, 36*(3), 277–284.

Zwahlen, H. T., Adams, C. C., & De Bald, D. P. (1988). Safety aspects of CRT touch panel controls in automobiles. In *Proceedings of the Second International Conference on Vision in Vehicles* (pp. 335–344).

Index